JIM RECHTIEN

# ELECTRODIAGNOSIS IN DISEASES OF NERVE AND MUSCLE:
## PRINCIPLES AND PRACTICE

# ELECTRODIAGNOSIS IN DISEASES OF NERVE AND MUSCLE:
## PRINCIPLES AND PRACTICE

## JUN KIMURA, M.D.

Professor of Neurology
Chief, Division of Clinical Electrophysiology
Department of Neurology
The University of Iowa College of Medicine
Iowa City, Iowa

F.A.Davis / Philadelphia

**Library of Congress Cataloging in Publication Data**

Kimura, Jun.
   Electrodiagnosis in diseases of nerve and muscle.
   Bibliography: p.
   Includes index.
   1. Neuromuscular diseases—Diagnosis.  2. Elec-
tromyography.   3. Electrodiagnosis.   I. Title.
[DNLM:  1.  Electrodiagnosis.  2.  Neuromuscular
diseases—Diagnosis. WE 550 K49e]
RC925.7.K55 1983    616.7'407547    82-17973
ISBN 0-8036-5341-7

**TO JUNKO
AND
OUR PARENTS**

# FOREWORD

I found particular pleasure in preparing this foreword to the work of a colleague whose professional development and scientific accomplishments I have followed very closely indeed for some twenty years.

Dr. Kimura, very early after his training in neurology, expressed an interest in clinical electrophysiology. His energy and talents led to full-time assignment and responsibility for the development and application of electrodiagnostic techniques in our laboratory of electromyography and then to direction of the Division of Clinical Electrophysiology.

From his early assignment, Dr. Kimura has exploited the possibilities for the applications of clinical electrophysiologic techniques to their apparent limits, which, however, seem to continually advance to the benefit of us all. This volume is based on very extensive personal experience with application of all of the now recognized procedures.

The beginner will be able to follow this discipline from its historical roots to the latest techniques with the advantage of an explanatory background of the clinical, physiologic, anatomic, and pathologic foundations of the methods and their interpretation. The instrumentation, so essential to any success in application of techniques, is further described and explained. The more experienced diagnostician will both appreciate and profit from this pragmatic, well-organized, and authoritative source with its important bibliographic references; the beginner will find it a bible.

There are few areas in electrodiagnosis that Dr. Kimura does not address from his own extensive experience, backed by clinical and pathologic confirmation. The sections on the blink reflex and the F-wave reflect his own pioneering work. He has closely followed the application of new techniques to the study of disease of the central nervous system by evoked cerebral potentials from the beginning. These sections reflect a substantial personal experience in establishment of standards and in interpretation of changes in disease.

So important are the findings of electrodiagnostic methods that the clinical neurologist must himself be an expert in their interpretation. Preferably he should perform tests on his own patients or closely supervise such tests. Only in this way can he best derive the data that he needs or direct the examination in progress to secure important information as unexpected findings appear. To acquire the knowledge to guide him either in supervised training or in self-teaching, he needs first an excellent and comprehensive guide such as this text by Dr. Kimura.

Dr. Kimura is justifiably regarded as a leader in clinical electrophysiology both nationally and internationally. Those of us who profit from daily contact with him should be pardoned for our pride in this substantial and authoritative work.

Maurice W. Van Allen, M.D.

# PREFACE

This book grew out of my personal experience in working with fellows and residents in our electromyography laboratory. It is intended for clinicians who perform electrodiagnostic procedures as an extension of their clinical examination. As such, it emphasizes the electrical findings in the context of the clinical disorder. Although the choice of material has been oriented toward neurology, I have attempted to present facts useful to practicing electromyographers regardless of their clinical disciplines. I hope that the book will also prove to be of value to neurologists and physiatrists who are interested in neuromuscular disorders and to others who regularly request electrodiagnostic tests as an integral part of their clinical practice.

The book is divided into seven parts and three appendices. Part 1 provides an overview of basic anatomy and physiology of the neuromuscular system. Nerve conduction studies, tests of neuromuscular transmission, and conventional and single fiber electromyography are described in the next three parts. Part 5 covers supplemental methods designed to test less accessible regions of the nervous system. The last two parts are devoted to clinical discussion. The appendices consist of a historical review, electronics and instrumentation, and a glossary of terms.

The selection of technique is necessarily influenced by the special interest of the author. Thus, in Part 5, the blink reflex, F-wave, H-reflex, and somatosensory evoked potential have been given more emphasis than is customary in other texts. I hope that I am not overestimating their practical importance and that these newer techniques will soon find their way into routine clinical practice. This is, of course, not to de-emphasize the conventional methods, which I hope are adequately covered in this text. The ample space allocated for clinical discussion in Parts 6 and 7 reflects my personal conviction that clinical acumen is a prerequisite for meaningful electrophysiologic evaluations. Numerous references are provided to document the statements made in the text. I hope that use of these references will promote interest and research in the field of electrodiagnosis.

J.K.

# ACKNOWLEDGMENTS

I came from the Island of the Rising Sun, where English is not the native language. It was thus with trepidation that I undertook the task of writing an English text. Although its completion gives me personal pride and satisfaction, I hasten to acknowledge that the goal could not have been achieved without help from others.

Dr. M. W. Van Allen has provided me with more than a kind foreword. I wish to thank him for his initial encouragement and continued support and advice. He was one of the first to do electromyography in Iowa. During my early years of training I had the pleasure of using his battery operated amplifier and a homemade loudspeaker (which worked only in his presence). I am indebted to Dr. A.L. Sahs, who initiated me into the field of clinical neurology and Dr. J.R. Knott, who taught me clinical neurophysiology. I am grateful to Drs. T. Yamada and E. Shivapour for attending the busy service of the Division of Clinical Electrophysiology while I devoted myself to writing. Dr. Yamada also gave me most valuable assistance in preparing the section on central somatosensory evoked potentials, which includes many of his original contributions. Drs. R.L. Rodnitzky, E.P. Bosch, J.T. Wilkinson, A.M. Brugger, F.O. Walker, and H.C. Chui read the manuscript and gave most helpful advice. Peter J. Seaba, M.S.E.E. and D. David Walker, M.S.E.E., our electrical engineers, contributed Appendix 2 and reviewed the text.

My special thanks go to the technicians and secretaries of the Division of Clinical Electrophysiology. Sheila R. Mennen, the senior technician of our electromyography laboratory, typed (and retyped time and time again) all the manuscript with devotion and dedication. Deborah A. Gevock, Cheri L. Doggett, Joanne M. Colter, Lauri Longnecker, Jane Austin, Sharon S. Rath, Lori A. Garwood, and Allen L. Frauenholtz have all given me valuable technical or secretarial assistance. Linda C. Godfrey and her staff in the Medical Graphics Department have been most helpful in preparing illustrations.

I owe my gratitude to Mr. Robert H. Craven, Sr., Mr. Robert H. Craven, Jr., Dr. Sylvia K. Fields, Miss Agnes A. Hunt, Ms. Sally Burke, Miss Lenoire Brown,

Mrs. Christine H. Young, and two anonymous reviewers of the F.A. Davis Company for their interest and invaluable guidance. A number of previously published figures and tables have been reproduced with permission from the publishers and authors. I wish to express my sincere appreciation for their courtesy. The sources are acknowledged in the legends. The *Glossary of Terms Commonly Used in Electromyography* of the American Association of Electromyography and Electrodiagnosis is reprinted in its entirety as Appendix 3, with kind permission from the Association and the members of the Nomenclature Committee.

My sons asked if the book might be dedicated to them for having kept mostly, though not always, quiet during my long hours of writing at home. However, the honor went to their mother instead, a decision enthusiastically approved by the children, in appreciation for her effort to keep peace at home. In concluding the acknowledgment, my heart goes to the members of my family in Nagoya and those of my wife's in Takayama, who have given us kind and warm support throughout our prolonged stay abroad. The credit is certainly theirs for my venture finally coming to fruition.

# CONTENTS

# PART 2 NERVE CONDUCTION STUDIES

# PART 4   ELECTROMYOGRAPHY

# PART 6 DISORDERS OF THE SPINAL CORD AND PERIPHERAL NERVOUS SYSTEM

# APPENDICES

# PART
# 1

## BASICS OF
## ELECTRODIAGNOSIS

# 1

## ANATOMIC BASIS FOR LOCALIZATION

Electrodiagnosis may be considered an extension of the neurologic examination. Both employ the same anatomic principles of localization, searching for evidence of motor and sensory compromise. Electrophysiologic studies supplement the clinical examination by providing additional precision, detail, and objectivity, and delineate a variety of pathologic changes that are clinically either obscure or undetectable. Atrophic, deeply situated, or paretic muscles, difficult to evaluate clinically, can be located and examined. The neuromuscular junction and nerve segments can be isolated and tested separately. Electrical studies also allow quantitative assessment of reflex amplitude and latencies as well as complex motor phenomena.

Because individual tests evaluate different groups of overlapping neural circuits, meaningful analysis of electrophysiologic findings is possible only with an understanding of neuroanatomy. In addition, superficial anatomy is important for locating skeletal muscles and peripheral nerves for accurate placement of recording and stimulating electrodes. The first section of this book contains a review of peripheral neuroanatomy important for the performance and interpretation of electrodiagnostic studies. It is a concise summary of clinically useful information that serves as a framework for the rest of the text.

Although the anatomy of skeletal muscles and peripheral nerves is an interesting subject, written descriptions tend to be complicated and rather dry. To compensate for this inherent problem, I have attempted to simplify the discussion by using schematic illustrations. Existing texts should be consulted for more detailed accounts of the superficial anatomy of skeletal muscles[3, 5, 9] or of general peripheral neuromuscular anatomy.[1, 2, 6, 7, 8, 10, 12, 13, 14]

## CRANIAL NERVES

The cranial nerves are the peripheral nerves of the brain. Nine cranial nerves innervate voluntary muscles as summarized in Table 1-1. The oculomotor, trochlear, and abducens nerves control the movements of the eyes. The trigeminal and facial nerves innervate the muscles of mastication and those of facial expression, respectively. The laryngeal muscles are innervated by the glossopharyngeal and vagal nerves and the cranial root of the accessory nerve. The hypoglossal nerve supplies the tongue. The spinal root

**TABLE 1-1 Muscles innervated by cranial nerves and cervical plexus**

| Nerve | Mesencephalon | Pons | Medulla | C-2 | C-3 | C-4 |
|---|---|---|---|---|---|---|
| Oculomotor | Levator palpebrae Superior rectus Medial rectus Inferior rectus Inferior oblique | | | | | |
| Trochlear | Superior oblique | | | | | |
| Trigeminal | Masseter Temporalis Pterygoid | | | | | |
| Abducens | | Lateral rectus | | | | |
| Facial | | Frontalis Orbicularis oculi Orbicularis oris Platysma Other muscles of facial expression | | | | |
| Glosso-pharyngeal | | | Laryngeal muscles | | | |
| Vagus | | | Laryngeal muscles | | | |
| Accessory (cranial root) | | | Laryngeal muscles | | | |
| Hypoglossal | | | Tongue | | | |
| Accessory (spinal root) and Cervical plexus | | | | Sternocleidomastoid | | |
| | | | | | Trapezius-upper, middle, & lower | |
| Phrenic | | | | | Diaphragm | |

of the accessory nerve innervates the sternocleidomastoid and upper portion of the trapezius. Of these, the most commonly tested in an electromyographic laboratory are the facial, trigeminal, and accessory nerves.

## Facial nerve

The course of the facial nerve, from the nucleus to the distal trunk, can be artificially subdivided into four segments (Fig. 1-1). The most central portion may be referred to as the intrapontine segment, which is initially directed posteriorly to hook around the sixth nerve nucleus. Because of its elongated course, it is vulnerable to various pontine lesions, which cause a peripheral, rather than central, type of facial palsy. The facial nerve complex exits the brain stem ventrolaterally at the caudal pons in the area generally designated as the cerebellopontine angle. This segment may be compressed by acoustic neuromas or other masses. After traversing the subarachnoid space, it enters the internal auditory meatus. Here the facial nerve begins the longest and most complex intraosseous course of any nerve in the body. The intraosseous segment is the presumed site of lesion in Bell's palsy. Upon exiting from the skull through the stylomastoid foramen, the facial nerve may be damaged by diseases affecting the superficial and deep lobes of the parotid gland. It then branches with some variation into five distal segments (Fig. 1-2).

## Trigeminal nerve

The trigeminal nerve subserves all superficial sensation to the face and buccal and nasal mucosa. It also supplies the muscles of mastication which consist of the masseters, temporalis, and pterygoids. The ophthalmic and maxillary divisions of the trigeminal nerve supply sensation to the upper and middle parts of the face, respectively,

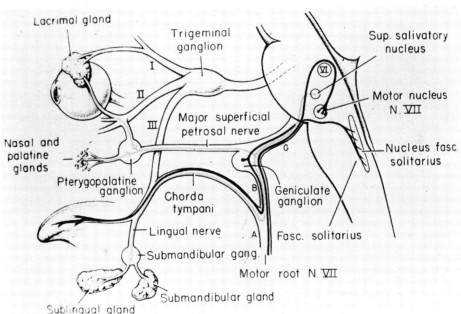

Figure 1-1
Diagram shows the various functional components of the facial nerve (n VII), which may be affected at the stylomastoid foramen (A), distal (B), or proximal to the geniculate ganglion (C), either extra- or intrapontine. The three major divisions of the trigeminal nerve are also shown. (From Carpenter,[2] with permission.)

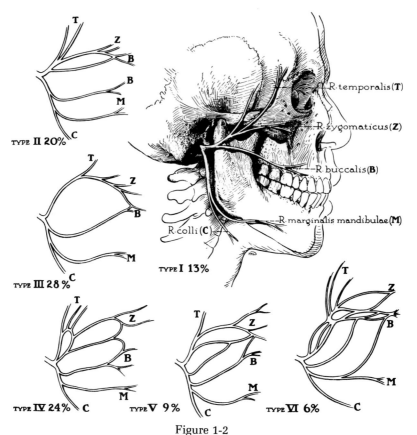

Figure 1-2

Major types of branching and intercommunication with percentage occurrence of each pattern in 350 recordings. (From Anson,[1] with permission.)

whereas the mandibular division carries the sensory fibers to the lower portion of the face as well as the motor fibers (see Fig. 1-1). The first order neurons concerned primarily with tactile sensation have their cell bodies in the gasserian ganglion. Their proximal branches enter the lateral portion of the pons and ascend to reach the main sensory nucleus. Those fibers subserving pain and temperature sensation also have cell bodies in the gasserian ganglion. However, upon entering the pons, their fibers descend to reach the spinal nucleus of the trigeminal nerve.

The first order afferent fibers concerned with proprioception from the muscles of mastication have their cell bodies in the mesencephalic nucleus. They make monosynaptic connection with the motor nucleus of the trigeminal nerve located in the midpons, medial to the main sensory nucleus. This pathway provides the anatomic substrate for the masseter reflex. The first component of the blink reflex is probably subserved by a disynaptic pathway from the main sensory nucleus to the ipsilateral facial nucleus, whereas the second component is relayed through polysynaptic connections via the spinal nucleus to the facial nuclei on both sides (see Fig. 16-1).

## Accessory nerve

The cell bodies of the cranial accessory nerve are located in the nucleus ambiguus. The fibers join the vagus nerve and are distributed through it to the striated muscles of the pharynx and larynx. Thus, despite the traditional name, the cranial portion of the accessory nerve is functionally a part of the vagus nerve. The spinal accessory nerve

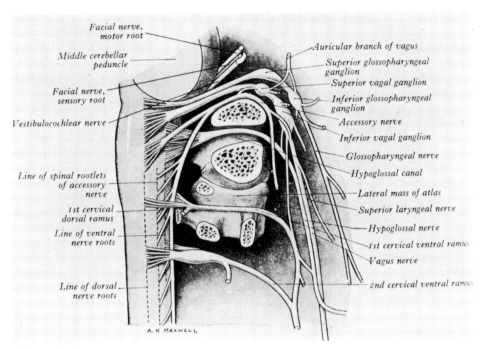

Figure 1-3
Diagram shows the communication between the last four cranial nerves on the right side viewed from the dorsolateral aspect. Note the division of the accessory nerve into the cranial accessory nerve, which joins the vagal nerve, and the spinal accessory nerve, which supplies the trapezius and sternocleidomastoid muscles. (From Williams and Warwick,[14] with permission.)

has its cells of origin in the spinal nucleus located in the first five or six cervical segments of the spinal cord (Figs. 1-3 and 1-4). The fibers ascend in the spinal canal to enter the cranial cavity through the foramen magnum and then leave by the jugular foramen to end in the upper portion of the trapezius and the sternocleidomastoid muscles. Although these two muscles receive additional nerve supply directly from C-2 through C-4 roots, it has been suggested that the spinal accessory nerve is the sole motor supply. The innervation from the cervical roots is felt to be purely proprioceptive in nature (Fig. 1-5). Since the accessory nucleus consists of several separate portions, a lesion in the spinal cord may affect it only in part, causing partial paralysis of the muscle groups innervated by this nerve. This central dissociation could be mistaken for a peripheral lesion affecting separate individual branches.

# ANTERIOR AND POSTERIOR RAMI OF THE SPINAL NERVE

The anterior and posterior roots, each composed of several rootlets, emerge from the spinal cord carrying motor and sensory fibers, respectively (Fig. 1-6). They join to form the spinal nerves that exist from their respective spinal canal through their respective intervertebral foramina. A small ganglion, containing the cell bodies of sensory fibers, lies on each posterior root in the intervertebral foramina just proximal to its union with the anterior root but distal to the cessation of the dural sleeve. There are 31 spinal nerves on each side: 8 cervical, 12 thoracic, 5 lumbar, 5 sacral, and 1 coccygeal nerve. After passing through the foramina, the spinal nerve branches into two divisions, the anterior and posterior primary rami.

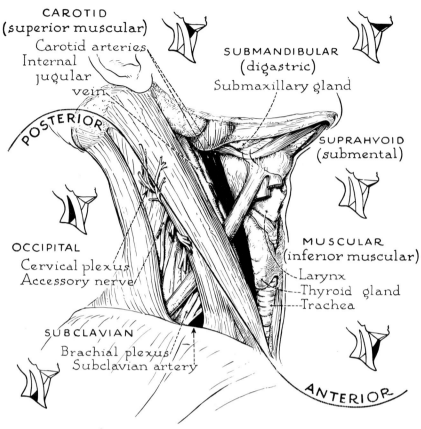

**CAROTID**
(superior muscular)
Carotid arteries
Internal
jugular
vein

POSTERIOR

**SUBMANDIBULAR**
(digastric)
Submaxillary gland

**SUPRAHYOID**
(submental)

**OCCIPITAL**
Cervical plexus
Accessory nerve

**MUSCULAR**
(inferior muscular)
Larynx
Thyroid gland
Trachea

**SUBCLAVIAN**
Brachial plexus
Subclavian artery

ANTERIOR

## CERVICAL TRIANGLES

Figure 1-4

The field bounded by the trapezius, mandible, midline of neck, and clavicle is divided into anterior and posterior triangles by the sternocleidomastoid. The posterior triangle is further subdivided into occipital and subclavian triangles by the obliquely coursing omohyoid. The contents of the occipital and subclavian triangles include the cervical plexus, spinal accessory nerve, and brachial plexus. The spinal accessory nerve becomes relatively superficial in the middle portion of the sternocleidomastoid along its posterior margin, where it is accessible to percutaneous stimulation. (From Anson,[1] with permission.)

The posterior rami supply the posterior part of the skin and the paraspinal muscles, which include the rectus capitis posterior, oblique capitis superior and inferior, semispinalis capitis, splenius capitis, longus capitis, and sacrospinalis. These muscles extend the head, neck, trunk, and pelvis, respectively. The anterior rami supply the skin of the anterolateral portion of the trunk and the extremities. They also form the brachial and lumbosacral plexuses, which, in turn, give rise to peripheral nerves in the upper and lower extremities. The anterior rami of the thoracic spinal nerves become 12 pairs of intercostal nerves supplying the intercostal and abdominal muscles. At least two adjoining intercostal nerves supply each segmental level in both the thoracic and abdominal regions.

The diagnosis of a root lesion is established if abnormalities are confined to a single spinal nerve without affecting adjacent higher or lower levels. Since the paraspinal muscles are supplied by the posterior rami which branch off the spinal nerve just distal to the intervertebral foramen, denervation found at this level may be used to differentiate radiculopathy from more distal lesions of the plexus or peripheral nerve.

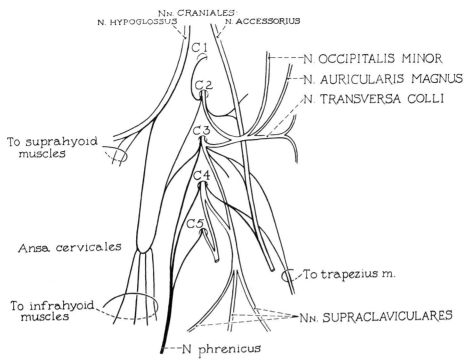

Figure 1-5

Diagram shows the anterior rami of the cervical spinal nerves, forming the cervical plexus. Note the phrenic nerve supplying the diaphragm, and the branches from C-2, C-3, and C-4 roots and the accessory nerve, both innervating the trapezius muscle. (From Anson,[1] with permission.)

However, radiculopathy does not necessarily affect the paraspinal muscles in early stages of the disease, when the compressing lesions may only irritate the root without causing structural damage. Furthermore, even if the axons are injured, spontaneous discharges do not appear immediately in the denervated muscles. Similar to the innervation of the intercostal muscles by the anterior rami, there is substantial overlap in innervation of the paraspinal muscles by the posterior rami. Therefore, the level of a radicular lesion must be established based on the distribution of abnormalities in the extremities even if the paraspinal muscles are involved.

## CERVICAL AND BRACHIAL PLEXUSES

The cervical plexus is formed by the anterior rami of the upper four cervical nerves, C-1 through C-4 (see Fig. 1-5). It innervates the lateral and anterior flexors of the head which consist of the rectus capitis lateralis, anterior longus capitis, and anterior longus colli. The brachial plexus is formed by the anterior rami of C-5 through T-1 spinal nerves. Occasional variations of innervation include the prefixed brachial plexus with contributions mainly from C-4 through C-8, and the postfixed brachial plexus derived primarily from C-6 through T-2. Tables 1-1 and 1-2 present a summary of the anatomic relationship between the nerves derived from cervical and brachial plexuses and the muscles of the shoulder and upper extremities.

Topographically, the brachial plexus may be divided into four segments: root, trunk, cord, and peripheral nerve (Fig. 1-7). The roots combine to form three trunks. The upper and lower trunks are formed by the union of C-5 and C-6, and C-8 and T-1 roots, respectively, whereas the middle trunk is derived from the C-7 root alone. Each of the three trunks is divided into anterior and posterior divisions. The posterior cord is

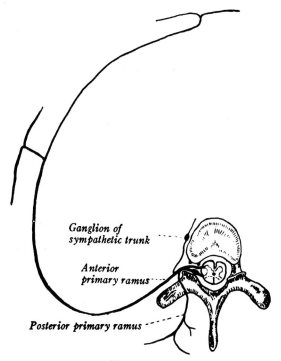

*Ganglion of sympathetic trunk*

*Anterior primary ramus*

*Posterior primary ramus*

Figure 1-6

Diagram shows the ventral and dorsal roots forming the spinal nerve, which divides into the anterior and posterior rami. The sensory ganglion of the dorsal root is located within the respective intervertebral foramen. (From Ranson and Clark,[11] with permission.)

**TABLE 1-2 Muscles of the shoulder girdle and upper extremity**

| Nerve | C-4 | C-5 | C-6 | C-7 | C-8 | T-1 |
|---|---|---|---|---|---|---|
| Dorsal scapular | Rhomboideus— major & minor Levator scapulae | | | | | |
| Supra scapular | | Supraspinatus Infraspinatus | | | | |
| Subscap- ular | | Teres major | | | | |
| Axillary | | Teres minor | | | | |
| | | Deltoid—anterior, middle, & posterior | | | | |
| Musculo- cutaneous | | Biceps Brachialis | | | | |
| | | | Coraco brachi- alis | | | |
| Long thoracic | | Serratus anterior | | | | |

**TABLE 1-2 (*Continued*) Muscles of the shoulder girdle and upper extremity**

| Nerve | C-4 | C-5 | C-6 | C-7 | C-8 | T-1 |
|---|---|---|---|---|---|---|
| Anterior thoracic | Pectoralis major (clavicular part) | | | Pectoralis major (sternocostal part) Pectoralis minor | | |
| Thoraco dorsal | | | | Latissimus dorsi | | |
| Radial | | Brachioradialis Extensor carpi radialis longus & brevis | | Triceps—long, lateral, & medial heads Anconeus | | |
| posterior inter- osseus | | | Supinator | | | |
| | | | | Extensor carpi ulnaris Extensor digitorum Extensor digiti minimi Abductor pollicis longus Extensor pollicis longus Extensor pollicis brevis Extensor indicis | | |
| Median | | | Pronator teres Flexor carpi radialis | | | |
| | | | | Palmaris longus | | |
| | | | | Flexor digitorum sublimis | | |
| | | | | | Abductor pollicis brevis Flexor pollicis brevis (superficial head) Lumbricals I & II Opponens pollicis | |
| anterior inter- osseus | | | | Flexor pollicis longus Flexor digitorum profundus I & II Pronator quadratus | | |
| Ulnar | | | | Flexor carpi ulnaris Flexor digitorum profundus III & IV | | |
| | | | | | Adductor pollicis Flexor pollicis brevis (deep head) Abductor digiti minimi Opponens digiti minimi Flexor digiti minimi Volar interossei Dorsal interossei Lumbricals III & IV | |

formed by the union of all three posterior divisions. At the axilla it gives off the axillary nerve and continues as the radial nerve. The anterior divisions of the upper and middle trunks form the lateral cord, which gives off the musculocutaneous nerve and the outer branch of the median nerve. The anterior division of the lower trunk, forming the medial cord, gives off the ulnar nerve, the inner branch of the median nerve, and cutaneous nerves.

The trunks pass through the supraclavicular fossa under the cervical and scalenus muscles, forming the cords just above the clavicle at the level of the first rib. Accompanied by the subclavian artery, the cords traverse the space known as the thoracic outlet between the first rib and the clavicle. Consequently, the trunks are likely to be affected if the lesion is above the clavicle, whereas the cords tend to be

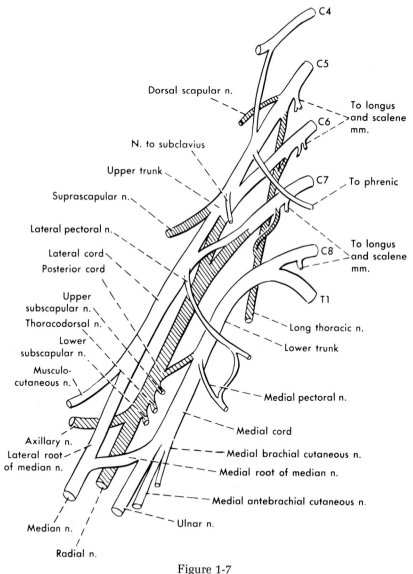

Figure 1-7
Anatomy of the brachial plexus with eventual destination of all root components. The posterior divisions are shaded. (From Hollinshead,[7] with permission.)

involved by a lesion below the clavicle. The peripheral nerves that emerge from the cords between the clavicle and axilla are affected by a more distal lesion.

## Phrenic nerve

The phrenic nerve is perhaps one of the most important branches of the cervical plexus. It arises from C-3 and C-4 roots and innervates the ipsilateral hemidiaphragm (see Table 1-1).

## Dorsal scapular nerve

The dorsal scapular nerve is derived from C-4 and C-5 roots through the upper trunk of the brachial plexus and supplies the rhomboid major and minor and a portion of the levator scapulae, which keeps the scapula attached to the posterior chest wall during arm motion.

## Suprascapular nerve

The suprascapular nerve is derived from C-5 and C-6 roots through the upper trunk of the brachial plexus. It reaches the upper border of the scapula behind the brachial plexus to enter the suprascapular notch where the nerve may be entrapped. The nerve supplies the supraspinatus and infraspinatus (see Fig. 1-7).

## Musculocutaneous nerve

The musculocutaneous nerve is a mixed nerve that derives from the lateral cord of the brachial plexus near the lower border of the pectoralis minor (Fig. 1-8). Its axons chiefly originate from C-5 and C-6 roots and innervate the biceps, brachialis, and coracobrachialis, although there are some variations in the nerve supply of the last two muscles. Its terminal branch is a sensory nerve called the lateral cutaneous nerve, which supplies the skin over the lateral aspect of the forearm.

## Axillary nerve

The axillary nerve arises from the posterior cord of the brachial plexus originating from C-5 and C-6 roots. It supplies the skin of the lateral aspect of the arm and the deltoid and teres minor muscles (Fig. 1-9).

# PRINCIPAL NERVES OF THE UPPER EXTREMITY

## Radial nerve

The radial nerve is a continuation of the posterior cord of the brachial plexus (see Fig. 1-7). The radial nerve derives its axons from C-5 through T-1; that is, all the spinal roots contributing to the plexus. After giving off its supply to the three heads of the triceps and the anconeus, which originates from the lateral epicondyle of the humerus as a continuation of the medial head of the triceps, the radial nerve enters the spiral groove winding around the humerus posteriorly from the medial to the lateral side (Fig. 1-9). As the radial nerve emerges from the spiral groove, it supplies the brachioradialis muscle and the extensor carpi radialis longus slightly more distally. As it enters the forearm at the level of the lateral epicondyle, it is located lateral to the biceps, between the brachialis and brachioradialis. At this point, it divides into a motor branch, the posterior interosseous nerve, and a sensory branch, which becomes superficial in the distal third of the forearm. The motor nerve innervates the supinator, the abductor

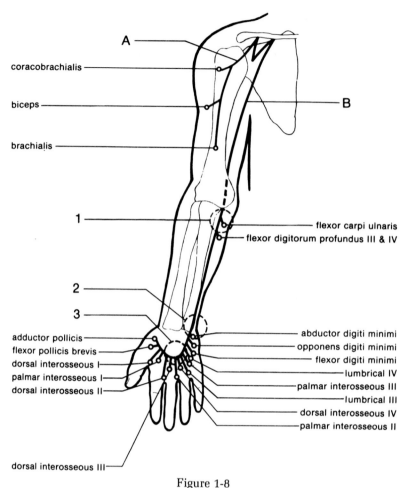

coracobrachialis

biceps

brachialis

A

B

1 — flexor carpi ulnaris
— flexor digitorum profundus III & IV

2

3

adductor pollicis
flexor pollicis brevis
dorsal interosseous I
palmar interosseous I
dorsal interosseous II

abductor digiti minimi
opponens digiti minimi
flexor digiti minimi
lumbrical IV
palmar interosseous III
lumbrical III
dorsal interosseous IV
palmar interosseous II

dorsal interosseous III

Figure 1-8

Musculocutaneous nerve (A) and ulnar nerve (B), and the muscles they supply. The common sites of lesion include ulnar groove and cubital tunnel (1), Guyon's canal (2), and midpalm (3). (Modified from: Medical Research Council: *Aids to the Examination of the Peripheral Nervous System.*[9])

pollicis longus, and all the extensor muscles in the forearm: extensor carpi radialis brevis, extensor carpi ulnaris, extensor digitorum, extensor digiti minimi, extensor pollicis longus and brevis, and extensor indicis. The sensory fibers originate from C-6 and C-7 roots, pass through the upper and middle trunks and the posterior cord, and then supply the skin over the lateral aspect of the dorsum of the hand.

## Median nerve

The median nerve arises from the lateral and median cords of the brachial plexus (see Fig. 1-7). It is a mixed nerve derived from C-6 through T-1 roots. The median nerve supplies most flexor muscles in the forearm and the muscles of the thenar eminence. It also subserves sensation to the skin over the lateral aspect of the palm and the dorsal surfaces of the terminal phalanges, along with the volar surfaces of the thumb, the index and middle fingers, and half of the ring finger. The sensory fibers of the middle finger enter the C-7 root through the lateral cord and middle trunk, whereas the skin of the thumb and the index finger is supplied by the C-6 or C-7 root through the lateral cord and upper or middle trunk. The median nerve innervates no muscles in the upper

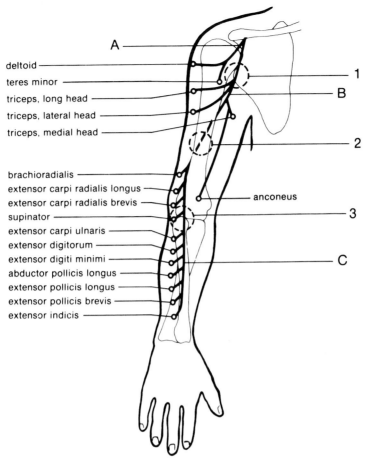

deltoid

teres minor

triceps, long head

triceps, lateral head

triceps, medial head

brachioradialis

extensor carpi radialis longus

extensor carpi radialis brevis

supinator

extensor carpi ulnaris

extensor digitorum

extensor digiti minimi

abductor pollicis longus

extensor pollicis longus

extensor pollicis brevis

extensor indicis

anconeus

A

B

1

2

3

C

Figure 1-9

Axillary nerve (A) and radial nerve (B) with its terminal branch, posterior interosseous nerve (C), and the muscles they supply. The nerve may be injured at the axilla (1), spiral groove (2) or at the elbow (3) as in the posterior interosseous nerve syndrome. (Modified from: Medical Research Council: *Aids to the Examination of the Peripheral Nervous System.*[9])

arm (Fig. 1-10). It enters the forearm by passing between the two heads of the pronator teres, which it supplies along with the flexor carpi radialis, palmaris longus, and flexor digitorum superficialis. It then gives rise to a pure motor branch called the anterior interosseous nerve, which innervates the flexor pollicis longus, pronator quadratus, and flexor digitorum profundus I and II. The main branch descends the forearm and passes through the carpal tunnel between the wrist and palm. It supplies lumbricals I and II after giving off the recurrent thenar nerve at the distal edge of the carpal ligaments. This motor branch to the thenar eminence innervates the abductor pollicis brevis, the lateral half of the flexor pollicis brevis, and the opponens pollicis.

## Ulnar nerve

The ulnar nerve is a continuation of the medial cord of the brachial plexus, which derives its fibers from C-8 and T-1 roots (see Fig. 1-7). It lies in close proximity to the median nerve and brachial artery at the axilla. In this position the ulnar nerve passes between the biceps and triceps, then deviates posteriorly at the midportion of the upper arm and becomes superficial behind the medial epicondyle (see Fig. 1-8). After entering

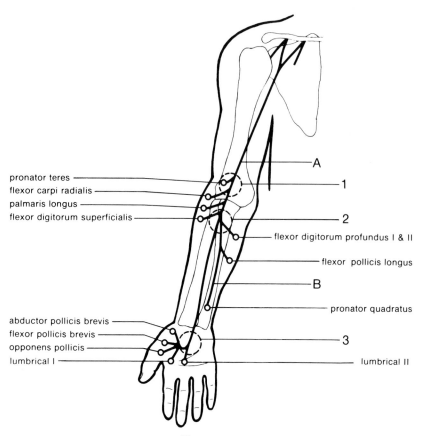

Figure 1-10

Median nerve (A) with its branch, anterior interosseous nerve (B), and the muscles they supply. The nerve may be affected at the elbow between the two heads of pronator teres (1), or slightly distally (2) as in the anterior interosseous syndrome, or at the palm (3) as in the carpal tunnel syndrome. (Modified from: Medical Research Council: *Aids to the Examination of the Peripheral Nervous System.*[9])

the forearm, it supplies the flexor carpi ulnaris and flexor digitorum profundus III and IV. It passes along the medial aspect of the wrist to enter the hand, where it divides into a superficial branch and a deep branch. The superficial branch, a sensory nerve, supplies the skin over the medial aspect of the hand from the wrist distally, including the hypothenar eminence, the fifth digit, and half of the fourth digit. The deep branch is a pure motor nerve which, near its origin, supplies hypothenar muscles: the abductor, opponens, and flexor digiti minimi. It then deviates laterally around the hamate to reach the lateral aspect of the hand, where it supplies the adductor pollicis and medial half of the flexor pollicis brevis. Along its course from hypothenar to thenar eminence the deep branch also innervates the interossei and lumbricals III and IV.

## GENERAL RULES AND ANOMALIES

The pattern of innervation in the upper extremities has been shown in Table 1-2. It may be difficult to memorize the exact innervation for all the individual muscles. Instead, it is more realistic to remember certain rules that may be used to broadly categorize muscles innervated by the median, ulnar, and radial nerves as follows.

The radial nerve innervates the brachioradialis, triceps, and all the extensors in the forearm, but none of the intrinsic hand muscles. The posterior interosseous nerve is the continuation of the radial nerve motor fibers below the elbow. All the muscles innervated by the ulnar nerve are intrinsic hand muscles with the exception of the flexor carpi ulnaris and the flexor digitorum profundus III and IV. In contrast, the median nerve innervates most flexors in the forearm, the muscles of the thenar eminence, and lumbricals I and II. The anterior interosseus nerve branches off the median nerve trunk in the forearm to innervate the flexor digitorum profundus I and II, flexor pollicis longus, and pronator quadratus.

The most common anomaly of innervation in the upper limb is the presence of a communicating branch from the median to the ulnar nerve in the forearm. The fibers involved in this anomaly, called the Martin-Gruber anastomosis, usually supply the ordinarily ulnar-innervated intrinsic hand muscles. Thus, the communicating fibers may be regarded as a portion of the ulnar nerve which, instead of coming from the medial cord of the brachial plexus, takes an anomalous route distally along with the median nerve and then reunites with the ulnar nerve proper in the distal forearm. Other anomalies reported in the literature include communication from the ulnar to median nerve in the forearm, and all median or all ulnar hands, in which one or the other nerve supplies all the intrinsic hand muscles. These are extremely rare when compared with the high incidence of the median-to-ulnar anastomosis. Failure to recognize an anomaly is a common source of error in clinical electrophysiology as discussed in Chapter 7.

# THE LUMBAR PLEXUS AND ITS MAJOR NERVES

The spinal cord ends at the level of L-1 to L-2 intervertebral space as the preconus (L-5 and S-1 cord level) and conus medullaris (S-2 through S-5). The cauda equina is formed by the lumbar and sacral roots which assume a downward direction from the conus toward their respective exit foramina. The filum terminale interna is a fibrous band which extends from the lowermost end of the spinal cord to the bottom of the dural sac at the level of the S-2 vertebra. The nerves derived from the lumbar plexus and the muscles they innervate are summarized in Table 1-3.

**TABLE 1-3 Muscles of the pelvic girdle and lower extremity**

| Nerve | L-2 | L-3 | L-4 | L-5 | S-1 | S-2 |
|---|---|---|---|---|---|---|
| Femoral | Iliopsoas Sartorius | | | | | |
| | Quadriceps femoris—rectus femoris, vastus lateralis, vastus intermedius, & vastus medialis | | | | | |
| | | Pectineus | | | | |
| Obturator | Gracilis Adductor longus, brevis, & magnus Obturator externus | | | | | |
| Sacral plexus | | | Obturator internus Superior & inferior gemelli Quadratus femoris | | | |
| | | | | | Piriformis | |
| Superior gluteal | | | Gluteal medius & minimus Tensor fascia latae | | | |
| Inferior gluteal | | | | Gluteus maximus | | |

TABLE 1-3 (*Continued*) Muscles of the pelvic girdle and lower extremity

| Nerve | L-2 | L-3 | L-4 | L-5 | S-1 | S-2 |
|---|---|---|---|---|---|---|
| Sciatic | | | | | | |
| peroneal division | | | | Biceps femoris-short head | | |
| tibial division | | | | Biceps femoris-long head Semitendinosus Semimembranosus | | |
| Common peroneal | | | | | | |
| deep peroneal | | | Tibialis anterior | | | |
| | | | | Extensor digitorum longus Extensor hallucis longus Extensor digitorum brevis Peroneus tertius | | |
| superficial peroneal | | | | Peroneus longus Peroneus brevis | | |
| Tibial | | | Tibialis posterior | | | |
| | | | | Popliteus | | |
| | | | | Flexor digitorum longus Flexor hallucis longus | | |
| | | | | | Gastrocnemius—median & lateral heads Soleus | |
| medial plantar | | | Flexor digitorum brevis | | | |
| | | | | Flexor hallucis brevis | | |
| | | | | | Abductor hallucis Lumbricals I | |
| lateral plantar | | | | | Abductor digiti minimi Adductor hallucis Flexor digiti minimi Interossei Quadratus plantae Lumbricals II, III, & IV | |

The anterior rami of the first three lumbar spinal nerves from L-1, L-2 and L-3, and part of L-4 roots unite to form the lumbar plexus within the psoas major muscle (Figs. 1-11 to 1-13). The iliohypogastric and ilioinguinal nerves arise from L-1 root and supply the skin of the hypogastric region and medial thigh, respectively. The genitofemoral nerve, which is derived from L-1 and L-2 roots, supplies the cremasteric muscle and the skin of the scrotum. The lateral femoral cutaneous nerve originates from L-2 and L-3 roots. It leaves the psoas muscle laterally to supply the lateral and anterior thigh. The anterior divisions of the L-2 through L-4 anterior rami join to form the obturator nerve which exits the psoas muscle medially and innervates the adductor muscles of the thigh. The posterior divisions of the same rami give rise to the femoral nerve which leaves the psoas muscle laterally. It then descends under the iliacus fascia

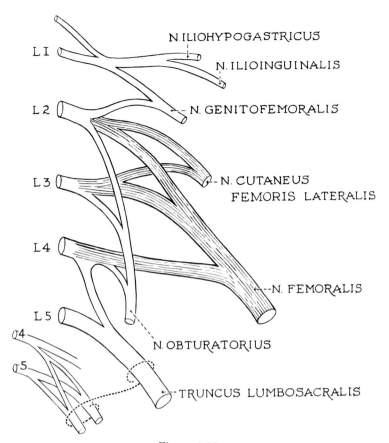

Figure 1-11

Diagram shows the anterior rami of the lumbar spinal nerve forming the lumbar plexus. The major nerves derived from this plexus are indicated. The dorsal divisions are shaded. (From Anson,[1] with permission.)

to reach the femoral triangle beneath the inguinal ligament. This is primarily a motor nerve but there are also sensory branches—the intermediate and medial cutaneous nerves and the saphenous nerve.

## Iliohypogastric nerve

The iliohypogastric nerve arises from L-1 root and supplies the skin of the upper buttock and hypogastric region.

## Ilioinguinal nerve

The ilioinguinal nerve, arising from L-1 and L-2 roots, supplies the skin over the upper and medial part of the thigh, the root of the penis, and the upper part of the scrotum or labium major. It also innervates the transversalis and internal oblique muscles. The nerve follows the basic pattern of an intercostal nerve, winding around the inner side of the trunk to the medial anterior iliac spine.

## Genitofemoral nerve

The genitofemoral nerve, arising from L-1 and L-2 roots, branches into lumboinguinal and external spermatic nerves. The lumboinguinal nerve supplies the skin over the

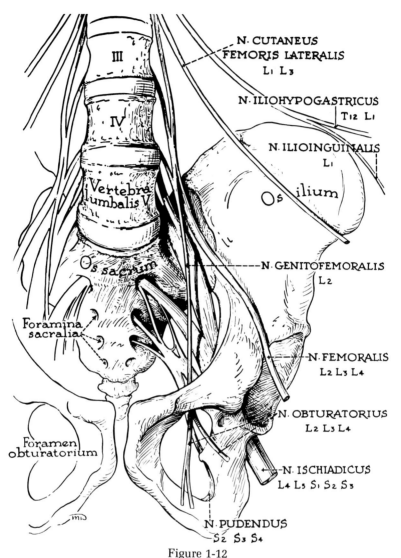

Figure 1-12

Diagram shows the lumbosacral plexus and the courses of the femoral, obturator, and sciatic nerves. (From Anson,[1] with permission.)

femoral triangle. The external spermatic nerve innervates the cremasteric muscle and the skin of the inner aspect of the upper thigh, scrotum, or labium.

## Lateral femoral cutaneous nerve

The lateral femoral cutaneous nerve, the first sensory branch of the lumbar plexus, is derived from L-2 and L-3 roots. It emerges from the lateral border of the psoas major muscle and runs forward, coursing along the brim of the pelvis to the lateral end of the inguinal ligament. The nerve reaches the upper thigh after going through a tunnel formed by the lateral attachment of the inguinal ligament and the anterior superior iliac spine. About 12 cm below its exit from the tunnel, the nerve divides into an anterior branch, which supplies the skin over the lateral and anterior surface of the thigh, and a posterior branch, which innervates the lateral and posterior portion of the thigh.

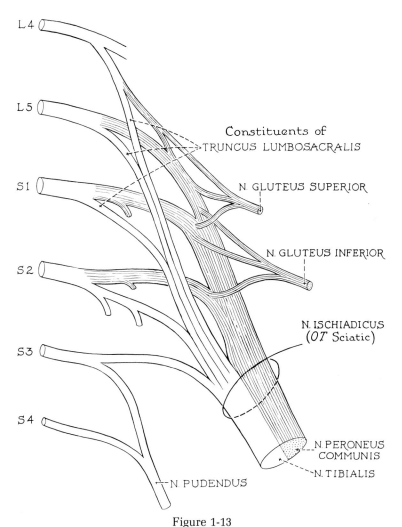

L4

L5

S1

S2

S3

S4

Constituents of
TRUNCUS LUMBOSACRALIS

N. GLUTEUS SUPERIOR

N. GLUTEUS INFERIOR

N. ISCHIADICUS
(*OT* Sciatic)

N. PERONEUS
COMMUNIS

N. TIBIALIS

N. PUDENDUS

Figure 1-13

Diagram shows the anterior rami of the lumbosacral spinal nerve forming the sacral plexus. The major nerves derived from this plexus are indicated. The dorsal divisions are shaded. (From Anson,[1] with permission.)

## Femoral nerve

The femoral nerve is formed near the vertebral canal from the anterior rami of the L-2 through L-4 roots (Fig. 1-14). It reaches the front of the leg passing along the lateral edge of the psoas muscle, which it supplies together with the iliacus, and exits the pelvis under the inguinal ligament just lateral to the femoral artery and vein. Its sensory branches supply the skin of the anterior thigh and medial aspect of the calf. The motor branch innervates the pectineus, sartorius, and quadriceps femoris, which consists of the rectus femoris, vastus lateralis, vastus intermedius, and vastus medialis. Of the muscles innervated by this nerve, the iliopsoas flexes the hip at the thigh, the quadriceps femoris extends the leg at the knee, the sartorius flexes the leg and the thigh, and the pectineus flexes the thigh.

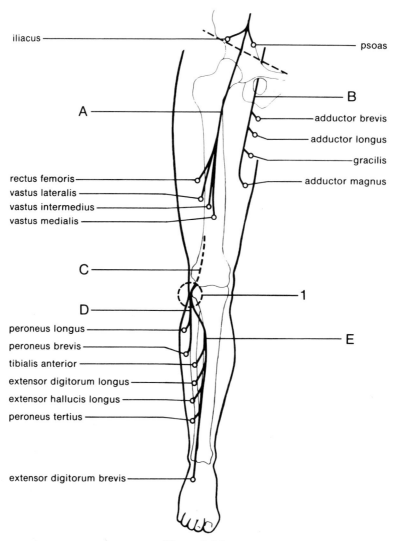

Figure 1-14
Femoral nerve (A), obturator nerve (B), and common peroneal nerve (C) branching into superficial (D) and deep peroneal nerve (E) and the muscles they supply. The peroneal nerve is commonly compressed at the fibular head (1). (Modified from: Medical Research Council: *Aids to the Examination of the Peripheral Nervous System.*[9])

# Saphenous nerve

The saphenous nerve, the largest and longest sensory branch of the femoral nerve, supplies the skin over the medial aspect of the thigh, leg, and foot. It is accompanied by the femoral artery in the femoral triangle, then descends medially under the sartorius muscle and gives off the infrapatellar branch at the lower thigh, which supplies the medial aspect of the knee. The main terminal branch descends along the medial aspect of the leg, accompanied by the long saphenous vein. It passes just anterior to the medial malleolus supplying the medial side of the foot.

## Obturator nerve

The obturator nerve arises from the anterior divisions of L-2 through L-4 roots (Fig. 1-14). It is formed within the psoas muscle and enters the pelvis immediately anterior to the sacroiliac joint. As it passes through the obturator canal, the obturator nerve divides into an anterior branch, which supplies the adductor longus and brevis and the gracilis, and a posterior branch, which innervates the obturator externus and half of the adductor magnus muscle. The sensory fibers supply the skin of the upper thigh over the medial aspect and give off a branch that anastomoses with the saphenous nerve.

# SACRAL PLEXUS AND ITS MAJOR NERVES

The sacral plexus, derived from L-5, S-1, and S-2 roots, is formed in front of the sacroiliac joint (see Figs. 1-12 and 1-13). The sacral plexus is usually connected to the lumbar plexus, and together they are sometimes designated as the lumbosacral plexus. Anomalous derivation is common, being either prefixed with a major contribution of the L-4 spinal nerve to the sacral plexus or postfixed with the L-5 spinal nerve supplying mainly the lumbar plexus. The sacral plexus gives rise to the superior gluteal nerve, which arises from L-4, L-5, and S-1 roots, and the inferior gluteal nerve, which arises from L-5, S-1, and S-2 roots. The sciatic nerve, the largest nerve in the body, arises from L-4 through S-2 roots. After giving off branches to the hamstring muscles, it divides into the tibial and the common peroneal nerves. The nerves derived from the sacral plexus, and the muscles that they innervate, are summarized in Table 1-3.

### Superior and inferior gluteal nerves

The superior gluteal nerve, derived from the L-4 through S-1 roots, innervates the gluteus medius and minimus, which abduct and rotate the thigh internally. The inferior gluteal nerve, arising from the L-5 through S-2 roots, innervates the gluteus maximus, which extends, abducts, and rotates the thigh externally.

### Sciatic nerve

All the anterior rami of L-4 through S-2 roots join to give rise to the sciatic nerve, which leaves the pelvis through the greater sciatic foramen (Fig. 1-15). The anterior and posterior divisions of the rami constitute the tibial and peroneal portions of the sciatic nerve, respectively. They split to form individual nerves in the lower third of the thigh. In the posterior aspect of the thigh, the tibial component of the sciatic trunk gives rise to a series of short branches to innervate the bulk of the hamstring muscles, which consist of the long head of the biceps femoris, semitendinosus, and semimembranosus. The peroneal component supplies the short head of the biceps femoris. The adductor magnus, primarily supplied by the obturator nerve, is also in part innervated by the sciatic trunk.

### Tibial nerve

The tibial or posterior tibial nerve is the extension of the medial popliteal nerve that arises at the bifurcation of the sciatic nerve in the popliteal fossa (Fig. 1-15). It gives off branches to the medial and lateral heads of the gastrocnemius and soleus. Further distally in the leg it supplies the tibialis posterior, flexor digitorum longus, and flexor hallucis longus. It enters the foot passing through the space between the medial malleolus and the flexor retinaculum, where it splits into medial and lateral plantar nerves after giving off a small calcaneal nerve.

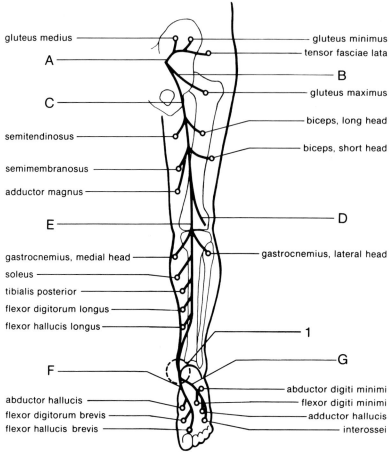

gluteus medius — 
A — 
C — 
semitendinosus — 
semimembranosus — 
adductor magnus — 
E — 
gastrocnemius, medial head — 
soleus — 
tibialis posterior — 
flexor digitorum longus — 
flexor hallucis longus — 
F — 
abductor hallucis — 
flexor digitorum brevis — 
flexor hallucis brevis — 

— gluteus minimus
— tensor fasciae lata
— B
— gluteus maximus
— biceps, long head
— biceps, short head
— D
— gastrocnemius, lateral head
— 1
— G
— abductor digiti minimi
— flexor digiti minimi
— adductor hallucis
— interossei

Figure 1-15

Superior gluteal nerve (A), inferior gluteal nerve (B), and sciatic nerve trunk (C), and the muscles they supply. The sciatic nerve bifurcates to form the common peroneal nerves (D) and the tibial nerve (E). The tibial nerve in turn gives rise to the medial (F) and lateral plantar nerve (G). The tibial nerve may be compressed at the medial malleolus in the tarsal tunnel syndrome (1). (Modified from: Medical Research Council: *Aids to the Examination of the Peripheral Nervous System.*[9])

The medial plantar nerve is accompanied by the medial plantar artery, which may be used to locate the nerve just below the medial malleolus. After giving off the motor branches that innervate the abductor hallucis, flexor digitorum brevis, and flexor hallucis brevis, the sensory fibers of the medial plantar nerve supply the medial anterior two-thirds of the sole and the plantar skin of the first three toes and part of the fourth toe. The lateral plantar nerve winds around the heel to the lateral side of the sole to innervate the abductor digiti minimi, the flexor digiti minimi, the abductor hallucis, and the interossei. It supplies the skin over the lateral aspect of the sole, lateral half of the fourth toe and the fifth toes.

## Common peroneal nerve

The common peroneal nerve is also called the lateral popliteal nerve as it branches off laterally from the sciatic trunk in the politeal fossa (see Fig. 1-14). It consists of fibers derived from L-4, L-5, and S-1 roots. Immediately after its origin the nerve becomes superficial as it winds around the head of the fibula laterally. After entering the leg at this position, it gives off a small recurrent nerve that supplies sensation to the patella. It then bifurcates into the superficial and deep peroneal nerves.

The superficial peroneal nerve, also known as the musculocutaneous nerve, supplies the peroneus longus and brevis, which plantarflex and evert the foot. The nerve descends between the peroneal muscles, which it innervates, then divides into medial and intermediate dorsal cutaneous nerves. These sensory branches pass anterior to the extensor retinaculum and supply the anterolateral aspect of the lower half of the leg and dorsum of the foot and toes.

The deep peroneal nerve, sometimes called the anterior tibial nerve, innervates the muscles that dorsiflex and evert the foot. These muscles include the tibialis anterior, extensor digitorum longus, extensor hallucis longus, peroneus tertius, and extensor digitorum brevis. The last muscle may be anomalously innervated by a communicating branch called the accessory deep peroneal nerve. This anomalous branch derived from the superficial peroneal nerve at the knee will be discussed in Chapter 7. The deep peroneal nerve also supplies the skin over a small, wedge-shaped area between the first and second toes.

## Sural nerve

The sural nerve is a pure sensory nerve that is formed by the union of the medial sural cutaneous branch of the tibial nerve and the sural communicating branch of the common peroneal nerve. It arises below the popliteal space, descends between the two bellies of the gastrocnemius, winds behind the lateral malleolus, and reaches the dorsum of the fifth toe. It supplies the skin over the posterolateral aspect of the distal leg and lateral aspect of the foot. The sural nerve is one of the few readily accessible sensory nerves in the lower extremities. The nerve is suited for biopsy studies because the sensory changes produced by its removal are minimal. As will be discussed in Chapter 4, a fascicular biopsy of the sural nerve allows in vitro recording of nerve action potentials. In vivo studies of the sural nerve are of particular interest as the data obtained may be directly correlated with in vitro conduction characteristics, as well as histologic findings, if the nerve is biopsied.[4]

# REFERENCE SOURCES

1. ANSON, BJ: *An Atlas of Human Anatomy*, ed 2. WB Saunders, Philadelphia, 1963.

2. CARPENTER, MB: *Human Neuroanatomy*, ed 7. Williams & Wilkins, Baltimore, 1976.

3. DELAGI, EF, ET AL: *Anatomic Guide for the Electromyographer: The Limbs.* Charles C Thomas, Springfield, Ill, 1975.

4. DYCK PJ, LAMBERT, EH, AND NICHOLS, PC: *Quantitative measurement of sensation related to compound action potential and number and size of myelinated fibres of sural nerve in health, Friedreich's ataxia, hereditary sensory neuropathy and tabes dorsalis.* In REMOND, A (ED): *Handbook of Electroencephalography and Clinical Neurophysiology,* Vol 9. Elsevier, Amsterdam, 1971, pp 83–118.

5. GOODGOLD, J: *Anatomical Correlates of Clinical Electromyography.* Williams & Wilkins, Baltimore, 1974.

6. HAYMAKER, W AND WOODHALL, B: *Peripheral Nerve Injuries: Principles of Diagnosis,* ed 2. WB Saunders, Philadelphia, 1953.

7. HOLLINSHEAD, WH: *Anatomy for Surgeons,* Volume 3: *The Back and Limbs,* ed 2. Harper & Row, New York, 1969.

8. HOLLINSHEAD, WH: *Functional Anatomy of the Limbs and Back,* ed 3. WB Saunders, Philadelphia, 1969.

9. MEDICAL RESEARCH COUNCIL: *Aids to the Examination of the Peripheral Nervous System.* Memorandum No. 45, Her Majesty's Stationery Office, London, 1976.

10. PATTEN, J: *Neurological Differential Diagnosis.* Harold Starke Ltd, London, 1977.

11.   RANSON, SW AND CLARK, SL: *The Anatomy of the Nervous System: Its Development and Function;* ed 10. WB Saunders, Philadelphia, 1959.

12.   ROMANES, GJ: *Cunningham's Textbook of Anatomy,* ed 11. Oxford University Press, London, 1972.

13.   SUNDERLAND, S: *Nerves and Nerve Injuries,* ed 2. Churchill Livingstone, New York, 1978.

14.   WILLIAMS, PL AND WARWICK, R: *Gray's Anatomy,* ed 36 (British). Churchill Livingstone, Edinburgh, 1980.

# 2

# ELECTRICAL PROPERTIES OF NERVE AND MUSCLE

The primary function of the nervous system is to convey information from one part of the body to another. This is achieved by propagating nerve action potentials from the cell body to the axon terminal. For determination of sensory or mixed nerve conduction velocities, this electrical signal can be recorded after stimulation of the nerve, through surface or needle electrodes. Similarly, the conduction of motor fibers is tested by recording the muscle action potential elicited by stimulation of the motor or mixed nerves. Electromyography permits analysis of electrical properties in the skeletal muscle at rest and during voluntary contraction. Thus, an understanding of the electrical properties of nerve and muscle is essential for proper interpretations of electrodiagnostic data in the clinical domain.

Despite different anatomic substrates subserving electrical impulses, the same basic membrane physiology applies to both nerve and muscle. Excitability of the membrane is determined by the magnitude of the transmembrane potential in a steady state. When stimulated electrically or chemically, the membrane becomes depolarized. Depolarization beyond the critical level, called threshold, results in generation of an action potential, which then propagates across the membrane. These electrical events can be recorded intracellularly in animal experiments. During clinical electrodiagnostic procedures, however, the potentials are recorded extracellularly by surface or needle electrodes, with the interstitial tissues acting as a volume conductor. Therefore, it is imperative to take into account the effect of volume conduction when analyzing electrical potentials recorded in a clinical setting.

## TRANSMEMBRANE POTENTIAL

To properly appreciate the electrical activity recorded during a clinical electrophysiologic examination, a brief review of membrane physiology at the cellular level is in order. This section deals with the ionic concentration of cell plasma and its role in maintaining transmembrane potentials. The next sections summarize the basic physiology of the propagating action potential and how it is recorded through volume conductors. The following discussion is intended merely as a background for subsequent discussion and covers only the fundamental principles relevant to clinical electrophysiology. Readers interested in a more detailed account of basic cell physiology are referred to established texts.[2, 10, 11, 12, 14, 16, 19, 22, 23, 24]

## Ionic concentration of cells

The muscle membrane is the boundary between intracellular (cell plasma) and extracellular (interstitial) fluids. Intracellular and extracellular fluids are similar in that both contain approximately equal numbers of ions dissolved in water. However, there are two major differences. First, there is an electrical potential difference, with the cell being negatively charged inside as compared with outside (transmembrane potential). The value of this steady potential is about $-90$ mV in human skeletal muscle cells,[21] but it varies from one tissue to another, ranging from $-20$ to $-100$ mV. Second, intracellular fluid consists of a much higher concentration of potassium ($K^+$), and lower concentration of sodium ($Na^+$) and chloride ($Cl^-$), relative to extracellular fluid (Table 2-1).

Since, in the steady state, the influx of an ion is the same as the efflux, various factors, which together determine the rate of the ionic flow, must be balanced or in equilibrium. Since the transmembrane concentration difference can be measured, the transmembrane potential theoretically required to maintain the balance (equilibrium potential) can be calculated for each ion (Fig. 2-1).

## Nernst equation

In the case of potassium, for example, the transmembrane concentration difference tends to push potassium from inside to outside the cell, since potassium concentration is higher inside. This force per mole of potassium is the chemical work ($W_c$), which is proportional to the logarithm of the ratio between internal and external concentration of the cation $(K^+)_i$ and $(K^+)_o$, and may be calculated as

$$W_c = RT \log_e (K^+)_i/(K^+)_o,$$

where R is the universal gas constant and T the absolute temperature.

The energy required to counter this force must be provided by the negative equilibrium potential ($E_k$) pulling the positively charged potassium from outside to inside

**TABLE 2-1 Compositions of extracellular and intracellular fluids of mammalian muscle**

|  | Extracellular (mmol/1) | Intracellular (mmol/1) | Equilibrium Potential (mV) |
|---|---|---|---|
| Cations |  |  |  |
| $Na^+$ | 145 | 12 | 66 |
| $K^+$ | 4 | 155 | $-97$ |
| Others | 5 | - | — |
| Anions |  |  |  |
| $Cl^-$ | 120 | 4 | $-90$ |
| $HCO_3^-$ | 27 | 8 | $-32$ |
| Others | 7 | 155 | — |
| Potential | 0 mV | $-90$ mV |  |

From Patton,[18] with permission.

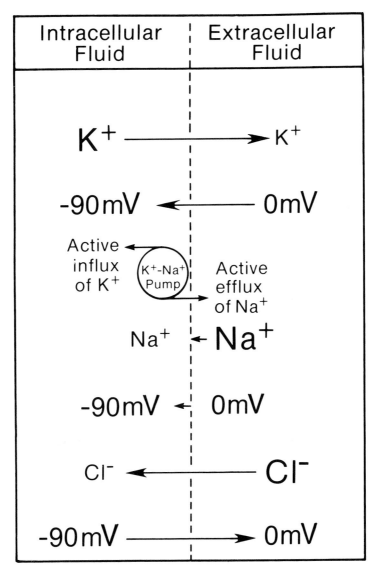

Figure 2-1

Simplified scheme of active and passive fluxes of K+, Na+ and Cl− in the steady state. Driving force on each ion is shown by vectors. For K+, the efflux due to concentration gradient equals the influx due to electrical force plus the active influx by Na+-K+ pump. For Na+, the influxes due to electrical and chemical gradient are both small because of membrane resistance. The sum of the two equals the active efflux by the Na+-K+ pump. For Cl−, the influx due to concentration gradient is the same as the efflux due to electrical force. The ratio of Na+ and K+ exchange is usually about 3:2, although this diagram illustrates a neutral pump with an exchange ratio of 1:1.

the cell. This force per mole of potassium is the electrical work ($W_e$), which is proportional to the transmembrane voltage $E_k$, and may be calculated as

$$W_e = Z_k \, F \, E_k,$$

where F is the number of coulombs per mole of charge and $Z_k$ the valence of the ion.

In the steady state, the sum of these two energies $W_c$ and $W_e$ must equal zero, since they are forces with opposite vectors. Therefore,

$$Z_k \, F \, E_k \, + \, RT \, \log_e \, (K^+)_i/(K^+)_o \, = \, 0.$$

The theoretical potassium equilibrium potential $E_k$ is thus calculated by the Nernst equation,

$$E_k = -(RT/Z_k F) \, \log_e \, (K^+)_i/(K^+)_o.$$

Similarly, the sodium and chloride equilibrium potentials, $E_{na}$ and $E_{cl}$, respectively, can be obtained as follows:

$$E_{na} = -(RT/Z_{na} \, F) \, \log_e \, (Na^+)_i/(Na^+)_o \text{ and}$$

$$E_{cl} = -(RT/Z_{cl}F) \, \log_e \, (Cl^-)_i(Cl^-)_o$$

The values of $E_k$, $E_{na}$, and $E_{cl}$ calculated on the basis of the ionic concentrations shown in Table 2-1 are $-97$ mV, $+66$ mV, and $-90$ mV, respectively. These compare with the actual measurement of the transmembrane potential ($E_m$), which is about $-90$ mV in the example under consideration. Thus, chloride is the only ion that is at equilibrium if only the transmembrane concentration and potential differences are taken into consideration.

## Sodium–potassium pump

In the case of potassium, the small discrepancy between $E_k$ ($-97$ mV) and $E_m$ ($-90$ mV) can be explained by an additional factor: the active transport of potassium by an energy-dependent pump. Thus, there are two forces pulling potassium from outside to inside the cell, transmembrane potential ($-90$ mV) and active potassium transport (approximately equivalent to $-7$ mV), which add up to be $-97$ mV, to counter almost exactly the transmembrane concentration gradient pushing potassium from inside to outside the cell. In the case of sodium, both the transmembrane concentration gradient and potential difference ($-90$ mV) tend to pull the ion from outside to inside the cell. This cation remains in equilibrium because of its impermeability due to a mechanical barrier imposed by the structure of the cell membrane. The small amount of sodium that does move inside of the cell is countered by active transport of sodium from inside to outside.

This energy-dependent process is referred to as the sodium–potassium pump, since the outward transport of sodium is in exchange for actively transported potassium in the opposite direction, a process required to maintain potassium equilibrium as mentioned earlier. In Figure 2-1, it is assumed that for every potassium ion actively transported inward, one sodium ion is pumped out. However, such a neutral pump is rarely seen. Instead, the ratio of sodium and potassium exchange is about 3:2 in most tissues.[18] Such an imbalanced arrangement is called an electrogenic sodium–potassium pump, since this type of exchange directly contributes to the membrane potential, although its effect is minimal compared with that of changes in membrane permeability.

## Goldman-Hodgkin-Katz equation

The Nernst equation closely predicts the membrane potential for chloride and potassium ions that are highly diffusible to the membrane. However, it does not fit well with much less permeable sodium ions, because, as indicated above, relative membrane permeability is not taken into consideration in the equation. When this factor is added, a more comprehensive formula can be derived based on the concentration gradients and membrane permeabilities of all ions. This is known as the Goldman-Hodgkin-Katz equation,

$$EM = (RT/F) \log_e \frac{P_{Na}(Na_o^+) + P_K(K_o^+) \text{ ------ } + P_{Cl}(Cl_i^-)}{P_{Na}(Na_i^+) + P_K(K_i^+) \text{ ------ } + P_{Cl}(Cl_o^-)}$$

where $P_{Na}$, $P_K$, and $P_{Cl}$ are permeabilities of the respective ions.

In this equation it is evident that the transmembrane potential is primarily determined by the concentration gradient of the most permeable ions. In the resting membrane, $P_K$ is very high relative to $P_{Na}$. If $P_{Na}$ is assumed to be negligible, then the Goldman-Hodgkin-Katz equation would approximate the Nernst equation using the potassium concentration gradients. The transmembrane potential calculated using either equation would be $-80$ to $-90$ mV. Conversely, the Goldman-Hodgkin-Katz potential would be close to the Nernst potential for sodium, if $P_K$ is made negligible relative to $P_{Na}$. In this situation, the calculated membrane potentials range from $+50$ to $+70$ mV. This reversal of potential is in fact seen during the generation of an action potential as outlined below.

# GENERATION OF ACTION POTENTIAL

Generation of the action potential can be divided into two phases: subthreshold and threshold events. Essential characteristics of subthreshold activation include a graded response that produces local changes in transmembrane potential. Subthreshold activation generates no action potential and is self-limiting because of the diminution of the local potential change with distance. The membrane potential reaches the critical level with about 15 to 25 mV of depolarization from $-90$ mV to $-65$ to $-75$ mV in the case of human muscle cells.[21] The action potential then develops in an all-or-none fashion; that is, the same maximal response is elicited regardless of the kind or magnitude of the stimulus (Fig. 2-2). This is a complex energy-dependent process.

## All-or-none response

In the intrinsic membrane, there are molecular channels that regulate the conductance of sodium ($Na^+$) and potassium ($K^+$) ions across the membrane. One set of channels is used for movement of sodium ions and another set for potassium ions. The channels may be open or closed, depending on the transmembrane potential. When open, the channels provide adequate pathways for that specific ion to cross the membrane. In the resting membrane, the channels for potassium ions are open, whereas those controlling movement of sodium ions are closed and inaccessible. When depolarization reaches the critical level, the molecular structure of the cell membrane changes in such a way that the channels for sodium ions are now open, giving rise to a 500-fold increase in its permeability to sodium ions.

This change is an intrinsic property of the nerve and muscle cells that underlie the all-or-none response: regardless of the nature of the stimulus, the action potential generated is the same as long as depolarization to the critical level occurs. Because of the increased conductance or permeability of the membrane, sodium ions now enter the cell seeking a new steady state. Increasing sodium entry further depolarizes the cell, which in turn accelerates sodium entry, thus changing the membrane toward the sodium equilibrium potential. Because of this regenerative sequence, an action potential develops explosively to its full size. According to the Goldman-Hodgkin-Katz equation, the transmembrane potential can be controlled by alterations in membrane permeability to ions without change in ionic concentration gradients. Thus, dramatic change in sodium permeability during the course of the action potential results in a reversal of membrane potential from $-80$ or $-90$ mV to $+20$ or $+30$ mV. In other words, the

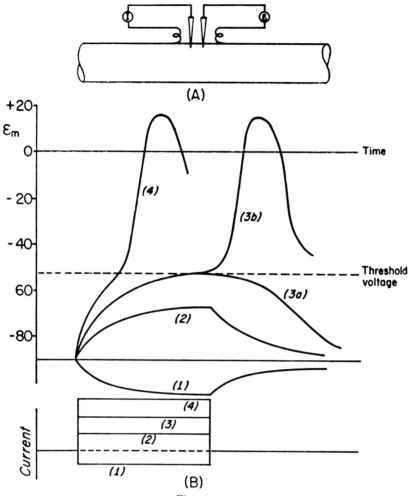

Figure 2-2

Schematic diagram of graded response after subthreshold stimuli and generation of action potential after suprathreshold stimuli. Experimental arrangement with intracellular stimulation (I) and recording electrodes (E) is shown on top (A) and polarity, strength, and duration of a constant current on bottom (B): hyperpolarizing (1) and subthreshold depolarizing current (2) produce nonpropagating local response. Current of just threshold strength will produce either local change (3a) or an action potential (3b). Suprathreshold stimulation (4) also generates an action potential but with a more rapid time course of depolarization. (From Woodbury,[23] with permission.)

membrane potential changes from a level near the potassium equilibrium potential (−80 to −90 mV) to one near sodium equilibrium potential (+50 to +70 mV).

When the membrane is depolarized the permeability to potassium ions also increases as a result of a change in the molecular structure, but only after a delay of about one millisecond. At about the same time, the increased permeability to sodium falls again to near the resting value. This is called inactivation of sodium conductance. These two factors, increased potassium conductance and inactivation of sodium conductance, are responsible for rapid recovery of the cell membrane from depolarization. After the potential falls rapidly towards the resting level, the membrane is transiently hyperpolarized because of the increase in potassium conductance, which then returns slowly to the resting value, completing the cycle of repolarization. It should be noted that the amount of sodium efflux and potassium efflux during the course of an action potential is too small to alter the concentration gradients of these two ions. Although repolarization is primarily the result of a delayed increase in potassium conductance in squid giant axon,[13] this may not be the case with mammalian peripheral or central myelinated axons. Voltage clamp experiments indicate that potassium conductance may be minimal or absent for intact mammalian peripheral myelinated axons[5] or mammalian dorsal column axons.[15]

## Local current

If an action potential is initiated at one point on the cell membrane, rendering the inside of the cell positive in that local region, intracellular current flows (according to a definition by convention) from the active area to the inside of the adjacent inactive region, where the inside of the cell membrane is negatively charged. The current is completed by a return flow through the extracellular fluid from the inactive to active region.[6] In other words, a current enters the cell at the site of depolarization and passes out in adjacent regions of the polarized membrane (see Fig. 4-3). This local current tends to depolarize inactive regions on both sides of the active area. When the depolarization reaches threshold, an action potential is generated, giving rise to a new local current further distally and proximally. Thus, once an impulse is generated in the nerve axon it is conducted in both directions from the original site of depolarization, initiating orthodromic as well as antidromic propagation of the action potential. The physiology underlying propagation of nerve action potentials will be further discussed in Chapter 4.

## After-potential

In an extracellular recording, an action potential is represented as a negative spike of about one millisecond duration (Fig. 2-3). There is an externally negative deflection grafted onto the declining phase of the negative spike (negative after-potential) followed by a prolonged externally positive deflection (positive after-potential). The negative after-potential, which is a super-normal period of excitability, is probably due to extracellular accumulation of potassium ions associated with the generation of an action potential. The positive after-potential is a subnormal period of excitability. This may be caused by elevated potassium conductance at the end of the action potential and an increased rate of ionic flux across the cell membrane via the sodium–potassium pump to counter the increased internal sodium concentration. However, the exact mechanism is unknown.

# VOLUME CONDUCTION
## Diphasic recording of action potential

A pair of electrodes placed on the surface of a nerve or muscle at rest register no difference of potential between them, since both electrodes are equally positive relative to the inside of the cell. If the tissue is activated at one end and the propagating action potential reaches the nearest electrode ($G_1$), then $G_1$ becomes negative relative to the distant electrode ($G_2$). This results in an upward deflection of the tracing according to the convention of clinical electrophysiology (although the oscilloscope could also be set to display negativity of $G_1$ as a downward deflection if so desired). With further passage of the action potential, the point is reached at which both $G_1$ and $G_2$ are equally affected by the depolarized zone. Here the trace returns to the baseline, since there is no longer any potential difference between the two electrodes. When the action potential moves further away from $G_1$ and toward $G_2$, $G_2$ becomes negative relative to $G_1$ (or $G_1$ is positive relative to $G_2$). Therefore, the trace now shows a downward deflection. It

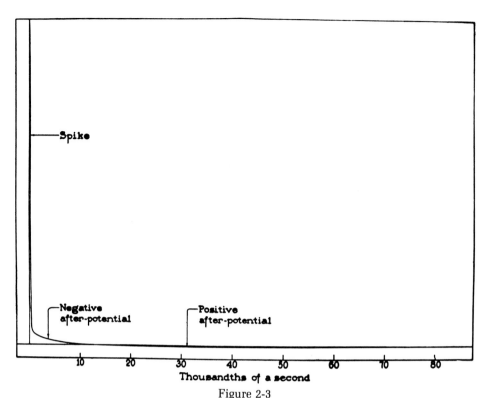

Figure 2-3

Diagrammatic representation of an action potential in A fibers of the cat. The spike and negative and positive after potentials are drawn in their correct relative size and true relationships. (From Gasser,[8] with permission.)

then returns to the baseline as the nerve activity becomes too distant to affect the electrical field near the recording electrodes. This produces a diphasic action potential as shown in Figure 2-4.[20]

## Effect of volume conduction

In the above discussion it was assumed that the recording electrodes were placed directly on the nerve or muscle with no intervening external conduction medium. During the clinical study of an action potential, this assumption is invalid, since the generator source is surrounded by connective tissue and interstitial fluid which act as a conduction medium or a volume conductor.[6, 9] The transmembrane potential recorded at a particular point in a volume conductor is difficult to analyze, because the resulting current flow is complicated. It is known, however, that variation of recorded potential at a given point in the volume conductor can be closely predicted by the solid angle subtended by the generator source. The theory of solid angle approximation will be briefly described below as it pertains to the analysis of an action potential recorded through a volume conductor.

An electrical field in a volume conductor is best illustrated if the source potential is represented as a dipole; that is, a pair of positive and negative charges.[1] In a volume conductor, currents move into an infinite number of pathways between the positive and negative ends of the dipole, although their densities (the number of charges passing through a unit area per unit time) are greatest along the straight path. The current flow decreases in proportion to the square of the distance from the generator source. Thus

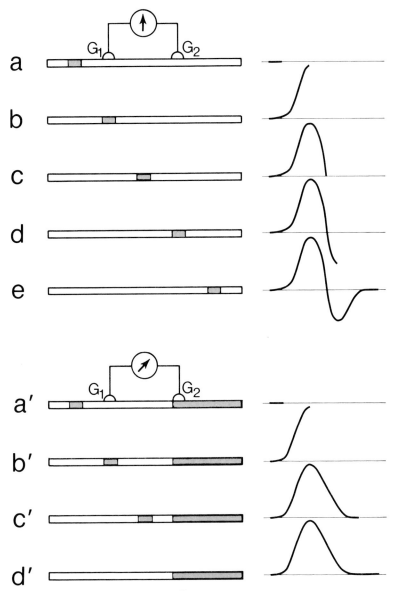

Figure 2-4

Diphasic (top) and monophasic recording (bottom). Action potential represented by the shaded area propagates from left to right. In the top series, the two electrodes are isopotential in (a), (c), and (e). The active electrode ($G_1$) is negative to the reference electrode ($G_2$) in (b), and $G_1$ is positive to $G_2$ in (d), resulting in a diphasic potential. In the bottom, the darkened area on the right indicates the killed end with permanent depolarization. Thus, $G_1$ is positive to $G_2$ in (a'), (c'), and (d'). In (b'), $G_1$ and $G_2$ are isopotential, causing upward deflection from the positive baseline to 0 potential.

the effect of the dipole at any point in a volume conductor may be recorded with an active recording electrode in the area of high current density and a reference electrode at a distance. Whether the electrode records positive or negative potentials depends on its spatial orientation to the opposing charges of the dipole. No potential is registered if the active electrode near the source is located at a point equidistant from the positive and negative charges. The amplitude of the recorded potential is determined by the charge density (the net charge per unit area) and the surface areas of the dipole, as well as its proximity to the active recording electrode.[7]

The resting transmembrane potential can be viewed as a series of dipoles arranged with positive charges on the outer surface and negative charges on the inner surface. When dealing with a dipole of the transmembrane potential it is convenient to use solid angle approximation.[3, 21] The solid angle subtended by an object is defined as the area of its surface divided by the squared distance from a specific point to the surface. In the context of our present discussion, the solid angle is proportional to the area of the polarized membrane viewed by the electrode and inversely proportional to the squared distance between the electrode and the membrane surface. Thus, the potential derived from a dipole layer can be predicted solely on the basis of the solid angle subtended by the membrane at the recording electrode. This relationship is schematically shown in Figure 2-5. The propagating action potential can then be visualized as a positively charged wave front representing depolarization at the cross-section of the nerve at which the transmembrane potential reverses.[17] This is followed by a negatively charged wave front representing repolarization of the activated zone.

## Clinical implications

These observations have practical implications for clinical diagnosis in which analyzing the waveform is of great importance in the assessment of nerve or muscle action potential. A sequence of potential changes arises as the two sufficiently close wave fronts travel in the volume conductor from left to right. As in Figure 2-6, this can be shown to be a positive-negative-positive triphasic wave as the moving fronts of depolarization and repolarization approach, then reach, and finally pass beyond the point of the recording electrode. In practice, a triphasic wave is seen when recording a propagating action potential from a deeply situated nerve using a pair of surface electrodes. If the potential is recorded at its entry into the volume conductor, or if the potential

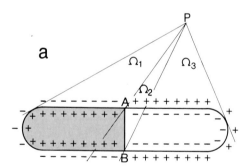

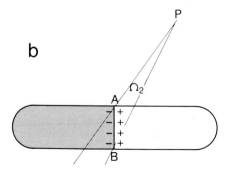

Figure 2-5
Potential recorded at P from a cell with active (dark area) and inactive region. In (a), total solid angle consists of $\Omega_1$, $\Omega_2$, and $\Omega_3$. Potential at P due to solid angles $\Omega_1$ and $\Omega_3$ is zero, since the nearer and farther membranes are dipoles of equal magnitude but opposite polarity. In $\Omega_2$, however, the nearer and farther membranes are dipoles of the same polarity because of depolarization. In (b), charges of the nearer and farther membranes due to solid angle $\Omega_2$ are placed on the axial section through a cylindrical cell to show that propagating action potential may be represented by a positively charged wave front moving from left to right. (Adapted from Patton,[17].)

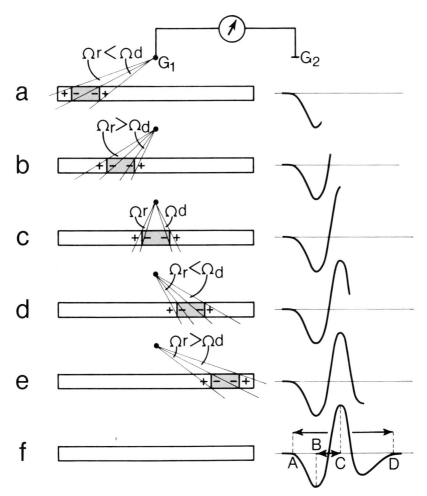

Figure 2-6

Triphasic potential due to a pair of wave fronts of opposite polarity representing depolarization and repolarization. The action potential travels from left to right in a volume conductor. The recording electrode, ($G_1$), is near the active region and reference electrode ($G_2$) on a remote inactive point. Initially (a), $G_1$ primarily sees the positivity of the first dipole, which has a greater solid angle ($\Omega d$) than the second dipole of negative front ($\Omega r$). As the active region approaches $G_1$, this relationship reverses, since $\Omega d$ becomes progressively smaller compared with $\Omega r$ (b). The maximal negativity is recorded when the active region is directly under $G_1$, which now sees only negative ends of the dipoles (c). With further progression of the action potential, the negativity declines as $G_1$ begins to register the positive end of the second dipole (d). The polarity reverses again as $\Omega r$ becomes greater than $\Omega d$ (e). The trace then returns to the baseline when the active region moves further away from the recording electrode (f). The last positive phase is smaller and longer than the first, indicating a slower time course of repolarization as compared with depolarization. A triphasic potential may be characterized by amplitude, duration (A-D), and rise time (B-C).

originates in the region near the electrode, the initial positivity is not seen. Thus, a negative-positive diphasic waveform is expected with the electrode near the end-plate region of the muscle fiber, which is activated by the action potential of the nerve terminal. In contrast, a positive-negative diphasic potential arises if an impulse approaches but does not leave the recording electrode.

The motor unit potential recorded in electromyography is basically the combination of triphasic potentials recorded from single muscle fibers. Because of the effect of volume conduction, the waveform of the recorded potential varies with the location of the recording tip relative to the source of the muscle potential.[4] Thus, the same motor unit has multiple profiles as represented by the different appearance of the motor unit potential recorded from different sites. On moving the recording electrode various distances away from the muscle fibers, one of the obvious changes is the reduction in amplitude. Additionally, the duration of the positive-to-negative rising phase (rise time) becomes greater as the electrode is moved further away. This is an important clue in determining whether or not the recording electrode is sufficiently near the muscle fiber generating the potential. Amplitude may not be used for this purpose, because it may be small owing to smaller muscle fibers or lower fiber density. The waveforms of spontaneous potentials are also determined by the location of the needle relative to the source of the discharges as discussed in Chapter 13.

# REFERENCE SOURCES

1. BOYD, DC, LAWRENCE, PD, AND BRATTY, P: *On modeling the single motor unit action potential.* IEEE Trans Biomed Eng 25:236, 1978.

2. BRAZIER, MAB: *Electrical Activity of the Nervous System,* ed 4. Pitman Medical, Kent, Great Britain, 1977.

3. BROWN, BH: *Theoretical and experimental waveform analysis of human compound nerve action potentials using surface electrodes.* Med Biol Eng 6:375, 1968.

4. BUCHTHAL, F, GULD, C, AND ROSENFALCK, P: *Volume conduction of the spike of the motor unit potential investigated with a new type of multielectrode.* Acta Physiol Scand 38:331, 1957.

5. CHIU, SY, ET AL: *A quantitative description of membrane currents in rabbit myelinated nerve.* J Physiol (Lond) 292:149, 1979.

6. CLARK, J AND PLONSEY, R: *The extracellular potential field of the single active nerve fiber in a volume conductor.* Biophys J 8:842, 1968.

7. DELISA, JA, KRAFT, GH, AND GANS, BM: *Clinical electromyography and nerve conduction studies.* Orthop Rev 7:75, 1978.

8. GASSER, HS: *The classification of nerve fibers.* Ohio J Science 41:145, 1941.

9. GATH, I AND STÅLBERG, E: *On the volume conduction in human skeletal muscle: In situ measurements.* Electroenceph Clin Neurophysiol 43:106, 1977.

10. HILLE, B: *Ionic basis of resting and action potentials.* In GEIGER, SR (ED): *Handbook of Physiology: Section 1: The Nervous System,* Vol 1. American Physiological Society, Bethesda, 1977, pp 99–136.

11. HODGKIN, AL: *Ionic movements and electrical activity in giant nerve fibres.* Proc R Soc (Lond) Series B, 148:1, 1958.

12. HODGKIN, AL: *The Conduction of the Nervous Impulse.* The Sherrington Lectures, Vol 7, Liverpool University Press, Liverpool, 1965.

13. HODGKIN, AL AND HUXLEY, AF: *A quantitative description of membrane current and its application to conduction and excitation in nerve.* J Physiol (Lond) 117:500, 1952.

14. KATZ, B: *Nerve, Muscle and Synapse.* McGraw-Hill, New York, 1966.

15. KOCSIS, JD AND WAXMAN, SG: *Absence of potassium conductance in central myelinated axons.* Nature 287:348, 1980.

16. LORENTE DE NO, R: *Analysis of the distribution of the action currents of nerve in volume conductors.* In: *Studies from the Rockefeller Institute for Medical Research: A Study of Nerve Physiology,* Vol 132. The Rockefeller Institute for Medical Research, New York, 1947, pp 384–482.

17. PATTON, HD: *Special properties of nerve trunks and tracts.* In RUCH, TC, ET AL (EDS): *Neurophysiology,* ed 2. WB Saunders, Philadelphia, 1965, pp 73–94.

18. PATTON, HD: *Resting and action potentials of neurons.* In PATTON, HD, ET AL (EDS): *Introduction to Basic Neurology.* WB Saunders, Philadelphia, 1976, pp 49–68.

19. PATTON, HD, ET AL: *Introduction to Basic Neurology.* WB Saunders, Philadelphia, 1976.

20. ROSENFALCK, P: *Intra and extracellular potential fields of active nerve and muscle fibres.* Acta Physiol Scand (Suppl 321) 1, 1969.

21. RUCH, TC AND FULTON, JF: *Medical Physiology and Biophysics,* ed 20. WB Saunders, Philadelphia, 1973.

22. RUCH, TC, ET AL (EDS): *Neurophysiology,* ed 2. WB Saunders, Philadelphia, 1965.

23. WOODBURY, JW: *Action potential: Properties of excitable membranes.* In RUCH, TC, ET AL (EDS): *Neurophysiology,* ed 2. WB Saunders, Philadelphia, 1965, pp 26–57.

24. WOODBURY, JW: *The cell membrane: Ionic and potential gradients and active transport.* In RUCH, TC, ET AL (EDS): *Neurophysiology,* ed 2. WB Saunders, Philadelphia, 1965, pp 1–25.

# 3

# ELECTRODES AND RECORDING APPARATUS

The apparatus required in the performance of routine electromyography include electrodes, amplifier, oscilloscope, time base, loudspeaker, and tape recorder. The electrical activity associated with muscle contraction may be recorded using either a surface electrode placed on the skin over the muscle or a needle electrode inserted into the muscle. Surface electrodes register a summated electrical activity. They are satisfactory for recording compound muscle or nerve action potentials in nerve conduction studies. For electromyography, needle electrodes are better suited, since they allow discrimination of individual motor unit potentials, which can be adequately recorded only if the electrode is placed very close to the generator site. The electrical and physical characteristics of recording electrodes significantly influence the amplitude and other aspects of the potentials under study.[16]

Amplified up to one million times, action potentials are displayed on an oscilloscope and played through a loudspeaker for simultaneous visual and auditory analysis. For optimal results, amplifier settings must be adjusted depending upon the kind of information desired and the type of activities being recorded. A visual display on the oscilloscope screen may be photographed or signals may be fed through a fiberoptic system to sensitive paper for permanent recordings. The potentials may also be stored using a magnetic tape recorder or digital storage for later analysis. Some means of providing amplitude and time calibration is required for verifying the accuracy of the cathode ray display. Although detailed discussion of electronics will be found in Appendix 2 practical aspects of instrumentation will be dealt with briefly in the following sections.

## ELECTRODES

The action potential recorded during voluntary muscle contraction depends to a great extent on the type of recording electrode.[7, 15] Surface electrodes placed over the muscle register summated activities from many motor units. With the use of a needle electrode, isolated motor unit potentials can be recorded. Commonly used in routine electromyography are the standard and bipolar concentric needle electrodes,[1] as well as monopolar needle electrodes.[18] The electrode described by Ekstedt and Stålberg[11] has a leading-edge small enough to allow recording of potentials derived from single muscle fibers in isolation. Less commonly used special purpose electrodes include the multielectrode and flexible wire electrode. As in animal experiments, the action potentials of a muscle fiber can also be recorded in man with a microelectrode placed intracellularly, but this technique is not suited for routine clinical examination.[6]

## Proper application of electrodes

Before application of surface electrodes, the skin should be cleaned with alcohol, and calloused surfaces should be lightly scraped to reduce the impedance. As described below, these precautions are particularly important if the input impedance of the amplifier is low. Needle electrodes should be sterilized before each use to prevent the transmission of infection. The electrodes may simply be washed and boiled in distilled water. Most commercially available electrode sterilizers bring the water temperature to 100°C and maintain that temperature without excessive boiling. It is recommended that needles be completely covered by boiling water for at least 20 minutes. The metal and plastic components of most needle electrodes will withstand the time and temperature of steam autoclaving. However, some connectors and lead wires must be disconnected before the sterilization procedure. Gas sterilization is also used successfully but may sometimes cause defects in electrode insulation due to the sensitivity of the plastic to the sterilizing agents. Thorough outgassing of electrodes minimizes the amount retained in the plastic material. Optimal sterilization methods can be found in the instructions provided by the electrode manufacturer.

After studying a patient with hepatitis or other potentially contagious disorders with serious consequences it is wise to discard the needle. Patients with Jakob-Creutzfeldt disease pose special problems because the transmissible agent responsible for the disease is resistant to conventional sterilization procedures.[14, 19] The American Association of Electromyography and Electrodiagnosis recommends that needle electrodes be discarded after use in all patients with dementia.[22] Before disposal, such needles and blood-contaminated materials should be incinerated or properly sterilized by autoclaving for one hour at 120°C and 15 PSI.[2] Disposal is financially feasible only with monopolar needles, which are much less expensive than standard or bipolar concentric electrodes.

Needle electrodes should be examined periodically for their structural integrity. The inner concentric shaft may become corroded. The Teflon coating of monopolar needles may peel off, exposing the insulated portion of the conductor. There may be a slight bend in the shaft or a crack in the tip. These defects are best detected with a dissecting microscope with a magnifying factor of ten. The needle insulation can be easily tested using an ammeter (continuity tester or volt-ohm meter) and a battery. One terminal of a battery is connected to the lead of a needle and the other terminal to an ammeter which is in turn connected to a small exploring metal hook or moist cotton. A current flow should be registered only if the exploring hook touches the exposed tip of the needle. The insulation is defective if any current is registered while exploring the shaft of the needle. Standard or bipolar concentric needles are tested by connecting the two leads to the battery through an ammeter. A current flow, if registered, indicates a short circuit at the needle tip. Current normally flows if the needle tip is immersed in water.

## Types of available electrodes

Common electrodes used in electromyography will be briefly described below and shown in Figure 3-1.

**SURFACE ELECTRODES.** Surface electrodes are square or round metal plates which are usually made of platinum or silver. They come in different sizes, but the dimension

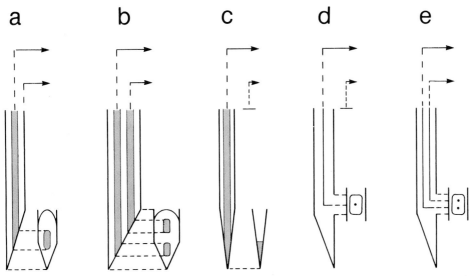

Figure 3-1

Schematic illustration of standard concentric (a), bipolar concentric (b), monopolar (c), and single fiber needles (d, e). Dimensions vary but the diameters of the outside cannulas shown are similar to 26-gauge hypodermic needles (460 μm) for (a), (d), and (e), 23-gauge needle (640 μm) for (b), and 28-gauge needle (360 μm) for (c). The exposed tip areas are about 150 μm × 600 μm for (a), 150 μm × 300 μm with spacing between wires of 200 μm center to center for (b), 0.14 mm² for (c), and 25 μm in diameter for (d) and (e). A separate reference electrode is necessary with monopolar needles (c) and (d) to complete the circuit. (Modified from Stålberg and Trontelj.[23])

is ordinarily about 1 by 1 cm. They are usually applied with adhesive tape to the skin over the muscle under study, although collodion may be used for long-term monitoring. To reduce the impedance, the skin may be cleansed with alcohol and the surface scraped if necessary. Electrolyte cream is applied under the electrode. Electrode offset voltage at the interface is a steady potential not recorded by the amplifier. However, an artifact is generated when movement causes a sudden mechanical change in the metal-electrolyte interface. To reduce this type of artifact some surface electrodes are designed to allow most movement to occur between electrolyte and skin rather than at the metal-electrolyte interface.

A surface electrode may be suitable for recording summated muscle action potentials, especially in monitoring an exercise for kinesiologic studies.[3] However, high frequency components are usually lost and individual motor unit potentials are difficult to discern. They are primarily used for recording compound nerve or muscle action potentials, for stimulation of the peripheral nerves, as a ground lead, and as a reference with monopolar needle electrodes.

**STANDARD CONCENTRIC (COAXIAL) NEEDLE.** This has been the most commonly used electrode for recording from inside the muscle since its introduction by Adrian and Bronk.[1] Coaxial electrodes are pointed, stainless steel cannulas similar to hypodermic needles, but with a wire in the center of the shaft of the needle. The wire is usually made of nichrome silver or platinum and is typically 0.1 mm or slightly larger in diameter. The outside diameter of the shaft is about 0.3 mm. Both the wire and shaft are bare at the tip. The potential difference between the needle tip and the shaft is recorded when the needle is near a source of electrical activity. The exposed surface is oval in shape with an exposed tip area of about 150 μm × 600 μm, and an impedance of around 50 Kohms. A separate ground electrode is required.

**BIPOLAR CONCENTRIC NEEDLE.** Bipolar needles contain two fine stainless steel or platinum wires within the cannula. If the same size wires are embedded, the cannula is larger for a bipolar than for a standard concentric needle. With this arrangement the potential difference between the two inside wires is recorded. The bipolar electrode thus detects potentials from a much smaller volume than the coaxial needle. Either wire may be considered active. If the cannula is grounded no separate ground is required. There are three terminals in the connecting cable, two active terminals and the ground terminal. Since a very localized area serves as the source for electrical activity, it is possible to record from a small number of single motor units. However, this restricted recording range is a major disadvantage when used for routine electromyography. Bipolar concentric needles may also be used as stimulating electrodes.

**MONOPOLAR NEEDLE.** Monopolar electrodes are thin needles ground to a fine point. They are insulated except at the distal 0.2 to 0.4 mm. They are usually made of stainless steel because of its mechanical properties. The wire, with an average diameter of about 0.8 mm, is insulated with a sleeve of Teflon. Monopolar needles are used with a surface electrode or a second needle in the subcutaneous tissue which serves as a reference lead. The voltage changes are recorded between the electrode and the reference. A separate surface electrode placed on the skin serves as a ground. The monopolar needle is considerably sharper and consequently causes much less pain than other needle electrodes. It is less expensive than the concentric electrode. The monopolar electrode, however, is less stable electrically, and hence noisier. Electronic noise can be reduced by lowering the electrode impedance. In one study,[25] the average impedance magnitudes of monopolar electrodes ranged from 1.4 megohms at 10 Hz to 6.6 Kohms at 10 KHz. Presoaking the electrodes with a small concentration of a wetting agent in saline solution reduces the impedance by 6- to 20-fold. Therefore, this pretreatment appears advantageous when recording low amplitude potentials. The amplitude of a motor unit potential is approximately twice as large when recorded by a monopolar needle as compared with a standard concentric needle. The recording characteristics, of course, differ considerably from one type of monopolar needle to another.

**SINGLE FIBER NEEDLE.** A much smaller leading-edge is used for single fiber electromyography.[10, 11] A 25-$\mu$m diameter electrode mounted on the side of a needle has been found optimal for the maximal amplitude discrimination between near and distant muscle fiber potentials.[12, 13] As in concentric electrodes, single fiber needles may contain two or more wires exposed along the shaft, serving as the leading-edge. The most commonly used, however, is made by inserting one wire into a cannula and exposing the wire end along the side of the cannula, a few millimeters behind the tip.[23] This type of electrode enables one to achieve selective recordings of discharge from single muscle fibers rather than single motor units as discussed in Chapter 15.

**MULTIELECTRODES.** Multielectrodes contain at least three insulated wires within a common cannula. One developed by Buchthal, Guld, and Rosenfalck[8] consisted of multiple wires exposed through the side of the cannula. One of the wires served as the indifferent electrode. Each wire was insulated from the others and from the cannula, which was connected to ground. The separation between the leads along the side of the multielectrode was either 0.5 mm or 1.0 mm, depending upon whether they were used for measurement of motor unit territory in myopathic or neuropathic disorders. The outside cannula of the electrode was 1 mm in diameter. The single fiber needle described above may also contain multiple wires exposed along the shaft.

**FLEXIBLE WIRE.** A flexible wire electrode[9] is used for kinesiologic examination, as it permits freedom of movement. The wires are usually introduced into the muscle with a hypodermic needle which is then withdrawn, leaving the wire within the muscle.[5]

Basmajian[4] has also developed a bipolar electrode made of nylon coated Evanohm alloy wire, 25 $\mu$m in diameter. Although they come in different sizes, the most commonly used are 50 to 100 $\mu$m diameter insulated platinum wires with the tip bare. Smaller lead-off surfaces in the order of 10 to 20 $\mu$m may be obtained if a small hole is made in the insulation of the wire.[17] These electrodes are, however, difficult to standardize and are not suited for quantitative studies of action potential.[23]

**GLASS MICROELECTRODES.** Glass microelectrodes are used to penetrate the cell membrane for cellular recording. They are made of fine glass tubing filled with potassium chloride solution. Because they are very fragile, a micromanipulator is used to insert them into the exposed muscle. If the skin needs to be penetrated, a cannula is used as a carrier. They have a very fine tip, less than 1 $\mu$m in diameter, and consequently a very high impedance, on the order of 5 megohms. Therefore, amplifiers of exceedingly high input impedance are used for recording from glass microelectrodes.[6]

# ELECTRODE AMPLIFIERS

Potentials assessed during electrodiagnostic examinations range in amplitude from microvolts to millivolts. For ordinary oscilloscope display, the signal voltages required for a vertical deflection of 1 cm are on the order of 1 to 100 V. If the oscilloscope display is set at 1 V per cm, signals of 1 $\mu$V and 1 mV have to be amplified 1,000,000 and 1000 times, respectively, to cause a 1 cm deflection. To accomplish this range of amplification, the amplifier usually consists of several stages. One system uses a preamplifier with a gain of 500, followed by several amplifier and attenuator stages to produce a variable gain of 2 to 2000. This arrangement is advantageous in increasing the signal-to-noise ratio, since it allows significant amplification of the signal near the source and little noise develops in the following circuits. To achieve this goal the preamplifier must have a high input impedance, a low noise level, and a large dynamic range.

## Differential amplifier

During electromyographic examination, a major source of interference comes from the coupled potential of the alternating current power line. Since the magnitude of this field is on the order of 100,000 times greater than the evoked potential of individual muscle fibers, proper assessment of the signal is impossible if the interference potential is amplified along with the action potential. This would be the case if the voltage appearing between an input terminal and ground terminal were amplified. The differential amplifiers used in most electromyographic apparatus, however, amplify only the voltage difference between the two input terminals connected to the recording electrodes. With this arrangement, any other voltages appearing between the input terminals and common ground, referred to as common mode voltages, are rejected. Common mode voltages include not only the power line interference but also distant muscle action potentials which affect the two recording electrodes equally.

## Common mode rejection ratio

Rejection of the common mode voltage is not perfect because of the inherent imbalance in the electrical system of the amplifier. The extent of differential amplification between the signal and the common mode voltage is termed common mode rejection ratio. Good differential amplifiers should have rejection ratios close to 100,000. In other words, the signals are amplified 100,000 times more than unwanted potentials appearing as a common mode voltage. A very high rejection ratio, however, will not guarantee the complete elimination of external interference caused by undesired distant potentials. The reasons are twofold. First, the effect of the electromagnetic interference is almost but not quite the same on the two recording electrodes, depending on their relative positions. Second, the contact impedances inevitably differ between the two recording electrodes, leading to unequal distribution of the common mode voltage. Interference occurs if the common mode voltage is too large to be perfectly balanced.

## Means to reduce interference

In addition to reducing and balancing contact impedances of the two electrodes, other precautions helpful in reducing electromagnetic interference include the use of short, well-shielded electrode cables. It is important to have effective grounding of not only the patient but also the instrument and, if necessary, the patient's bed or chair as well as the examiner. Unshielded power cords running to other appliances in the vicinity of the recording apparatus should be removed even if they are not being used at the time. If care is taken, a shielded room is usually unnecessary with most modern equipment. In case the interference cannot be adequately reduced by ordinary means, however, a properly constructed Faraday shield is of great help. To be effective it should enclose the examining room as one continuous conductor and be grounded only at one point. The patient may then be disconnected from the ground electrode, which might register unintended distant potentials. The power line interference can also be reduced by the use of a 50 to 60 Hz filter available for some instruments. Since the use of such filters also distorts electromyographic signals, it should be limited to special situations, such as portable recording, in which all other attempts to reduce interference have failed.

## Input impedance

Analogous to the resistance in a DC circuit, the impedance in an AC circuit determines the current flow for a given alternating voltage source. For recording muscle action potentials, the impedances of the tissue and electrode wires are negligible compared with those at the needle tip and at the input terminal of the amplifier. In this circuit, the muscle action potential is in effect divided into voltage changes at the needle tip and at the input terminals. Thus, if the impedance is equally divided between these two, only one-half of the original muscle potential will appear across the input terminals. To minimize the loss of this potential, the impedance should be considerably higher at the input of the amplifier than at the electrode tip. The input impedances of most amplifiers range from 100 kilohms to hundreds of megohms.

An amplifier with a high input impedance also improves the common mode rejection ratio because the higher the input impedance, the smaller the effect of electrical asymmetry of the recording electrodes. Higher electrode impedances increase amplifier noise and external interference.

## Frequency response

Most commercially available apparatus are equipped with variable high and low frequency filters so that the frequency response can be adjusted according to the type of potentials under study. Complex waveforms encountered in electromyography have rapid rises and are of long duration. If these waveforms are analyzed mathematically (for example, Fourier analysis), it is possible to assign sine waves of different frequencies as their harmonic constituents. The significant sine wave frequencies of muscle action potentials range from 10 Hz to 10 KHz. For clinical electromyography, the frequency band of the amplifier should ideally cover this range. However, in the interfering presence of high frequency noise or low frequency drift, a frequency band extending from 50 Hz to 5 KHz is acceptable. If the high frequency filter is set too low, the amplitude of high frequency components is disproportionately reduced. Extending the high frequency response beyond the band required for proper recording of muscle potentials results in an unnecessary increase in background noise. If the low frequency filter is set too high it causes a distortion of the recorded potential that approximates the rate of change (that is, first derivative) rather than the actual waveform of the original potential. If the frequency response is too low, the baseline becomes unstable, exhibiting the effect of slowly changing biopotentials.

Calibration signals are essential for accurately determining the latency, amplitude, and duration of the recorded potentials. Most commonly used are square wave pulses of known amplitude and duration. The degree of distortion of the calibration waveform indicates the effects of high and low frequency filters. The rise time of the recorded calibration signal is an index of the high frequency response, whereas the slope of the flat top indicates the degree of low frequency response (see App. Fig. 2-8). Other calibration signals include sine waves from the power line or discontinuous waveforms of known frequency and amplitude.

# OSCILLOSCOPE

Following appropriate amplification, action potentials are displayed on an oscilloscope for visual analysis. For a display of rapidly changing amplitude against time, the cathode ray tube is most suitable because it has no mechanical limitations in dynamic high frequency response.

## Cathode ray tube

An electron beam is discharged from an electron gun towards the inside surface of the glass screen of the cathode ray tube. When struck by a beam of electrons the phosphor coating on the inside surface of the screen emits light. This bright spot can be positioned horizontally by adjusting the voltage between a pair of horizontal deflection plates. The spot is made to sweep at a constant speed by applying a ramp voltage to the plates. The vertical position of the electron beam is controlled by a pair of vertical deflection plates, which are connected to the signal voltage from the amplifier. The waveform displayed on the face of the oscilloscope, therefore, represents changing amplitude of the action potential in time. The vertical axis provides a scale for amplitude, whereas the horizontal axis shows units of time. For electromyographic examination, the time base is usually in a free running mode such that, when the spot reaches the end of the screen, it returns rapidly to the beginning to repeat. Many manufacturers now provide digital circuitry to process and store the potentials before displaying them on the cathode ray tube as discussed in Appendix 2B.

## Delay line

The free running mode may be interrupted to generate each sweep on command. In this mode of operation, it is possible to trigger the sweep by a recurring motor unit potential itself. This is convenient for the detailed analysis of a given motor unit potential, since it can be displayed successively at the beginning of each sweep. However, the portion of the waveform preceding the trigger point is not displayed. An electronic delay line circumvents this difficulty by storing the recorded motor unit potential for a short period. After a predetermined delay following the onset of a sweep triggered by the real-time potential, the stored signal leaves the delay line to appear on the screen. With this arrangement, the potential in question occurs repetitively and in its entirety on the same spot of the screen, allowing precise determination of its amplitude and duration.[21]

## Multiple channel recording

Some electromyographic apparatus have multiple channels to allow simultaneous recording from two or more sets of electrodes. This can be achieved by using more than one electron gun and individual deflection plates for each channel with a common time base. Alternatively, a beam from a single gun may be shared by switching the point vertically between the base lines of different traces as it sweeps horizontally across the screen. This electrical switching is done extremely fast, so that each trace appears to be continuous despite the sharing of a single electron beam among various traces.

## Storage oscilloscope

Storage oscilloscopes have a different cathode ray tube that retains traces on the face of the screen for several hours. One type uses a special phosphor that changes its color when electrons strike it. It is erased by applying heat to the phosphor, a process that takes about 30 seconds. In a second type, the trace is retained as electrostatic charges on a mesh behind the screen. The latter is more expensive as it requires a second electron gun which floods the screen to visualize the stored pattern. In this type of storage scope, however, the pattern may be erased quickly by electrically discharging the mesh.

# OTHER RECORDING APPARATUS

## Loudspeaker

The electrical potential recorded from the muscle may be converted into sound through a loudspeaker. This is an essential part of clinical electromyography because of the characteristic sounds produced by different kinds of spontaneous or voluntarily activated muscle potentials during needle examination. Acoustical information is also important because potentials from a motor unit near the recording electrode have a clear, crisp sound, reflecting a short rise time, compared with the dull sound of distant units. In fact an experienced electromyographer can detect the difference between near and distant units by sound better than by oscilloscope display. Thus, the acoustical characteristics of a motor unit potential help to accomplish proper positioning of the needle for accurate assessment of its amplitude and duration.

## Magnetic tape recorder

Magnetic tape recordings may be used to store electrical potentials for later analysis. Direct recording, or the amplitude modulation (AM) method, impresses the signal itself on the tape, whereas in the frequency modulation (FM) method, the signal is converted to a varying frequency of constant amplitude and this is recorded on the tape. The direct type of recording reproduces high frequency potentials well but is limited in low frequency responses from 10 to 15 Hz. In contrast, the FM method can record low frequency potentials but requires a very high tape speed to achieve sufficiently high frequency response for electromyography. The amplitude of the recorded response is more accurately retained with the FM than the AM method. The former is thus preferred for recording compound action potentials.

# ARTIFACTS

Not all electrical potentials registered during an electromyographic examination originate in skeletal muscle. Any voltage not representing the muscle potential sought is considered an artifact. Artifacts can usually be detected relatively easily because of their peculiar discharge pattern. They cause unusual sounds on the loudspeaker in conjunction with bizarre waveforms on the oscilloscope. However, some artifacts are nearly indistinguishable from muscle activity, even by a trained examiner.

Most artifacts originate outside the muscle under study and consequently are unaffected by the position of the recording electrode. These exogenous artifacts may

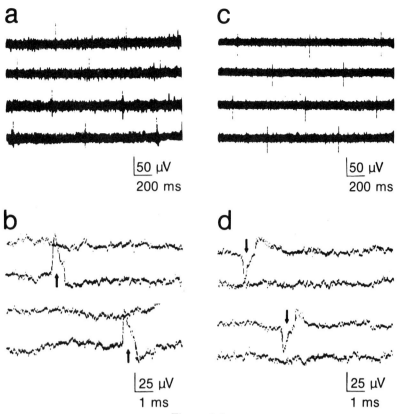

Figure 3-2

Artifacts induced by a cardiac pacemaker recorded by a monopolar needle electrode from the gluteus medius (a, b) and paraspinal muscle (c, d). Note opposite polarity of the sharp discharge in the two recording sites. The interval between the successive impulses is 800 ms, corresponding to 75 impulses/minute. In (a) and (c), trains were recorded continuously from top to bottom, whereas those in (b) and (d) were interrupted between each sweep.

result from an event peculiar to the patient such as the activities induced by the cardiac pacemaker (Fig. 3-2) or transcutaneous stimulator (Fig. 3-3). More commonly, they are related to 60 Hz interference from an electrostatic or electromagnetic field induced by nearby electrical appliances. Characteristic patterns of interference have been described for different generator sources, but none is considered specific (Fig. 3-4). The artifacts may originate in the recording apparatus or a more remote generator site such as a hammer drill (Fig. 3-5). Some are caused by electrical activity derived from impedance variability within the muscle tissue and are dependent upon the location of the needle tip. Still others are genuine biologic potentials generated in the muscle. They include end-plate noises and end-plate spikes, which are considered artifacts by definition, because they are not the intended signals sought during the electromyographic examination. These potentials will be further considered in Chapter 12 (see Figs. 12-3 and 12-4).

## Electrode noise

Potentials may arise from two active metals or the metal-fluid junction when the needle electrode is located intramuscularly. If the electrode-fluid potential is constant, the electrode is said to be polarized and may not receive the signals properly. If the potential is changing, it will result in electrode noise. A smaller electrode tip is associated

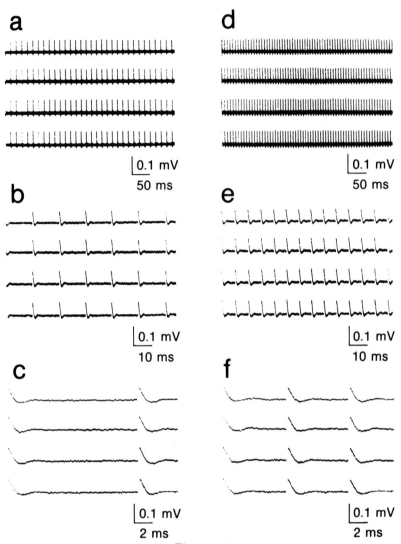

Figure 3-3
Artifact induced by a transcutaneous stimulator. The interval between the successive impulses is 14 ms (a, b, c) and 7 ms (d, e, f), corresponding to approximate rates of 70 and 140 impulses/second, respectively.

with higher impedance, which in turn results in a greater voltage drop during the passage of current. Thus, the smaller the electrode surface, the greater the interference due to electrode polarization or electrode noise. Therefore, the type of metal is more important for needle electrodes than for surface electrodes. In fact, the effects of potentials from active metals are insignificant with skin electrodes. They are very significant for small intramuscular electrodes, unless relatively inert metals, such as stainless steel or platinum, are used.

## Amplifier noise

A certain amount of electrical noise is inherent in an amplifier. It originates from all components, including resistors, transistors, and integrated circuits. Noise arises from the thermal agitation of electrons in the resistor. In the input stage, it is proportional to

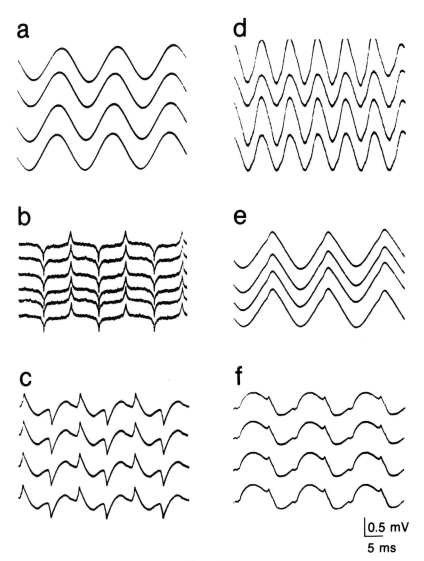

0.5 mV

5 ms

Figure 3-4

Various patterns of 60 Hz interference induced by nearby electrical appliance. They include common 60 Hz interference (a), 60 Hz interference with spikes probably induced by high impedance of the recording electrode (b), typical 60 Hz interference from fluorescent light (c), 120 Hz interference from a diathermy unit (d), and 60 Hz interference from a heat lamp (e and f).

the electrode impedance. Microphonic noise results from mechanical vibration of various components. Noise in the cathode ray tube results from nonuniform electron emissions. The internal noise of transistors tends to be slightly higher than that of vacuum tubes. Low frequency noise from these and other sources in amplifier circuits is usually filtered out. High frequency noise potentials, however, appear as a thickening of the baseline as it sweeps across the screen. This is associated with a hissing noise on the loudspeaker. The level of amplifier noise as perceived on the oscilloscope increases in proportion to amplifier gain and frequency response. Thus, this component of noise seen on the screen will be substantially reduced if the system is operated at lower gains and with narrower filter band widths.

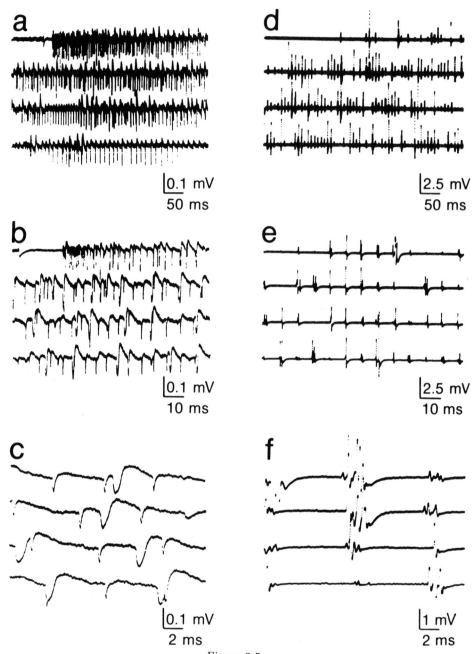

Figure 3-5

Effect of hammer drill operated nearby (a, b, c), and oscillation of the amplifier circuits probably induced by an excessively high impedance of the electrode tip (d, e, f). Both superficially resemble the complex repetitive discharge, but the recordings with a fast sweep speed (c, f) uncover the waveform and pattern of recurrence not usually associated with a biologic discharge.

# Defective apparatus

A broken wire causes bizarre artifacts. This may not be suspected if the insulating cover appears intact. A partially severed conductor may cause movement-induced artifacts, which are very deceptive. Other common causes of needle artifacts include defective insulation of the monopolar needle and a short-circuited tip of the concentric needle. According to a two-year study on the durability of monopolar electrodes,[20] the average number of patients that could be examined ranged from 20 to 63, depending on the manufacturer. Common causes of failure were, in order of frequency, Teflon retraction, dull or burred tip, break in wire or pin, electrical artifacts, and bend of the needle shaft.

The potential will also be distorted if the electrode tip is inadvertently insulated by blood protein which is "baked on" in the process of autoclaving. Careful cleaning of the needle tip prior to autoclaving will alleviate this problem. An ultrasonic cleaner may be used to loosen dried material from the needle. Improper or inadequate grounding results in electromagnetic interference from the nearby alternating current source. A loose connection in some parts of the recording circuit may be associated with generation of electrical activity similar to the muscle action potential.

# Movement artifact

When the patient contracts a muscle, the surface electrode may slide over the skin. This causes a movement artifact primarily because of the change in impedence between the surface electrode and the skin. Movement-induced potentials are also caused by existing fields near the surface of the skin, particularly those originating from sweat glands.[24] Movement of electrode wires may produce artifacts resembling muscle activity mostly owing to changing capacitance. Rubbing the lead of the needle electrode with the finger or cloth sometimes produces friction artifacts due to a static charge. This type of interference may be reduced if the needle is adequately insulated, ideally with the use of driven shields.

# Electrostatic and electromagnetic interference

The sources of 60 Hz interference are many (see Fig. 3-4). They include electric fans, lamps, fluorescent lights, electric motors, light dimmers, and even unused power cords plugged into wall outlets. The examiner, acting as an antenna, may increase 60 Hz interference simply by touching the needle. This can be avoided if the examiner is properly grounded. The interference is especially noticeable if such appliances are on the same circuit as the electromyographic apparatus. Strong interference may be detected from a nearby diathermy apparatus, which produces a characteristic wave pattern. Modern diathermy units now must fulfill Federal regulations, which restrict their interference with other equipment. The 60 Hz interference may also be carried by radio frequency (electromagnetic) waves.

There is no simple way to reduce electromagnetic interference. The problem may be solved by the relocation of electrode wires relative to the patient or recording apparatus, or repositioning the patient and recording apparatus within the room. If the interference cannot be adequately controlled by these simple means, it may then be necessary to remove all the electrical appliances from the room and shield the examining area.

# Radio interference

High frequency interference or audio interference may be seen on the screen of the oscilloscope from radio broadcasts, television, or radio paging systems. This type of artifact is often transient and difficult to identify, unless it is associated with sounds also heard through the loudspeaker. Relocation or screening of the electromyographic apparatus may be necessary to avoid this type of interference.

# REFERENCE SOURCES

1. ADRIAN, ED AND BRONK, DW: *The discharge of impulses in motor nerve fibres. Part II. The frequency of discharge in reflex and voluntary contractions.* J Physiol (Lond) 67:119, 1929.

2. BARINGER, JR, ET AL: *Transmissible dementias: Current problems in tissue handling.* Neurology (New York) 30:302, 1980.

3. BASMAJIAN, JV: *Electrodes and electrode connectors.* In DESMEDT, JE (ED): *New Developments in Electromyography and Clinical Neurophysiology,* Vol 1. Karger, Basel, 1973, pp 502–510.

4. BASMAJIAN, JV: *Muscles Alive: Their Functions Revealed by Electromyography,* ed 4. Williams & Wilkins, Baltimore, 1978.

5. BASMAJIAN, JV AND STECKO, G: *A new bipolar electrode for electromyography.* J Appl Physiol 17:849, 1962.

6. BERÁNEK, R: *Intracellular stimulation myography in man.* Electroenceph Clin Neurophysiol 16:301, 1964.

7. BUCHTHAL, F, GULD, C, AND ROSENFALCK, P: *Action potential parameters in normal human muscle and their dependence on physical variables.* Acta Physiol Scand 32:200, 1954.

8. BUCHTHAL, F, GULD, C, AND ROSENFALCK, P: *Volume conduction of the spike of the motor unit potential investigated with a new type of multielectrode.* Acta Physiol Scand 38:331, 1957.

9. CLAMANN, HP: *Activity of single motor units during isometric tension.* Neurology (Minneap) 20:254, 1970.

10. EKSTEDT, J: *Human single muscle fiber action potentials.* Acta Physiol Scand (Suppl 226) 61:1, 1964.

11. EKSTEDT, J AND STÅLBERG, E: *A method of recording extracellular action potentials of single muscle fibres and measuring their propagation velocity in voluntarily activated human muscle.* Bull Am Assoc Electromyogr Electrodiagn 10:16, 1963.

12. EKSTEDT, J AND STÅLBERG, E: *How the size of the needle electrode leading-off surface influences the shape of the single muscle fibre action potential in electromyography.* Computer Prog Biomed 3:204, 1973.

13. EKSTEDT, J AND STÅLBERG, E: *Single fibre electromyography for the study of the microphysiology of the human muscle.* In DESMEDT, JE (ED): *New Developments in Electromyography and Clinical Neurophysiology,* Vol 1. Karger, Basel, 1973, pp 89–112.

14. GAJDUSEK, DC, ET AL: *Precautions in medical care of, and in handling materials from, patients with transmissible virus dementia (Creutzfeldt-Jakob disease).* N Engl J Med 297:1253, 1977.

15. GEDDES, LA, BAKER, LE, AND McGOODWIN, M: *The relationship between electrode area and amplifier input impedance in recording muscle action potentials.* Med Biol Engin 5:561, 1967.

16. GULD, C, ROSENFALCK, A, AND WILLISON, RG: *Report of the committee on EMG instrumentation. Technical factors in recording electrical activity of muscle and nerve in man.* Electroenceph Clin Neurophysiol 28:399, 1970.

17. HANNERZ, J: *An electrode for recording single motor unit activity during strong muscle contractions.* Electroenceph Clin Neurophysiol 37:179, 1974.

18. JASPER, H AND NOTMAN, R: *Electromyography in peripheral nerve injuries.* National Research Council of Canada, Report C 6121, N.R.C. Grant No. Army Med. 28 From the Montreal Neurological Institute, Vol IV, McGill University, Montreal, Quebec, 1944.

19. MANUELIDIS, EE, ET AL: *Experimental Creutzfeldt-Jakob disease transmitted via the eye with infected cornea.* N Engl J Med 296:1334, 1977.

20. MIKOLICH, LM AND WAYLONIS, GW: *Durability of monopolar Teflon-coated electromyographic needles.* Arch Phys Med Rehabil 58:448, 1977.

21. NISSEN-PETERSEN, H, GULD, C, AND BUCHTHAL, F: *A delay line to record random action potentials.* Electroenceph Clin Neurophysiol 26:100, 1969.

22. SKAGGS, H, ET AL: *Guidelines in EMG.* Professional Standards Committee, American Association of Electromyography and Electrodiagnosis, 1979.

23. STÅLBERG, E AND TRONTELJ, JV: *Single Fibre Electromyography.* The Mirvalle Press Limited, Old Woking, Surrey, U.K., 1979.

24. TAM, HW AND WEBSTER, JG: *Minimizing electrode motion artifact by skin abrasion.* IEEE Trans Biomed Engin 24:134, 1977.

25. WIECHERS, DO, BLOOD, JR, AND STOW, RW: *EMG needle electrodes: Electrical impedance.* Arch Phys Med Rehabil 60:364, 1979.

# PART
# 2

# NERVE CONDUCTION STUDIES

# 4

# ANATOMY AND PHYSIOLOGY OF THE PERIPHERAL NERVE

Understanding of peripheral nerve function in health and disease has advanced considerably during the last decade with the advent of newer histologic techniques. Many pathologic processes have now been clearly defined by means of fiber diameter spectrum and quantitative assessment of single teased fiber preparations under electronmicroscopy. Electrophysiologic methods have made equally significant contributions to the understanding of the pathophysiology of peripheral nerve disorders. In particular, in vitro recordings of compound nerve action potentials from the sural nerve have been helpful in delineating the types of fibers predominantly affected in certain neuropathic processes. In addition, close relationships between histologic and physiologic findings have now been demonstrated in many disease entities.

With traumatic lesions of the nerve, there may or may not be structural changes in the axon. Damage to the axon may occur with or without separation of its supporting connective tissue sheath. Nontraumatic disorders of the peripheral nerve may primarily affect the nerve cell body, axon, Schwann cell, connective tissue, or vascular supply. These components may be involved either singly or in combination. The electrophysiologic abnormalities depend on the kind and degree of nerve damage. Hence, the results of nerve conduction studies can be closely correlated to the structural abnormalities of the nerve. Based on histologic changes in the nerve and the nature of conduction abnormalities, two principal types of peripheral nerve lesions can be identified: axonal degeneration and segmental demyelination.

This chapter will deal with fundamentals in the anatomy and physiology of the peripheral nerve together with various types of conduction abnormalities. For a more detailed review of the subject, excellent texts are available elsewhere.[2, 10, 24, 50, 65, 91, 97] The clinical aspects of peripheral nerve disorders will be discussed in Chapters 20 through 23.

## ANATOMY OF PERIPHERAL NERVES

### Gross anatomy

The axons in the nerve trunks are surrounded by three kinds of connective tissue: endoneurium, perineurium, and epineurium (Fig. 4-1). The endoneurium is the supporting structure found around individual axons within each fascicle. The perineurium is collagenous tissue binding each fascicle with elastic fibers and mesothelial cells. Strictly speaking, perineurium is neither a connective tissue nor a simple supporting structure, since it probably provides a diffusion barrier to regulate intrafascicular fluid.[85,102] Individual fascicles are bound tightly together by the epineurium, which is composed of collagen tissue, elastic fibers, and fatty tissue. This is the outermost layer of supporting structure for the peripheral nerve and is continuous with the dura mater of the spinal roots.[43] Endoneurial collagen is sparse at the roots as compared with the nerve trunk. This may be why the roots are selectively involved in some disease processes, although this relationship has not been proven. The vasa nervorum, located in the epineurium, branch into arterioles that penetrate the perineurium to form capillary anastomoses in the fascicles. The perineurium probably acts as a blood-nerve barrier, but its detailed function remains to be elucidated.[102]

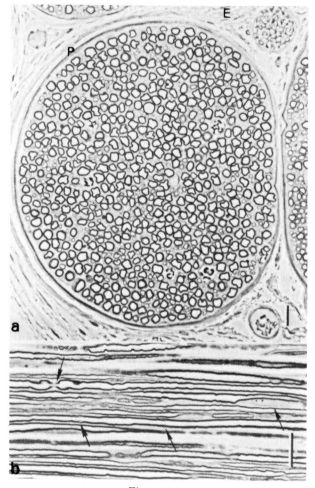

Figure 4-1

Transverse (a) and longitudinal (b) sections of the sciatic nerve shown at low magnification. Vertical scales at lower right represent 20 $\mu$m. In (a), the epineurium (E) contains vessels, fibroblasts, and collagen. The perineurium (P) surrounds fascicles of nerve fibers which are separated by endoneurial connective tissue. The longitudinal section (b) includes a node of Ranvier (upper arrow), a Schwann cell nucleus (right arrow), and Schmidt-Lantermann clefts (lower arrows). (From Webster,[111] with permission.)

## Myelinated and unmyelinated fibers

The nerve trunks contain myelinated and unmyelinated axons. In myelinated fibers, the surface membrane of a Schwann cell spirals around the axon to provide the myelin sheath (Fig. 4-2). Each myelinated axon is surrounded by its own Schwann cell. The junctions between adjacent Schwann cells are called the nodes of Ranvier, which represent uninsulated gaps along the myelinated fiber. Unmyelinated fibers are closely associated with Schwann cells as well. However, several unmyelinated axons share a single Schwann cell, which gives rise to many separate processes, each surrounding one axon.[34]

In myelinated fibers, the internodal distance is determined by the spacing of the Schwann cells at the time of myelination. As the nerve grows in length, the internodal distance increases, since there is no proliferation of Schwann cells. Thus, the fibers myelinated early achieve larger diameters and wider spacing of the nodes of Ranvier.[105] The larger the diameter of the fiber is, the greater is the internodal distance. As discussed later in this chapter, action potentials are generated only at the nodes of Ranvier in myelinated fibers, and the rate of propagation is approximately proportional to the internodal length and fiber diameter. In unmyelinated nerves, conduction velocity is proportional to the square root of the fiber diameter.

In general, nerve fiber diameter is closely correlated to function, although there are some exceptions. The largest and fastest conducting fibers include the sensory fibers transmitting proprioceptive, positional, and touch sensations to the spinal cord and the alpha motor neurons. Among small myelinated and unmyelinated fibers are those conducting pain and temperature sense and those subserving autonomic functions. Types of nerve fibers are further described later in this chapter.

## Axonal transport

In the peripheral nervous system, the motor and sensory axons are up to 1 m in length, and their cell bodies are in the order of 50 to 100 $\mu$m in diameter. The metabolic needs of the terminal axon segments are provided by a complicated system of axonal transport. Thus, axons are not only conductors of the propagating electrical potential but also active participants in the maintenance of metabolic integrity, conveying nutrient and other trophic substances.[41] The velocity of transport varies from several hundred to a few millimeters per day.[12, 66] The major flow appears to be centrifugal, but centripetal movement of particles has also been observed.

Axonal transport in the peripheral nerve plays a complex role in the maintenance not only of the peripheral nerve itself, but also of muscle tissue innervated by the nerve. Histochemical and electrophysiologic properties of muscle fibers depend at least in part on the axonal flow of trophic substances. However, with the exception of acetylcholine (ACh), actual transfer of particles across the neuromuscular junction has not been proven. Acetylcholine molecules may have a trophic influence on muscle in addition to its role as a neurotransmitter. If separated from the cell body, the axon degenerates centrifugally and the muscle fibers atrophy. Neuromuscular transmission fails and the nerve terminals degenerate faster if the length of the remaining distal segment is shorter. Similarly, membrane changes in denervated muscle appear more rapidly if the nerve is cut close to the muscle than if it is cut far away.[44]

# PHYSIOLOGY OF NERVE CONDUCTION

## Transmembrane potential

The electrical properties common to the membranes of all excitable cells have been discussed in Chapter 2. Measured transmembrane steady state potentials in different

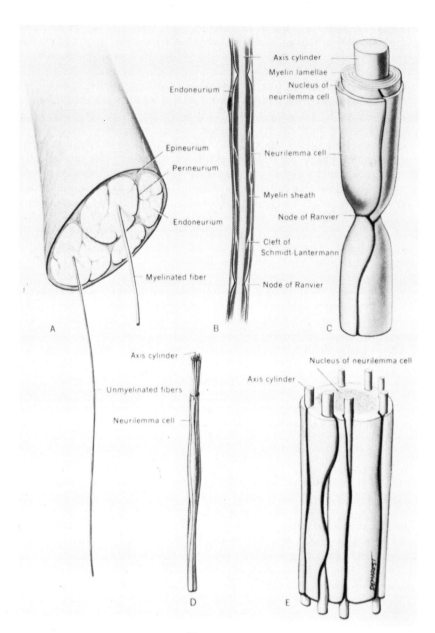

Figure 4-2

Fine structures of the peripheral nerve as visualized with the light microscope (A, B, D) and as reconstructed from electron micrographs (C, E). (A) The entire nerve is covered by epineurium, whereas the perineurium and endoneurium surround individual fascicles and nerve fibers, respectively. (B) The myelinated fiber consists of axis cylinder, myelin sheath, and Schwann (neurilemma) cells. The myelin sheath is absent at the node of Ranvier. (C) The helically laminated myelin sheath is an extension of the Schwann cell. (D) Several unmyelinated nerve fibers are surrounded by one Schwann cell. (E) Several axis cylinders of unmyelinated fibers are located around the nucleus of the Schwann cell. (From Noback,[73] with permission.)

tissues vary from about $-20$ to $-100$ mV, but the basic mechanism of their generation is probably the same. In neurons the magnitude of polarization is less in the soma membrane ($-70$ mV) than in the axon ($-90$ mV). The measured soma membrane potential, however, may not represent a true resting potential owing to continuous subliminal synaptic influences. As in any excitable element, generation of the nerve action potential can be divided into two steps: subliminal excitation and suprathreshold activation. Subthreshold depolarization is graded and can be caused by an externally applied stimulus, which may be chemical, mechanical, or electrical in nature. It produces a local nonpropagating change in the transmembrane potential, which rapidly diminishes with distance. In contrast, threshold depolarization produces an all-or-none action potential whose magnitude is determined by the inherent nature of the cell membrane, irrespective of the type of stimulus applied.

## Generation and propagation of action potential

If a weak current is applied to a nerve, negative charges from the negative pole of the stimulating electrode (cathode) accumulate on the outside of the membrane, making the inside of the cell relatively more positive (cathodal depolarization). The process is reversed in the nerve segment under the positive pole (anode), where the negative charges tend to leave the outside of the membrane, making the inside of the cell relatively more negative (anodal hyperpolarization). Because of cell plasma resistance and membrane conductance and capacitance, local changes in the form of depolarization or hyperpolarization can be detected only within a few millimeters of the point of origin. After about 10 to 30 mV of depolarization, the membrane potential reaches the critical level and an action potential develops with the same maximal response regardless of the kind or magnitude of the stimulus. This is an energy-dependent process involving complex molecular changes of the cell membrane as described in Chapter 2.

The threshold intensity, of course, depends on the duration of the current. It is high with a short-duration stimulus and much lower with a long-lasting shock. The strength-duration curve is obtained by plotting the relationship between the intensity (Y axis) and duration (X axis) of a stimulus applied at a motor point which will elicit a constant muscle response. A long-duration shock excites both nerve and muscle, whereas a short stimulus will be effective only for the nerve. On the basis of this and other excitability characteristics of the nerve and muscle, strength-duration curves indicate whether a muscle is normally innervated, or partially or totally denervated. Attempts have also been made to formulate numerical indices of excitability. Rheobase is defined as the minimal current strength below which no response can be elicited, even if the current is applied for an infinite period. In practice a duration of at least 300 ms is used to determine the rheobase. Chronaxie is the minimal duration of a current required to excite the cell at twice the rheobase strength. Although of historical interest, neither rheobase nor chronaxie has proven satisfactory as a test in clinical practice. The strength-duration curve itself has lost popularity because of the length of time required for its determination and the complexity of its interpretation. These excitability tests have now been largely replaced by nerve conduction studies and electromyography.

An action potential initiated along the course of the axon is propagated in both directions from its point of origin (Fig. 4-3). Intracellular current flows from the active area, where the interior of the cell is positively charged, to the adjacent inactive region, where the inside of the cell membrane is negatively charged. An opposing current flows through the extracellular fluid from the inactive to active region. Because of this local current, the inactive regions on both sides of the active area become depolarized. When depolarization reaches the critical level, an action potential is generated, initiating a new local current further distally and proximally. Although an action potential initiated by external stimulation at one point along the axon is propagated bidirectionally,

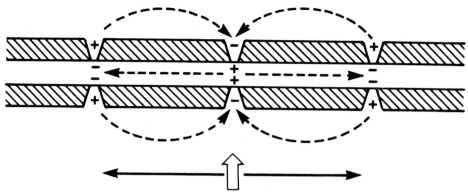

Figure 4-3

Saltatory conduction along the myelinated fiber. The internodal segment is effectively insulated by the myelin sheath, whereas the axon is bare at the node of Ranvier, where the current flows between intracellular and extracellular fluid. A local current (dotted arrows) produced by an action potential at one node (open arrow) depolarizes the axis cylinder at the adjacent nodes on either side. The impulse is propagated in both directions (solid arrows). This type of excitation is called saltatory, since it jumps from one node to the next.

physiologic impulses arising at one end of the axon, that is, the cell body or sensory terminal, are conducted only orthodromically. In pathologic situations, however, impulses may arise in the midportion of nerve fibers. One such example is the generation of impulses in the spinal root axons of dystrophic mice, either spontaneously or as a result of ephaptic transmission (cross-talk) between single fibers.[81]

## Factors determining the conduction velocity

Various factors affect the time necessary for generation of action potentials, which in turn determines the conduction velocity of an axon. Faster propagation is associated with (1) faster rates of action potential generation, which more rapidly depolarize the adjacent segment; (2) larger diameter fibers with decreased axoplasmic resistance, which increases the current flow along the axon and decreases the time required to excite the adjacent segment; (3) lower depolarization thresholds of the cell membrane, which allow the local current to depolarize the adjacent membrane in a shorter time; and (4) higher temperature, which, by increasing sodium conductance, facilitates depolarization. The relationship between temperature and conduction velocity is nearly linear from 29 to 38°C.[45] Since the velocity increases by about 5 percent per degree centigrade over this temperature range, a change of 2 to 3 m/s occurs per degree in a normal nerve conducting at 40 to 60 m/s.[51] Temperature and other factors of clinical importance for nerve conduction velocity will be discussed further in Chapter 5.

Conduction is much faster in myelinated fibers in which action potentials occur only at the nodes of Ranvier. This induces a local current which, in effect, jumps from one node to the next producing saltatory conduction (see Fig. 4-3), instead of continuous propagation as in unmyelinated fibers. For rapid conduction, the internodal distance must be great enough to maximize the jump of the action potential, while at the same time small enough to minimize loss of current through the internodal membrane. Typically the internodal distance and conduction time are about 1 mm and 20 $\mu$s, respectively. The conduction velocity would then be 50 m/s.

In myelinated fibers, the time required for local current to excite the next node is determined not only by the longitudinal resistance of axoplasm but also by the capacitance and conductance of the internodal membrane. With larger values of these three parameters, more current is dissipated before the impulse reaches the next node. Longer time is then required for local current to depolarize the adjacent nodal membrane, resulting in slower conduction. Both internodal capacitance and conductance decrease with myelin thickness. Thus, for a fixed axon diameter, conduction velocity increases with myelin thickness up to a certain point. For a fixed total fiber diameter, there is an optimal ratio between axon diameter and myelin thickness, since axoplasm resistance increases with smaller axon diameter.[108] Theoretical considerations indicate that the anatomic characteristics of myelinated fibers fulfill all the conditions required for optimization of conduction velocity.

In segmental demyelination, or during partial remyelination, myelin sheath is thin and the internodal capacitance and conductance are increased. More local current is lost to charge the capacitors and by leakage through the internodal membrane before reaching the next node of Ranvier. Failure to activate the next node results in conduction block. Even if the conduction itself is maintained, impulse propagation is slowed, since it takes longer for the dissipated current to generate an action potential.[61, 82, 83] Thus, conduction in demyelinated axons is characterized by conduction failure, slowing of conduction velocity, and temporal dispersion of impulses.[107] Conduction may become continuous rather than saltatory in smaller diameter fibers after segmental demyelination.[9] This continuous mode of conduction requires the presence of a sufficient number of sodium channels in the demyelinated region. Conduction past focally demyelinated zones may be facilitated by reduction in length of the adjacent internodes.[109]

Conduction also slows in the absence of demyelination if fiber diameter is decreased, as is known to occur during focal compression. Reduced fiber diameter is associated with decreased capacitance of the internodal membrane, which tends to facilitate conduction. However, this is more than offset by increased resistance of the axoplasm, which delays generation of an action potential at the next node. Most mechanisms known to decrease nerve conduction velocity affect local current as described above. Additionally, altered characteristics of the nodal membrane itself may interfere with generation of the action potential and slow conduction. This possibility has not been identified experimentally, however.[63]

# TYPES OF NERVE FIBERS AND IN VITRO RECORDING

## Classification of nerve fibers

The compound action potential recorded after supramaximal stimulation of a mixed nerve consists of several peaks, each representing a group of fibers with a different conduction velocity. Erlanger and Gasser[28] in their original study of what is now referred to as the A fibers designated successive peaks using the Greek letters, $\alpha$, $\beta$, $\gamma$, and $\delta$ in order of decreasing velocity. Subsequent studies have revealed two additional components: B and C. Both are of very slow conduction velocity and the B fibers are not found in mammalian peripheral nerves. The designation B is now used for preganglionic fibers in mammalian autonomic nerves. There has been some confusion with the terminology for various peaks of the A fibers.[64] The initial peak was referred to as either A-alpha[35] or A-beta.[27] The subsequent peak, originally called A-gamma, was shown to be an artifact of recording by Gasser.[35] Current practice designates the two peaks in the A potential of cutaneous nerves as A-alpha and A-delta.

Thus, there are three types of nerve fibers known as A, B, and C, which are histologically and electrophysiologically distinctive (Table 4-1). The A fibers are myelinated somatic axons, either afferent or efferent. The B fibers are myelinated efferent axons which constitute the preganglionic axons of the autonomic nerves. The C fibers are unmyelinated and may be subdivided into the efferent postganglionic axons of autonomic nerve and the small afferent axons of the dorsal root and peripheral nerves. Histologic distinction between the B fibers and small A fibers is difficult, but the two can be differentiated on the basis of their physiologic characteristics. For instance, the B fibers lack negative after-potentials and consequently have no super-normal period of excitability after generation of an action potential. Spike duration is more than twice as long in B as in A fibers. The compound action potential of the B fibers is smooth without discrete peaks, because the velocity spectrum is evenly distributed. The C fibers are easily recognized histologically by the absence of myelin sheaths. Unlike A and B fibers, which are individually bound by Schwann cells, several C fibers share a single Schwann cell. The C fibers are also distinguished physiologically by high thresholds of activation, long spike duration, and slow conduction velocity.

The A fibers may be subdivided into those found in cutaneous nerves and those found in muscle nerves. Afferent fibers of the cutaneous nerves show a bimodal diameter distribution, with one component ranging between 6 to 12 $\mu$m and the other between 1 to 5 $\mu$m. Using the Greek letter designation, these two components are customarily referred to as A-alpha and A-delta fibers. The A fibers in muscle nerves are either efferent or afferent. The efferent fibers consist of the axons of alpha and gamma motor neurons. In Lloyd's Roman numeral classification, the afferent fibers are divided into three groups based on fiber diameter. They are designated groups I, II, and III, consisting of fibers with diameters ranging from 12 to 21 $\mu$m, 6 to 12 $\mu$m, and 1 to 6 $\mu$m, respectively. The C fibers are sometimes called group IV. The A-alpha fibers of cutaneous nerve (6 to 17 $\mu$m) approximately correspond in size to groups I and II, and the A-delta fibers (1 to 6 $\mu$m) to group III of afferent fibers in muscle nerves.

## In vitro recording of sural nerve potentials

An in vitro method for obtaining compound action potentials of the sural nerve has been described by Dyck and Lambert.[23] In most instances, the electrophysiologic study is combined with a quantitative morphometric assessment of the excised nerve to compare the fiber diameter spectrum with the range of conduction velocities and the different components of the sensory nerve action potential. A fascicular nerve biopsy is obtained above the lateral malleolus. A bundle of several fascicles is dissected for a total length of approximately 10 cm. The distal half is used for histologic studies and the proximal half for the in vitro electrophysiologic study. The portion of the nerve

---

**TABLE 4-1 Types of nerve fibers**

I. A fibers
  Myelinated fibers of somatic nerves
  a) Muscle nerve
    afferent—Group I (12–21 $\mu$)
             II ( 6–12 $\mu$)
             III ( 1–6 $\mu$)
             IV (C fiber)
    efferent—alpha motor neuron
             gamma motor neuron
  b) Cutaneous nerve
    afferent—alpha (6–17 $\mu$)
           delta (1–6 $\mu$)
II. B fibers
  Myelinated preganglionic fibers of autonomic nerve
III. C fibers
  Unmyelinated fibers of somatic or autonomic nerve
  a) sC fibers
    efferent postganglionic fibers of autonomic nerve
  b) d.r.C fibers
    afferent fibers of the dorsal root and peripheral nerve

---

used for conduction studies is immediately immersed in cool Tyrode's solution which is continuously aerated by 5 percent carbon dioxide in oxygen.

For physiologic studies, the nerve is transferred to a sealed chamber filled with 5 percent carbon dioxide in oxygen and saturated with water vapor. In the chamber, a series of silver electrodes support the nerve, which is held under slight tension by the pull of a 0.5 to 0.9 gm weight attached to each end. The temperature of the chamber is kept constant by immersing it in a water bath maintained at 37°C. The nerve is stimulated at the distal end and the compound nerve action potential is recorded with a wire electrode placed 20 to 30 mm proximally. The reference electrode is located 10 mm proximally. A maximal stimulus is used for each component under study. To obtain monophasic recordings, the nerve is crushed between the recording electrodes and 0.1 percent procaine applied at the distal electrode (see Fig. 2-4). The compound nerve action potential recorded in vitro consists of three distinct peaks: A-alpha, A-delta, and C components (Fig. 4-4). The average conduction velocity is approximately 60 m/s for the onset of A-alpha, 20 m/s for the peak of A-delta, and 1 to 2 m/s for the peak of C components. The onset of the last two peaks may be difficult to define.

The corresponding fiber diameter histogram for the first two components is shown in Figure 4-5, where increasing fiber diameter is plotted from left to right on the abscissa. The first peak on the left corresponds to A-delta and the second smaller peak to A-alpha fibers. The opposite arrangement with decreasing diameter plotted from left to right may also be used. In this instance, fiber groups appear in order of decreasing conduction velocity, just as they are represented in the tracings of compound action potentials. In normal fiber groups, fiber diameter histograms show a continuous distribution between the large and small myelinated fibers with no clear separation between the two. Similarly there is no discontinuity between A-alpha and A-delta peaks, which simply reflects a high concentration of fibers within the continuous spectrum.[5] Since the largest fibers are close to 12 $\mu$m in diameter in normal fiber groups, the ratio of conduction velocity to fiber diameter is approximately 5:1.

In addition to fiber diameter histogram, the distribution of histologic abnormalities can be assessed quantitatively by determining the internodal length spectra in

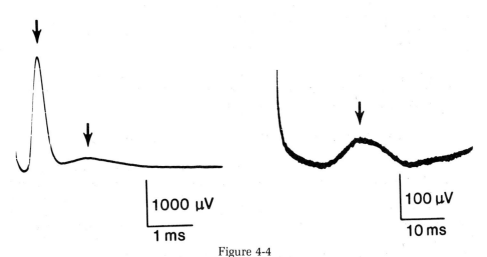

Figure 4-4

Compound nerve action potential of a normal sural nerve recorded in vitro from an 11-year-old boy who had an above-knee amputation for osteogenic sarcoma. Three distinct peaks indicated by arrows are, from left to right: A-alpha, A-delta, and C components. They are 2.6 mV, 0.22 mV, and 70 $\mu$V in amplitude and 42 m/s, 16 m/s, and 1 m/s in conduction velocity as calculated using the peak latency, respectively. (Courtesy of E. Peter Bosch, M.D., Department of Neurology, University of Iowa Hospitals and Clinics.)

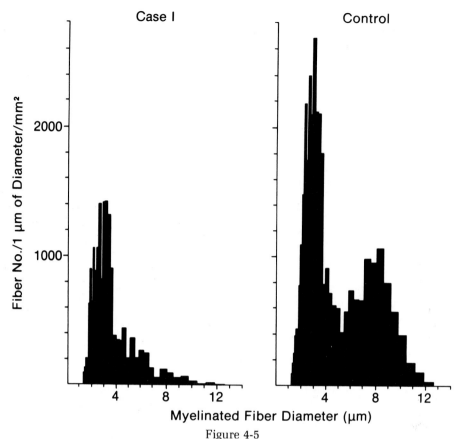

Figure 4-5

Myelinated fiber size-frequency histogram plotting the number of fibers with increasing diameter from left to right. The first large peak on the left corresponds to A-delta and the second smaller peak to A-alpha. Note a bimodal distribution of myelinated fiber diameter in a normal subject (control). An abnormal unimodal pattern with preferential loss of the larger myelinated fibers is seen in a patient (case 1) with familial pressure-sensitive neuropathy. (Courtesy of E. Peter Bosch, M.D., Department of Neurology, University of Iowa Hospitals and Clinics.)

teased fiber preparation (Fig. 4-6). Significant correlations have been reported between teased fiber changes and conduction abnormalities affecting both motor and sensory nerves in patients with sensory motor polyneuropathies.[8]

## Analysis of compound nerve action potentials

The amplitude of a compound action potential E, recorded over the surface of a nerve, is proportional to current flow and external resistance. This is expressed by Ohm's Law as $E = IR$, where I and R represent current and resistance, respectively. Larger nerves have a greater number of fibers and would generate larger currents, since each fiber contributes an approximately equal amount. However, nerves with greater cross-sectional areas would be associated with smaller resistances. The overall effect of large nerve size on amplitude may therefore be negligible. In fact, Lambert and Dyck[64] have shown that a whole nerve composed of many fascicles does not necessarily give rise to an action potential larger than the one recorded from a single dissected fascicle.

Since current is proportional to fiber number and resistance is inversely proportional to square diameter, amplitude of an action potential is an expression of fiber

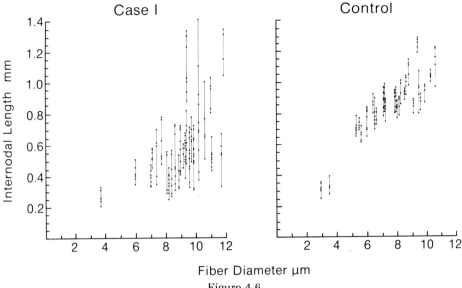

Figure 4-6

Internodal length spectra of the same nerves shown in Figure 4-5. Each vertical line indicates internodal lengths measured on a given myelinated fiber. The marked variability of internodal length in the patient reflects the effects of chronic demyelination and remyelination. (Courtesy of E. Peter Bosch, M.D., Department of Neurology, University of Iowa Hospitals and Clinics.)

density or fiber number per unit cross-sectional area. In diseased nerves the waveform of compound action potentials may be significantly altered by increased temporal dispersion. In these cases, the area under the waveform is a better indicator of fiber density than the amplitude. The action potential may also be affected by conduction block or diminution of current in individual nerve fibers. If a pathologic process affects different groups of fibers selectively, the waveform is distorted. If fibers of different size are involved uniformly, amplitude is decreased for all components. Thus, fiber density and distribution of fiber spectrum can be estimated from the amplitude and waveform of compound nerve action potentials.

# CLASSIFICATION OF NERVE INJURIES

Seddon[90, 91] defined three degrees of nerve injury: neurapraxia, axonotmesis, and neurotmesis. Neurapraxia is characterized by conduction loss without structural change in the axon. Fibers usually regain function promptly, although the conduction velocity may be slowed for a time if there is associated demyelination. Conduction velocity returns to normal when remyelination is completed. With axonotmesis, axonal continuity is lost and there is subsequent Wallerian degeneration of the distal segment. Recovery depends on regeneration of nerve fibers, a process which takes place slowly over months or years at a rate of 1 to 3 mm per day. Neurotmesis is injury that results in separation of the entire nerve, including the supporting connective tissue. Regeneration, if possible at all, is incomplete and poorly organized.

Seddon's classification was originally used in the assessment of nerve lesions due to external trauma, such as superficial nerve injuries or penetrating wounds of deeply located nerves. Similar distinctions may be applied in categorizing the severity of compression neuropathies such as the carpal tunnel syndrome, tardy ulnar palsy, and Saturday night palsy, as well as experimentally induced tourniquet paralysis.

# Neurapraxia

The mildest form of nerve block results from local injection of procaine or the transient loss of circulation that may occur with leg crossing. These injuries are not associated with structural changes in the axon and consequently are immediately reversible when the effect of the anesthetic agent is lost or when circulation is re-established. Transient paralysis can be experimentally induced by an inflated cuff around the arm. During ischemia, despite the absence of demonstrable nerve fiber lesions, conduction velocity may be decreased by as much as 30 percent. A complete conduction block usually occurs after 25 to 30 minutes of compression. The site of conduction block can be delineated by serial stimulation along the course of the nerve, since the excitability is essentially normal in the segment distal to the lesion, so long as the proximal lesion remains neurapraxic in nature. These short-term changes in nerve conduction are probably caused by anoxia secondary to ischemia.[67] Chronic nerve ischemia, as may be induced by a bovine shunt, may result in axonal degeneration of sensory fibers initially, and of motor fibers later.[7]

In most acute compression neuropathies, such as a Saturday night palsy or crutch palsy of the radial nerve, conduction recovers across the affected segment within a few weeks. A neurapraxic state, however, could persist for a few months or longer under certain circumstances. In these cases incomplete and comparatively short-lived paralysis due to neurapraxia is usually associated with localized demyelination.[18, 19] Similarly the prolonged application of a tourniquet causes sustained conduction block with paranodal demyelination.[77] Conduction may return immediately after decompression, but it is markedly slowed until remyelination takes place. Prognosis for complete recovery is excellent.

Tourniquet palsy was once considered analogous to a physiologic nerve block, and the underlying demyelination was attributed to anoxia secondary to ischemia.[18, 19] However, recent studies of experimental acute pressure neuropathy and chronic entrapment neuropathy have stressed the importance of mechanical factors[33, 38, 75, 76, 87] with the initial displacement of axoplasm and myelin in opposite directions under the edges of the compressed region (Figs. 4-7 and 4-8). Part of one myelin segment invaginates the next with occlusions of the nodal gaps. Demyelination of the stretched portions of myelin follows. Severe conduction block of sensory and motor fibers localized to the presumed lower margin of the compression has been described in human pneumatic tourniquet paralysis.[6, 86]

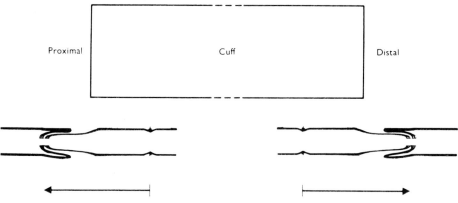

Figure 4-7

Diagram showing the direction of displacement of the nodes of Ranvier in relation to the cuff. Proximal and distal paranodes are invaginated by the adjacent one. (From Ochoa, Fowler, and Gilliatt,[75] with permission.)

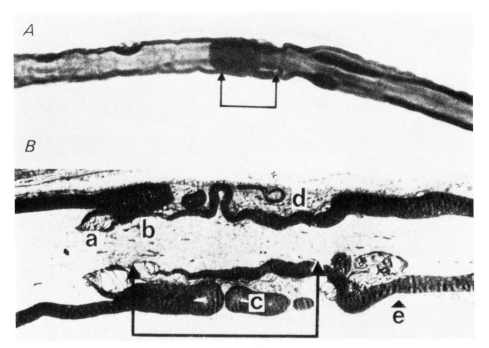

Figure 4-8

(A) Part of a single teased fiber showing an abnormal node. (B) Electron micrograph of nodal region shown in A. a = terminal myelin loops of ensheathing paranode; b = terminal myelin loops of ensheathed paranode; c = myelin fold of ensheathing paranode cut tangentially; d = Schwann cell cytoplasm; e = microvilli indicating site of Schwann cell junction. Large arrows show length of ensheathed paranode (approx. 20 μm). (From Ochoa, et al,[77] with permission.)

Chronic entrapment states such as carpal tunnel syndrome or tardy ulnar palsy are also characteristically associated with focal demyelination.[59, 74] As with neurapraxia seen in acute compression, local demyelination in chronic entrapment can best be explained as a result of mechanical forces rather than ischemia, although microscopic findings of single fibers are not the same in acute and chronic compression. Chronic subclinical entrapment is rather common, as evidenced by unexpected abnormalities of nerve conduction studies when using increasingly sensitive electrophysiologic techniques. In fact corresponding focal anatomic abnormalities have been documented at routine autopsies in patients without known disease of the peripheral nerve.[72]

Associated neurapraxia is a major cause of paralysis in demyelinating neuropathy, since reduced strength is primarily consequent to the loss of functional axons and not to slowing of conduction. It is debated whether fibrillation potentials and positive sharp waves may be seen in the paralyzed muscles due to a lack of neural influence alone, even if there is no axonal damage. This was found to be the case in 25 percent of 31 patients studied by Trojaborg[103] following a conduction block lasting more than 14 days. In the remaining 75 percent, spontaneous discharges were attributed to axonal damage.

## Axonotmesis

In this condition, damage results in loss of continuity of the axons which then become fragmented in the distal segment (Fig. 4-9). Immediate conduction block occurs across the site of nerve injury. Although there is considerable variability among different species,[42] it is usually not until four or five days following acute interruption that the distal segment becomes inexcitable due to degeneration of nerve fibers.[40] Little information is available about nerve conduction during wallerian degeneration in man. In two cases studied serially after traumatic transection of the digital nerve, action potentials became unobtainable only at 185 hours in one case and 168 hours in the other. There was no change in the conduction velocity during wallerian degeneration prior to the loss of recorded response.[79] During the first few days after nerve injury, therefore, it is not possible to distinguish axonotmesis from neurapraxia on the basis of distal nerve excitability.

Gilliatt and Hjorth[39] have shown in the baboon that the muscle response to nerve stimulation disappears four or five days after nerve section, but an ascending nerve action potential may be recorded in the segment distal to the section for two or three more days. Preceding conduction failure, there is no change in the maximal conduction velocity of either the descending motor potential or ascending nerve action potential. Histologically, degeneration occurs in the terminal portion of the intramuscular nerve at a time when the proximal parts of the same fibers are relatively intact. The central stump of a transected nerve fiber remains excitable, but the nerve action potentials and conduction velocity may all be slightly reduced, possibly due to retraction of the myelin sheath.[42, 56, 100] Transverse section at this level shows a marked reduction in the number of myelinated fibers present.[1]

An electrical study of the entire nerve, as opposed to individual nerve fibers, does not allow precise definition of the category of injury, since not all the axons are affected to the same degree. Indeed, different types of abnormalities coexist in the majority of nerve injuries and neuropathies. Nerve conduction studies only across the site of the lesion are of limited value in distinguishing neurapraxia from axonotmesis; a complete conduction block may occur in either condition, whereas the conduction velocity may remain normal in partial axonotmesis if uninjured axons are functionally intact. Stimulation of the nerve segment distal to the lesion is useful in the differential diagnosis, since injured axons undergoing wallerian degeneration lose distal excitability, and the evoked action potential declines steeply after the first few days of injury. Electromyog-

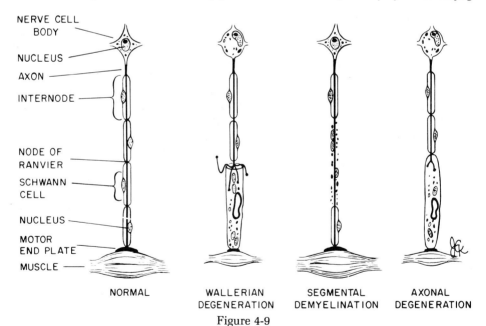

Figure 4-9

Schematic representation of nerve axon and myelin sheath. From left to right, normal structures, wallerian degeneration following transection of the fiber, segmental demyelination, and axonal degeneration secondary to disorders of the nerve cell. (From Asbury and Johnson,[2] with permission.)

raphy shows positive sharp waves one to two weeks and fibrillation potentials two to three weeks after axonotmesis.

During the process of regeneration, structural proteins newly synthesized in the cell body are transported down the axon to supply multiple sprouts derived from the parent axon. Once the axon successfully reaches the periphery and re-establishes the physiologic connections, an orderly sequence of maturation takes place and fiber diameter progressively increases.[112] The remaining sprouts that fail to make functional reconnection will eventually degenerate. If the Schwann cell basement membrane and the remaining connective tissues are intact, regeneration of the nerve axon occurs in an orderly manner along the intact nerve sheath. The axons regenerate at a rate of approximately 1 to 3 mm per day, nearly restoring the normal number and size of fibers when fully regenerated.

## Neurotmesis

Sunderland[97] has proposed three subdivisions of Seddon's neurotmesis. In the first type, the perineurium and architecture of the nerve sheath is preserved, although the axon and surrounding connective tissue are damaged. Regeneration is fairly effective, but less complete than in axonotmesis, and may be misdirected, leading to innervation of muscle fibers previously not supplied by the nerve. The clinical phenomenon of synkinesis probably indicates an antecedent nerve injury of at least this severity.[60, 98] In the second type, the perineurium is also damaged, but the nerve maintains continuity and remains grossly intact. Some regeneration may occur, but it is poorly oriented and requires surgical intervention. The last type represents a complete separation of the nerve with loss of continuity, even microscopically. The nerve must be sutured, often requiring a nerve graft to bridge the gap. Regeneration is poorly oriented with frequent neuroma formation. There may be spontaneous discharges of nerve impulses reflecting changes in membrane properties. This may be the source of pain associated with neuromas.[106]

Following re-anastomosis of the nerve, regenerating nerve fibers do not regain their original number or diameter. The diameter of regenerating fibers increases gradually over many years following nerve repair. The conduction velocity also increases slowly, reaching 60 percent of the normal value within four years[47] and a mean value of 85 percent after 16 years.[94] Distal latencies may remain prolonged presumably because only a limited number of fibers are present. In detailed sequential studies of the median nerve after complete section and suture, Buchthal and Kühl[13] showed that the average growth rate was 1.5 to 2.0 mm per day in three patients. When the sensory potential was first recorded three to four months after the injury, the nerve conduction velocity was 10 to 25 percent of normal. It then increased at 3 percent per month during the first two years, and 10 times slower thereafter. By 40 months, the sensory potential was still dispersed five times more than normal, when the amplitude and tactile sensibility had returned to normal. Conduction velocity had reached 65 to 75 percent of normal in the adults. In children, the same degree of recovery in conduction velocity was achieved 13 to 19 months after anastomosis. The sensory potential recovered five times faster after a compressive nerve lesion than after section and repair.

Few studies have dealt with the neurophysiologic recovery of human peripheral nerves after repair with an autogenous nerve graft.[3] In one study,[99] motor and sensory nerve conduction velocities showed sustained improvement following sural nerve grafts of the ulnar and median nerves. Two years after surgery the motor conduction velocity across the graft itself reached, in most cases, 40 to 50 percent of the normal conduction velocity obtained in the contralateral limb. Sensory nerve action potentials were present in 44 percent of nerves after 18 months, although they were greatly reduced in amplitude and conduction velocity. In author study[20] based on experience with 67 injured nerves, voluntary motor unit activity became apparent 7 months after repair and 12 months after grafting. A compound muscle action potential was measurable by 10 months after suture and 14 months after graft. Motor unit potentials steadily increased in amplitude with time, but both clinical and electrophysiologic recovery were poor in sensory fibers.

# INVOLVEMENT OF AXON VERSUS MYELIN

The preceding section has dealt with types of conduction abnormalities associated with nerve injuries. Electrophysiologic abnormalities found in other disease processes will be discussed in this section. Conduction disturbances of the peripheral nerve may be localized, as in entrapment syndromes or following nerve trauma, or more diffuse as in polyneuropathies. On the basis of histologic[52] and electrophysiologic characteristics, disorders of peripheral nerves may be divided into three relatively distinct categories (see Fig. 4-9): (1) wallerian degeneration due to focal interruptions of axons as in vasculitis; (2) centripetal axonal degeneration (dying back) as a result of metabolic derangement of the neuron; and (3) segmental demyelination.[2, 57, 68, 71] Of these, wallerian and axonal degeneration are associated with reduction in amplitude of compound action potential and electrical evidence of denervation, whereas demyelination is characterized by slowing of nerve conduction.

## Axonal degeneration

Axonal degeneration may occur in neuropathies, from mechanical compression of the nerve, following application of toxic substances, or after the death of the cell body. In the absence of demyelination, mild neuropathies of this type may be present without abnormalities of nerve conduction velocities, especially if the disease primarily affects the small fibers. More commonly, selective loss of the large, fast conducting fibers results in some slowing of conduction, but the velocity is seldom reduced by more than 20 to 30 percent. In these cases, the compound muscle action potential is also reduced in amplitude due to loss of nerve fibers. These two changes are intercorrelated. In regenerating nerves, conduction velocities are slower than normal because nerve fibers are small and have thin myelin sheaths.

Selective loss of the fastest fibers may also occur in anterior horn cell diseases. Thus, motor conduction velocity in patients with poliomyelitis is less than 75 percent of the average normal value and is proportional to the decrease in total amplitude.[46] Slightly slow motor conduction velocities are occasionally found in patients with motor neuron disease. Slower conduction in patients with more severe atrophy may be in part related to lowered temperature of the wasted extremities.[62]

Electromyography characteristically shows a reduced number of motor unit potentials during the acute stage. In the chronic phase, they are not only reduced in number but also polyphasic in waveform and increased in duration and amplitude. Fibrillation potentials and positive sharp waves develop in 2 to 3 weeks after the onset of axonal degeneration. These electromyographic abnormalities are commonly seen in neuropathies secondary to alcoholism, uremia, polyarteritis nodosa, acute intermittent porphyria, some cases of diabetic and carcinomatous neuropathies, and most toxic and nutritional neuropathies.[37]

In neuropathies secondary to chronic alcoholism, carcinoma, and uremia, axonal degeneration appears to initially involve the most terminal segment of the longest peripheral nerve fibers. The distal predominance of pathology and its centripetal progression led to the term dying back neuropathy. Less commonly encountered conditions associated with the dying back phenomenon include thiamine deficiency,[17] triorthorcresyl phosphate neuropathy,[15] acute intermittent porphyria,[16] and experimental acrylamide neuropathies.[32, 80, 96] In these conditions, it is tempting to postulate that axoplasmic flow is most impaired in the segment of the nerve furthest from the perikaryon.

Primary involvement of the neurons leads to axonal degeneration that is more prominent in the distal segment, further removed from the trophic influence of the nerve cell.[93]

Single unit recording has confirmed that the earliest functional change in dying back axons is a failure of impulse generation in the terminal axon when impulse propagation throughout the remainder of the axon is normal.[95] In acrylamide dying back neuropathy in rats,[104] a sequential morphometric study of the end-plate region showed initial enlargement of the nerve terminal area due to distension by neurofilaments. The postsynaptic regions eventually became denuded as more than half of all nerve terminals subsequently disappeared.

Whereas the concept of dying back has been clearly demonstrated in experimental acrylamide neuropathy,[31, 49, 89] not all the peripheral neuropathies with a distal predominance may qualify as truly dying back in type. Bradley and Thomas[11] have suggested that the same pattern may be produced with selective loss of the perikarya and axons of the longest and largest fibers. Distally predominant symptoms do not necessarily indicate a distal pathologic process, since probabilistic models can reproduce a distal sensory deficit on the basis of randomly distributed axonal lesions.[110] In some neuropathies, studies fail to reveal the exact site of the primary damage responsible for axonal degeneration.

## Segmental demyelination

In the second group, disturbance of the Schwann cells causes segmental demyelination associated with substantial reduction of nerve conduction velocity, commonly, though not always, by more than 30 to 40 percent.[14] This degree of slowing is not seen with axonal degeneration, even if the fast conducting fibers are selectively affected, leaving the slow conducting fibers relatively intact. In experimental demyelination, transmission of nerve impulses may be blocked in some fibers through the demyelinated zone. However, the conduction velocity is decreased, primarily because nerve impulses are delayed passing through the lesion and not simply because of selective block of transmission in the fast conducting fibers.[69, 70] In focal segmental demyelination, the nerve conduction is slowed locally across the demyelinated segment but is normal below the lesion.[83, 84] In addition to various toxins, removal of a small piece of perineurium in amphibian nerve also causes a lesion consistent with demyelination and may be used in studying the pathophysiology of this condition.[78]

The course of experimental demyelination and remyelination may be summarized as follows. In Kaeser's series[53, 54] using diphtheria toxin, the maximal conduction velocity decreased progressively beginning one week after inoculation, reached a plateau during the sixth to eighth week, and recovered to the original level between the 18th and 20th week. The degree of slowing was positively correlated with the severity of paralysis and the dose of toxin administered. However, the amplitude of the compound muscle action potential, an indication of conduction block, reflected the degree of weakness even more accurately than the conduction velocity. In a more recent study, Saida and associates[88] outlined the relationship between remyelination and functional recovery following antiserum-mediated focal demyelination in male Wistar rats. Conduction block and paralysis of the foot muscles were apparent within a few hours of injection and persisted until about the seventh day, when low amplitude, long latency muscle action potentials could be recorded for the first time. The strength gradually recovered thereafter, returning to normal by 16 days. There was morphologic evidence of remyelination with 2 to 8 myelin lamellae around each axon coincident with the onset of clinical and electrophysiologic recovery. Conduction velocities returned to pre-injection values by the 37th day, when the myelin layer of remyelinating fibers was only about one third that of control nerves.

Common demyelinating diseases of the peripheral nerve include Guillain-Barré syndrome, chronic relapsing polyradiculoneuropathies, myelomatous polyneuropathies, hypertrophic type of Charcot-Marie-Tooth disease or hereditary motor and sensory neuropathy Type I,[22] metachromatic leukodystrophy,[30] and Krabbe's leukodystrophy.[21] Some cases of diabetic and carcinomatous neuropathies also belong to this category,[36, 37] although the vast majority of the latter group are axonal rather than demyelinating in type. Diphtheritic polyneuritis has rarely been studied in man, but alterations in conduction velocity are similar to those seen in animal experiments, in which there is usually a marked reduction in conduction velocity diffusely or, in the case of focal demyelination, over a relatively restricted region. A proximal demyelinating lesion may escape detection by the conventional nerve conduction studies, which are basically designed for assessment of the more distal segments.[58] Despite well-established concepts of segmental demyelination associated with chronic lead intoxication in animals, the nerve conduction velocity in lead poisoning in humans is either normal[92] or only mildly slowed.[29]

In addition to slowed nerve conduction, there may be a reduction of amplitude from localized conduction block in demyelinating polyneuropathy. Increased range of conduction velocity may be seen if thinner fibers are affected exclusively or disproportionately to larger fibers. The evoked action potential broadens because of increased temporal dispersion. Desynchronization of the nerve volley may also result from repetitive discharges after the passage of a single impulse if the nerve excitability is significantly altered at the site of lesion. Unless axonal degeneration occurs secondary to damage of the myelin sheath, electromyography reveals little or no evidence of denervation. The motor unit potentials tend to be normal, although they may be reduced in number if conduction block occurs in severely demyelinated fibers.

## Mixed pattern

The division into axonal and demyelinating neuropathies is somewhat arbitrary, and few cases fall precisely into one group or the other. A neuropathy with extensive demyelination is often associated with axonal degeneration.[26, 36, 37, 101] Conversely, axonal neuropathy may cause secondary paranodal demyelination.[25, 48] Nonetheless, the electrophysiologic finding of any true axonal or demyelinating component is an important and major contribution in the differential diagnosis. The pathologic observation of secondary paranodal demyelination in axonal neuropathies often has limited clinical or electrophysiologic correlation. Thus, a substantial reduction in conduction velocity with essentially normal amplitude of the evoked potential supports the diagnosis of a predominantly demyelinating neuropathy, even when superimposed upon moderate axonal degeneration as demonstrated on needle electromyography. In contrast, the absence of a significant conduction delay does not necessarily rule out the beginning of a demyelinating process. In fact, this is often the case with the Guillain-Barré syndrome at the onset.

The dichotomy into axonal and demyelinating neuropathies provides a simple and practical means of correlating electrophysiologic abnormalities with major pathologic changes in the nerve fibers. Beyond such a broad classification, electrical studies have limited value in distinguishing one variety of neuropathy from another. In particular, little can be said regarding specific etiology on the basis of the conduction studies and electromyography. In some cases, slowing in conduction cannot be accounted for either by the slight loss of fibers or the mild degree of demyelination demonstrated histologically in the same nerve.[4]

# REFERENCE SOURCES

1. ANDERSON, MH, ET AL: *Changes in the forearm associated with median nerve compression at the wrist in the guinea-pig.* J Neurol Neurosurg Psychiatry 33:70, 1970.

2. ASBURY, AK AND JOHNSON, PC: *Pathology of Peripheral Nerve*, Vol 9. In BENNINGTON, JL (ED): *Major Problems in Pathology*. WB Saunders, Philadelphia, 1978.

3. BALLANTYNE, JP AND CAMPBELL, MJ: *Electrophysiological study after surgical repair of sectioned human peripheral nerves.* J Neurol Neurosurg Psychiatry 36:797, 1973.

4. BEHSE, F AND BUCHTHAL, F: *Sensory action potentials and biopsy of the sural nerve in neuropathy.* Brain 101:473, 1978.

5. BISHOP, GH: *My life among the axons.* In HALL, VE (ED): *Annual Review of Physiology*, Vol 27. Annual Reviews, Inc, Palo Alto, California, 1965, pp 1–18.

6. BOLTON, CF AND MCFARLANE, RM: *Human pneumatic tourniquet paralysis.* Neurology (New York) 28:787, 1978.

7. BOLTON, CF, DRIEDGER, AA, AND LINDSAY RM: *Ischaemic neuropathy in uraemic patients caused by bovine arteriovenous shunt.* J Neurol Neurosurg Psychiatry 42:810, 1979.

8. BOLTON, CF, ET AL: *Nerve and muscle biopsy: Electrophysiology and morphology in polyneuropathy.* Neurology (New York) 29:354, 1979.

9. BOSTOCK, H AND SEARS, TA: *Continuous conduction in demyelinated mammalian nerve fibres.* Nature 263:786, 1976.

10. BRADLEY, WG: *Disorders of Peripheral Nerves.* Blackwell Scientific Publications, Oxford, 1974.

11. BRADLEY, WG AND THOMAS, PK: *The pathology of peripheral nerve disease.* In WALTON, JN (ED): *Disorders of Voluntary Muscle*, ed 3. Churchill Livingstone, Edinburgh, 1974, pp 234–273.

12. BRADLEY, WG, MURCHISON, D, AND DAY MJ: *The range of velocities of axoplasmic flow. A new approach, and its application to mice with genetically inherited spinal muscular atrophy.* Brain Res 35:185, 1971.

13. BUCHTHAL, F, AND KÜHL, V: *Nerve conduction, tactile sensibility, and the electromyogram after suture or compression of peripheral nerve: A longitudinal study in man.* J Neurol Neurosurg Psychiatry 42:436, 1979.

14. BUCHTHAL, F, ROSENFALCK, A, AND BEHSE, F: *Sensory potentials of normal and diseased nerves.* In DYCK, PJ, THOMAS, PK, AND LAMBERT, EH (EDS): *Peripheral Neuropathy*, Vol 1. WB Saunders, Philadelphia, 1975, pp 442–464.

15. CAVANAGH, JB: *Peripheral nerve changes in ortho-cresyl phosphate poisoning in the cat.* J Pathol Bacteriol 87:365, 1964.

16. CAVANAGH, JB AND MELLICK, RS: *On the nature of the peripheral nerve lesions associated with acute intermittent porphyria.* J Neurol Neurosurg Psychiatry 28:320, 1965.

17. DENNY-BROWN, D: *The neurological aspects of thiamine deficiency.* Proc Fed Am Soc Exper Biol (suppl 2) 17:35, 1958.

18. DENNY-BROWN, D AND BRENNER, C: *Paralysis of nerve induced by direct pressure and by tourniquet.* Arch Neurol Psychiatry 51:1, 1944.

19. DENNY-BROWN, D AND BRENNER, C: *Lesion in peripheral nerve resulting from compression by spring clip.* Arch Neurol Psychiatry 52:1, 1944.

20. DONOSO, RS, BALLANTYNE, JP, AND HANSEN, S: *Regeneration of sutured human peripheral nerves: An electrophysiological study.* J Neurol Neurosurg Psychiatry 42:97, 1979.

21. DUNN, HG, ET AL: *The neuropathy of Krabbe's infantile cerebral sclerosis (Globoid cell leukodystrophy).* Brain 92:329, 1969.

22. DYCK, PJ: *Inherited neuronal degeneration and atrophy affecting peripheral motor, sensory, and autonomic neurons.* In DYCK, PJ, THOMAS, PK, AND LAMBERT, EH (EDS): *Peripheral Neuropathy*, Vol 2. WB Saunders, Philadelphia, 1975, pp 825–867.

23. DYCK, PJ AND LAMBERT, EH: *Compound nerve action potentials and morphometry.* Electroenceph Clin Neurophysiol 36:573, 1974.

24. DYCK, PJ, THOMAS, PK, AND LAMBERT, EH: *Peripheral Neuropathy*, Vols I and II. WB Saunders, Philadelphia, 1975.

25. DYCK, PJ, ET AL: *Segmental demyelination secondary to axonal degeneration in uremic neuropathy.* Mayo Clin Proc 46:400, 1971.

26. DYCK, PJ, ET AL: *Histologic and teased-fiber measurements of sural nerve in disorders of lower motor and primary sensory neurons.* Mayo Clin Proc 43:81, 1968.

ANATOMY AND PHYSIOLOGY OF THE PERIPHERAL NERVE

27. ERLANGER, J: *The interpretation of the action potential in cutaneous and muscle nerves.* Am J Physiol 82:644, 1927.

28. ERLANGER, J AND GASSER, HS: *Electrical Signs of Nervous Activity.* University of Pennsylvania Press, Philadelphia, 1937.

29. FELDMAN, RG, HADDOW, J, AND CHISOLM, JJ: *Chronic lead intoxication in urban children.* In DESMEDT, JE (ED): *New Developments in Electromyography and Clinical Neurophysiology,* Vol 2. Karger, Basel, 1973, pp 313–317.

30. FULLERTON, PM: *Peripheral nerve conduction in metachromatic leucodystrophy (sulphatide lipidosis).* J Neurol Neurosurg Psychiatry 27:100, 1964.

31. FULLERTON, PM: *Electrophysiological and histological observations on peripheral nerves in acrylamide poisoning in man.* J Neurol Neurosurg Psychiatry 32:186, 1969.

32. FULLERTON, PM AND BARNES, JM: *Peripheral neuropathy in rats produced by acrylamide.* Br J Industr Med 23:210, 1966.

33. FULLERTON, PM AND GILLIATT, RW: *Median and ulnar neuropathy in the guinea-pig.* J Neurol Neurosurg Psychiatry 30:393, 1967.

34. GAMBLE, HJ AND EAMES, RA: *An electron microscope study of the connective tissues of human peripheral nerve.* J Anat (Lond) 98:655, 1964.

35. GASSER, HS: *Effect of the method of leading on the recording of the nerve fiber spectrum.* J Gen Physiol 43:927, 1960.

36. GILLIATT, RW: *Nerve conduction in human and experimental neuropathies.* Proc R Soc Med 59:989, 1966.

37. GILLIATT, RW: *Recent advances in the pathophysiology of nerve conduction.* In DESMEDT, JE (ED): *New Developments in Electromyography and Clinical Neurophysiology,* Vol 2. Karger, Basel, 1973, pp 2–18.

38. GILLIATT, RW: *Peripheral nerve compression and entrapment.* In LANT, AF (ED): *Eleventh Symposium on Advanced Medicine.* Pitman Medical, Kent, Great Britain, 1975, pp 144–163.

39. GILLIATT, RW AND HJORTH, RJ: *Nerve conduction during Wallerian degeneration in the baboon.* J Neurol Neurosurg Psychiatry 35:335, 1972.

40. GILLIATT, RW AND TAYLOR, JC: *Electrical changes following section of the facial nerve.* Proc R Soc Med 52:1080, 1959.

41. GRAFSTEIN, B AND FORMAN, DS: *Intracellular transport in neurons.* Physiol Rev 60:1167, 1980.

42. GUTMANN, E AND HOLUBÁR, J: *The degeneration of peripheral nerve fibres.* J Neurol Neurosurg Psychiatry 13:89, 1950.

43. HALLER, FR AND LOW, FN: *The fine structure of the peripheral nerve root sheath in the subarachnoid space in the rat and other laboratory animals.* Am J Anat 131:1, 1971.

44. HARRIS, JB AND THESLEFF, S: *Nerve stump length and membrane changes in denervated skeletal muscle.* Nature New Biol 236:60, 1972.

45. HENRIKSEN, JD: *Conduction velocity of motor nerves in normal subjects and patients with neuromuscular disorders.* Thesis, University of Minnesota, Minneapolis, 1966.

46. HODES, R: *Selective destruction of large motoneurons by poliomyelitis virus. I. Conduction velocity of motor nerve fibers of chronic poliomyelitis patients.* J Neurophysiol 12:257, 1949.

47. HODES, R, LARRABEE, MG AND GERMAN, W: *The human electromyogram in response to nerve stimulation and the conduction velocity of motor axons. Studies on normal and injured peripheral nerves.* Arch Neurol Psychiatry 60:340, 1948.

48. HOPKINS, A: *Toxic neuropathy due to industrial agents.* In DYCK, PJ, THOMAS, PK AND LAMBERT, EH (EDS): *Peripheral Neuropathy,* Vol II. WB Saunders, Philadelphia, 1975, pp 1207–1226.

49. HOPKINS, AP AND GILLIATT, RW: *Motor and sensory nerve conduction velocity in the baboon: Normal values and changes during acrylamide neuropathy.* J Neurol Neurosurg Psychiatry 34:415, 1971.

50. HUBBARD, JI: *Neuromuscular transmission—Presynaptic factors.* In HUBBARD, JI (ED): *The Peripheral Nervous System.* Plenum Press, New York, 1974, pp 151–180.

51. JOHNSON, EW AND OLSON, KJ: *Clinical value of motor nerve conduction velocity determination.* JAMA 172:2030, 1960.

52. JOHNSON, PC AND ASBURY, AK: *The pathology of peripheral nerve.* Muscle and Nerve 3:519, 1980.

53. KAESER, HE: *Neurophysiologische Erkenntnisse zum Problem der Neuritis.* Bull Schweiz Akad Med Wiss 18:196, 1962.

54. KAESER, HE: *Funktionsprüfungen peripherer Nerven bei experimentellen Polyneuritiden und bei der Wallerschen Degeneration.* Deutsche Z Nervenheilk 183:268, 1962.

55. KAESER, HE: *Zur Diagnose des Karpaltunnelsyndroms.* Praxis 40:991, 1962.

56. KAESER, HE: *Diagnostische Probleme beim Karpaltunnelsyndrom.* Deutsche Z Nervenheilk 185:453, 1963.

57. KAESER, HE AND LAMBERT, EH: *Nerve function studies in experimental polyneuritis.* Electroenceph Clin Neurophysiol (suppl 22)29, 1962.

58. KIMURA, J: *F-wave velocity in the central segment of the median and ulnar nerves. A study in normal subjects and in patients with Charcot-Marie-Tooth disease.* Neurology (Minneap) 24:539, 1974.

59. KIMURA, J: *The carpal tunnel syndrome. Localization of conduction abnormalities within the distal segment of the median nerve.* Brain 102:619, 1979.

60. KIMURA, J, RODNITZKY, R AND OKAWARA, S: *Electrophysiologic analysis of aberrant regeneration after facial nerve paralysis.* Neurology (Minneap) 25:989, 1975.

61. KOLES, ZJ AND RASMINSKY, M: *A computer simulation of conduction in demyelinated nerve fibres.* J Physiol (Lond) 227:351, 1972.

62. LAMBERT, EH: *Neurophysiological techniques useful in the study of neuromuscular disorders.* In ADAMS, RD, EATON, LM AND SHY, GM (EDS): *Neuromuscular Disorders,* Vol 38. Williams & Wilkins, Baltimore, 1960, pp 247–273.

63. LAMBERT, EH: *Pathophysiology of focal nerve lesions.* Am Acad Neurol (Spec Course #15), Clinical Electromyography, 1977.

64. LAMBERT, EH AND DYCK, PJ: *Compound action potentials of sural nerve in vitro in peripheral neuropathy.* In DYCK, PJ, THOMAS, PK, AND LAMBERT, EH (EDS): *Peripheral Neuropathy,* Vol 1. WB Saunders, Philadelphia, 1975, pp 427–441.

65. LANDON, DN (ED): *The Peripheral Nerve.* Chapman and Hall, London, 1976.

66. LASEK, R: *Axoplasmic transport in cat dorsal root ganglion cells: As studied with [3H]-L-leucine.* Brain Res 7:360, 1968.

67. LEWIS, T, PICKERING, GW AND ROTHSCHILD, P: *Centripetal paralysis arising out of arrested bloodflow to the limb, including notes on a form of tingling.* Heart 16:1, 1931.

68. McDONALD, WI: *Conduction in muscle afferent fibres during experimental demyelination in cat nerve.* Acta Neuropathol 1:425, 1962.

69. McDONALD, WI: *The effects of experimental demyelination on conduction in peripheral nerve: A histological and electrophysiological study. 1. Clinical and histological observations.* Brain 86:481, 1963.

70. McDONALD, WI: *The effects of experimental demyelination on conduction in peripheral nerve: A histological and electrophysiological study. II. Electrophysiological observations.* Brain 86:501, 1963.

71. McLEOD, JG, PRINEAS, JW, AND WALSH, JC: *The relationship of conduction velocity to pathology in peripheral nerves. A study of the sural nerve in 90 patients.* In DESMEDT, JE (ED): *New Developments in Electromyography and Clinical Neurophysiology,* Vol 2. Karger, Basel, 1973, pp 248–258.

72. NEARY, D, OCHOA, J, AND GILLIATT, RW: *Sub-clinical entrapment neuropathy in man.* J Neurol Sci 24:283, 1975.

73. NOBACK, CR: *The Human Nervous System.* McGraw-Hill, New York, 1967.

74. OCHOA, J AND MAROTTE, L: *The nature of the nerve lesion caused by chronic entrapment in the guinea-pig.* J Neurol Sci 19:491, 1973.

75. OCHOA, J, FOWLER, TJ AND GILLIATT, RW: *Anatomical changes in peripheral nerves compressed by a pneumatic tourniquet.* J Anat 113:433, 1972.

76. OCHOA, J, FOWLER, TJ, AND GILLIATT, RW: *Changes produced by a pneumatic tourniquet.* In DESMEDT, JE (ED): *New Developments in Electromyography and Clinical Neurophysiology,* Vol 2. Karger, Basel, 1973, pp 174–180.

ANATOMY AND PHYSIOLOGY OF THE PERIPHERAL NERVE

77. OCHOA, J, ET AL: *Nature of the nerve lesion caused by a pneumatic tourniquet.* Nature 233:265, 1971.

78. PENCEK, TL, ET AL: *Disruption of the perineurium in amphibian peripheral nerve: Morphology and physiology.* Neurology (New York) 30:593, 1980.

79. PILLING, JB: *Nerve conduction during Wallerian degeneration in man.* Muscle and Nerve 1:81, 1978.

80. PRINEAS, J: *The pathogenesis of dying-back polyneuropathies. Part II. An ultrastructural study of experimental acrylamide intoxication in the cat.* J Neuropathol Exper Neurol 28:598, 1969.

81. RASMINSKY, M: *Ectopic generation of impulses and cross-talk in spinal nerve roots of "dystrophic" mice.* Ann Neurol 3:351, 1978.

82. RASMINSKY, M: *Physiological consequences of demyelination.* In SPENCER, PS AND SCHAUMBURG, HH (EDS): *Experimental and Clinical Neurotoxicology.* Williams & Wilkins, Baltimore, 1980, pp 257–271.

83. RASMINSKY, M AND SEARS, TA: *Internodal conduction in undissected demyelinated nerve fibres.* J Physiol (Lond) 227:323, 1972.

84. RASMINSKY, M AND SEARS, TA: *Saltatory conduction in demyelinated nerve fibres.* In DESMEDT, JE (ED): *New Developments in Electromyography and Clinical Neurophysiology,* Vol 2. Karger, Basel, 1973, pp 158–165.

85. ROSS, MH AND REITH, EJ: *Perineurium: Evidence for contractile elements.* Science 165:604, 1969.

86. RUDGE, P: *Tourniquet paralysis with prolonged conduction block. An electrophysiological study.* J Bone Joint Surg 56B:716, 1974.

87. RUDGE, P, OCHOA, J, AND GILLIATT, RW: *Acute peripheral nerve compression in the baboon.* J Neurol Sci 23:403, 1974.

88. SAIDA, K, ET AL: *Antiserum-mediated demyelination: Relationship between remyelination and functional recovery.* Ann Neurol 8:12, 1980.

89. SCHAUMBURG, HH, WIŚNIEWSKI, HM, AND SPENCER, PS: *Ultrastructural studies of the dying-back process. I. Peripheral nerve terminal and axon degeneration in systemic acrylamide intoxication.* J Neuropathol Exp Neurol 33:260, 1974.

90. SEDDON, HJ: *Three types of nerve injury.* Brain 66:237, 1943.

91. SEDDON, H: *Surgical Disorders of the Peripheral Nerves,* ed 2. Churchill Livingstone, Edinburgh, 1975.

92. SIMPSON, JA: *Conduction velocity of peripheral nerves in human metabolic disorders.* Electroenceph Clin Neurophysiol (suppl 22)36, 1962.

93. SPENCER, PS AND SCHAUMBURG, HH: *Central-peripheral distal axonopathy—The pathology of dying-back polyneuropathies.* In ZIMMERMAN, HM (ED): *Progress in Neuropathology,* Vol III. Grune & Stratton, New York, 1976, pp 253–295.

94. STRUPPLER, A AND HUCKAUF, H: *Propagation velocity in regenerated motor nerve fibres.* Electroenceph Clin Neurophysiol (suppl 22)58, 1962.

95. SUMNER, A: *Physiology of dying-back neuropathies.* In WAXMAN, SG (ED): *Physiology and Pathobiology of Axons.* Raven Press, New York, 1978, pp 349–359.

96. SUMNER, AJ AND ASBURY, AK: *Physiological studies of the dying-back phenomenon. Muscle stretch afferents in acrylamide neuropathy.* Brain 98:91, 1975.

97. SUNDERLAND, S: *Nerves and Nerve Injuries,* ed 2. Churchill Livingstone, Edinburgh, 1978.

98. SWIFT, TR, LESHNER, RT, AND GROSS, JA: *Arm-diaphragm synkinesis: Electrodiagnostic studies of aberrant regeneration of phrenic motor neurons.* Neurology (New York) 30:339, 1980.

99. TALLIS, R, STANIFORTH, P, AND FISHER, TR: *Neurophysiological studies of autogenous sural nerve grafts.* J Neurol Neurosurg Psychiatry 41:677, 1978.

100. THOMAS, PK: *Motor nerve conduction in the carpal tunnel syndrome.* Neurology (Minneap) 10:1045, 1960.

101. THOMAS, PK: *The morphological basis for alterations in nerve conduction in peripheral neuropathy.* Proc R Soc Med 64:295, 1971.

102. THOMAS, PK AND OLSSON, Y: *Microscopic anatomy and function of the connective tissue components of peripheral nerve.* In DYCK, PJ, THOMAS, PK, AND LAMBERT, EH (EDS): *Peripheral Neuropathy,* Vol 1. WB Saunders, Philadelphia, 1973, pp 168–189.

103. TROJABORG, W: *Early electrophysiologic changes in conduction block.* Muscle and Nerve 1:400, 1978.

104. TSUJIHATA, M, ENGEL, AG, AND LAMBERT, EH: *Motor end-plate fine structure in acrylamide dying-back neuropathy: A sequential morphometric study.* Neurology (Minneap) 24:849, 1974.

105. VIZOSO, AD AND YOUNG, JZ: *Internode length and fibre diameter in developing and regenerating nerves.* J Anat (Lond) 82:110, 1948.

106. WALL, PD AND GUTNICK, M: *Properties of afferent nerve impulses originating from a neuroma.* Nature 248:740, 1974.

107. WAXMAN, SG: *Conduction in myelinated, unmyelinated, and demyelinated fibers.* Arch Neurol 34:585, 1977.

108. WAXMAN, SG: *Determinants of conduction velocity in myelinated nerve fibers.* Muscle and Nerve 3:141, 1980.

109. WAXMAN, SG AND BRILL, MH: *Conduction through demyelinated plaques in multiple sclerosis: Computer simulations of facilitation by short internodes.* J Neurol Neurosurg Psychiatry 41:408, 1978.

110. WAXMAN, SG, ET AL: *Probability of conduction deficit as related to fiber length in random-distribution models of peripheral neuropathies.* J Neurol Sci 29:39, 1976.

111. WEBSTER, H: *Peripheral nerve structure.* In HUBBARD, JI (ED): *The Peripheral Nervous System.* Plenum Press, New York, 1974, pp 3–26.

112. YOUNG, JZ: *Growth and differentiation of nerve fibres.* In *Symposia of the Society for Experimental Biology. II: Growth in Relation to Differentiation and Morphogenesis.* University Press, Cambridge, 1948, pp 57–74.

# PRINCIPLES OF NERVE CONDUCTION STUDIES

Conduction velocity of motor fibers was originally measured by Helmholtz[39] who recorded the mechanical response of a muscle. Piper[68] was the first to use the muscle action potential for this purpose, but it was the animal experiment of Berry, Grundfest, and Hinsey[2] and the human study of Hodes, Larrabee, and German[44] that popularized the technique as a clinical test. Eichler[26] was first to successfully record nerve potentials percutaneously from mixed nerves in man. The reliable technique of determining mixed nerve conduction was developed by Dawson and Scott[19] who obtained better resolution, initially by photographic superimposition and later by electrical averaging. Pure sensory nerve action potentials were first recorded by Dawson[18] through surface electrodes placed over the nerve trunk after stimulating the digital nerves using ring electrodes.

With steady improvement of recording apparatus, nerve conduction studies have become a simple and reliable test of peripheral nerve function. The method has now been adequately standardized and is widely used as a means of not only objectifying the lesion but also precisely localizing the site of maximal involvement.[50] With this technique the nerve is electrically stimulated to initiate an impulse, which travels along motor, sensory, or mixed nerves. The conduction time can be measured by recording evoked potentials either from the muscle innervated by the motor nerve or from the nerve itself in the case of the sensory or mixed nerve conduction. The same principles apply for all the peripheral nerves, although the exact technique used for testing a given nerve is dictated by its anatomic course and pattern of innervation. Electrical shocks are most convenient for clinical studies, but nerve action potentials can also be elicited by tactile stimulation.[1, 3, 64, 71]

## ELECTRICAL STIMULATION OF THE NERVE

### Cathode and anode

Either surface or needle electrodes may be used to stimulate the nerve. Surface electrodes are usually made of silver plate and are round in shape. They come in different sizes, but the most commonly used are 0.5 to 1.0 cm in diameter. Stimulating electrodes consist of a cathode (negative pole) and anode (positive pole), so called because they attract cations and anions, respectively. As the current flows from the anode to the cathode, negative charges that accumulate between the cathode and the nerve surface tend to depolarize the nerve. Conversely, the nerve is hyperpolarized under the anode. With bipolar stimulation, the usual practice is to place both electrodes over the nerve trunk, with the cathode closer to the recording site than the anode to avoid possible anodal block of the propagated impulse. Anodal hyperpolarization can be prevented simply by locating the anode away from the nerve. In calculating conduction velocities the distance is measured between the consecutive cathodal points or from the cathode to the recording electrode if the nerve potential is recorded. The cathode and anode must be clearly labeled to avoid anodal block and inadvertent surface measurement from the cathode at one stimulus site to the anode at another.

## Types of stimulators

Most commercially available stimulators provide a probe to which the cathode and anode are mounted at a fixed distance, usually 2 to 3 cm apart, for bipolar stimulation. The control for stimulus intensity may be located in the insulated handle. Although it is a convenient arrangement, especially if the test is done by a single examiner, this type of stimulus probe is necessarily bulky. A satisfactory alternative is the use of ordinary banana plugs connected by shielded cable to the stimulator. The nerve may also be stimulated in a monopolar fashion using a small cathode placed on the nerve trunk and a large anode some distance away in the same extremity. The conduction velocities obtained with monopolar stimulation differ slightly but randomly from those determined by bipolar stimulation.[42] If a needle electrode is inserted subcutaneously over and perpendicular to the nerve, the current required to elicit a response is, of course, significantly less than that of surface stimulation. The anode may be a surface electrode located nearby for monopolar stimulation, or a second needle electrode for bipolar stimulation.

Two basically different kinds of electric stimulators are used in nerve conduction studies: constant voltage and constant current units. In the former, the stimulus output is regulated in voltage so that the actual current varies inversely with the impedance of the electrode, skin, and subcutaneous tissues. In constant current units, the voltage changes according to the impedance, so that a specified amount of current can be delivered to the nerve as long as the skin resistance is within certain limits. Either type is satisfactory for clinical use, provided that the range of stimulus output is adequate for eliciting maximal muscle and nerve action potentials in all patients. However, a constant current unit is better suited for serially assessing the level of shock intensity as a measure of nerve excitability.

## Stimulus intensity and duration

The output impulse is usually a square wave of variable duration, ranging from 0.05 to 1.0 ms. In general, full activation of a healthy nerve can be achieved by surface stimulation of 0.1 ms duration and 150 to 300 V or 20 to 40 mA intensity. A maximal output of up to 500 to 600 V or 60 to 75 mA may be required in some diseased nerves with decreased excitability. Electrical stimulation within the above intensity range may be delivered to any ordinary patients with no particular risk. One possible exception may be patients with cardiac pacemakers. No experimental data are available, but the pacemaker could be inhibited if a current of sufficient amplitude is induced near the implantation site.[72] It is recommended that special care be given to proper grounding and that the stimulator be used with extreme caution near the pacemaker.[75] In patients with indwelling cardiac catheters or central venous pressure lines inserted directly into the heart, all the current may be directed to the cardiac tissue. Routine nerve conduction studies are contraindicated in these electrically sensitive patients. This and other problems related to general electrical safety will be discussed in Appendix 2C.

It is common to qualify electrical stimuli based on the magnitude of the evoked potential. A threshold stimulus is just sufficient to trigger a response in some but not all of the axons contained in the nerve. A maximal stimulus activates the entire group of axons, so that further increase in shock intensity causes no additional increase in the amplitude of the evoked potential. The current required for maximal stimulation varies greatly from one subject to the next and from one nerve to another in the same individual. A supramaximal stimulus is any stimulus that has an intensity greater than the maximal stimulus.

If large diameter fibers are always activated initially, as has been shown to occur in animal experiments,[28, 77] then a submaximal stimulus should theoretically suffice for determining the onset latency of the fastest conducting fibers. This is usually the case in man, especially with sensory nerves.[70] However, the exact order of activation seems to depend to some extent on the spatial relationship of various fibers to the stimulating electrode.[31] Thus, the first axons excited may have the longest latencies.[45, 48] Further, latency is partially determined by the lengths of the axon terminals, which may vary within a given nerve. Thus with submaximal stimuli, the onset latency could vary considerably from one trial to the next, depending on which axons within a nerve are activated. The contribution of latency variability due to those factors can be substantially reduced if the responses are elicited by supramaximal stimuli, which activate all the axons.[69]

Most commercial stimulators are designed to provide a pair of stimuli at variable intervals and a train of stimuli of different rates and duration. It is convenient if each stimulus of a pair can be independently regulated as to its duration and intensity. The stimulator should have a trigger output for the oscilloscope sweep which precedes the stimulus by a variable delay. This provides clear display of the exact stimulus point on the oscilloscope.[74]

## Stimulus artifact

A major technical problem encountered in nerve stimulation techniques is the control of stimulus artifact. Most electrode amplifiers recover from an overloading input in 5 to 10 ms, depending on the amplifier design and the amount of overload. When the stimulus is of sufficient magnitude to cause overloading artifact, short latency responses cannot be accurately recorded. This may be improved with better stimulus isolation.[11] The stimulator can be isolated from the ground by delivering the stimulus through an isolating transformer. Not only does this serve to reduce excessive shock artifact and eliminate amplifier overloading, but it also protects the patient from unexpected current leakage. The transformer must be designed so that the waveform of the original stimulus is faithfully preserved. Stimulus artifacts are also minimized by the use of a radio-frequency isolation unit, which also preserves the shape of the stimulus better than the transformer. Unfortunately, high frequency stimulus isolation units generally fail to deliver adequate intensity of supramaximal stimulation. Finally, stimulus artifact may also be effectively circumvented by the use of a fast-recovery amplifier.[81]

Shock artifacts are particularly large when stimulating and recording electrodes are located in close proximity and the active ($G_1$) and reference ($G_2$) recording electrodes are widely separated. Even if the stimulus is a square pulse of 0.1 ms duration, with excessive surface spread the volume-conducted stimulus duration at the active electrode site may be several milliseconds at the signal level of recording. Thus, care in reducing the surface spread of stimulus current is important for optimal recording of short latency responses. If the skin surface between the stimulating and recording electrodes is moist with perspiration, it should be wiped with alcohol and dried before the stimulus is delivered. The stimulating and recording sites must also be adequately prepared to reduce skin resistance. Surface grease can be dissolved by cleaning the skin with ether. If necessary, calloused skin may be abrased gently with a dull knife or fine sandpaper. Rubbing the skin with a cream or solvent of high conductance is also helpful in reducing the impedance between the electrode and underlying tissue. To reduce the size of the stimulus artifact, the ground electrode is placed between the stimulating and recording electrode whenever possible. This is not, however, an absolute requirement, especially if a fast recovery amplifier is in use.[81]

# RECORDING OF MUSCLE AND NERVE POTENTIALS

## Surface and needle electrodes

Surface electrodes, in general, are better suited than needle electrodes for recording evoked muscle action potentials. The response recorded by surface electrodes is a compound action potential with contributions from all the muscle fibers innervated by the nerve. Thus, its onset latency indicates the conduction time of the fastest fiber, whereas its amplitude is approximately proportional to the number of available axons. This is in contrast to recording from a needle electrode, which registers only a small portion of the muscle action potential. With the needle electrode, however, the onset of the muscle action potential is more abrupt and easier to discern, and interference from the neighboring muscles is less conspicuous. Therefore, the needle electrode may be preferred in recording from small atrophic muscles or from proximal muscles that cannot be activated in isolation. It is also helpful in isolating an action potential from the intended muscle when a stimulus inadvertently activates more than one nerve simultaneously.

Sensory and mixed nerve action potentials can be recorded by either surface or needle electrodes. The latter are preferred by some, because of the higher amplitude of the recorded potential when placed close to the nerve. According to Rosenfalck,[70] advantages of the needle electrode over the surface electrode are twofold: first, the amplitude of the potential is 2 to 3 times larger, and second, the noise from the electrode tissue surface is 2 to 3 times lower. This increases the signal-to-noise ratio by about 5 times and, if the averaging technique is used, the time required to reach the same resolution is considerably reduced. Antidromic sensory potentials may be recorded from digital nerves using ring electrodes placed around the proximal and distal interphalangeal joints. For routine clinical use, electronic averaging is unnecessary, because in the upper extremities the individual sensory potentials recorded by this means are of sufficient amplitude.

## Optimal recording of intended signals

The principles of amplification and display have already been described in Chapter 3. Instead of continuous runs, the sweep is intermittently triggered by a prepulse followed, after a short delay, by the stimulus. This arrangement allows precise measurement of the time interval between the stimulus and the onset of the evoked potential. Amplifier gain must be adjusted according to the size of the potential under study. Adequate gain is necessary for accurate determination of the latency. Overamplification, however, results in truncation of the recorded response which precludes assessment of its amplitude and waveform. The muscle action potentials are normally on the order of 1.0 mV or greater. This signal must be amplified 1000 times to cause a 1 cm vertical deflection on the oscilloscope when it is set at the commonly used display of 1 V per cm. A much higher gain is required for sensory or mixed nerve conduction studies in which the total amplification is about 100,000 times, since the signal is on the order of 10 $\mu$V. With such a high gain it is important that the inherent noise level of the amplifier be very low. The use of high frequency (low-pass) filters is helpful in further reducing the noise level. In our laboratory, the frequency response used is 10 Hz to 2 KHz for sensory nerves compared with 10 Hz to 32 KHz for muscle action potentials. It is recommended that the electrode amplifier provide differential amplification with a signal-to-noise discrimination ratio close to 100,000 to 1 and an input impedance greater than 1 megohm. It should respond to frequencies of wide bandwidth ranging from 10 Hz to 10 KHz without undue distortion.

## Averaging technique

Signals within the expected noise level of the system cannot be accurately recorded using conventional techniques. The signal-to-noise ratio may be improved by interposing a step-up transformer between the recording electrodes and the amplifier.[4] It is also advantageous to have the first stage of the amplifier in a remote preamplifier box that can be placed near the electrode site.[81] An alternative approach is the use of digital averaging, which represents an improvement over the photographic superimposition[19] and early averager of Dawson[17] with its motor driven switch and multiple storage capacitors. The electronic devices now in use sum consecutive samples of waveforms stored digitally as they are triggered by repetitive stimulation. Since the voltage due to noise is unrelated to stimulation, the potentials accumulated from successive tracings will average close to zero at each point in time after stimulus onset. In contrast, signals time-locked to the stimulus will sum at a constant latency and appear as an evoked potential, distinct from the background noise. The summated potential will then be electrically divided by the number of trials to obtain an average value of the signal under consideration. With averaging, the degree of enhancement is proportional to the square root of the number of trials—four trials give twice as big a response, nine trials give three times, 16 trials give four times, and so forth. In other words, the signal-to-noise ratio improves by a factor of the square root of two every time the number of trials is doubled.

## Display and storage of recorded signals

The evoked response is displayed on an oscilloscope with a frequency range of 10 Hz to 2 to 10 KHz. The responses may be photographed (using Polaroid film) for latency determination. A more convenient arrangement is to use an oscilloscope with a storage tube. If a series of responses is displayed with a stepwise vertical shift of the baseline, it facilitates the comparison of successively elicited potentials in waveform and latency. The latency is most accurately determined using an automatic device that digitally displays the value when the marker is manually positioned to the desired spot of the waveform. The time base of modern oscilloscopes is so stable that the marking of calibration signals on the second beam is no longer essential. Consequently, a single channel is satisfactory for most routine nerve conduction studies. Dual channels are, however, a distinct asset, as they allow simultaneous recording of related events. Oscilloscopes with four or more channels are also available for multichannel analysis.

For a permanent record, the display of the storage scope is photographed by a 35 mm or Polaroid camera. The original potentials may be fed into a magnetic tape recorder using either frequency (FM) or amplitude modulation (AM). The FM method is better suited for analysis of evoked muscle or nerve potentials, since it preserves the amplitude of the recorded potential very accurately. The FM mode is limited in high frequency response but can adequately record the frequency range of the compound action potential, including DC changes. In contrast, the AM modulation is responsive to high frequency bands but may distort the amplitude of the recorded response. As mentioned in Chapter 3, the AM method is preferred for recording motor unit potentials with needle electrodes to preserve the high frequency components.

# MOTOR NERVE CONDUCTION

## Stimulation and recording

For motor nerve conduction studies, the nerve is stimulated at two or more points along its course. The stimulating electrodes are placed with the anode 2 to 3 cm proximal to the cathode, which is closer to the recording electrode. This arrangement is essential, since the nerve is depolarized under the cathode and hyperpolarized under the anode. Depolarization results in the generation of a nerve action potential, whereas hyperpolarization tends to block the propagation of the nerve impulse. A series of pulses of moderate intensity is applied and the position of the cathode is adjusted until further movements cause no increase in the size of the muscle action potential. With the cathode at the best stimulating site, stimulus intensity is gradually increased until the maximal potential is obtained. This intensity is defined as the maximal stimulus for that nerve. Increasing the stimulus further should result in no change in the size of the muscle potential. The use of 20 to 30 percent supramaximal intensity guarantees the activation of all of the nerve axons innervating the recorded muscle.

The compound muscle action potentials are recorded using a pair of surface electrodes (Fig. 5-1). The active electrode ($G_1$) is placed on the belly of the muscle and the

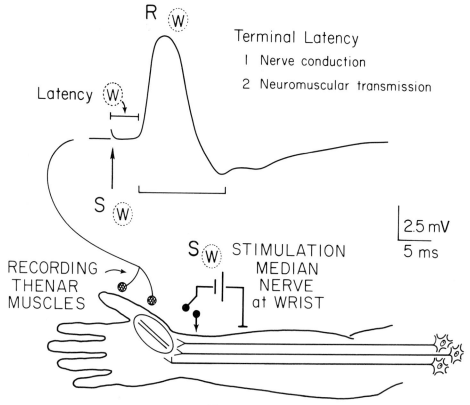

Figure 5-1

Compound muscle action potential recorded from the thenar eminence following stimulation of the median nerve at the wrist. The distal or terminal latency includes (1) nerve conduction from the stimulus point to the axon terminal; and (2) neuromuscular transmission including the time required for generation of the muscle action potential after depolarization of the end-plate.

indifferent electrode ($G_2$) on the tendon (belly-tendon recording). With this arrangement, the propagating muscle action potential originates under $G_1$ located near the motor point. As discussed in Chapter 2, the recorded response is a simple biphasic potential with initial negativity and maximal amplitude. If a small positive potential precedes the negative peak, the recording electrode should be repositioned until the appropriate shape of the evoked potential is obtained. The amplitude is determined from the baseline to the negative peak or between negative and positive peaks. The duration is measured from the onset to the negative or positive peak or to the final return to the baseline. The latency is measured from the stimulus artifact to the onset of the negative response. This time interval consists of two components: (1) nerve conduction from the stimulus point to the nerve terminal and (2) neuromuscular transmission including the time required for the muscle membrane to generate an action potential consequent upon depolarization of the end-plate. Since the latency is determined to the onset of the negative potential, it is a measure of the fastest conducting motor fibers.

## Calculation of conduction velocity

To calculate the motor nerve conduction velocity, the latency of the second component mentioned above must be eliminated. This can be achieved indirectly if the nerve is stimulated at two separate points and the latency difference between the two responses calculated (Fig. 5-2). Since the time required for neuromuscular transmission and generation of the muscle action potential is common to the two stimulations, the value thus obtained represents the time required for the nerve impulse to travel between the two stimulus points. The conduction velocity can now be obtained simply by dividing the nerve length between the two stimulation points by the latency difference. The length of the nerve segment is estimated by the surface distance between the two cathodal points along the course of the nerve. Accurate determination of the conduction distance is essential for reliable results. The nerve conduction velocity is calculated as

$$\frac{D \text{ mm}}{L_p - L_d \text{ ms}} = \frac{D}{L_p - L_d} \text{ m/s,}$$

where D is the distance between the two stimulus points in millimeters, and $L_p$ and $L_d$ the proximal and distal latencies in milliseconds, respectively. If a nerve can be stimulated at multiple points along its length, then the velocity can be assessed for a total number of nerve segments equal to the number of stimulus points minus one. Accurate determination of conduction velocity is possible only if the two stimulation points are separated by at least several, and preferably more than ten, centimeters.

The conduction time from the most distal stimulus point to the muscle is generally referred to as the distal or terminal latency. As mentioned earlier, the conduction velocity cannot be calculated over this segment, since the distal latency includes not only the nerve conduction time, but also neuromuscular transmission time. The actual conduction time in the terminal segment is slightly longer than would be expected for the same distance based on the conduction velocity of the more proximal segment. The difference is referred to as the residual latency, which is a measure of the conduction delay at the fine nerve terminals and at the neuromuscular junction.[44, 51, 52]

## Possible sources of error

In normal subjects, the compound muscle action potentials are nearly identical in waveform, regardless of the site of nerve stimulation, provided, of course, that each stimulus is of supramaximal intensity. The impulses of the slow conducting fibers lag further behind those of the fast conducting fibers over a longer conducting path. Hence, the duration of the evoked potential may be slightly greater with a more proximal

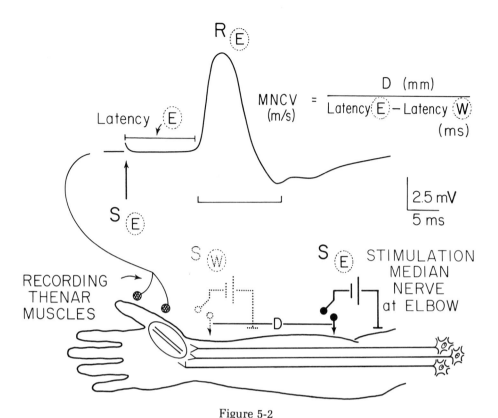

$$\text{MNCV (m/s)} = \frac{D \text{ (mm)}}{\text{Latency } E - \text{Latency } W \text{ (ms)}}$$

Figure 5-2

Compound muscle action potential recorded from the thenar eminence following stimulation of the median nerve at the elbow. The nerve conduction time from the elbow to the wrist can be determined as the latency difference between the distal and proximal stimulations. The motor nerve conduction velocity (MNCV) is then calculated by dividing the surface distance between the stimulus points by the latency difference.

stimulation, as compared with a more distal one. This physiologic temporal dispersion does not drastically alter the waveform of the recorded potentials, however. If the evoked potentials are dissimilar in shape, the two onset latencies cannot be compared, since they may represent fibers of different conduction characteristics. This may occur in diseased nerves in which the impulse from a proximal site of stimulation fails to propagate in some fibers because of conduction block. More commonly, however, distorted waveforms result if the stimulus intensity is inappropriately low. In this case, the latency of the evoked response does not necessarily represent that of the fastest conducting fibers, since the largest fibers are not always stimulated first by a threshold stimulus.[31] The error is even greater if the nerve is stimulated submaximally at one point and supramaximally at a second site. On the other hand, an excessive stimulus intensity can cause an erroneously short latency due to depolarization of the nerve a few millimeters away from the stimulating cathode.[67] In this case, the surface length between the two stimulus points does not accurately measure the conduction distance of the nerve segment under study.[82]

If a muscle action potential is recorded with a high gain, a small negative peak is sometimes seen to precede the main negative component.[5, 37, 74] This small potential should be disregarded when determining the latency, as it likely represents a nerve action potential originating from small nerve fibers near the motor point. Awareness of this possibility is particularly important if the nerve action potential precedes the muscle response with stimulation at one point but not at a second point. This is sometimes the case when a different gain is required for recording the muscle potential with distal and proximal stimulation.

## Types of abnormalities

Conduction abnormalities of diseased nerve fibers have already been mentioned in Chapter 4. In general, axonal damage or dysfunction results in loss of amplitude, whereas demyelination leads to prolongation of conduction time. Assessment of a nerve as a whole, as opposed to individual nerve fibers, is more complicated because different types of abnormalities tend to coexist. Nonetheless, there are three basic types of abnormalities commonly encountered in motor nerve conduction studies, when the nerve is stimulated at a site proximal to the presumed lesion. They are (1) reduced amplitude with normal or slightly increased latency; (2) increased latency with relatively normal amplitude; and (3) absent response (Fig. 5-3).

In the first variety, the compound muscle action potential may be reduced in amplitude when the nerve is stimulated above but not below the site of the lesion (Fig. 5-4). This is commonly seen with a partial nerve lesion causing neuropraxia or early axonotmesis before the onset of distal degeneration. Distinction between the two possibilities can be made by stimulating the nerve below the lesion several days after injury when degenerating axons are no longer excitable. If the muscle response is still signif-

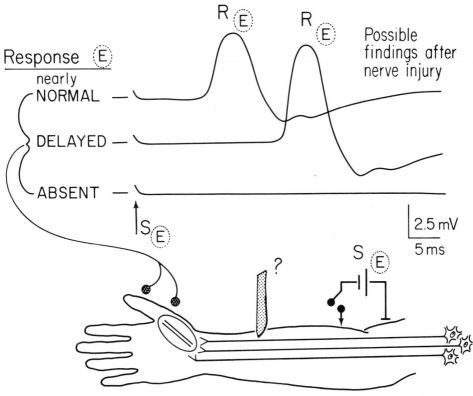

Figure 5-3

Three basic types of alteration in the compound muscle action potential occur after a presumed nerve injury distal to the site of stimulation. The response may be mildly reduced in amplitude but nearly normal in latency (top). It may be essentially normal in amplitude but substantially increased in latency (middle). Or it may be absent or markedly reduced in amplitude even with a shock of supramaximal intensity (bottom).

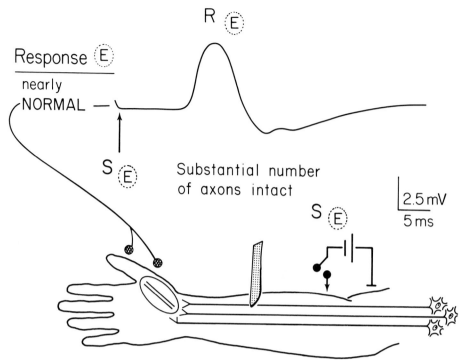

Figure 5-4

Mild reduction in amplitude of the compound muscle action potential with nearly normal latency. This type of abnormality is seen when a substantial number of axons remain functional. Conduction block in the affected axons may be secondary to neurapraxia or axonotmesis. The latency is nearly normal because the surviving axons conduct normally. Because of inherent individual variability, minor changes in amplitude may not be detected as a sign of significant abnormality.

icantly larger with distal stimulation, the presence of partial neurapraxia should be considered. If the size of the muscle response is reduced to the same degree with stimulation above and below the point of the lesion, it may be concluded that the failure of conduction is due to axonotmesis.

The amplitude of the muscle response varies considerably from one normal subject to another. Thus, minor diminution in the recorded potential may be difficult to substantiate, when the response is the same with proximal and distal stimulation. This type of abnormality often escapes undetected, especially if the onset latency of the remaining axons is normal.

In the second variety, amplitude is relatively normal, but the conduction is slowed when the nerve is stimulated above the lesion (Fig. 5-5). These changes are generally attributed to segmental demyelination affecting a majority of the nerve fibers. A prolonged latency or slowing of conduction velocity, however, also occurs in axonal neuropathy if the fastest conduction fibers are lost. In this case, amplitude would be significantly reduced as well. Slowing of motor conduction velocity associated with reduced amplitude usually occurs in the peripheral nerve disorders. However, in myelopathies, if the amplitude of the compound action potential is reduced to less than 10 percent of normal, the motor conduction velocity can be reduced by as much as 30 percent of the mean normal value.[60] Significant slowing due to axonal loss does not occur if the amplitude is greater than 40 to 50 percent of the mean normal value. The presence of peripheral nerve disease is suggested, regardless of the amplitude, if the velocity is reduced to less than 60 percent of normal.[61]

In mild demyelination proximal stimulation above the lesion ordinarily activates a compound muscle action potential similar in waveform to the one elicited by a distal

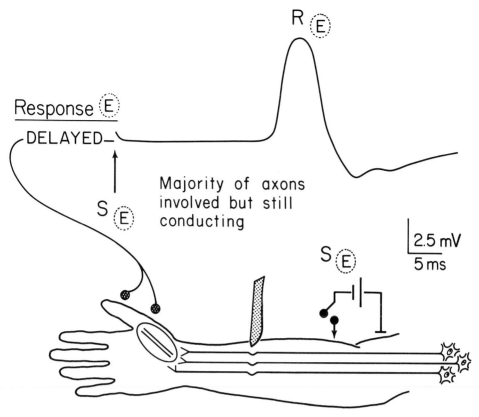

Figure 5-5

Increased latency of the compound muscle action potential with normal amplitude. This type of abnormality is commonly seen with demyelination affecting the majority of nerve fibers as in a compression neuropathy. The amplitude may be reduced if the demyelination is associated with conduction block affecting some of the axons.

stimulus below the lesion. However, the recorded compound muscle action potentials show abnormal temporal dispersion in a severe demyelinative neuropathy (Fig. 5-6). If this is associated with neurapraxia of a substantial number of nerve fibers, conduction velocity cannot be calculated accurately, since the onset latencies of the distal and proximal responses may represent two groups of motor fibers with different conduction characteristics.

Absent responses indicate that a majority of the nerve fibers are not conducting across the site of the presumed lesion (Fig. 5-7). This is commonly seen in neurotmesis. However, for the first four to seven days, one cannot differentiate a completely neurapraxic lesion from nerve transection, since, in either case, nerve stimulation distal to the lesion elicits an entirely normal muscle action potential. During the second week this distinction becomes possible based on distal nerve excitability, which remains normal only with neurapraxic lesions. With neurotmesis, stimulation below the point of the lesion produces little or no muscle action potentials (Fig. 5-8).

# SENSORY NERVE CONDUCTION

## Stimulation and recording

For sensory conduction studies in the upper extremities, the digital nerves may be stimulated to record an orthodromic sensory potential from a more proximal site, or

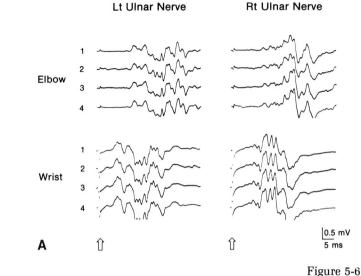

Lt Ulnar Nerve        Rt Ulnar Nerve

Elbow
1
2
3
4

Wrist
1
2
3
4

A        ⇧        ⇧

0.5 mV
5 ms

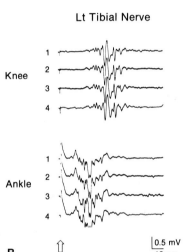

Lt Tibial Nerve

Knee
1
2
3
4

Ankle
1
2
3
4

B        ⇧

0.5 mV
10 ms

Figure 5-6

Delayed and temporally dispersed compound muscle action potentials in a 31-year-old man with the Guillain-Barré syndrome. (*A*) The right and left ulnar nerves were stimulated at the elbow and wrist, and the muscle responses were recorded using surface electrodes placed at the belly ($G_1$) and tendon ($G_2$) of the abductor digiti minimi. Four consecutive trials are shown at each stimulus site to show consistency of the evoked potentials. (*B*) The tibial nerve was stimulated at the knee and ankle, and the compound muscle action potentials were recorded using surface electrodes placed over the belly ($G_1$) and tendon ($G_2$) of the abductor hallucis. The recorded potentials are not only increased in latency and duration but are also very irregular in waveform, regardless of the site of stimulation.

alternatively, the nerve may be stimulated proximally and the digital potential recorded antidromically.

The latency can also be measured by stimulating the trunk of a mixed nerve and recording the nerve potential from a second point on the same nerve trunk. For example, the ulnar or median nerve may be stimulated at the wrist and the action potential recorded through surface electrodes placed over the nerve trunk at the elbow. Large diameter sensory fibers have lower thresholds and conduct faster than motor fibers by about 5 to 10 percent.[18] Thus mixed nerve potentials allow determination of the fastest sensory nerve conduction velocity. However, this relationship may not hold for peripheral nerve diseases with relatively selective involvement of sensory fibers. In these circumstances, it would be difficult to differentiate the sensory and motor components of mixed nerve potentials.

For routine clinical recordings surface electrodes suffice, since they are noninvasive yet provide adequate and reproducible information. As discussed earlier, needle electrodes are preferred by some because of their greater signal-to-noise ratio.[70] Needle electrodes often permit recordings of nerve potentials from the proximal segment. Assessment of temporal dispersion is also more accurate with needle than with surface

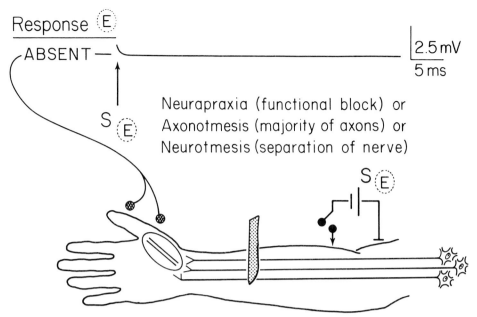

Figure 5-7

No evoked potential with supramaximal stimulation of the nerve proximally. This type of abnormality is seen whenever the majority of axons fail to conduct, as a result of neurapraxia, axonotmesis, or neurotmesis.

electrodes, especially when combined with signal averaging. This technique has proven to be a sensitive measure of nerve damage, since it defines small late components originating from demyelinated, remyelinated, or regenerated fibers.[6, 7, 32, 70]

## Amplitude, duration, and waveform

When using surface electrodes, the digital potential recorded antidromically is larger than the orthodromic response from the nerve trunk, since the digital nerves are nearer to the surface.[5] The opposite is true, however, if the potentials are recorded with needle electrodes placed near the nerve. In studying the mixed nerve, antidromically recorded sensory potentials may be obscured by the superimposition of action potentials from distal muscles, since some motor axons have thresholds similar to those of large myelinated sensory axons.[36] However, overlap of muscle action potentials is ordinarily easily recognizable by the greater latency and characteristic waveform of the elicited response.[56]

The amplitude of the sensory potential may be measured either from the baseline to the negative peak or between the negative and positive peaks. The variability in amplitude of the nerve action potential is essentially the same whether the response is recorded with surface or needle electrodes.[5] The amplitude of the digital nerve potential expresses the density of sensory innervation in each finger. Since degeneration of sensory fibers occurs only with a lesion distal to the sensory ganglion, this can be used as a criterion to differentiate preganglionic root avulsion and plexopathy.[35] Although the digital nerve potential may also be affected in postganglionic root lesion, its differentiation from plexopathy is usually possible based on the relatively selective radicular innervation of the first and second digits by C-6, the third digit by C-7, and the fourth and fifth digits by C-8 roots. Relative amplitude values of the sensory action potential have been determined for each digit.[15, 16]

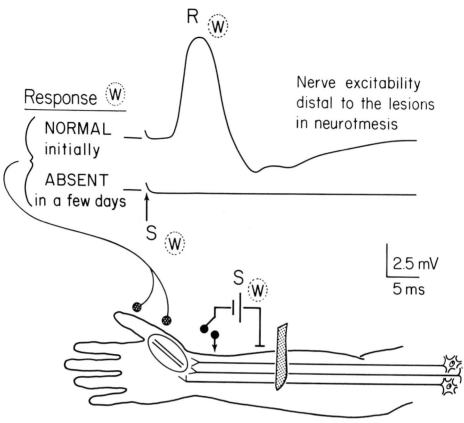

Figure 5-8

Nerve excitability distal to the lesion in neurotmesis or substantial axonotmesis. Distal stimulation elicits a normal compound muscle action potential during the first few days after the nerve injury, even if all the axons are completely severed. Consequent to wallerian degeneration subsequent to transection, the distal nerve segment becomes inexcitable in three or four days. In contrast, distal excitability remains normal if the proximal conduction block is chiefly caused by neurapraxia.

The duration of the nerve action potential may be measured from the initial deflection of the baseline to the intersection of the descending phase and the baseline, or to the negative or positive peak. Less commonly, it is measured to the point at which the tracing finally returns to baseline, but this point of reference is sometimes difficult to define.

The waveform of a sensory nerve action potential is markedly affected by the position of the recording electrodes within the volume conductor. The orthodromic potential recorded with an active electrode ($G_1$) on the nerve and a reference electrode ($G_2$) at a remote site is triphasic with initial positivity. A separate late phase may appear if the response is recorded at a more proximal site where temporal dispersion is greater. If $G_2$ is also placed near the nerve with a distance of more than 3 cm between the electrodes, the recorded potential may be tetraphasic, although the initial deflection is still positive.[5] In contrast, digital potentials recorded antidromically with a pair of ring electrodes around the finger are usually biphasic with initial negativity.

## Calculation of conduction velocity

Unlike a motor latency, which includes neuromuscular transmission, sensory latency is equivalent to the nerve conduction time from the stimulus point to the recording electrode. The sensory nerve conduction velocity can therefore be calculated after stimulation of the nerve at a single site. The latency of the orthodromically recorded sensory potential may be measured to the initial positive peak or to the subsequent negative peak. If the sensory nerve is stimulated at several points and the waveforms of the recorded potentials are compared, the interval between the positive and negative peaks becomes greater as the stimulating electrodes are moved further away from the recording site. Because of this dispersion of fast and slow conducting impulses, the conduction velocity calculated with the latency to the negative peak is not a measure of the fastest conducting sensory fibers.[18]

Nonetheless the negative peak is frequently used as the point of reference, if the preceding smaller positive peak is difficult to identify, which may be especially true in diseased nerves.[33] When this is done, the usual practice has been to measure the conduction distance to the midpoint of $G_1$ and $G_2$ to compensate for the discrepancy between the arrival of the impulse and the appearance of the negative peak.[25] Using modern amplifiers with high resolution, however, it is now feasible in most cases to measure the sensory latency to the initial positive peak. Determinations of the conduction distance from the stimulus point to $G_1$ then allows accurate calculation of conduction velocity for the fastest fibers.[5] With the biphasic digital potential recorded antidromically, the onset latency is measured to the initial take-off of the negative peak from the baseline, and the conduction distance from the cathode to $G_1$. In this situation, it is rarely, if at all, necessary to resort to the determination of the peak latency, because antidromically recorded digital potentials are considerably larger than orthodromic potentials. Antidromic and orthodromic conduction times are nearly identical, although the standard deviation is slightly higher in the former.[5]

# VARIABILITY
# IN NERVE CONDUCTION MEASUREMENT

The validity of the nerve conduction velocity calculation depends on the accuracy in determining the latencies and the conduction distance. Sources of error in measuring latencies include unstable or incorrect triggering of the sweep; poorly defined take-off of the evoked response; and inappropriate stimulus strength and inaccurate calibration.[61, 74] Errors in measurement of the conduction distance by surface measurement result from uncertainty as to the exact site of stimulation and the exact course of the nerve trunk. Surface determination of the nerve length is particularly imprecise when the nerve takes a nonlinear path, as in the brachial plexus, or across the elbow or knee.

Because of these uncontrollable variables, the calculated velocities are not absolute values of nerve conduction.[63] On repeated testing, the values might vary, occasionally as much as 10 m/s, because of the limitations inherent in the technique.[62] If standard procedures are adhered to, however, the results are sufficiently reproducible. Since the range of normal is small, the use of nerve conduction studies as a clinical diagnostic test is justified. In general, the results expressed as latency are more difficult to use in comparison studies, unless the distance between electrodes can be maintained at a constant interval. As listed below, a number of factors have been investigated with regard to their role in modifying motor and sensory conduction studies. Familiarity with these factors is essential for proper interpretation.

## Effect of temperature

It is well known that nerve impulses conduct faster at a higher body temperature.[20, 40, 66] The conduction velocity increases almost linearly, by 2.4 m/s or approximately 5 percent per degree, as the temperature measured near the nerve increases from 29 to 38°C.[42, 47] Similarly, the wrist-to-muscle latencies increase by 0.3 ms per degree for both median and ulnar nerves upon cooling the hand.[9] The effect of localized cooling on the amplitude of nerve and muscle potential is less well known. Hodgkin and Katz[46] demonstrated an increase in amplitude of action potential after cooling the squid axon. This observation was confirmed by a more recent human study in which cooling was associated with significant increases in the amplitude and area under the negative component.[21, 22]

To reduce temperature-related variability, studies should be done in a warm room with the temperature maintained between 21 and 23°C. A warmer room at 26 to 28°C is recommended by some to reduce the temperature gradient along the course of a nerve. This gradient is minimal if room temperature is elevated to 30°C[53] but this is impractical and unnecessary.

It is possible to check the intramuscular temperature using a thermometer inserted through the skin. This procedure, however, is neither convenient nor practical, since it requires an additional skin puncture for each muscle tested. The more common practice is to measure the skin temperature with a plate thermistor. There is a linear correlation between skin temperature and subcutaneous and intramuscular temperatures.[38] If the skin is 34°C or above, it may be assumed that the muscle is close to 37°C.[23] If the skin temperature is below 34°C, the limbs should be warmed with an infrared heat lamp or by immersion in warm water. If not, an appropriate conversion factor should be applied to normalize the result by adding 5 percent of the calculated conduction velocity for each degree below 34°C. However, the use of a conversion factor based upon an average of many subjects may be misleading in certain individuals.

## Variation among different nerves and segments

Both proximal and distal conduction velocities are significantly slower in the lower than in the upper extremities. The small reduction in temperature in the lower limb as compared with the upper limb does not account for the recorded differences which range between 7 to 10 m/s.[58, 79] One may postulate that longer nerves generally conduct more slowly than shorter nerves. An inverse relationship between height and nerve conduction velocity is consistent with this view.[8] Conduction velocities are comparable in the median and ulnar nerves, but tibial nerve conduction may be slightly slower than peroneal conduction.[49]

Conduction velocity is generally considered to be faster in the more proximal than in the distal nerve segment.[34, 41] Small differences in velocity may be due to the progressive reduction in axonal diameter, to the shorter internodal distances, or to colder temperature found more distally. Distal slowing of conduction has not been a universal finding. Some authors have reported no difference when compared with a proximal segment, whereas others have noted a slower conduction proximally.[43, 76] In an experiment using a baboon, the conduction velocity of single motor axons was slower in the brachial plexus than in the peripheral nerve trunk.[13] In man, the most proximal portion of a peripheral nerve is not accessible by conventional nerve conduction techniques.

Using the F-wave, it is possible to calculate the ratio between motor nerve conduction time from the spinal cord to the stimulus site and that of the remaining nerve segment to the muscle.[55] As will be discussed in Chapter 17, this ratio is normally close to unity for the median and ulnar nerves stimulated at the elbow and for the peroneal and tibial nerves stimulated at the knee. Thus, the time required for the passage of impulses from the cord to the site of stimulation is approximately the same as that from the stimulus site to the muscle. This finding indicates faster conduction proximally, since the cord-to-elbow segment is longer than the elbow-to-muscle segment. Likewise, the cord-to-knee segment is substantially longer than the knee-to-muscle segment, whether estimated by surface determination or measured directly in cadavers.[57] The most proximal motor nerve conduction velocity determined by F-wave latency is faster than the conventionally derived most distal conduction velocity.[14, 27, 54, 57, 59] However, there is no significant difference between cord-to-axilla and axilla-to-elbow segments.[54]

# Effects of age

It is well known that nerve conduction velocities in full-term infants are roughly half those in adults.[78] The velocity increases rapidly as the process of myelination advances during the first few years of life, reaching the adult range in 3 to 5 years (Fig. 5-9). Table 5-1 summarizes the results of one series showing the rapid increase in conduction of the peroneal nerve through infancy and the slower maturation of the median nerve during early childhood.[30] The conduction velocities are even slower in premature infants, ranging from 17 to 25 m/s in the ulnar nerve and from 14 to 28 m/s in the peroneal nerve.[12] Conduction velocities decrease slightly in higher age groups. The reduction occurs after 30 to 40 years of age, but the change is normally less than 10 m/s by the 60th year[80] or even by the 80th year.[65] Table 5-2 shows the results of Mayer,[63] indicating a reduction in the mean conduction rate of about 10 percent at 60 years of age. Aging also causes a decrement in sensory conduction and changes in the shape of the evoked potential, especially at the common sites of compression.[15] Evoked amplitude also declines with older age. The F-wave and peaks of the somatosensory evoked potentials have been shown to gradually increase in latency with advancing age.[24]

# Other factors

It has long been known that nerve excitability is significantly altered during ischemia induced by a pneumatic tourniquet.[73] During ischemia, there is progressive slowing in conduction velocity, decrease in amplitude, and increase in duration of the sensory action potential. The effect of ischemia on conduction of the median nerve has been shown to be more rapid in the carpal tunnel syndrome than in normal controls.[29] Con-

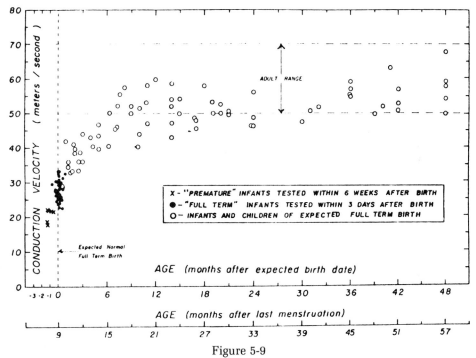

Figure 5-9

Relation of age to conduction velocity of motor fibres in the ulnar nerve between the elbow and wrist. Velocities in normal young adults range from 47 to 73 m/s with the majority of values between 50 and 70 m/s. Age has been plotted in relation to the date on which infant would have been considered full term on the basis of calculation from the first day of last menstruation. (From Thomas and Lambert,[78] with permission.)

**TABLE 5-1 Normal motor nerve conduction velocities in different age groups**

| Age | Ulnar | Median | Peroneal |
|---|---|---|---|
| 0–1 week | 32 (21–39) | 29 (21–38) | 29 (19–31) |
| 1 week–4 months | 42 (27–53) | 34 (22–42) | 36 (23–53) |
| 4 months–1 year | 49 (40–63) | 40 (26–58) | 48 (31–61) |
| 1–3 years | 59 (47–73) | 50 (41–62) | 54 (44–74) |
| 3–8 years | 66 (51–76) | 58 (47–72) | 57 (46–70) |
| 8–16 years | 68 (58–78) | 64 (54–72) | 57 (45–74) |
| Adults | 63 (52–75) | 63 (51–75) | 56 (47–63) |

From Gamstorp,[30] with permission.

**TABLE 5-2 Normal motor and sensory conduction velocities in different age groups**

| Nerve | Age groups | | | | | |
|---|---|---|---|---|---|---|
| | 10 to 35 years (30 cases) | | 36 to 50 years (16 cases) | | 51 to 80 years (18 cases) | |
| | Sensory | Motor | Sensory | Motor | Sensory | Motor |
| Median nerve | | | | | | |
| digit-wrist | 67.5±4.7 | | 65.8±5.7 | | 59.4±4.9 | |
| wrist-muscle | | 3.2± .3* | | 3.7± .3* | | 3.5± .2* |
| wrist-elbow | 67.7±4.4 | 59.3±3.5 | 65.8±3.1 | 55.9±2.6 | 62.8±5.4 | 54.5±4.0 |
| elbow-axilla | 70.4±4.8 | 65.9±5.0 | 70.4±3.4 | 65.1±4.2 | 66.2±3.6 | 63.6±4.4 |
| Ulnar nerve | | | | | | |
| digit-wrist | 64.7±3.9 | | 66.5±3.4 | | 57.5±6.6 | |
| wrist-muscle | | 2.7± .3* | | 2.7± .3* | | 3.0±.35* |
| wrist-elbow | 64.8±3.8 | 58.9±2.2 | 67.1±4.7 | 57.8±2.1 | 56.7±3.7 | 53.3±3.2 |
| elbow-axilla | 69.1±4.3 | 64.4±2.6 | 70.6±2.4 | 63.3±2.0 | 64.4±3.0 | 59.9± .7 |
| Common peroneal nerve | | | | | | |
| ankle-muscle | | 4.3± .9* | | 4.8± .5* | | 4.6± .6* |
| ankle-knee | 53.0±5.9 | 49.5±5.6 | 50.4±1.0 | 43.6±5.1 | 46.1±4.0 | 43.9±4.3 |
| Posterior tibial nerve | | | | | | |
| ankle-muscle | | 5.9±1.3* | | 7.3±1.7* | | 6.0±1.2* |
| ankle-knee | 56.9±4.4 | 45.5±3.8 | 49.0±3.8 | 42.9±4.9 | 48.9±2.6 | 41.8±5.1 |
| H reflex, popliteal fossa | | 71.0±4.0 | | 64.0±2.1 | | 60.4±5.0 |
| | | 27.9±2.2* | | 28.2±1.5* | | 32.0±2.1* |

From Mayer,[63] with permission.
*Latency in milliseconds
†Mean values±one standard deviation

versely, a greater resistance to ischemia has been found in peripheral nerves of diabetic and uremic patients, as well as elderly subjects.[10]

There is no significant difference in the mean conduction velocities and the range of values before and after a fast of 2 to 3 weeks' duration.[62]

# REFERENCE SOURCES

1.  BANNISTER, RG AND SEARS, TA: *The changes in nerve conduction in acute idiopathic poly-neuritis.* J Neurol Neurosurg Psychiatry 25:321, 1962.
2.  BERRY, CM, GRUNDFEST, H, AND HINSEY, JC: *The electrical activity of regenerating nerves in the cat.* J Neurophysiol 7:103, 1944.

3. BUCHTHAL, F: *Action potentials in the sural nerve evoked by tactile stimuli.* Mayo Clin Proc 55:223, 1980.

4. BUCHTHAL, F AND ROSENFALCK, A: *Action potentials from sensory nerve in man: Physiology and clinical application.* Acta Neurol Scand (suppl 13) 41:263, 1965.

5. BUCHTHAL, F AND ROSENFALCK, A: *Evoked action potentials and conduction velocity in human sensory nerves.* Brain Res 3:1, 1966.

6. BUCHTHAL, F AND ROSENFALCK, A: *Sensory potentials in polyneuropathy.* Brain 94:241, 1971.

7. BUCHTHAL, F, ROSENFALCK, A AND BEHSE, F: *Sensory potentials of normal and diseased nerves.* In DYCK, PJ, THOMAS, PK, AND LAMBERT, EH (EDS): *Peripheral Neuropathy,* Vol 1. WB Saunders Company, Philadelphia, 1975, pp 442–464.

8. CAMPBELL, WW, WARD, LC, AND SWIFT, TR: *Nerve conduction velocity varies inversely with height.* Muscle and Nerve 3:436, 1980.

9. CARPENDALE, MTF: *Conduction time in the terminal portion of the motor fibers of the ulnar, median, and peroneal nerves in healthy subjects and in patients with neuropathy.* Thesis, University of Minnesota, Minneapolis, 1956.

10. CARUSO, G, LABIANCA, O AND FERRANNINI, E: *Effect of ischemia on sensory potentials of normal subjects of different ages.* J Neurol Neurosurg Psychiatry 36:455, 1973.

11. CASEY, EB AND LE QUESNE, PM: *Digital nerve action potentials in healthy subjects, and in carpal tunnel and diabetic patients.* J Neurol Neurosurg Psychiatry 35:612, 1972.

12. CERRA, D AND JOHNSON EW: *Motor nerve conduction velocity in premature infants.* Arch Phys Med Rehabil 43:160, 1962.

13. CLOUGH, JFM, KERNELL, D AND PHILLIPS, CG: *Conduction velocity in proximal and distal portions of forelimb axons in the baboon.* J Physiol (Lond) 198:167, 1968.

14. CONRAD, B, ASCHOFF, JC AND FISCHLER, M: *Der Diagnostische Wert der F-Wellen-Latenz.* J Neurol 210:151, 1975.

15. CRUZ MARTÍNEZ, A, ET AL: *Electrophysiological aspects of sensory conduction velocity in healthy adults. 1. Conduction velocity from digit to palm, from palm to wrist, and across the elbow, as a function of age.* J Neurol Neurosurg Psychiatry 41:1092, 1978.

16. CRUZ MARTÍNEZ, A, ET AL: *Electrophysiological aspects of sensory conduction velocity in healthy adults. 2. Ratio between the amplitude of sensory evoked potentials at the wrist on stimulating different fingers in both hands.* J Neurol Neurosurg Psychiatry 41:1097, 1978.

17. DAWSON, GD: *A summation technique for the detection of small evoked potentials.* Electroenceph Clin Neurophysiol 6:65, 1954.

18. DAWSON, GD: *The relative excitability and conduction velocity of sensory and motor nerve fibres in man.* J Physiol (Lond) 131:436, 1956.

19. DAWSON, GD AND SCOTT, JW: *The recording of nerve action potentials through skin in man.* J Neurol Neurosurg Psychiatry 12:259, 1949.

20. DEJESUS, PV, HAUSMANOWA-PETRUSEWICZ, I, AND BARCHI, RL: *The effect of cold on nerve conduction of human slow and fast nerve fibers.* Neurology (Minneap) 23:1182, 1973.

21. DENYS, EH: *The effect of temperature on the compound action potential in neuromuscular disease and normal controls.* Electroenceph Clin Neurophysiol 43:598, 1977.

22. DENYS, EH: *The role of temperature in electromyography.* Minimonograph #14, American Association of Electromyography and Electrodiagnosis, 1980.

23. DESMEDT, JE: *The neuromuscular disorder in myasthenia gravis. 1. Electrical and mechanical response to nerve stimulation in hand muscles.* In DESMEDT, JE (ED): *New Developments in Electromyography and Clinical Neurophysiology,* Vol 1. Karger, Basel, 1973, pp 241–304.

24. DORFMAN, LJ AND BOSLEY, TM: *Age-related changes in peripheral and central nerve conduction in man.* Neurology (New York) 29:38, 1979.

25. DOWNIE, AW AND NEWELL, DJ: *Sensory nerve conduction in patients with diabetes mellitus and controls.* Neurology (Minneap) 11:876, 1961.

26. EICHLER, W: *Über die Ableitung der Aktionspotentiale vom menschlichen Nerven in situ.* Z Biol 98:182, 1937.

27. EISEN, A, SCHOMER, D, AND MELMED, C: *The application of F-wave measurements in the differentiation of proximal and distal upper limb entrapments.* Neurology (Minneap) 27:662, 1977.

28.  ERLANGER, J AND GASSER, HS: *Electrical Signs of Nervous Activity.* University of Pennsylvania Press, Philadelphia, 1937.

29.  FULLERTON, PM: *The effect of ischaemia on nerve conduction in the carpal tunnel syndrome.* J Neurol Neurosurg Psychiatry 26:385, 1963.

30.  GAMSTORP, I: *Normal conduction velocity of ulnar, median and peroneal nerves in infancy, childhood and adolescence.* Acta Paediatrica (suppl 146) 68, 1963.

31.  GASSEL, MM: *A study of femoral nerve conduction time.* Arch Neurol 9:607, 1963.

32.  GILLIATT, RW: *Sensory conduction studies in the early recognition of nerve disorders.* Muscle and Nerve 1:352, 1978.

33.  GILLIATT, RW AND SEARS, TA: *Sensory nerve action potentials in patients with peripheral nerve lesions.* J Neurol Neurosurg Psychiatry 21:109, 1958.

34.  GILLIATT, RW AND THOMAS, PK: *Changes in nerve conduction with ulnar lesions at the elbow.* J Neurol Neurosurg Psychiatry 23:312, 1960.

35.  GILLIATT, RW, ET AL: *Wasting of the hand associated with a cervical rib or band.* J Neurol Neurosurg Psychiatry 33:615, 1970.

36.  GILLIATT, RW, ET AL: *A study of normal nerve action potentials using an averaging technique (barrier grid storage tube).* J Neurol Neurosurg Psychiatry 28:191, 1965.

37.  GUTMANN, L: *The intramuscular nerve action potential.* J Neurol Neurosurg Psychiatry 32:193, 1969.

38.  HALAR, EM, DeLISA, JA AND BROZOVICH, FV: *Nerve conduction velocity: Relationship of skin, subcutaneous and intramuscular temperatures.* Arch Phys Med Rehabil 61:199, 1980.

39.  HELMHOLTZ, H: *Vorläufiger Bericht über die Fortpflanzungsgeschwindigkeit der Nervenreizung.* Arch Anat Physiol Wiss Med 71, 1850.

40.  HELMHOLTZ, H: *Mitteilung betreffend Versuch uber die Fortpflanzungsgeschwindigkeit der Reizung in den motorischen Nerven des Menschen, welche Herr N Baxt aus Petersburg im Physiologischen Laboratorium zu Heidelbert ausgefuhrt hat.* Mber Akad Wiss (Berlin) 228, 1867.

41.  HELMHOLTZ, H AND BAXT, N: *Neue Versuche Über die Fortpflanzungsgeschwindigkeit der Reizung in den motorischen Nerven der Menschen.* Mber Konigl Preus Akad Wiss 184, 1870.

42.  HENRIKSEN, JD: *Conduction velocity of motor nerves in normal subjects and in patients with neuromuscular disorders.* Thesis, University of Minnesota, Minneapolis, 1966.

43.  HODES, R: *Selective destruction of large motoneurons by poliomyelitis virus. I. Conduction velocity of motor nerve fibers of chronic poliomyelitis patients.* J Neurophysiol 12:257, 1949.

44.  HODES, R, LARRABEE, MG, AND GERMAN, W: *The human electromyogram in response to nerve stimulation and the conduction velocity of motor axons.* Arch Neurol Psychiatry 60:340, 1948.

45.  HODES, R, ET AL: *Low threshold associated with slow conduction velocity.* Arch Neurol 12:510, 1965.

46.  HODGKIN, AL AND KATZ, B: *The effect of temperature on the electrical activity of the giant axon of the squid.* J Physiol (Lond) 109:240, 1949.

47.  JOHNSON, EW AND OLSEN, KJ: *Clinical value of motor nerve conduction velocity determination.* JAMA 172:2030, 1960.

48.  KADRIE, HA, ET AL: *Multiple point electrical stimulation of ulnar and median nerves.* J Neurol Neurosurg Psychiatry 39:973, 1976.

49.  KAESER, HE: *Veränderungen der Leitgeschwindigkeit bei Neuropathien und Neuritiden.* Fortschr Neurol Psychiatr 33:221, 1965.

50.  KAESER, HE: *Nerve conduction velocity measurements.* In VINKEN, PJ AND BRUYN, BW (EDS): *Handbook of Clinical Neurology,* Vol 7. North Holland Publishing Company, Amsterdam, 1970, pp 116–196.

51.  KAPLAN, PE: *Sensory and motor residual latency measurements in healthy patients and patients with neuropathy. Part I.* J Neurol Neurosurg Psychiatry 39:338, 1976.

52.  KAPLAN, P AND SAHGAL, V: *Residual latency: New applications of an old technique.* Arch Phys Med Rehabil 59:24, 1978.

53.  KATO, M: *The conduction velocity of the ulnar nerve and the spinal reflex time measured by means of the H-wave in average adults and athletes.* Tohoku J Exper Med 73:74, 1960.

54. KIMURA, J: *F-wave velocity in the central segment of the median and ulnar nerves: A study in normal subjects and in patients with Charcot-Marie-Tooth disease.* Neurology (Minneap) 24:539, 1974.

55. KIMURA, J: *A method for determining median nerve conduction velocity across the carpal tunnel.* J Neurol Sci 38:1, 1978.

56. KIMURA, J: *The carpal tunnel syndrome. Localization of conduction abnormalities within the distal segment of the median nerve.* Brain 102:619, 1979.

57. KIMURA, J, BOSCH, P, AND LINDSAY, GM: *F-wave conduction velocity in the central segment of the peroneal and tibial nerves.* Arch Phys Med Rehabil 56:492, 1975.

58. KIMURA, J, YAMADA, T, AND STEVLAND, N: *Distal slowing of motor nerve conduction velocity in diabetic polyneuropathy.* J Neurol Sci 42:291, 1979.

59. KING, D AND ASHBY, P: *Conduction velocity in the proximal segments of a motor nerve in the Guillain-Barré syndrome.* J Neurol Neurosurg Psychiatry 39:538, 1976.

60. LAMBERT, EH: *Neurophysiological techniques useful in the study of neuromuscular disorders.* In ADAMS, RD, EATON, LM AND SHY, GM (EDS): *Neuromuscular Disorders.* Williams & Wilkins, Baltimore, 1960, pp 247–273.

61. LAMBERT, EH: *Diagnostic value of electrical stimulation of motor nerves.* Electroenceph Clin Neurphysiol (suppl 22) 9, 1962.

62. MATTSON, RH AND LECOCQ, FR: *Nerve conduction velocities in fasting patients.* Neurology (Minneap) 18:335, 1968.

63. MAYER, RF: *Nerve conduction studies in man.* Neurology (Minneap) 13:1021, 1963.

64. MCLEOD, JG: *Digital nerve conduction in the carpal tunnel syndrome after mechanical stimulation of the finger.* J Neurol Neurosurg Psychiatry 29:12, 1966.

65. NORRIS, AH, SHOCK, NW, AND WAGMAN, IH: *Age changes in the maximum conduction velocity of motor fibers of human ulnar nerves.* J Appl Physiol 5:589, 1953.

66. PAINTAL, AS: *Effects of temperature on conduction in single vagal and saphenous myelinated nerve fibres of the cat.* J Physiol (Lond) 180:20, 1965.

67. PINELLI, P: *Physical, anatomical and physiological factors in the latency measurement of the M response.* Electroenceph Clin Neurophysiol 17:86, 1964.

68. PIPER, H: *Weitere Mitteilungen über die Geschwindigkeit der Erregungsleitung im markhaltigen menschlichen Nerven.* Pflugers Arch Ges Physiol 127:474, 1909.

69. PRESWICK, G: *The effect of stimulus intensity on motor latency in the carpal tunnel syndrome.* J Neurol Neurosurg Psychiatry 26:398, 1963.

70. ROSENFALCK, A: *Early recognition of nerve disorders by near-nerve recording of sensory action potentials.* Muscle and Nerve 1:360, 1978.

71. ROSENFALCK, A AND BUCHTHAL, F: *Sensory potentials and threshold for electrical and tactile stimuli.* In DESMEDT, JE (ED): *New Developments in Electromyography and Clinical Neurophysiology,* Vol 2. Karger, Basel, 1973, pp 45–51.

72. SCRANTON, PE, JR, HASIBA, U, AND GORENC, TJ: *Intramuscular hemorrhage in hemophiliacs with inhibitors. A medical emergency.* JAMA 241:2028, 1979.

73. SENEVIRATNE, KN AND PEIRIS, OA: *The effect of ischaemia on the excitability of human sensory nerve.* J Neurol Neurosurg Psychiatry 31:338, 1968.

74. SIMPSON, JA: *Fact and fallacy in measurement of conduction velocity in motor nerves.* J Neurol Neurosurg Psychiatry 27:381, 1964.

75. SKAGGS, H, ET AL: *Guidelines in EMG.* Professional Standard Committee, American Association of Electromyography and Electrodiagnosis, 1979.

76. SPIEGEL, MH AND JOHNSON, EW: *Conduction velocity in the proximal and distal segments of the motor fibers of the ulnar nerve of human beings.* Arch Phys Med Rehabil 43:57, 1962.

77. TASAKI, I: *Electric stimulation and the excitatory process in the nerve fiber.* Am J Physiol 125:380, 1939.

78. THOMAS, JE AND LAMBERT, EH: *Ulnar nerve conduction velocity and H-reflex in infants and children.* J Appl Physiol 15:1, 1960.

79. THOMAS, PK, SEARS, TA, AND GILLIATT, RW: *The range of conduction velocity in normal motor nerve fibres to the small muscles of the hand and foot.* J Neurol Neurosurg Psychiatry 22:175, 1959.

80. WAGMAN, IH AND LESSE, H: *Maximum conduction velocities of motor fibers of ulnar nerve in human subjects of various ages and sizes.* J Neurophysiol 15:235, 1952.

81. WALKER, DD AND KIMURA, J: *A fast-recovery electrode amplifier for electrophysiology.* Electroenceph Clin Neurophysiol 45:789, 1978.

82. WIEDERHOLT, WC: *Threshold and conduction velocity in isolated mixed mammalian nerves.* Neurology (Minneap) 20:347, 1970.

CHAPTER
# 6

# ASSESSMENT OF INDIVIDUAL NERVES

Determination of the nerve conduction velocity is possible in any nerve accessible to surface or needle stimulation. The evoked potential can be recorded either from the nerve itself or from a muscle innervated by the nerve. The basic principles outlined in the previous section apply to the study of nerves in general. This section will discuss specific approaches to each of the commonly tested individual nerves. The common points of stimulation and recording sites will be described, together with the normal values as reported in the literature or established in our institution. However, it is recommended that each laboratory develop its own normal ranges using a standardized method, since the technique differs considerably from one center to the next.

For many of the measurements used in the tables, the upper and lower limits of normal are presented as a mean plus or minus two standard deviations. This is not always correct, since the data are not necessarily distributed in a gaussian manner. In our materials, however, the vast majority of individual values from the controls fell within the range defined above. An alternative approach would be to use a log transformation of the data and then, if the data are equally distributed, express the normal range in terms of plus or minus two standard deviation confidence intervals. Some of the tables are incomplete, because many early studies failed to record amplitude of evoked responses.

In the upper extremities, motor and sensory conduction velocities can be readily measured in the median, ulnar, and radial nerves. The brachial plexus, musculocutaneous nerve, and the other nerves innervating the muscles of the shoulder girdle are more difficult to study by nerve stimulation techniques, primarily because of their deep location and anatomic complexity. The most commonly tested in the lower extremities are motor conduction of the peroneal and tibial nerves and sensory conduction of the superficial peroneal and sural nerves. Less easily accessible are the lumbosacral plexus and the femoral and sciatic nerves. Other sensory nerve studies are more difficult, but techniques have been described to study the dorsal sensory branch of the ulnar nerve, the lateral cutaneous nerve of the forearm, the lateral femoral cutaneous nerve, and the saphenous nerve.

The central or most proximal nerve segment in the upper and lower extremities, including the radicular portion, cannot be tested by the usual nerve conduction studies. However, the motor and sensory conduction along the central segment can be assessed by the use of the F-wave, H-reflex, and somatosensory evoked potentials as described in Chapters 17, 18, and 19, respectively. Electrophysiologic evaluation of the facial nerve will be discussed in Chapter 7, and in Chapter 16 in conjunction with the blink reflex.

# COMMONLY TESTED NERVES IN THE UPPER LIMB

## Median nerve—Motor fibers

The median nerve is relatively superficial in its entire course from the axilla to the palm (Fig. 6-1). The conventional sites of stimulation include Erb's point, axilla, elbow, and wrist. Additionally, the nerve is accessible to percutaneous stimulation in the palm.[38, 51] Normal values are summarized in Tables 6-1 and 6-2. Selective stimulation of median motor fibers is difficult at Erb's point or the axilla, where it is found in close proximity to other nerves.[30] This problem can be circumvented by the use of the collision technique that will be described in Chapter 7. The nerve is stimulated at the elbow over the brachial pulse with the cathode at the volar crease. For stimulation at the wrist, the cathode is usually placed 3 cm proximal to the distal crease on the volar surface. At each stimulation site the anode is located 2 cm proximal to the cathode, and the ground electrode is around the forearm between the stimulating and recording electrodes whenever possible. But, in stimulating the thenar nerve at the palm,[35] the electrode position is reversed, with the anode placed distal to rather than proximal to the cathode. Otherwise the thenar nerve would sometimes be activated near the anode owing to spread of stimulating current as will be discussed in Chapter 7.

The compound muscle action potential is recorded with the active electrode ($G_1$) over the belly of the abductor pollicis brevis and the indifferent electrode ($G_2$) just distal to the metacarpophalangeal joint (Fig. 6-2a). The recorded response is not specific to this muscle, since, depending upon the electrode positioning, there is a varying degree of contribution from other muscles innervated by the median nerve. In the presence of an anomalous crossover between the median and ulnar nerve in the forearm, the waveform of the recorded potentials changes with distal and proximal stimulation, despite the use of supramaximal intensity at both sides. Recognition of this communication is important, since, in its presence, the latencies of distally and proximally activated compound muscle action potentials are not directly comparable for calculation of the nerve conduction velocity. This is one of the common sources of error in nerve conduction studies and will be discussed further in Chapter 7.

## Median nerve—Sensory fibers

Possible sites of stimulation for antidromic studies of the sensory fibers are the same as for the motor fibers.[46] In our laboratory, the stimulus site at the wrist is 3 cm proximal to the distal crease of the wrist, whereas the palmar stimulation site is 5 cm distal to the crease (see Fig. 6-1b). Alternatively, the stimulus site at the wrist may be standardized as a fixed distance from the recording electrode, most commonly 12 to 14 cm. The distal potentials are recorded with ring electrodes placed around the proximal ($G_1$) and distal ($G_2$) interphalangeal joints of the second digit (Fig. 6-2a). Normal values are summarized in Tables 6-1 and 6-2.

The sensory potential could also be recorded from the first or third digit (Fig. 6-2b), or lateral half of the fourth digit. These recording sites are useful when the symptoms are limited to or most severe in these digits. Because of mixed sensory innervation, stimulating the radial or ulnar nerve also elicits a sensory nerve potential over the first or fourth digit, respectively. This could be a source of error if these nerves are inadvertently activated by spread of stimulating current intended for the median nerve. The digital nerve potential of the middle finger is used to evaluate C-7 root, middle

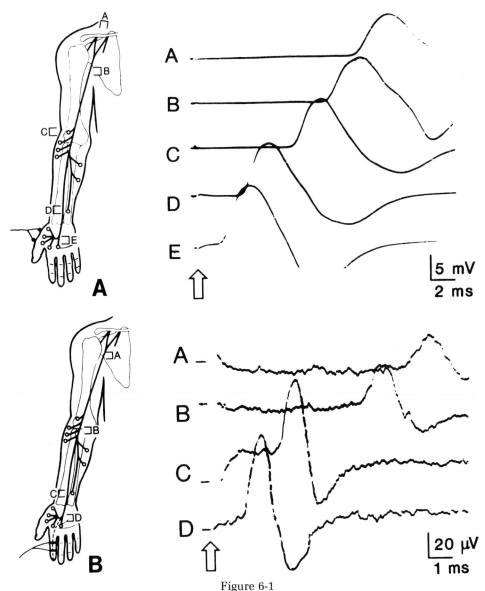

Figure 6-1

(A) Motor nerve conduction study of the median nerve. The sites of stimulation include Erb's point (A), axilla (B), elbow (C), wrist (D), and palm (E). Compound muscle action potentials are recorded percutaneously from the thenar eminence. (B) Sensory nerve conduction study of the median nerve. The sites of stimulation include axilla (A), elbow (B), wrist (C), and palm (D). Digital potentials are recorded antidromically, using the ring electrodes placed around the second digit.

trunk, and lateral cord, whereas that of the thumb provides assessment of C-6 or C-7 roots, upper or middle trunk, and lateral cord. In contrast to postganglionic lesions, which cause degeneration of the sensory axons, preganglionic root avulsion gives rise to no abnormalities of the sensory potential recorded from the anesthestic digits.

Unlike the compound muscle action potentials which are essentially the same in amplitude regardless of the site of stimulation, the antidromically activated digital potentials are significantly smaller with proximal as compared to more distal stimulation. Indeed, stimulation at Erb's point or the axilla often fails to elicit unequivocal digital potentials unless an averaging technique is used. This is, at least in part, because

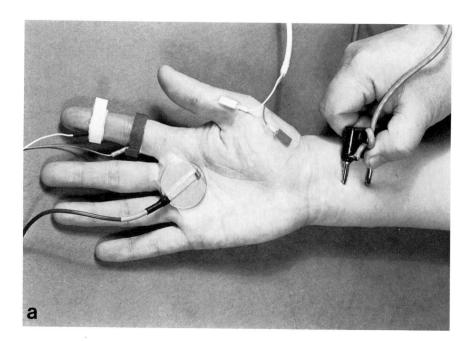

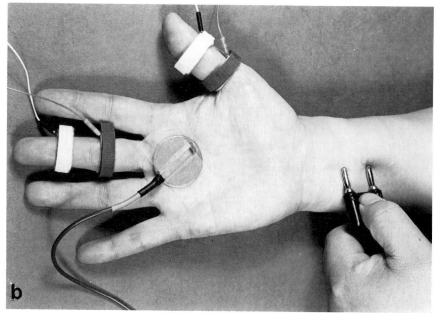

Figure 6-2

(a) Motor and sensory conduction studies of the median nerve. The nerve is stimulated at the wrist, 3 cm proximal to the distal crease. The recording electrodes are placed over the belly ($G_1$) and tendon ($G_2$) of the abductor pollicis brevis for motor conduction, and proximal ($G_1$) and distal ($G_2$) interphalangeal joints of the second digit for sensory conduction. The ground electrode is located between the stimulating and recording electrodes but may also be placed elsewhere if the shock artifact can be adequately controlled. (b) Alternative recording sites for sensory conduction study of the median nerve. The ring electrodes are placed around the proximal ($G_1$) and distal ($G_2$) interphalangeal joints of the third digit, or the base ($G_1$) and the interphalangeal joint ($G_2$) of the thumb.

## TABLE 6-1 Median Nerve[1]

| Site of stimulation | Amplitude[2] mV for motor µV for sensory | Latency[3] to recording site ms | Difference between right and left ms | Conduction time between two points ms | Conduction velocity m/s |
|---|---|---|---|---|---|
| **Motor Fibers** | | | | | |
| palm | 6.9±3.2 | 1.86±0.28 (2.4)[4] | 0.19±0.17 (0.5)[4] | 1.65±0.25 (2.2)[4] | 48.8±5.3 (38)[5] |
| wrist | 7.0±3.0 | 3.49±0.34 (4.2) | 0.24±0.22 (0.7) | 3.92±0.49 (4.9) | 57.7±4.9 (48) |
| elbow | 7.0±2.7 | 7.39±0.69 (8.8) | 0.31±0.24 (0.8) | 2.42±0.39 (3.2) | 63.5±6.2 (51) |
| axilla | 7.2±2.9 | 9.81±0.89 (11.6) | 0.42±0.33 (1.1) | | |
| **Sensory Fibers** | | | | | |
| digit | | | | | |
| palm | 39.0±16.8 | 1.37±0.24 (1.9) | 0.15±0.11 (0.4) | 1.37±0.24 (1.9) | 58.8±5.8 (47) |
| wrist | 38.5±15.6 | 2.84±0.34 (3.5) | 0.18±0.14 (0.5) | 1.48±0.18 (1.8) | 56.2±5.8 (44) |
| elbow | 32.0±15.5 | 6.46±0.71 (7.9) | 0.29±0.21 (0.7) | 3.61±0.48 (4.6) | 61.9±4.2 (53) |

1. Mean±standard deviation (SD) in 122 nerves from 61 patients, 11–74 years of age (average 40), with no apparent disease of the peripheral nerves.
2. Amplitude of the evoked response measured from the baseline to negative peak.
3. Latency measured to the onset of the evoked response.
4. Upper limits of normal calculated as mean + 2SD.
5. Lower limits of normal calculated as mean − 2SD.

TABLE 6-2 Latency comparison between two nerves in the same limb[1]

|  | Site of stimulation | Median nerve ms | Ulnar nerve ms | Difference ms |
|---|---|---|---|---|
| Motor Fibers | wrist | 3.34±0.32 (4.0)[2] | 2.56±0.37 (3.3)[2] | 0.79±0.31 (1.4)[2] |
|  | elbow | 7.39±0.72 (8.8) | 7.06±0.79 (8.6) | 0.59±0.60 (1.8) |
| Sensory Fibers | palm | 1.33±0.21 (1.8) | 1.19±0.22 (1.6) | 0.22±0.17 (0.6) |
|  | wrist | 2.80±0.32 (3.4) | 2.55±0.30 (3.2) | 0.29±0.21 (0.7) |

1. Mean±standard deviation (SD) in 70 nerves from 35 patients, 14 to 74 years of age (average 37), with no apparent disease of the peripheral nerve.
2. Upper limits of normal calculated as mean + 2SD.

of temporal dispersion between fast and slow conducting fibers.[4] In addition, the antidromic impulse may be partially extinguished by collision with ongoing orthodromic sensory impulses. These tendencies would be greater with a proximal as compared with a more distal stimulation in proportion to the nerve length between the stimulating and recording electrodes.

In studying the mixed nerve, the antidromically recorded sensory potential may be obscured by superimposition of action potentials from distal muscles, since some motor axons have a threshold similar to that of the large myelinated sensory axons. The sensory fibers of the median nerve can be selectively activated with palmar stimulation distal to the origin of the recurrent motor fibers. Moving more proximally, possible superimposition of muscle action potentials is easily recognized by a change in waveform of the elicited response.[39] Thus, a simple recording of the antidromic sensory potentials suffices for routine clinical purposes. Alternatively, the digital[5, 6, 7, 63] or palmar nerve[12, 22] may be stimulated to record the orthodromic sensory potential at the palm, wrist, and elbow. Either surface or needle electrodes may be used for recording. The orthodromic recording is technically more demanding than the antidromic approach. The averaging technique is of distinct advantage for detection of small nerve potentials, especially in a diseased nerve.

## Multiple stimulation across the carpal ligament

The use of palmar stimulation provides a simple means to establish whether the slowing of sensory or motor conduction is attributable to compression by the transverse carpal ligament or to a disease process of the most terminal segment. This distinction is sometimes important in differentiating the carpal tunnel syndrome from a distal neuropathy in which the median nerve may be more intensely affected in its terminal portions, as shown by Casey and LeQuesne[11] in digital nerves of diabetics. To further localize the point of maximal conduction delay within the distal segment of the median nerve,[38, 39] antidromic digital potentials may be recorded after stimulation of the median nerve at multiple sites across the wrist (Fig. 6-3A). The sensory axons normally show a predictable latency change of 0.16 to 0.20 ms per cm as the stimulus site is moved proximally from midpalm to distal forearm in 1 cm increments (Fig. 6-3B). A sharply localized latency increase across a 1 cm segment may be seen in focal abnormalities of the median nerve (Fig. 6-3C and D).

Unlike the sensory nerve, the median motor axons are difficult to activate in steps of 1 cm along the recurrent course of the thenar nerve off the median nerve trunk. Thus, unless the exposed nerve is directly stimulated,[3] palmar stimulation may inadvertently activate unintended portions of the thenar nerve as will be discussed in Chapter 7. Specifically, surface stimulation intended for the origin of the thenar nerve at the palm commonly depolarizes the thenar branch near the motor point, resulting in an erroneously short latency. An unreasonably large latency increase then occurs between the wrist and palm, thereby presenting a fallacious impression of the carpal tunnel syndrome. To avoid this error in the calculation of motor latency, it is essential to select carefully the most distal point of palmar stimulation that elicits an appropriate thumb twitch, indicating contraction of the abductor pollicis brevis. One can then be reasonably certain that the palmar stimulation activated the median nerve at or near the origin of the thenar nerve as intended. This problem is further compounded, because the recurrent branch may take an anomalous course in rare instances.[62]

## Ulnar nerve

Like the median nerve, the ulnar nerve takes a relatively superficial course along its entire length. It is readily accessible at multiple sites, including Erb's point, the axilla, above, below, and at the elbow, and in the wrist and palm (Fig. 6-4). For routine motor conduction studies, the muscle potential is recorded from the hypothenar muscles with surface electrodes placed over the belly of the abductor digiti minimi ($G_1$) and its tendon ($G_2$) 3 cm distally (Fig. 6-5A). In studying the deep palmar branch of the ulnar nerve, it is also helpful to record the muscle potential from the first dorsal interosseous or adductor pollicis (Fig. 6-5B). The latency difference between the hypothenar and thenar responses may be taken as a measure of conduction along the deep branch. Selective stimulation of the ulnar nerve may be difficult at Erb's point or in the axilla. Spread of stimulus current causes fewer problems in studying the ulnar, as compared with the median nerve, because the hypothenar eminence contains only ulnar-innervated muscles. Nonetheless, the collision technique may be required to eliminate inadvertent volume-conducted potentials from the thenar eminence, if the median nerve is simultaneously activated.[37] Normal values are shown in Tables 6-2 and 6-3.

The motor fibers are commonly tested with stimulation above and below the elbow to document a tardy ulnar palsy and a cubital tunnel syndrome. For accurate determination of conduction velocity in the segment across the elbow, the distance between the proximal and distal stimulus sites must be of adequate length. However, if the proximal site of stimulation is too high, the median nerve may also be activated. The ulnar nerve slides back and forth in the cubital tunnel as the position of the elbow joint is changed. Thus, for accurate calculation of conduction velocity, the arm must be held in the same position (usually flexed at 90 degrees) during stimulation of the nerve and measurement of the surface distance. At the wrist the nerve is stimulated a fixed distance away from either the distal crease of the wrist or the recording electrode. This is particularly important when comparing the distal motor latencies between the two sides in one individual and among different subjects. In our laboratory, the cathode is placed 3 cm proximal to the distal crease of the wrist and the anode 2 cm further, proximally.

With stimulation of the nerve at the palm, wrist, or elbow, an antidromic sensory potential may be recorded from the fourth or fifth finger (Fig. 6-5A and B). It is also possible to record a mixed nerve potential from the ulnar nerve proximally after stimulation of the nerve at the palm or wrist. For orthodromic sensory conduction, the digital nerve may be stimulated with ring electrodes placed around the proximal (cathode) and distal (anode) interphalangeal joints of the fifth finger. Sensory nerve action potentials can then be recorded at various sites along the course of the nerve. In our laboratory, antidromic sensory potentials are recorded from the fourth or fifth digit. The cathode is placed 3 cm proximal to the distal crease for stimulation at the wrist and 5 cm distal to the crease for palmar stimulation. In either case, the anode is located 2 cm further, proximally. This arrangement allows for a meaningful comparison between the median and ulnar nerve sensory conduction in the segment across the wrist. Studies of the digital nerve potentials from the fourth or fifth digit not only provide an evaluation of the ulnar nerve but also help differentiate lesions of C-8 and T-1 roots from those of

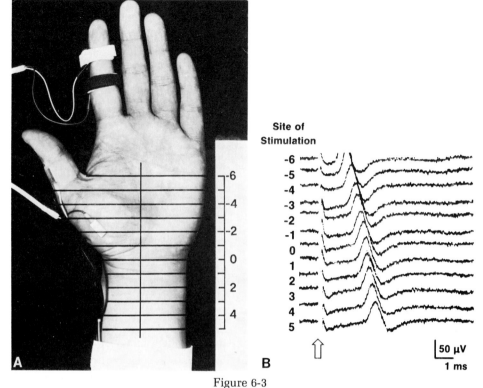

Figure 6-3

(A) Twelve sites of stimulation in 1 cm increments along the length of the median nerve. The 0 level is at the distal crease of the wrist, corresponding to the origin of the transverse carpal ligament. Sensory nerve and muscle action potentials are recorded from the second digit and abductor pollicis brevis, respectively. (B) Sensory nerve potentials in a normal subject recorded after stimulation of the median nerve at multiple points across the wrist. The site of each stimulus is indicated on the left (compare part A). The latency increased linearly as the stimulus site was moved proximally in 1 cm increments.

the lower trunk and medial cord of the brachial plexus. The sensory potential should be normal in preganglionic C-8 and T-1 root avulsion, despite the clinical sensory loss.

The forearm segment of the ulnar nerve can be tested by recording the nerve action potential from the dorsal sensory branch as it leaves the common trunk of the nerve 5 to 8 cm proximal to the ulnar styloid.[32, 36] The active recording electrode ($G_1$) is placed over the dorsum of the hand either between the fourth and fifth metacarpals or on the fifth metacarpal, with the reference electrode ($G_2$) at the base of the fifth digit (Fig. 6-5C). The dorsal sensory branch is stimulated as it becomes superficial between the tendon of the flexor carpi ulnaris and the ulna, at a fixed distance of 8 to 12 cm from the active recording electrode. The ulnar nerve trunk can, of course, be stimulated more proximally. The antidromic sensory potential is then masked by much larger action potentials from the ulnar-innervated intrinsic hand muscles, unless a lesion at the wrist has rendered them paretic. The hand may be either supinated or pronated to achieve maximal relaxation of the forearm muscles during the test. In one study,[32] the mean value for the latency recorded 8 cm from the point of stimulation was 2.0 ± 0.3 ms (mean ± SD), with the conduction velocity between elbow and forearm of 60 ± 4.0 m/s. The mean amplitude of the nerve action potential was 20 ± 6 µV with distal stimulation. This technique is useful in assessing the forearm segment of the ulnar nerve, especially in the presence of a severe lesion at the wrist, which precludes the conventional recording from the hypothenar muscles or digits. It is also of value in

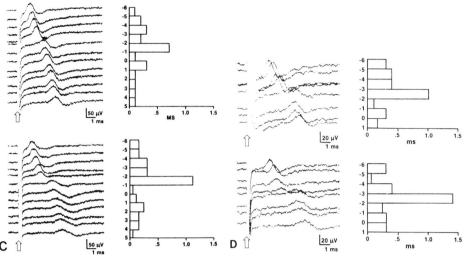

Figure 6-3 (*Continued*)
(*C*) Sensory nerve potentials in a patient with the carpal tunnel syndrome. A sharply localized slowing was found from −2 to −1 in both hands, representing a segmental conduction velocity of 14 m/s on the left (top) and 9 m/s on the right (bottom). Note a distinct change in waveform of the sensory potential at the point of localized conduction delay. Double humped appearance at −2 on the left suggests sparing of some sensory axons at this level. (*D*) Sensory nerve potential in a patient with the carpal tunnel syndrome. A sharply localized slowing was found from −3 to −2 in both hands, representing a segmental conduction velocity of 10 m/s on the left (top) and 7 m/s on the right (bottom). Note a change in waveform of the sensory potential at the point of localized conduction delay. (From Kimura,[39] with permission.)

localizing a lesion within the forearm, since the dorsal sensory branch is affected only if the ulnar nerve is damaged above the take-off of this branch.

## Radial nerve

The motor axons are accessible to electrical stimulation at Erb's point, in the axilla near the spinal groove, above the elbow, and in the forearm (Fig. 6-6). At the axilla the electrode is placed in the groove between the coracobrachialis and medial edge of the triceps, about 18 cm proximal to the medial epicondyle. The stimulus point above the elbow is between the brachioradialis and the tendon of the biceps, 6 cm proximal to the lateral epicondyle. In the forearm, the nerve is accessible over the dorsal aspect of the ulna, 8 to 10 cm proximal to the styloid process, where it becomes superficial between the extensor carpi ulnaris and extensor digiti minimi. Muscle action potentials may be obtained from the extensor digitorum communis or extensor indicis using needle or surface electrodes (Fig. 6-7A).

There are a number of problems in measuring motor nerve conduction velocities of the radial nerve. These include difficulty in maintaining a supramaximal stimulation, especially with an obese or muscular limb, activation of more than one extensor muscle simultaneously, and an initial positive deflection of the compound muscle action potential, indicating the presence of a volume conducted response from distant muscles. Further, the waveform of the recorded potentials usually changes because distal stimulation activates fewer muscles than does proximal stimulation. Consequently, a comparison between distally and proximally activated muscle potentials is difficult and not always valid. Surface recording is much more difficult than needle recording in this regard. Needle electrodes are also preferred when recording from more proximal mus-

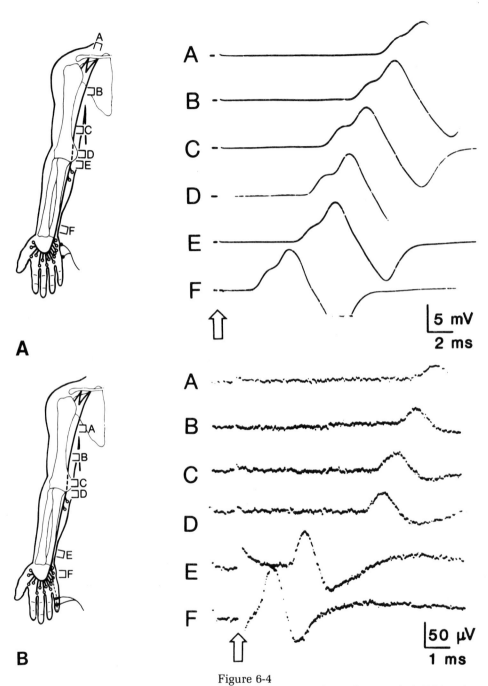

Figure 6-4

(A) Motor nerve conduction study of the ulnar nerve. The sites of stimulation include Erb's point (A), axilla (B), above the elbow (C), elbow (D), below the elbow (E), and wrist (F). Compound muscle action potentials are recorded percutaneously from the hypothenar eminence. (B) Sensory nerve conduction study of the ulnar nerve. The sites of stimulation include axilla (A), above the elbow (B), elbow (C), below the elbow (D), wrist (E), and palm (F). Digital potentials are recorded antidromically using the ring electrodes placed around the fifth digit.

cles such as the anconeus, brachioradialis, or triceps, because of the relative selectivity.[28, 34]

The sensory fibers may be studied antidromically with the application of ring electrodes around the base of the thumb for recording (Fig. 6-7B). Alternatively, the disc electrode (G$_1$) may be placed over the radial nerve, where it is palpable as it crosses the extensor pollicis longus at the base of the thumb.[17, 18] In this case, the reference electrode (G$_2$) is placed 2 to 3 cm distally, near the first dorsal interosseous muscle. The stimulating electrode is located at the lateral edge of the radius in the distal forearm, where the sensory nerve becomes superficial. The usual distance between the stimulating and recording electrodes is 10 to 14 cm, but this may be adjusted according to individual arm length. The nerve may be stimulated at the elbow under the brachioradialis muscle lateral to the biceps tendon (see Fig. 6-6B). Conduction velocities can then be determined in the segments between the elbow and wrist and the wrist and thumb.[24, 53, 55]

Orthodromic sensory potentials can be recorded from the axilla or elbow after stimulation of the radial nerve at the thumb or the wrist. However, since the thumb is in part supplied by the median nerve, 25 percent of the sensory potential recorded over the radial nerve at the wrist or elbow and 50 percent at the axilla may be due to spread from median nerve fibers.[59] The radial nerve can be more selectively activated with stimulation at the wrist, especially if needle electrodes are placed along the nerve. Table 6-4 summarizes the results by Trojaborg and Sindrup.[59] Studies of the digital nerve potential from the thumb provide an evaluation of not only the radial nerve itself but also C-6 and C-7 roots, and upper and middle trunk and posterior cord of the brachial plexus. Preganglionic C-6 and C-7 root avulsion gives rise to a clinical sensory loss associated with no abnormalities of the sensory potentials.

# OTHER NERVES DERIVED FROM THE CERVICAL OR BRACHIAL PLEXUS

## Phrenic nerve

Conduction studies of the phrenic nerve, though described early, have not been widely used.[13, 48] This is in part because percutaneous stimulation in the cervical area requires shocks of a relatively high intensity, which may be painful. Further, some patients tolerate the esophageal electrode used for recording the diaphragmatic potentials poorly. In an alternative method recommended by some investigators, the phrenic nerve is tested with the use of needle electrodes for stimulating the nerve and surface electrodes for recording the response.

A standard monopolar needle electrode is inserted medially from the lateral aspect of the neck at the level of the cricoid cartilage (Fig. 6-8). After traversing the posterior margin of the sternocleidomastoid muscle, the needle tip comes to lie between the carotid artery anteriorly and the anterior scalene muscle posteriorly. In this position, the needle tip is within a few millimeters of the phrenic nerve and adequately distant from the carotid artery or the apex of the lung. The anode is a metal plate placed on the manubrium. With this method, shocks of very low intensity suffice for supramaximal stimulation and are far better tolerated than the high intensity required for surface stimulation. If the needle is placed appropriately, selective stimulation of the phrenic nerve is possible without simultaneously activating the brachial plexus, which is located posterior to the anterior scalene muscle.

The compound muscle action potential is recorded from the diaphragm, using surface electrodes. The most consistent results are obtained with the active electrode (G$_1$) placed on the xiphoid process and the indifferent electrode (G$_2$) at the eighth intercostal space near the costochondral junction. The mean values and standard deviations in 30 normal subjects studied, using this recording arrangement, were 7.4 $\pm$ 0.59

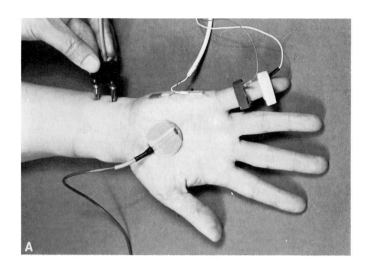

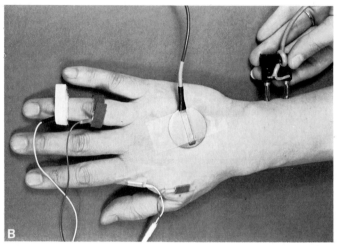

Figure 6-5

(A) Motor and sensory conduction study of the ulnar nerve. The nerve is stimulated at the wrist, 3 cm proximal to the distal crease. The recording electrodes are placed over the belly ($G_1$) and tendon ($G_2$) of the abductor digiti minimi for motor conduction, and proximal ($G_1$) and distal ($G_2$) interphalangeal joints of the fifth digit for sensory conduction. (B) Alternative recording sites for motor and sensory conduction studies of the ulnar nerve. The recording electrodes are placed over the belly ($G_1$) and tendon ($G_2$) of the first dorsal interosseous muscle for motor conduction and around the proximal ($G_1$) and distal ($G_2$) interphalangeal joints of the fourth digit for sensory conduction.

ms for latency with the difference between right and left of 0.08 ± 0.42 ms; 8.45 ± 40.5 μV for amplitude; and 48.1 ± 12.2 ms for duration.[43] The mean latency is very close to the earlier results (Table 6-5) obtained by surface stimulation.[13, 48]

## Brachial plexus

The brachial plexus is most easily accessible to electrical stimulation at Erb's point, which is located in the angle formed by the clavicle and the posterior borders of the sternocleidomastoid muscle at the level of the sixth cervical vertebra (see Fig. 1-4). The trunks traverse the supraclavicular fossa at Erb's point before branching into posterior and anterior divisions, which in turn form the posterior cord, and medial and lateral

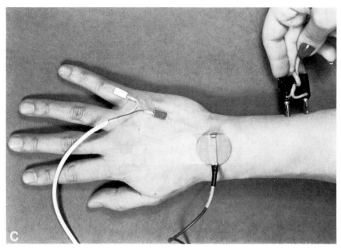

Figure 6-5 (Continued)

(C) Sensory conduction study of the dorsal cutaneous branch of the ulnar nerve. The nerve is stimulated along the medial aspect of the forearm between the tendon of the flexor carpi ulnaris and the ulna, 14–18 cm from the active electrode. The recording electrodes are placed over the dorsum of the hand between the fourth and fifth metacarpals ($G_1$) and the base of the fifth digit ($G_2$).

cords, respectively. With stimulation of the brachial plexus at Erb's point, muscle action potentials may be recorded from the proximal muscles of the shoulder girdle and their latencies determined. Evoked potentials can also be detected in the distal muscles, including those of the thenar and hypothenar eminence. With stimulation at Erb's point, as opposed to more distal sites of stimulation, muscles innervated by different peripheral nerves are simultaneously activated. The presence of volume conducted potentials from distant muscles then interferes with the accurate recording of the potential from the intended muscle. This difficulty can be largely circumvented with the use of the collision technique, if a second stimulus can be applied distally to the nerve not being tested as will be described in Chapter 7.

In the triceps, the end-plate zone is vertically oriented with the distal portion of the muscle innervated by longer nerve branches. Thus, the latency of a recorded response becomes greater as the distance from the stimulus point increases. The latency change, however, is not linearly related to the distance, presumably because the points of innervation are irregular. In the biceps and deltoid, the end-plates are mostly located in the middle of the muscle, directed horizontally. The latency of the response from these muscles, therefore, is not affected by the point of recording as much as in the triceps. The same probably applies to the infraspinatus and supraspinatus. The use of needle recording electrodes, which register from a more limited area, provides a preferred method of obtaining reliable latencies, especially if many nerves are activated.[40] However, intramuscular recordings do not allow precise determination of the compound muscle action potential in amplitude or waveform, because of restricted recording area.

Nerve conduction times from Erb's point to the muscles of the shoulder girdle (Table 6-6) have been described by Gassel.[26] The trunks of the brachial plexus are stimulated at Erb's point, and muscle action potentials are recorded from the biceps, deltoid, triceps, supraspinatus, and infraspinatus, individually or simultaneously, using a multichannel recorder. When testing a unilateral involvement of the brachial plexus, it is best to compare the affected and normal sides. For a meaningful assessment, the distance between the stimulating and recording electrodes should be the same on both sides. This is particularly important when studying the triceps for the reasons stated

## TABLE 6-3 Ulnar Nerve[1]

| | Site of stimulation | Amplitude[2] mV for motor μV for sensory | Latency[3] to recording site ms | Difference between right and left ms | Conduction time between two points ms | Conduction velocity m/s |
|---|---|---|---|---|---|---|
| Motor Fibers | wrist | 5.7±2.0 | 2.59±0.39 (3.4)[4] | 0.28±0.27 (0.8)[4] | | |
| | below elbow | 5.5±2.0 | 6.10±0.69 (7.5) | 0.29±0.27 (0.8) | 3.51±0.51 (4.5)[4] | 58.7±5.1 (49)[5] |
| | above elbow | 5.5±1.9 | 8.04±0.76 (9.6) | 0.34±0.28 (0.9) | 1.94±0.37 (2.7) | 61.0±5.5 (50) |
| | axilla | 5.6±2.1 | 9.90±0.91 (11.7) | 0.45±0.39 (1.2) | 1.88±0.35 (2.6) | 66.5±6.3 (54) |
| Sensory Fibers | digit wrist | 35.0±14.7 | 2.54±0.29 (3.1) | 0.18±0.13 (0.4) | 2.54±0.29 (3.1) | 54.8±5.3 (44) |
| | below elbow | 28.8±12.2 | 5.67±0.59 (6.9) | 0.26±0.21 (0.5) | 3.22±0.42 (4.1) | 64.7±5.4 (53) |
| | above elbow | 28.3±11.8 | 7.46±0.64 (8.7) | 0.28±0.27 (0.8) | 1.79±0.30 (2.4) | 66.7±6.4 (54) |

1. Mean±standard deviation (SD) in 130 nerves from 65 patients, 13–74 years of age (average 39), with no apparent disease of the peripheral nerves.
2. Amplitude of the evoked response measured from the baseline to negative peak.
3. Latency measured to the onset of the evoked response.
4. Upper limits of normal calculated as mean + 2SD.
5. Lower limits of normal calculated as mean − 2SD.

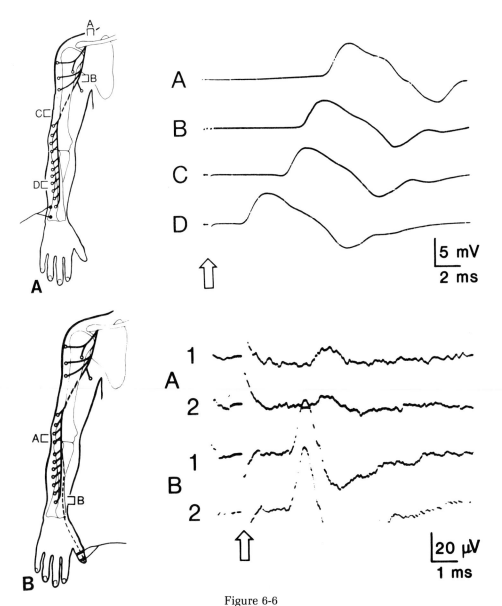

Figure 6-6

(A) Motor nerve conduction study of the radial nerve. The sites of stimulation include Erb's point (A), axilla (B), above the elbow (C), and mid-forearm (D). Compound muscle action potentials are recorded from the extensor indicis, with either needle or surface electrodes. (B) Sensory nerve conduction study of the radial nerve. The sites of stimulation include elbow (A) and distal forearm (B). Digital potentials are recorded antidromically, using the ring electrodes placed around the thumb.

previously. However, the same practice should be adhered to no matter which muscle of the shoulder girdle is under consideration.

Alternatively, a localized stimulus may be applied directly to the nerve roots by means of a needle electrode inserted into the posterior paraspinal area.[43, 44] In this method, the cathode is a standard 50 to 75 mm monopolar needle insulated along the shaft, except for an exposed tip. The needle is inserted perpendicular to the skin surface, until the tip comes to rest directly on the vertebral transverse process. It is possible to

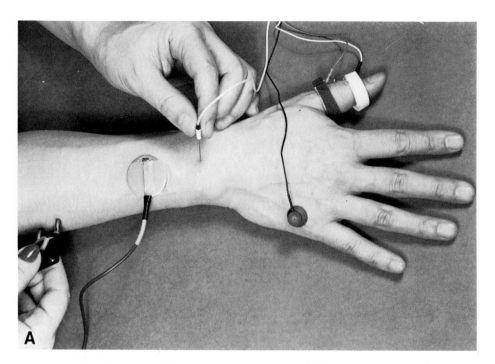

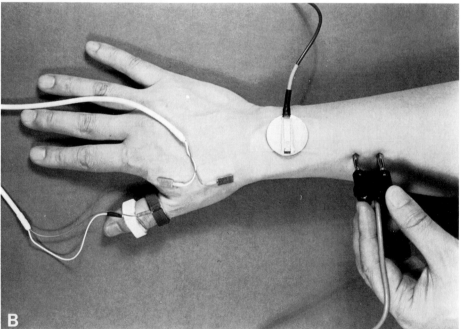

Figure 6-7

(A) Motor and sensory conduction studies of the radial nerve. The nerve is stimulated in the forearm with the cathode at the lateral edge of the extensor carpi ulnaris muscle, 8–10 cm proximal to the styloid process. The monopolar needle electrode ($G_1$) is inserted in the extensor indicis with a reference electrode ($G_2$) over the dorsum of the hand laterally for motor conduction studies. The recording electrodes are placed around the base ($G_1$) and interphalangeal joint ($G_2$) of the thumb for sensory conduction. (B) Alternative stimulation and recording sites for sensory nerve conduction study of the radial nerve. The cathode is placed at the lateral edge of the radius where the sensory nerve becomes superficial in the distal forearm, and the anode is placed 2 cm proximally. The recording electrodes are placed either around the base ($G_1$) and interphalangeal joint ($G_2$) of the thumb, or over the palpable nerve between the first and second metacarpals ($G_1$) and 2–3 cm distally ($G_2$).

TABLE 6-4 Radial nerve

| Motor conduction between | N | Conduction velocity (m/s) or conduction time (ms) | Amplitude (mV for motor) (μV for sensory) | Distance (cm) |
|---|---|---|---|---|
| axilla-elbow | 8 | 69±5.6 | 11±7.0 | 15.7±3.3 |
| elbow-forearm | 10 | 62±5.1 | 13±8.2 | 18.1±1.5 |
| forearm-muscle | 10 | 2.4±0.5 | 14±8.8 | 6.2±0.9 |
| **Sensory conduction between** | | | | |
| axilla-elbow | 16 | 71±5.2 | 4±1.4 | 18.0±0.7 |
| elbow-wrist | 20 | 69±5.7 | 5±2.6 | 20.0±0.5 |
| wrist-thumb | 23 | 58±6.0 | 13±7.5 | 13.8±0.4 |

From Trojaborg and Sindrup,[59] with permission.

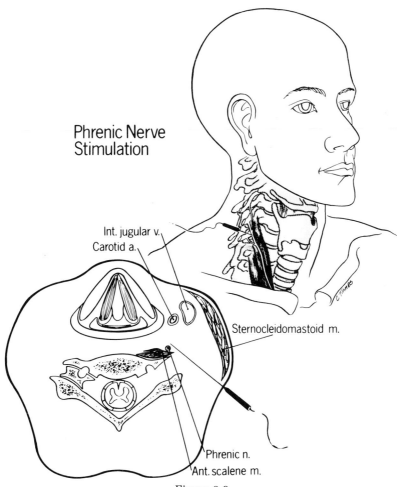

Figure 6-8

Motor conduction study of the phrenic nerve. The nerve is stimulated with needle inserted medially through the posterior margin of the sternocleidomastoid at the level of the cricoid cartilage. The recording electrodes are placed on the xiphoid process ($G_1$) and at the eighth intercostal space near the costochondral junction ($G_2$). (From MacLean and Mattioni,[43] with permission.)

**TABLE 6-5 Phrenic nerve**

| Authors | Stimulation point | Recording site | No. | Onset latency ms |
|---|---|---|---|---|
| Newsom Davis[48] | | | 18 | 7.7±0.80 |
| Delhez[13] | | | 30 on rt. | 7.5±0.53 |
| | | | 30 on lt. | 8.2±0.71 |
| MacLean and Mattioni[43] | Needle electrode placed posterior to sternocleidomastoid | Xiphoid process | 30 | 7.4±0.59 |

stimulate C-5 and C-6 roots jointly for testing the upper trunk and lateral cord by placing the needle 1 to 2 cm lateral to the C-5 spinous process (Fig. 6-9A). Similarly, the needle is placed slightly caudal to the C-7 spinous process to stimulate C-8 and T-1 roots simultaneously, for conduction across the lower trunk and medial cord (Fig. 6-9B). The needle is inserted between these two points to activate C-6, C-7, and C-8 roots together for evaluation of the posterior cord. The anode is a metal plate or disk electrode on the skin surface or a second needle electrode. The muscle action potential is recorded from the biceps and triceps to determine conduction time across the upper trunk and lateral cord, and the posterior cord, respectively. To evaluate the lower trunk and medial cord, the evoked potential is recorded from a distal ulnar-innervated muscle. In this case the conduction time across the brachial plexus is calculated by subtracting the distal latency obtained by stimulating the ulnar nerve at the axilla, 25 cm distal to the sternal notch. The normal values of MacLean are listed in Table 6-7. A latency difference between the right and left sides is considered abnormal if it exceeds 0.6 ms and is probably a more sensitive index for detecting unilateral lesions than the absolute latency.

## Musculocutaneous nerve

To determine motor conduction velocity,[47, 58] the nerve may be stimulated at two sites along its course; that is, at Erb's point[27, 40] and at the axilla.[50] The electrical stimulus is applied through an insulated stainless steel needle electrode, placed at the posterior cervical triangle, just behind the sternocleidomastoid muscle, approximately 3 to 6 cm above the clavicle (see Figs. 1-4 and 1-8). At the axilla it is located between the axillary artery medially and the coracobrachialis muscle laterally. The muscle action potentials

**TABLE 6-6 Nerve conduction times from Erb's point to muscle**

| Muscle | N | Distance (cm) | Latency (ms) |
|---|---|---|---|
| Biceps | 19 | 20 | 4.6±0.6 |
| | 15 | 24 | 4.7±0.6 |
| | 14 | 28 | 5.0±0.5 |
| Deltoid | 20 | 15.5 | 4.3±0.5 |
| | 17 | 18.5 | 4.4±0.35 |
| Triceps | 16 | 21.5 | 4.5±0.42 |
| | 23 | 26.5 | 4.9±0.45 |
| | 16 | 31.5 | 5.3±0.5 |
| Supraspinatus | 19 | 8.5 | 2.6±0.32 |
| | 16 | 10.5 | 2.7±0.27 |
| Infraspinatus | 20 | 14 | 3.4±0.4 |
| | 15 | 17 | 3.4±0.5 |

Modified from Gassell.[26]

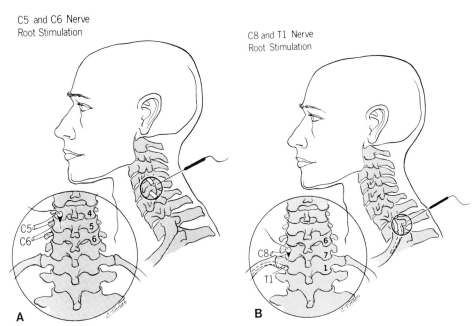

C5 and C6 Nerve
Root Stimulation

C8 and T1 Nerve
Root Stimulation

A

B

Figure 6-9

(A) C-5 and C-6 root stimulation. The needle is inserted perpendicular to the skin, 1–2 cm lateral to the C-5 spinous process. (B) C-8 and T-11 root stimulation. The needle is inserted slightly caudal to the C-7 spinous process. (From MacLean,[42] with permission.)

are recorded from the biceps brachii muscle with surface electrodes or concentric needle electrodes placed near the end-plate zone (Table 6-8).

The electrodes positioned to stimulate motor axons can be used to record sensory potentials at the posterior cervical triangle and the axilla. The sensory fibers of the musculocutaneous nerve are stimulated at the level of the elbow, just lateral to the tendon of the biceps as it emerges as the lateral cutaneous nerve. The nerve can be palpated between the tendon of the biceps medially and the brachioradialis laterally. The sensory potentials can also be recorded antidromically to evaluate the distal branch, the lateral cutaneous nerve of the forearm. For this purpose, surface stimulation is applied at the elbow, where the nerve becomes superficial (Fig. 6-10). Surface recordings are made 12 cm distally over the course of the nerve in the forearm, along

**TABLE 6-7 Brachial plexus latencies as determined by nerve root stimulation**

| Plexus | Site of stimulation | Recording site | Latency across plexus (ms) | | |
|---|---|---|---|---|---|
| | | | Range | Mean | SD |
| Brachial (upper trunk and lateral cord) | C-5 and C-6 | Biceps brachii | 4.8–6.2 | 5.3 | 0.4 |
| Brachial (posterior cord) | C-6, C-7, and C-8 | Triceps brachii | 4.4–6.1 | 5.4 | 0.4 |
| Brachial (lower trunk and medial cord) | C-8 and T-1<br><br>Ulnar nerve | Abductor digiti quinti | 3.7–5.5 | 4.7 | 0.5 |

From MacLean,[42] with permission.

**TABLE 6-8 Musculocutaneous nerve**

| Age | Motor nerve conduction between Erb's point and axilla | | | | Orthodromic sensory nerve conduction between Erb's point and axilla | | | Orthodromic sensory nerve conduction between axilla and elbow | | |
|---|---|---|---|---|---|---|---|---|---|---|
| | N | Range of conduction velocity (m/s) | Range of amplitude (µV) axilla | Erb's point | N | Range of conduction velocity (m/s) | Range of amplitude (µV) | N | Range of conduction velocity (m/s) | range of amplitude (µV) |
| 15–24 | 14 | 63–78 | 9–32 | 7–27 | 14 | 59–76 | 3.5–30 | 15 | 61–75 | 17–75 |
| 25–34 | 6 | 60–75 | 8–30 | 6–26 | 6 | 57–74 | 3–25 | 8 | 59–73 | 16–72 |
| 35–44 | 8 | 58–73 | 8–28 | 6–24 | 7 | 54–71 | 2.5–21 | 8 | 57–71 | 16–69 |
| 45–54 | 10 | 55–71 | 7–26 | 6–22 | 10 | 52–69 | 2–18 | 13 | 55–69 | 15–65 |
| 55–64 | 9 | 53–68 | 7–24 | 5–21 | 9 | 49–66 | 2–15 | 10 | 53–67 | 14–62 |
| 65–74 | 4 | 50–66 | 6–22 | 5–19 | 4 | 47–64 | 1.5–12 | 6 | 51–65 | 13–59 |

From Trojaborg,[58] with permission.

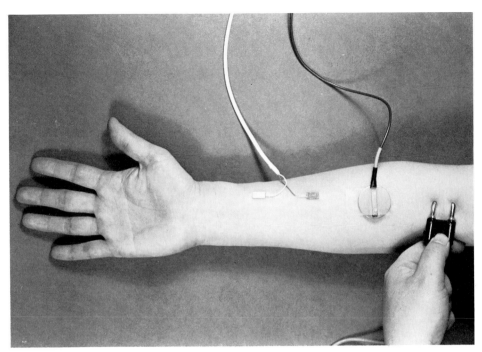

Figure 6-10
Sensory conduction study of the lateral cutaneous nerve of the forearm. The nerve is stimulated just lateral to the tendon of the biceps. The recording electrodes are placed 12 cm distal to the cathode along the straight line to the radial artery at the wrist ($G_1$) and 2–3 cm further distally ($G_2$).

the straight line from the stimulus point to the radial artery at the wrist. In one study[56] using this technique, the normal values were an onset and peak latency of the action potential of 1.8 $\pm$ 0.1 ms (mean $\pm$ SD) and 2.3 $\pm$ 0.1 ms, respectively, maximum conduction velocity of 65 $\pm$ 3.5 m/s, and amplitude of 24 $\pm$ 7.2 $\mu$V. Study of the musculocutaneous nerve allows evaluation of the C-6 root and the upper trunk and lateral cord of the brachial plexus. Thus, they may provide confirmatory information to median sensory studies recorded from the thumb.

# COMMONLY TESTED NERVES IN THE LOWER LIMB

## Tibial nerve

Motor conduction velocity can be measured by stimulating the tibial nerve at the popliteal fossa and again at the medial malleolus, while recording the evoked potentials from the abductor hallucis innervated by the medial plantar nerve or abductor digiti quinti supplied by the lateral plantar nerve (Figs. 6-11 and 6-12). Tables 6-9 and 6-10 summarize the normal values in our laboratory. It is also possible to stimulate the medial plantar branch of the tibial nerve above and below the medial malleolus to determine the conduction velocity in this short segment, in which the nerve runs through the so-called tarsal tunnel. Using needle electrodes, nerve action potentials can be recorded at the knee after stimulation of the tibial nerve at the ankle.[45] The recorded potential is a mixture of orthodromic sensory and antidromic motor impulses.

For sensory conduction studies of the medial and lateral plantar nerves, stimuli are applied to the first and fifth toes, respectively. The evoked sensory potentials are recorded, using surface or needle electrodes placed over the tibial nerve just below the

TABLE 6-9 Tibial Nerve[1]

| Site of stimulation | Amplitude[2] mV | Latency[3] to recording site ms | Difference between right and left ms | Conduction time between two points ms | Conduction velocity m/s |
|---|---|---|---|---|---|
| ankle | 5.8±1.9 | 3.96±1.00 (6.0)[4] | 0.66±0.57 (1.8)[4] | 8.09±1.09 (10.3)[4] | 48.5±3.6 (41)[5] |
| knee | 5.1±2.2 | 12.05±1.53 (15.1) | 0.79±0.61 (2.0) | | |

1. Mean±standard deviation (SD) in 118 nerves from 59 patients, 11–78 years of age (average 39), with no apparent disease of the peripheral nerves.
2. Amplitude of the evoked response measured from the baseline to negative peak.
3. Latency measured to the onset of the evoked response.
4. Upper limits of normal calculated as mean + 2SD.
5. Lower limits of normal calculated as mean − 2SD.

TABLE 6-10 Latency comparison between two nerves in the same limb[1]

| Site of stimulation | Peroneal nerve ms | Tibial nerve ms | Difference ms |
|---|---|---|---|
| ankle | 3.89±0.87 (5.6)[2] | 4.12±1.06 (6.2)[2] | 0.77±0.65 (2.1)[2] |
| knee | 12.46±1.38 (15.2) | 12.13±1.48 (15.1) | 0.88±0.71 (2.3) |

1. Mean±standard deviation (SD) in 104 nerves from 52 patients, 17 to 86 years of age (average 41), with no apparent disease of the peripheral nerve.
2. Upper limits of normal calculated as mean + 2SD.

medial malleolus. Alternatively, the tibial nerve may be stimulated below the medial malleolus and the antidromic sensory nerve potential recorded from the first or fifth toes, using a pair of ring electrodes. In either case, an averaging technique is required, because the elicited responses are otherwise too small to detect. Testing the plantar nerves may be useful in patients with footdrop to evaluate the involvement of post-ganglionic sensory fibers derived from L-4 and L-5 roots.[31]

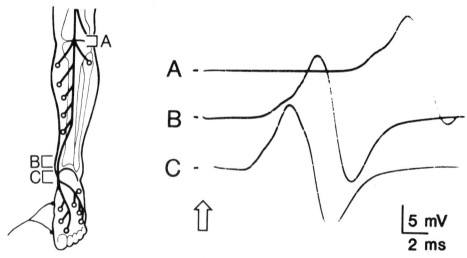

Figure 6-11
Motor nerve conduction study of the tibial nerve. The sites of stimulation include knee (A), above the medial malleolus (B), and below the medial malleolus (C). Compound muscle action potentials are recorded from the abductor hallucis.

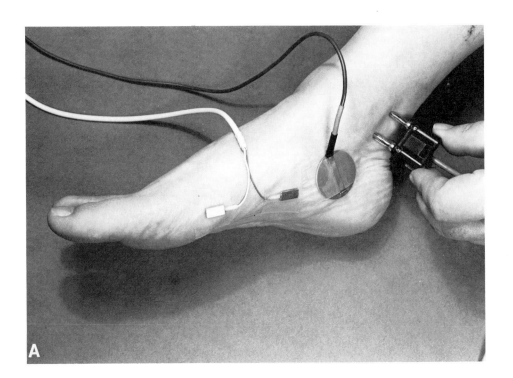

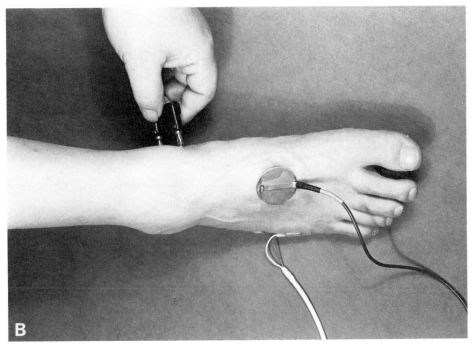

Figure 6-12

(A) Motor conduction study of the tibial nerve (medial plantar nerve). The nerve is stimulated above the medial malleolus, 10 cm from the recording electrodes placed over the belly ($G_1$) and tendon ($G_2$) of the abductor hallucis. (B) Alternative recording site for motor nerve conduction study of the tibial nerve (lateral plantar nerve). The nerve is stimulated below the medial malleolus. The recording electrodes are placed over the belly ($G_1$) and tendon ($G_2$) of the abductor digiti quinti.

## Common and deep peroneal nerve

The usual approach to determining motor conduction velocity is to stimulate the nerve above and below the head of the fibula and just above the ankle, while recording the muscle action potentials from the extensor digitorum brevis (Figs. 6-13 and 6-14). This muscle, primarily supplied by the deep peroneal nerve, may also receive anomalous innervation from the superficial peroneal nerve via the accessory deep peroneal nerve, which passes behind the lateral malleolus to reach the lateral portion of the muscle. In the presence of this anomaly the compound muscle action potential elicited by stimulation of the deep peroneal nerve at the ankle may be unusually small. This is a common source of error that will be further discussed in Chapter 7. For accurate determination of conduction velocity in the segment across the knee, the proximal and distal stimulus sites should ideally be at least 10 cm apart. If the extensor digitorum brevis muscle is atrophic, this segment can still be tested by recording the muscle potential from the tibialis anterior using either surface or needle electrodes.[14] Mixed nerve potentials can also be recorded with a needle electrode placed at the head of the fibula, after stimulation of the peroneal nerve at the ankle.[29] This potential is difficult to record with surface electrodes, unless an averaging technique is employed. The normal values are summarized in Tables 6-10 and 6-11.

## Superficial peroneal nerve

The superficial peroneal nerve is derived from the L-5 root branching off the common peroneal nerve below the fibular head. It gives rise to two sensory branches in the lower third of the leg, the medial dorsal cutaneous nerve and intermediate dorsal cutaneous nerve, which innervate the skin of the dorsum of the foot and the anterior and lateral aspects of the leg. A sensory nerve action potential can be recorded from either branch. For the medial dorsal cutaneous nerve, the recording electrodes are placed over the dorsum of the foot medially. The nerve is stimulated at the anterolateral aspect of the leg about 5 cm above and 2 cm medial to the lateral malleolus as it pierces the superficial fascia and becomes accessible.[10, 15] The position of the stimulating electrode may be adjusted so that the shocks will produce a sensation that radiates into the toes. The recorded antidromic sensory potential is approximately half the amplitude of that

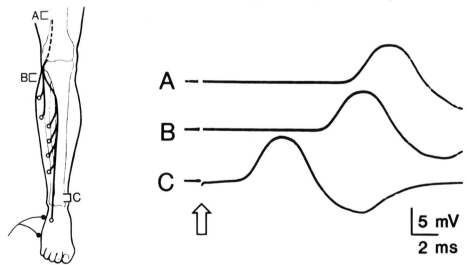

Figure 6-13

Motor nerve conduction study of the common peroneal nerve. The sites of stimulation include above the knee (A), below the knee (B), and ankle (C). Compound muscle action potentials are recorded from the extensor digitorum brevis.

TABLE 6-11 Peroneal Nerve[1]

| Site of stimulation | Amplitude[2] mV | Latency[3] to recording site ms | Difference between right and left ms | Conduction time between two point ms | Conduction velocity m/s |
|---|---|---|---|---|---|
| ankle | 5.1±2.3 | 3.77±0.86 (5.5)[4] | 0.62±0.61 (1.8)[4] | 7.01±0.89 (8.8)[4] | 48.3±3.9 (40)[5] |
| below knee | 5.1±2.0 | 10.79±1.06 (12.9) | 0.65±0.65 (2.0) | 1.72±0.40 (2.5) | 52.0±6.2 (40) |
| above knee | 5.1±1.9 | 12.51±1.17 (14.9) | 0.65±0.60 (1.9) | | |

1. Mean±standard deviation (SD) in 120 nerves from 60 patients, 16–86 years of age (average 41), with no apparent disease of the peripheral nerves.
2. Amplitude of the evoked response measured from the baseline to negative peak.
3. Latency measured to the onset of the evoked response.
4. Upper limits of normal calculated as mean + 2SD.
5. Lower limits of normal calculated as mean − 2SD.

recorded from the sural nerve. Electrical averaging is especially necessary in recording from a diseased nerve.

The antidromic nerve potential may be recorded from the intermediate dorsal cutaneous branch at the ankles,[33] as it crosses just medial to the lateral malleolus (Fig. 6-15). The stimulating electrodes are placed against the anterior edge of the fibula at a fixed distance of 12 cm from the active recording electrode at the ankle. The ground electrode is between the stimulating and recording electrodes. The proximal segment of the nerve may be tested by stimulating the nerve at a second point, 8 to 9 cm above the distal stimulation. This method has an advantage in that the amplitude of the recorded potential is on the average greater than that of the sural sensory potential in the same limb.[33] The normal values are shown in Table 6-12. Studies of this nerve are helpful in distinguishing L-5 radiculopathy from more distal lesions.

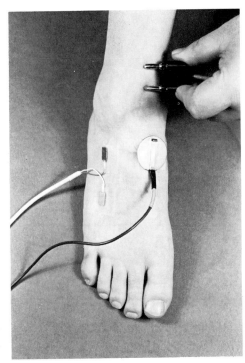

Figure 6-14
Motor conduction study of the common peroneal nerve. The nerve is stimulated over the dorsum of the foot near the ankle, 7 cm from the recording electrodes placed over the belly ($G_1$) and tendon ($G_2$) of the extensor digitorum brevis.

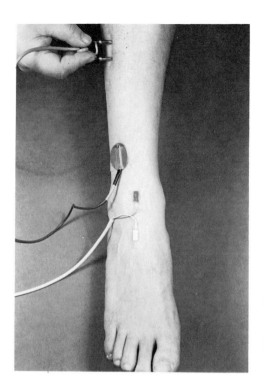

Figure 6-15
Sensory nerve conduction study of the superficial peroneal nerve. The nerve is stimulated against the anterior edge of the fibula, 12 cm from the active electrode ($G_1$), located just medial to the lateral malleolus at the ankle. Reference electrode ($G_2$) is placed 2–3 cm distally.

## Sural nerve

The sural nerve, primarily derived from the S-1 root via the medial sural branch of the tibial nerve, originates in the popliteal fossa. It becomes superficial at the junction of the mid and lower third of the leg, at which point it receives a sural communicating branch of the common peroneal nerve. In some cases, the communicating branch is larger than the main trunk of the sural nerve. The nerve continues to descend toward the ankle and turns anterolaterally along the inferior aspect of the lateral malleolus. Its terminal branch is the lateral dorsal cutaneous nerve, which supplies the lateral aspect of the dorsum of the foot. As discussed in Chapter 4, the sural nerve may be biopsied for in vitro conduction studies and histologic assessments.[19, 20, 21] The findings may then be directly correlated with the results of in vivo studies.

Sensory conduction in the sural nerve may be studied reliably without resorting to an averaging device.[8, 15, 16, 52] In this method, antidromic sensory potentials are recorded using surface electrodes placed on the nerve as it passes around the lateral malleolus (Figs. 6-16 and 6-17). The nerve is stimulated in the lower third of the leg, with surface electrodes placed over the posterior aspect slightly lateral to the midline. It is also possible to stimulate the nerve at three points, dividing the sural nerve into three contiguous nerve segments of 7 cm each. When this is done the mean velocity is significantly smaller in the most distal segment than in the middle or proximal segment, with no difference between the middle and proximal segments.[60]

In vivo measurement of orthodromic sural nerve action potentials has also been described using electronic averaging.[1, 2, 54] By this means, sensory potentials are recorded at the popliteal fossa and high at the ankle, 10 to 15 cm proximal to the lateral malleolus, following stimulation of the nerve over the lateral aspect of the foot. This allows comparison between distal and proximal segments of the nerve (Table 6-13). Sural nerve conduction is considered one of the most frequently abnormal electrophysiologic parameters in neuropathies of various etiologies. Studies of this nerve are helpful in distinguishing peripheral lesions from S-1 or S-2 radiculopathy or cauda equina

## TABLE 6-12 Superficial peroneal nerve

| Stimulation point | Recording site | N | Age | Amplitude (µV) | Peak latency (ms) | Conduction velocity m/s | |
|---|---|---|---|---|---|---|---|
| 5 cm above and 2 cm medial to lateral malleolus | dorsum of foot | 50 | 1–15 | 13.0±4.6 | 1.22±0.40 | 53.1±5.3 | distal segment |
| | | 50 | over 15 | 13.9±4.0 | 2.24±0.49 | 47.3±3.4 | distal segment |
| anterior edge of fibula, 12 cm above the active electrode | medial to lateral malleolus | 50 | 3–60 | 20.5±6.1 | 2.9±0.3 | 65.7±3.7 | proximal segment |

Modified from DiBenedetto[15] and Jabre.[33]

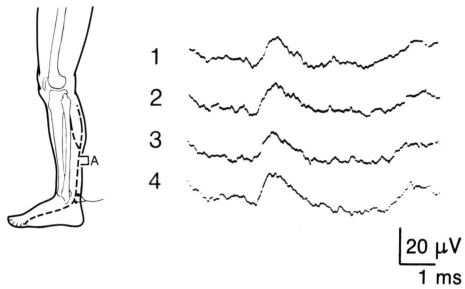

**Figure 6-16**
Sensory nerve conduction study of the sural nerve. The nerve is stimulated on the calf slightly lateral to the midline in the lower third of the leg. Sensory potentials are recorded antidromically using the surface electrodes placed over the nerve behind the lateral malleolus.

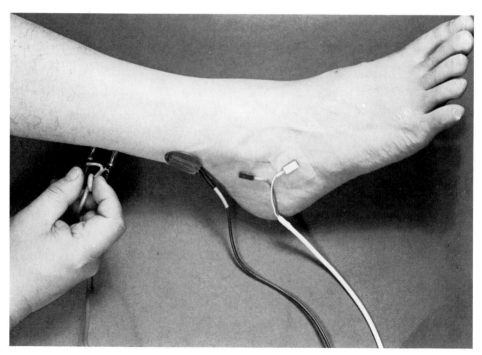

**Figure 6-17**
Sensory conduction study of the sural nerve. The nerve is stimulated along the posterior surface of the leg, slightly lateral to the midline and 7–10 cm from the active electrode ($G_1$). The recording electrodes are placed above ($G_1$) and below ($G_2$) the lateral malleolus as the nerve passes around it, or immediately posteroinferior to the lateral malleolus ($G_1$) and 2–3 cm distally along the lateral dorsum of the foot ($G_2$).

## TABLE 6-13 Sural nerve

| Authors | Stimulation point | Recording site | N | Age | Amplitude (μV) | Peak latency (ms) | Conduction velocity (m/s) |
|---------|-------------------|----------------|---|-----|----------------|-------------------|---------------------------|
| Shiozawa and Mavor[54] | foot | high ankle | 40 | 13–41 | 6.3 (1.9–17) | | 44.0±4.7 |
| DiBenedetto[15] | lower one third of leg | lateral malleolus | 38 | 1–15 | 23.1±4.4 | 1.46±0.43 | 52.1±5.1 |
| | | | 62 | over 15 | 23.7±3.8 | 2.27±0.43 | 46.2±3.3 |
| Behse and Buchthal[1] | 15 cm above lateral malleolus | dorsal aspect of foot | 71 | 15–30 | | | 51.2±4.5 |
| | | | | 40–65 | | | 48.3±5.3 |
| Schuchmann[52] | 14 cm above lateral malleolus | lateral malleolus | 101 | 13–66 | | 3.50±0.25 | 40.1 |
| Wainapel, Kim, and Ebel[61] | lower one third of leg | lateral malleolus | 80 | 20–79 | 18.9±6.7 | 3.7±0.3 | 41.0±2.5 |
| Truong, et al[60] | distal 10 cm | lateral malleolus | 102 | | | | 33.9±3.3 |
| | middle 10 cm | | 102 | | | | 51.0±3.8 |
| | proximal 10 cm | | 102 | | | | 51.6±3.8 |

lesions which consistently spare the sensory potential, since the involvement is proximal to the sensory ganglion. The effect of age on sural nerve conduction velocity has been delineated.[41]

# OTHER NERVES DERIVED FROM THE LUMBOSACRAL PLEXUS

## Lumbosacral plexus

The lumbosacral plexus consists of the lumbar plexus with fibers derived from L-2, L-3, and L-4 roots and the sacral plexus, which arises from L-5, S-1, and S-2 roots. Neither portion of the plexus is accessible to percutaneous electrical stimulation. Thus, conventional conduction studies are of limited value in the evaluation of this plexus. However, the propagation of impulses across this region can be measured indirectly with the use of the F-wave and H-reflex, as will be discussed in Chapters 17 and 18. An alternative method for direct measurement of conduction has been proposed.[42, 49] It involves direct stimulation of L-4, L-5, or S-1 root just proximal to the plexus and stimulation of the peripheral nerve just distal to the plexus. Conduction time through the plexus is then calculated by subtracting the distal latency from the proximal latency.

For evaluation of the lumbar plexus, the L-4 root is stimulated by a 75 mm standard monopolar needle, placed so as to lie just below the level of the iliac crest. The needle is inserted into the paraspinous muscle, perpendicular to the skin surface, until it reaches the periosteum of the articular process (Fig. 6-18). The needle position is adjusted, using a shock of very low intensity, until the maximal response is elicited. For calculation of conduction time across the lumbar plexus, the femoral nerve is stimulated just distal to the inguinal ligament, with either a surface or, preferably, a needle electrode (Fig. 6-18A). The nerve can be easily located, as it lies immediately lateral to the femoral artery, which is readily palpable. The compound muscle action potentials are recorded from the vastus medialis. The technique for studying the femoral nerve will be discussed later in this section.

To study the sacral plexus, a needle is placed between the spinous process and posterior iliac spine for the S-1 root and halfway in between the L-4 and S-1 levels for the L-5 root. Conduction time across the sacral plexus can be obtained if the sciatic nerve is stimulated with a needle electrode (Fig. 6-18B). The nerve is located at the level of the gluteal skin fold as it bisects a line drawn between the ischial tuberosity and the greater trochanter of the femur.[64] The position of the needle tip can be adjusted using shocks of very low intensity and observing muscle contraction distally. Compound muscle action potentials can be elicited in any muscle innervated by the sciatic nerve but are usually recorded from the tibialis anterior for evaluation of the L-5 root and abductor hallucis when studying the S-1 root. Common sources of error with this technique center on volume-conducted potentials from distant muscles, which are inadvertently activated as the stimulus spreads to an unintended portion of the plexus. This is particularly troublesome when recording from the tibialis anterior because the recording electrodes over this muscle regularly register a simultaneously activated action potential of the triceps surae. The results of MacLean are summarized in Table 6-14.

## Femoral nerve

If the femoral nerve is stimulated above and below the inguinal ligament, the response can be recorded from electrodes situated at various distances from the point of stimulation in the rectus femoris muscle. Because of the vertical orientation of the end-plate region of this muscle, the latency of the response increases progressively with the distance. Gassel[25] reported the mean value for the latency recorded at 14 and 30 cm from the point of stimulation (Table 6-15). The mean conduction velocity of the femoral nerve calculated between these points was 70 m/s. This determination of conduction velocity assumes that the femoral nerve branches supplying proximal and distal parts of the muscle are similar in their electrophysiologic characteristics and are directly comparable.

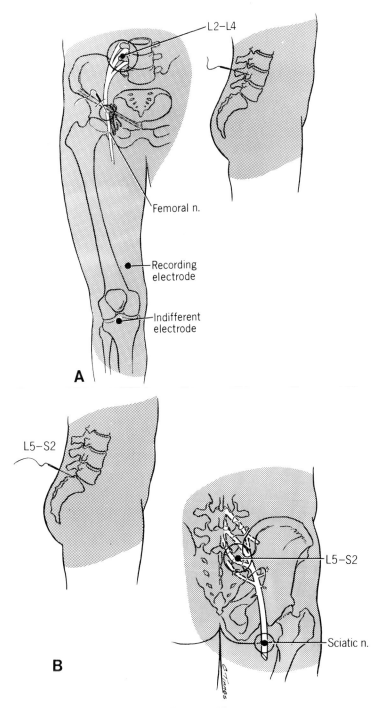

Figure 6–18

(A) Motor conduction study of the lumbar plexus. To stimulate the L-4 root, the needle is inserted perpendicular to the skin, until it reaches the articular process, just below the level of the iliac crest. The femoral nerve is stimulated just distal to the inguinal ligament immediately lateral to the femoral artery. The recording electrodes are placed over the vastus medialis ($G_1$) and patella ($G_2$). (B) Motor nerve conduction study of the sacral plexus. To stimulate the S-1 root, the needle is inserted at the level of the posterior iliac spine. The L-5 root is stimulated halfway in between the L-4 and S-1 roots. The sciatic nerve is stimulated at the level of gluteal skin fold midpoint between the ischial tuberosity and the greater trochanter of the femur. The recording electrodes (not shown) are placed on the belly ($G_1$) and tendon ($G_2$) of the tibialis anterior and of the abductor hallucis for L-5 and S-1 root study, respectively. (From MacLean,[42] with permission.)

**TABLE 6-14 Lumbosacral plexus latencies as determined by nerve root stimulation**

| Plexus | Site of stimulation | Recording site | Latency across plexus (ms) | | |
|---|---|---|---|---|---|
| | | | Range | Mean | SD |
| Lumbar | L-2, L-3, and L-4 Femoral nerve | Vastus medialis | 2.0–4.4 | 3.4 | 0.6 |
| Sacral | L-5 and S-1 Sciatic nerve | Abductor hallucis | 2.5–4.9 | 3.9 | 0.7 |

From MacLean,[42] with permission.

**TABLE 6-15 Femoral nerve**

| Stimulation point | Recording site | No. | Age | Onset latency (ms) | Conduction velocity (m/s) |
|---|---|---|---|---|---|
| just below inguinal ligament | 14 cm from stimulus point | 42 | 8–79 | 3.7±0.45 | 70±5.5 between the two recording sites |
| | 30 cm from stimulus point | 42 | 8–79 | 6.0±0.60 | |

Modified from Gassel,[25]

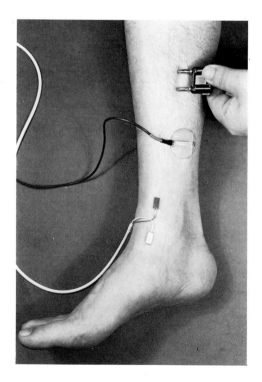

Figure 6-19
Sensory conduction study of the saphenous nerve. The nerve is stimulated 14 cm above the active electrode (G₁) along the medial surface of the leg with the electrode pressed firmly between the tibia and gastrocnemius muscle. The recording electrodes are placed at the ankle, 2–3 cm above (G₁) and just anterior to the medial malleolus (G₂).

**TABLE 6-16 Saphenous nerve**

| Authors | Method | Age | Inguinal ligament—Knee | | | Knee—Medial malleolus | | |
|---|---|---|---|---|---|---|---|---|
| | | | Number | Amplitude (µV) | Conduction velocity (m/s) | Number | Amplitude (µV) | Conduction velocity (m/s) |
| Ertekin[23] | Orthodromic | 17–38 | 33 | 4.2±2.3 | 59.6±2.3 | 10 | 4.8±2.4 | 52.3±2.3 |
| Stöhr, Schumm, and Ballier[57] | Orthodromic | < 40 | 28 | 5.5±2.6 | 58.9±3.2 | 22 | 2.1±1.1 | 51.2±4.7 |
| | | > 40 | 41 | 5.1±2.7 | 57.9±4.0 | 32 | 1.7±0.8 | 50.2±5.0 |
| Wainapel, Kim and Ebel[61] | Antidromic | 20–79 | | | | 80 | 9.0±3.4 | 41.7±3.4 |

# Saphenous nerve

The recording electrodes are placed on the nerve as it passes the medial malleolus just anterior to its highest prominence along the medial border of the tibialis anterior tendon (Fig. 6-19). The nerve is stimulated 12 to 14 cm above the proximal recording electrode ($G_1$). Since the nerve lies deep along the medial border of the tibia, the stimulating electrodes must be placed firmly between the medial gastrocnemius muscle and tibia. The technique of signal averaging is of considerable practical value in detecting small sensory potentials. In one study,[61] the mean latency recorded at 14 cm was 3.6 ± 0.4 ms (mean ± SD), measured to the peak of the first negative deflection. Table 6-16 summarizes the mean conduction velocity between the stimulating and recording sites and the mean amplitude of the evoked response, measured from negative to positive peaks.

Saphenous nerve conduction can also be determined orthodromically.[23, 57] The nerve is stimulated at two levels, anterior to the medial malleolus, and medial to the knee. The evoked potential is recorded from a needle electrode placed near the femoral nerve trunk at the inguinal ligament (Table 6-16). Signal averaging is necessary, since the orthodromic potentials are about one half the size of the antidromic potentials in amplitude. Studies of this nerve provide an evaluation of the sensory fibers of the femoral nerve. The saphenous nerve is the largest and longest branch of the femoral nerve and may be affected in lumbar plexopathy and femoral neuropathy. These are distinguished from L-3 and L-4 radiculopathy which spares the distal sensory nerve potentials.

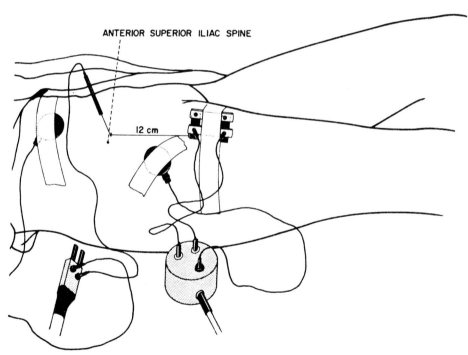

Figure 6-20
Sensory nerve conduction of the lateral femoral cutaneous nerve. The nerve is stimulated above the inguinal ligament. The recording electrodes are placed over the thigh, 12 cm below the anterior-superior iliac spine ($G_1$) and 2–3 cm distally ($G_2$). (From Butler, Johnson and Kaye,[9] with permission.)

## Lateral femoral cutaneous nerve

The nerve may be stimulated using a surface electrode 12 cm below the anterior superior iliac spine, where the nerve becomes superficial and divides into a large anterior and smaller lateral branches. The orthodromic sensory potential is recorded with a needle electrode inserted 1 cm medial to the lateral end of the inguinal ligament. Alternatively, the nerve may be stimulated at the inguinal ligament with a needle electrode and antidromic sensory potentials recorded from the thigh (Fig. 6-20). In one study[9] using specially constructed recording electrodes consisting of a pair of 1.2 × 1.9 cm lead strips fastened 4 cm apart, the normal values in 25 healthy adults included a latency of 2.6 ± 0.2 ms (mean ± SD), an amplitude of 10 to 25 $\mu$V, and a calculated velocity of 47.9 ± 3.7 m/s.

# REFERENCE SOURCES

1. BEHSE, F AND BUCHTHAL, F: *Normal sensory conduction in the nerves of the leg in man.* J Neurol Neurosurg Psychiatry 34:404, 1971.

2. BEHSE, F AND BUCHTHAL, F: *Sensory action potentials and biopsy of the sural nerve in neuropathy.* Brain 101:473, 1978.

3. BROWN, WF, ET AL: *The location of conduction abnormalities in human entrapment neuropathies.* Can J Neurol Sci 3:111, 1976.

4. BUCHTHAL, F AND ROSENFALCK, A: *Evoked action potentials and conduction velocity in human sensory nerves.* Brain Res 3:1,122, 1966.

5. BUCHTHAL, F AND ROSENFALCK, A: *Sensory potentials in polyneuropathy.* Brain 94:241, 1971.

6. BUCHTHAL, F AND ROSENFALCK, A: *Sensory conduction from digit to palm and from palm to wrist in the carpal tunnel syndrome.* J Neurol Neurosurg Psychiatry 34:243, 1971.

7. BUCHTHAL, F, ROSENFALCK, A, AND TROJABORG, W: *Electrophysiological findings in entrapment of the median nerve at wrist and elbow.* J Neurol Neurosurg Psychiatry 37:340, 1974.

8. BURKE, D, SKUSE, NF, AND LETHLEAN, AK: *Sensory conduction of the sural nerve in polyneuropathy.* J Neurol Neurosurg Psychiatry 37:647, 1974.

9. BUTLER, ET, JOHNSON, EW, AND KAYE, ZA: *Normal conduction velocity in the lateral femoral cutaneous nerve.* Arch Phys Med Rehabil 55:31, 1974.

10. CAPE, CA: *Sensory nerve action potentials of the peroneal, sural and tibial nerves.* Am J Phys Med 50:220, 1971.

11. CASEY, EB AND LE QUESNE, PM: *Digital nerve action potentials in healthy subjects, and in carpal tunnel and diabetic patients.* J Neurol Neurosurg Psychiatry 35:612, 1972.

12. DAUBE, JR: *Percutaneous palmar median nerve stimulation for carpal tunnel syndrome.* Electroenceph Clin Neurophysiol 43:139, 1977.

13. DELHEZ, L: *Modalités, chez l'homme normal, de la réponse électrique des piliers du diaphragme à la stimulation électrique des nerfs phréniques par des chocs uniques.* Arch Internat de Physiol Biochim 73:832, 1965.

14. DEVI, S, LOVELACE, RE, AND DUARTE, N: *Proximal peroneal nerve conduction velocity: Recording from anterior tibial and peroneus brevis muscles.* Ann Neurol 2:116, 1977.

15. DIBENEDETTO, M: *Sensory nerve conduction in lower extremities.* Arch Phys Med Rehabil 51:253, 1970.

16. DIBENEDETTO, M: *Evoked sensory potentials in peripheral neuropathy.* Arch Phys Med Rehabil 53:126, 1972.

17. DOWNIE, AW AND SCOTT, TR: *Radial nerve conduction studies.* Neurology (Minneap) 14:839, 1964.

18. DOWNIE, AW AND SCOTT, TR: *An improved technique for radial nerve conduction studies.* J Neurol Neurosurg Psychiatry 30:322, 1967.

19. DYCK, PJ AND LAMBERT, EH: *Numbers and diameters of nerve fibers and compound action potential of sural nerve: Controls and hereditary neuromuscular disorders.* Trans Am Neurol Assoc 91:214, 1966.

20. DYCK, PJ AND LOFGREN, EP: *Method of fascicular biopsy of human peripheral nerve for electrophysiologic and histologic study.* Mayo Clin Proc 41:778, 1966.

21. DYCK, PJ, LAMBERT, EH, AND NICHOLS, PC: *Quantitative measurement of sensation related to compound action potential and number and sizes of myelinated and unmyelinated fibers of sural nerve in health, Friedreich's ataxia, hereditary sensory neuropathy, and tabes dorsalis.* In: RÉMOND, A (ED): *Handbook of Electroencephalography and Clinical Neurophysiology,* Vol. 9. Elsevier, Amsterdam, 1972, pp 83–118.

22. EKLUND, G: *A new electrodiagnostic procedure for measuring sensory nerve conduction across the carpal tunnel.* Upsala J Med Sci 80:63, 1975.

23. ERTEKIN, C: *Saphenous nerve conduction in man.* J Neurol Neurosurg Psychiatry 32:530, 1969.

24. FEIBEL, A AND FOCA, FJ: *Sensory conduction of radial nerve.* Arch Phys Med Rehabil 55:314, 1974.

25. GASSEL, MM: *A study of femoral nerve conduction time.* Arch Neurol 9:57, 1963.

26. GASSEL, MM: *A test of nerve conduction to muscles of the shoulder girdle as an aid in the diagnosis of proximal neurogenic and muscular disease.* J Neurol Neurosurg Psychiatry 27:200, 1964.

27. GASSEL, MM: *Sources of error in motor nerve conduction studies.* Neurology (Minneap) 14:825, 1964.

28. GASSEL, MM AND DIAMANTOPOULOS, E: *Pattern of conduction times in the distribution of the radial nerve. A clinical and electrophysiological study.* Neurology (Minneap) 14:222, 1964.

29. GILLIATT, RW, GOODMAN, HV, AND WILLISON, RG: *The recording of lateral popliteal nerve action potentials in man.* J Neurol Neurosurg Psychiatry 24:305, 1961.

30. GINZBURG, M, ET AL: *Median and ulnar nerve conduction determinations in the Erb's point-axilla segment in normal subjects.* J Neurol Neurosurg Psychiatry 41:444, 1978.

31. GUILOFF, RJ AND SHERRATT, RM: *Sensory conduction in medial plantar nerve. Normal values, clinical applications, and a comparison with the sural and upper limb sensory nerve action potentials in peripheral neuropathy.* J Neurol Neurosurg Psychiatry 40:1168, 1977.

32. JABRE, JF: *Ulnar nerve lesions at the wrist: New technique for recording from the sensory dorsal branch of the ulnar nerve.* Neurology (New York) 30:873, 1980.

33. JABRE, JF: *The superficial peroneal sensory nerve revisited.* Arch Neurol 38:666, 1981.

34. JEBSEN, RH: *Motor conduction velocity in proximal and distal segments of the radial nerve.* Arch Phys Med Rehabil 47:597, 1966.

35. JOHNSON, RK AND SHREWSBURY, MM: *Anatomical course of the thenar branch of the median nerve—Usually in a separate tunnel through the transverse carpal ligament.* J Bone Joint Surg 52A:269, 1970.

36. KIM, DJ, ET AL: *Dorsal cutaneous ulnar nerve conduction: Diagnostic aid in ulnar neuropathy.* Arch Neurol 38:321, 1981.

37. KIMURA, J: *Collision technique—Physiological block of nerve impulses in studies of motor nerve conduction velocity.* Neurology (Minneap) 26:680, 1976.

38. KIMURA, J: *A method for determining median nerve conduction velocity across the carpal tunnel.* J Neurol Sci 38:1, 1978.

39. KIMURA, J: *The carpal tunnel syndrome. Localization of conduction abnormalities within the distal segment of the median nerve.* Brain 102:619, 1979.

40. KRAFT, GH: *Axillary, musculocutaneous and suprascapular nerve latency studies.* Arch Phys Med Rehabil 53:383, 1972.

41. LAFRATTA, CW AND ZALIS, AW: *Age effects on sural nerve conduction velocity.* Arch Phys Med Rehabil 54:475, 1973.

42. MACLEAN, IC: *Nerve root stimulation to evaluate conduction across the brachial and lumbosacral plexuses.* Third Annual Continuing Education Course, American Association of Electromyography and Electrodiagnosis, September 25, 1980, Philadelphia, Pennsylvania.

43. MACLEAN, IC AND MATTIONI, TA: *Phrenic nerve conduction studies: A new technique and its application in quadriplegic patients.* Arch Phys Med Rehabil 62:70, 1981.

44. MacLEAN, IC AND TAYLOR, RS: *Nerve root stimulation to evaluate brachial plexus conduction.* Abstracts of Communications of the Fifth International Congress of Electromyography, Rochester, Minnesota, 1975, p 47.

45. MAVOR, H AND ATCHESON, JB: *Posterior tibial nerve conduction. Velocity of sensory and motor fibers.* Arch Neurol 14:661, 1966.

46. MAVOR, H AND SHIOZAWA, R: *Antidromic digital and palmar nerve action potentials.* Electroenceph Clin Neurophysiol 30:210, 1971.

47. NELSON, RM AND CURRIER, DP: *Motor-nerve conduction velocity of the musculocutaneous nerve.* Phys Ther 49:586, 1969.

48. NEWSOM DAVIS, J: *Phrenic nerve conduction in man.* J Neurol Neurosurg Psychiatry 30:420, 1967.

49. PEIRIS, OA: *Conduction in the fourth and fifth lumbar and first sacral nerve roots: Preliminary communication.* NZ Med J 80:502, 1974.

50. REDFORD, JWB: *Conduction time in motor fibers of nerves which innervate proximal muscles of the extremities in normal persons and in patients with neuromuscular diseases.* Thesis, University of Minnesota, Minneapolis, 1958.

51. ROTH, G: *Vitesse de conduction motrice du nerf médian dans le canal carpien.* Annales de Médecine Physique 13:117, 1970.

52. SCHUCHMANN, JA: *Sural nerve conduction: A standardized technique.* Arch Phys Med Rehabil 58:166, 1977.

53. SHAHANI, B, GOODGOLD, J, AND SPIELHOLZ, NI: *Sensory nerve action potentials in the radial nerve.* Arch Phys Med Rehabil 48:602, 1967.

54. SHIOZAWA, R AND MAVOR, H: *In vivo human sural nerve action potentials.* J Appl Physiol 26:623, 1969.

55. SHIRALI, CS AND SANDLER, B: *Radial nerve sensory conduction velocity: Measurement by antidromic technique.* Arch Phys Med Rehabil 53:457, 1972.

56. SPINDLER, HA AND FELSENTHAL, G: *Sensory conduction in the musculocutaneous nerve.* Arch Phys Med Rehabil 59:20, 1978.

57. STÖHR, M, SCHUMM, F, AND BALLIER, R: *Normal sensory conduction in the saphenous nerve in man.* Electroenceph Clin Neurophysiol 44:172, 1978.

58. TROJABORG, W: *Motor and sensory conduction in the musculocutaneous nerve.* J Neurol Neurosurg Psychiatry 39:890, 1976.

59. TROJABORG, W AND SINDRUP, EH: *Motor and sensory conduction in different segments of the radial nerve in normal subjects.* J Neurol Neurosurg Psychiatry 32:354, 1969.

60. TRUONG, XT, ET AL: *Conduction velocity in the proximal sural nerve.* Arch Phys Med Rehabil 60:304, 1979.

61. WAINAPEL, SF, KIM, DJ, AND EBEL, A: *Conduction studies of the saphenous nerve in healthy subjects.* Arch Phys Med Rehabil 59:316, 1978.

62. WERSCHKUL, JD: *Anomalous course of the recurrent motor branch of the median nerve in a patient with carpal tunnel syndrome. Case report.* J Neurosurg 47:113, 1977.

63. WIEDERHOLT, WC: *Median nerve conduction velocity in sensory fibers through carpal tunnel.* Arch Phys Med Rehabil 51:328, 1970.

64. YAP, CB AND HIROTA, T: *Sciatic nerve motor conduction velocity study.* J Neurol Neurosurg Psychiatry 30:233, 1967.

# 7

# FACTS, FALLACIES, AND FANCIES OF NERVE STIMULATION TECHNIQUES

The clinical value of nerve conduction studies has long been established, and the technique for determining nerve conduction velocities is now well standardized. Although the method is simple, it is nonetheless subject to frequent technical errors.[20, 69] Commonly encountered, yet not widely appreciated, sources of error in the nerve stimulation techniques include (1) unexpected failure in the stimulating or recording system; (2) spread of the stimulating current to a nerve not under study; (3) recording a volume-conducted potential from distant muscles; (4) the presence of anomalous crossover between the median and ulnar nerves in the forearm; and (5) anomalous innervation of the extensor digitorum brevis by the accessory peroneal nerve. Under some of these circumstances, it may be desirable to block unwanted impulses in the nerve without affecting those under study. This can be achieved by collision, if a second stimulus is delivered distally to the nerve not being tested.

The principle of collision is also used in assessing other features of nerve conduction.[30, 34, 44, 45, 46, 49] Conventional studies primarily deal with the evaluation of the fastest conducting fibers, because the latency is measured to the onset of the evoked potential. It is conceivable that, in some clinical entities, measuring other aspects of nerve conduction may be more informative. Additional parameters being studied in some laboratories include conduction velocity of the slow conducting fibers and the time course of the absolute and relative refractory periods. The application of these methods appears promising as a supplement to the conventional technique, although their clinical value and limitations have not yet been clearly delineated.

## COMMON TECHNICAL ERRORS

Unexpected findings during routine nerve conduction studies are more often than not caused by technical problems. Possible sources of error must be carefully excluded before a finding is accepted as a manifestation of the disease. The difficulties may originate in the stimulating or recording system or both. If properly identified, most problems can be corrected with ease. The most commonly encountered will be reviewed briefly.

## Stimulating system

Absent or unexpectedly small responses may indicate that the nerve is being stimulated submaximally, or if the applied current is misdirected, not at all. The stimulating electrode should be relocated closer to the nerve and pressed more firmly, if necessary, using shocks of higher intensity and longer duration. The use of monopolar or concentric needle electrodes may be helpful especially in stimulating obese patients. A stimulating current will be ineffective if it is shunted between the cathode and anode, as is known to occur with profusely perspiring patients, or when there is an excessive amount of cream over the skin surface. Inadvertent reversal of the anode and cathode may cause anodal block of the propagating impulse. A submaximal activation may erroneously suggest a conduction block, especially if a larger response is elicited distally by supramaximal stimulation. Unintended compound muscle potentials may result from current spread to other nerves. Visual inspection of contracting muscles is often of value in determining whether activation is limited to the intended nerve.

## Recording system

Despite optimal stimulation, the recorded response may be of low amplitude if there is a faulty connection in the recording system. Common problems include inappropriate placement of the recording electrodes over the muscle, breaks in the electrode wires, connections to a wrong preamplifier, loss of power supply to the amplifier, and incorrect oscilloscope settings for gain, sweep, or filters. To test the integrity of the recording system the patient is asked to voluntarily contract the muscle with the electrode in position. Muscle action potentials are displayed on the oscilloscope, only if each step of the recording circuit is operational. A broken recording electrode is not always apparent, especially if the insulating sheath remains intact. With partial damage to the wire, stimulus-induced muscle twitches cause movement-related potentials, which may be mistaken for a compound muscle action potential.

An initial positivity preceding the negative peak of the compound muscle action potential usually suggests incorrect positioning of the active electrode. If so, it should be moved closer to the end-plate region. Alternatively, an initial positivity may represent a volume conducted potential from other muscles that are inadvertently activated by way of anomalous innervation or unintended stimulation of other nerves. The compound muscle action potential appears reversed in polarity if the active ($G_1$) and reference ($G_2$) electrodes are switched. Similarly, distortion of the recorded potential may occur if the reference electrode is located in an active rather than remote region in relation to the muscle action potential under consideration.

# INADVERTENT ACTIVATION OF UNINTENDED NERVES

Among a number of possible sources of error, spread of stimulating current to a nerve not under study is relatively frequent, but not commonly appreciated.[42] Failure to recognize this possibility may result in fallacious determination of latencies, because the recording electrodes often register a volume-conducted potential from distant muscles.[20] A few examples of this type of artifact will be illustrated later in this chapter. In some of these circumstances the collision technique may be used to block unwanted nerve stimulation.[44] Needle electrodes record from more limited areas and are valuable in studying the innervation of individual motor branches or patterns of anomalies. However, intramuscular electrodes do not reliably record the size of compound muscle action potentials, because they register electrical activity only from a restricted area in the muscle.

# Stimulation of the facial nerve

As will be discussed in Chapter 16, the facial nerve is accessible to surface or needle stimulation as it exits from the stylomastoid foramen (see Figs. 16-2 and 16-3). The excitability of the distal segment is tested by visual inspection of muscle contraction or by recording compound muscle action potentials from various facial muscles. Distal excitability remains normal for a few days, even after complete separation of the nerve at a proximal site, but is lost by the end of the first week coincident with the onset of nerve degeneration. Prognosis is generally good if excitability remains normal during the first week after injury.

With shocks of very high intensity, stimulating current may also activate the masseter at its motor point. A volume-conducted potential from this muscle may erroneously suggest a favorable prognosis when in fact the facial nerve has already degenerated (Fig. 7-1). In these instances, visual inspection of the contracting muscle is essential to verify that the recorded potential originates from the intended muscle. Surface stimulation of the facial nerve may also activate cutaneous fibers of the trigeminal nerve, causing reflexive contraction of the orbicularis oculi. The reflex response should not be mistaken for a late component of the compound muscle action potential or recurrent response due to antidromic activation of motor neurons.

## Axillary stimulation and collision technique

Unless shocks of an unusually high intensity are used,[42] stimulation of the median or ulnar nerve at the wrist or elbow ordinarily activates only the nerve in question. However, selective stimulation cannot be guaranteed at the axilla, where the two nerves lie in close proximity.[43] If stimulating current intended for the median nerve at the axilla spreads to the ulnar nerve, the electrodes placed on the thenar eminence record a potential originating from ulnar-innervated muscles. The measured latency will be erroneously short when the median nerve conducts slower than the ulnar nerve, as in the carpal tunnel syndrome (Fig. 7-2). In the same case, a stimulus at the elbow activates only the median nerve and the latency will be prolonged. Thus, the conduction velocity

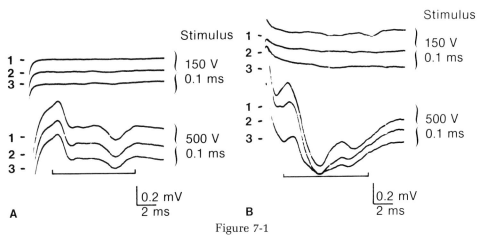

Figure 7-1

Direct response on the left (A) and right (B) sides in a patient with traumatic facial diplegia. Compound muscle potentials were recorded by surface electrodes over the orbicularis oculi ($G_1$) and the side of the nose ($G_2$). No response was obtained when the facial nerve was stimulated with shocks of an ordinary intensity (top three tracings). With shocks of a much higher intensity a definitive muscle response appeared (bottom three tracings). Close visual inspection revealed that the masseter muscle rather than the orbicularis oculi was contracting in response to the stimulation.

# Carpal Tunnel Syndrome

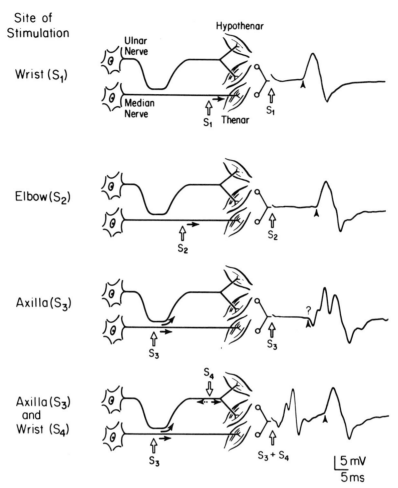

Figure 7-2

A 39-year-old man with the carpal tunnel syndrome. The median nerve was stimulated at the wrist ($S_1$), elbow ($S_2$), or axilla ($S_3$), and the muscle potential was recorded by surface electrodes from the thenar eminence. Spread of axillary stimulation ($S_3$) to the ulnar nerve (third tracing from top) activated ulnar-innervated thenar muscles with shorter latency, obscuring the onset (arrow head) of the muscle response under study. Another stimulus ($S_4$) applied to the ulnar nerve at the wrist (bottom tracing) blocked the proximal impulses by collision. The muscle action potential elicited by the distal stimulation occurred much earlier without overlapping with the muscle response under study. The figures on the left show diagrammatically the orthodromic (solid arrows) and antidromic (dotted arrows) impulses of each stimulation. (From Kimura,[44] with permission.)

from axilla to elbow would be calculated as being too fast. The latency of the recorded muscle response may even be shorter with stimulation of the median and ulnar nerves at the axilla than with selective stimulation of the median nerve at the elbow.

After median nerve stimulation, the surface electrodes on the hypothenar eminence nearly always register a potential (a positive wave of 1 to 5 mV in amplitude and 10 to 20 ms in duration), originating from thenar muscles or lumbricals or both. When studying the ulnar nerve in the conventional manner, inadvertent spread of stimulating current to the median nerve is not readily recognized, because a small volume-conducted potential from distant thenar muscles is usually buried in a much larger response of the hypothenar muscles. Spread of stimulus to the median nerve is more apparent if the ulnar nerve conducts slower than the median nerve, as in tardy ulnar palsy (Fig. 7-3). Precise definition of the onset of the electrical response originating from hypothenar muscles is then obscured by the earlier onset of a potential from thenar muscles. The latency measured to the onset of the latter potential is erroneously short. A stimulus at the elbow in the same case activates only the ulnar nerve with a prolonged latency. Again, the conduction velocity from axilla to elbow would be calculated as being too fast.

## Tardy Ulnar Palsy

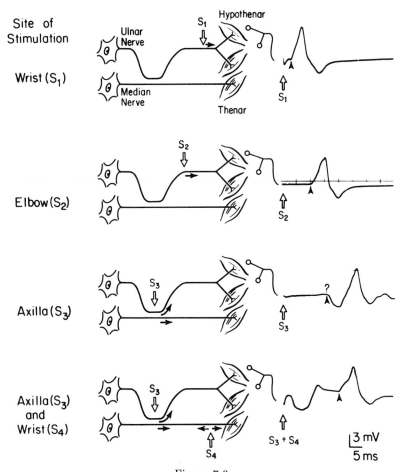

Figure 7-3

A 29-year-old man with tardy ulnar palsy. The ulnar nerve was stimulated at the wrist ($S_1$), elbow ($S_2$), or axilla ($S_3$); and the muscle potential was recorded by surface electrodes from the hypothenar eminence. Spread of axillary stimulation ($S_3$) to the median nerve (third tracing from top) activated median innervated thenar muscles with shorter latency. The potential originating from these muscles was registered through volume conduction as a positive wave obscuring the onset (arrow head) of the muscle response under study. Another stimulus ($S_4$) applied to the median nerve at the wrist (bottom tracing) blocked the proximal impulses by collision. The positive potential elicited by the wrist stimulus ($S_4$) occurred earlier without interfering with the muscle response under study. (From Kimura,[44] with permission.)

In studying the median or ulnar nerve under each of the aforementioned conditions, it is desirable to block impulses in one nerve without affecting those in the other. This can be achieved by delivering another stimulus at the wrist to the nerve not being tested. With this collision technique, the antidromic impulse activated in the nerve at the distal point extinguishes the orthodromically directed impulse from the proximal stimulation.[43] Of course, the orthodromic impulse induced by the distal stimulus itself elicits a muscle action potential. However, this response, which occurs much earlier, does not usually obscure the compound muscle action potential under study. Greater separation between these two responses can be accomplished by delivering the stimulus at the wrist a few milliseconds before the proximal stimulation. The time interval between these two stimuli must be chosen such that the antidromic impulse of the distal stimulation has not yet reached the point of proximal stimulation at the time the latter is delivered. Otherwise the proximal stimulus would escape antidromic collision.

As illustrated in Figures 7-2 and 7-3, the collision technique is helpful in clarifying otherwise confusing results of motor nerve conduction studies in conjunction with the carpal tunnel syndrome and tardy ulnar palsy. In each of these patients, spread of stimulus is obvious, because of the marked difference in waveform of the evoked potentials elicited by distal and proximal stimuli. In our experience, less apparent discrepancies commonly occur secondary to inadvertent spread of stimulating current. When this source of error is suspected, it is essential to block unwanted nerve stimulation so that the recorded response truly originates in the intended muscles. The collision technique is noninvasive and simpler than the procaine nerve block previously employed[20, 33] to identify the origin of the recorded muscle potentials. The method is of practical value in improving the accuracy of latency determination whenever selective stimulation of the median or ulnar nerve at a proximal point is technically difficult. The use of needle electrodes, recording from a more limited area, provides an alternative method of obtaining reliable latencies, if both nerves are activated simultaneously. However, intramuscular recording is less reliable for the assessment of a compound muscle action potential, as stated earlier.

## Palmar stimulation of the median nerve

As mentioned in Chapter 6, the median nerve may be stimulated not only at the wrist but also at the palm.[7, 15, ,47, 67, 81] With serial stimulation in 1 cm increments from palm to wrist, sensory latency increases almost linearly (see Fig. 6-3B). Unlike sensory axons, motor axons do not always show linear latency changes distal to the −1 level (see Fig. 6-3A). Indeed, the motor latency not uncommonly decreases as the stimulus site is moved proximally in the palm, because of the recurrent course of the thenar nerve. If one stimulus is inadvertently misdirected to a terminal portion of the thenar nerve, and another stimulus, delivered 1 cm proximally, activates only the median nerve trunk, an unreasonably large latency increase occurs between the two stimuli thereby presenting a fallacious impression of focal slowing (Fig. 7-4A). A disproportionate latency change is indicative of focal slowing, only if serial stimulation shows a linear latency increase in the segment proximal and distal to the site of lesion (Fig. 7-4B).

To avoid the same sort of error in the calculation of motor latency over the wrist-to-palm segment, it is essential to select a stimulation site that activates the median nerve at or near the origin of the thenar nerve as intended. In determining the origin of the thenar nerve at the palm, the anode must be placed distally rather than proximally to the cathode. This reversal of electrode position is necessary, since otherwise[47] the thenar nerve is sometimes activated near the anode from the spread of stimulating current, even if the cathode is clearly distal to the origin of the nerve. A surface distance measured to the cathodal point would then overestimate the nerve length, thereby resulting in an erroneously fast motor nerve conduction velocity. The stimulating

**Site of
Stimulation**

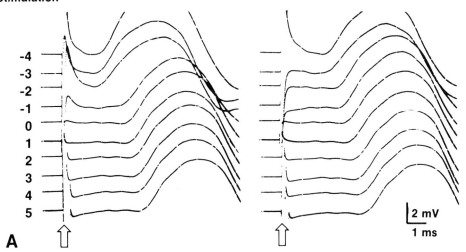

-4
-3
-2
-1
0
1
2
3
4
5

2 mV
1 ms

A

Figure 7-4

(A) Compound muscle action potentials in a normal subject recorded after stimulation of the median nerve at multiple points across the wrist. On the initial trial (left), the latency decreased as the cathode was moved proximally from −4 to −2, because of inadvertent spread of stimulating current to a distal portion of the thenar nerve. An apparent steep latency change from −2 to −1 gave an erroneous impression of a focal slowing at this level. This was shown not to be the case with a more careful placement of the cathode to avoid unintended activation of the thenar nerve when stimulating the median nerve proper. The 0 level was at the distal crease of the wrist, corresponding to the origin of the transverse ligament. (Compare Figure 6-3A.) (B) Sensory nerve (top) and muscle action potentials (bottom) in a symptomatic hand with the carpal tunnel syndrome. Serial stimulation showed a linear motor latency increase from −4 to −2 and from −1 to 5 with a localized slowing between −2 and −1. Note a temporally dispersed, double-peaked sensory nerve potential at the point of localized conduction delay from −4 to −3. (From Kimura,[47] with permission.)

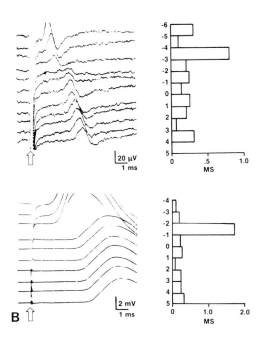

electrodes are moved in small increments from the distal palm towards the wrist, until an appropriate thumb twitch appears, indicating that the cathode is just over the origin of the thenar nerve. In most subjects, the median-innervated thenar muscles are first activated 3 or 4 cm distal to the distal crease of the wrist; that is, near the distal edge of the transverse carpal ligament.[40] Stimulation further distally either fails to produce a twitch or causes adduction of the thumb with activation of a deep branch of the ulnar nerve.

# ANOMALIES AS SOURCES OF ERROR

## Martin-Gruber anastomosis

Anatomic studies of Martin[59] and Gruber[24] demonstrated frequent communication from the median to the ulnar nerve at the level of the forearm. This anastomosis usually involves fibers supplying intrinsic hand muscles that are ordinarily ulnar-innervated, most notably the first dorsal interosseous, adductor pollicis, and abductor digiti minimi muscles.[57, 82] The number of axons taking the anomalous course varies widely. Adjusting the site and intensity of the electrical stimulus delivered at the elbow, it is often possible to activate the anomalous fibers, maximally and selectively, without activating the median nerve proper.[49] This observation suggests that the nerve fibers forming the anastomosis are grouped together in a separate bundle, rather than scattered within the median nerve. Anatomic studies and electrophysiologic data suggest that this anomaly occurs in 15 to 31 percent of subjects in an unselected population. When present, the anomaly tends to be bilateral.[49] The high incidence of the median to ulnar anastomosis indicates the phylogenetic origin of this communication.[9] In contrast, the reverse communication involving axons crossing from the ulnar to the median nerve is extremely rare.[73]

The presence of Martin-Gruber anomaly may be detected during routine nerve conduction studies by carefully analyzing the shape of the compound muscle action potentials. Stimulation of the median nerve at the elbow evokes a response not only from the median-innervated thenar muscle but also from thenar and hypothenar muscles anomalously innervated by fibers crossing to the ulnar nerve in the forearm. The response elicited by stimulation of the median nerve at the wrist is usually smaller, since the ulnar component is absent. Studying the ulnar nerve, the reverse discrepancy is noted in the amplitude of compound muscle action potentials elicited by proximal and distal stimulation. The response from ulnar-innervated thenar or hypothenar muscles is smaller with stimulation at the elbow than at the wrist because the distal stimulation activates additional anomalous fibers.

In equivocal cases, the presence of an anomaly may be confirmed if action potentials are recorded from the first dorsal interosseous, adductor pollicis, or hypothenar muscles, after stimulation of the median nerve at the elbow. Potentials recorded over these muscles, however, may be volume conducted from median-innervated distant muscles rather than originating from anomalously activated muscles.[8, 20, 44, 52, 69] Distinguishing between these two possibilities is sometimes difficult, although typically the volume-conducted potentials are initially positive and remain unchanged when the nerve is stimulated at the wrist or at the elbow. In contrast, anomalously innervated muscles are activated only with stimulation of the median nerve at the elbow. The recorded potential may be initially positive or negative, depending on the location of the contracting muscle relative to the recording electrode. In difficult cases, recording with a needle electrode in the muscle may clarify the origin of the recorded response, although intramuscular recordings do not entirely preclude volume-conducted potentials.

The collision technique may be used to separate these two types of responses by stimulating the median nerve simultaneously at the wrist and elbow (Fig. 7-5). Normally, antidromically directed impulses from the distal stimulation would collide with and block the orthodromic impulses from the proximal stimulation in the same nerve, thus eliminating the muscle potentials resulting from the latter.[30, 78] However, the orthodromic impulses traveling through an anastomotic branch to the ulnar nerve would bypass the antidromic impulses and escape collision.[44] By this means, it is also possible to assess the actual size of the anomalous response, which is clearly separated from the volume-conducted potentials.

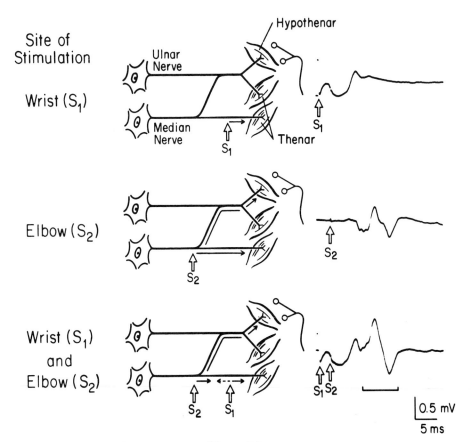

Figure 7-5

The median nerve was stimulated at the sites indicated, and muscle action potentials were record-ed from the hypothenar eminence. The top tracing shows a volume conducted potential from thenar muscles (U-shaped wave of positive polarity). In the middle tracing, a small negative poten-tial is seen superimposed upon the volume-conducted potential. The bottom tracing shows the anomalous response (bracket) clearly separated from the volume-conducted potential when the collision technique was used. The distal stimulus was given four milliseconds before the proximal stimulation. (From Kimura, Murphy, and Varda,[49] with permission.)

To determine whether thenar muscles are also innervated by fibers forming the median to ulnar anastomosis the collision technique is used to record an anomalous potential from the thenar, as opposed to hypothenar, eminence. In this case (Fig. 7-6), an anomalous response must be detected in the presence of a large compound muscle action potential from median-innervated thenar muscles activated by the distal stimu-lus. Separation of these two muscle potentials is in part accomplished by delivering the stimulus at the wrist a few milliseconds before the stimulation at the elbow. The time interval between the two stimuli must not exceed the latency difference between proxi-mal and distal stimuli. Otherwise, the nerve impulses produced by proximal stimula-tion would escape antidromic collision even in the absence of an anomalous route of transmission.

Under ordinary circumstances, the median or ulnar nerve can be selectively stimulated at the elbow, where these two nerves are located on opposite sides of the arm. However, in the presence of Martin-Gruber anastomosis, stimulation of the medi-an nerve at the elbow activates ulnar-innervated intrinsic hand muscles, including the

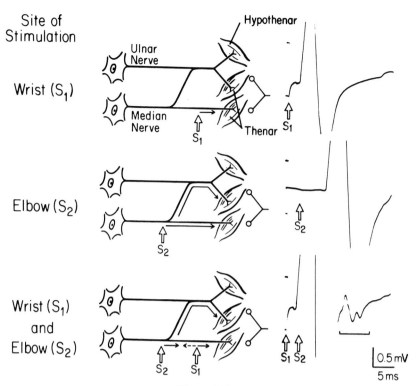

## Figure 7-6

The median nerve was stimulated at two points, and muscle action potentials were recorded from the thenar eminence. (Compare Figure 7-5.) The top and middle tracings show a compound action potential from median-innervated thenar muscles. In the middle tracing, this potential overlapped with an anomalous response mediated by the anastomosis. In the bottom tracing, these two muscle potentials were separated by the collision technique to detect the anomalous response (bracket). The distal stimulus was given four milliseconds before the proximal stimulation. (From Kimura, Murphy, and Varda,[49] with permission.)

adductor pollicis, through communicating fibers. If this anomaly is associated with the carpal tunnel syndrome, stimulation of the median nerve at the elbow may evoke two temporally dispersed potentials, the normal ulnar and delayed median response. If the latency is measured to the onset of the initial response, it is erroneously short and not consistent with the delayed distal latency obtained with stimulation at the wrist.[39, 44, 52] An unreasonably fast conduction velocity from elbow to wrist in some patients with the carpal tunnel syndrome has been attributed to this anomaly.[8, 44, 52] Since the anomalously innervated ulnar muscles are usually at some distance from the recording electrodes placed on the abductor pollicis brevis, the initial ulnar component is usually, though not always, a positive deflection.[26, 27] Under these circumstances, it is desirable to block impulses in the anomalous fibers without affecting those in the median nerve proper. This can be achieved by collision if a second stimulus is delivered distally to the nerve not being tested, as discussed earlier in this chapter. (Fig. 7-7).

If the ulnar nerve is severed or otherwise substantially injured at the elbow, the segment distal to the lesion becomes inexcitable consequent to wallerian degeneration. In the absence of the anomaly, therefore, stimulation of the degenerated nerve at the wrist fails to evoke muscle action potentials. In the presence of a median to ulnar communication in the forearm, however, a small but otherwise normal muscle action potential is elicited by stimulation of the anomalous fibers at the wrist. In extreme cases, separation of the ulnar nerve at the elbow may not appreciably affect the intrin-

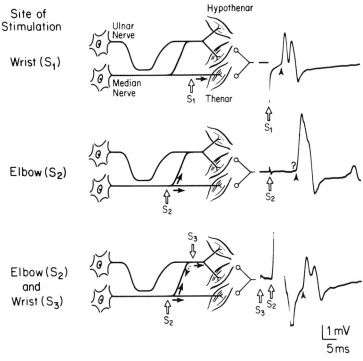

Figure 7-7

A 55-year-old man with the carpal tunnel syndrome in the presence of an anomalous communication from the median to ulnar nerve. The median nerve was stimulated at the wrist ($S_1$) or elbow ($S_2$), and the muscle potential was recorded by surface electrodes from the thenar eminence. Spread of the elbow stimulation ($S_2$) to the ulnar nerve through the anomalous communication (middle tracing) activated ulnar-innervated thenar muscles, obscuring the onset (arrow head) of the muscle response under study. Another stimulus ($S_3$) applied to the ulnar nerve at the wrist (bottom tracing) blocked the impulses transmitted through the communicating fibers. The stimulus at the wrist ($S_3$) was delivered four milliseconds before the stimulation at the elbow ($S_2$) to avoid an overlap of the muscle responses elicited by these two stimuli. (From Kimura,[44] with permission.)

sic hand muscles, because of substantial ulnar innervation via the communication. This rare condition is called the all median hand.[58] An anomaly of this type, if undetected, is a source of considerable confusion, since electromyography may reveal normal motor unit potentials in the ulnar-innervated muscles, despite severe damage to the ulnar nerve at the elbow. Conversely, an injury to the median nerve at the elbow could lead to the appearance of spontaneous discharges in the ulnar-innervated intrinsic hand muscles.

## Anomalies of the hand

Common anomalies of the peripheral nerves include variations in innervation of the intrinsic hand muscles. Although not as widely recognized as the median-to-ulnar communication, they constitute sources of error in the evaluation of nerve conduction velocity and electromyography. Electrophysiologic techniques are useful in determining the presence or absence of such anastomoses, but anatomic studies are necessary to precisely characterize and delineate the extent of each anomaly.[74]

Richie[66] and Cannieu[10] originally described various communications between motor branches of the median and ulnar nerves in the lateral portion of the hand. Variations may occur in any of the intrinsic hand muscles. In particular, the flexor pollicis brevis may be innervated by the median or ulnar nerve or may receive dual innervation.[68] In a small percentage of cases, thenar muscles, including the adductor pollicis, may be innervated exclusively by the median or ulnar nerve. In addition to neural anastomoses, congenital skeletal anomalies of the upper limb are well recognized. Absent thenar muscles have been described on this basis. Recognition of this possibility is important in the differential diagnosis of the carpal tunnel syndrome.[11]

## Accessory deep peroneal nerve

The most frequent anomaly of the lower extremity relates to the pattern of innervation for the extensor digitorum brevis, which is commonly used in conduction studies of the peroneal nerve. This muscle is usually supplied by the deep peroneal nerve, a major branch of the common peroneal nerve. In 20 to 28 percent of an unselected population, the extensor digitorum brevis is also innervated by the superficial peroneal nerve via an anomalous communication. This branch, called the accessory deep peroneal nerve (Fig. 7-8), usually supplies the lateral portion of the muscle.[37, 53, 83] Occasionally the extensor digitorum brevis is innervated exclusively by this anomalous communication.[61] The accessory deep peroneal nerve descends on the lateral aspect of the leg, after arising from the superficial peroneal nerve, then passes behind the lateral malleolus, and proceeds anteriorly to innervate the extensor digitorum brevis. The anomaly appears to be inherited in a dominant fashion.[12]

This anomaly should be suspected if the compound action potential of the extensor digitorum brevis is smaller with stimulation of the deep peroneal nerve at the ankle than with stimulation of the common peroneal nerve at the knee. The presence of the accessory deep peroneal nerve can be substantiated by stimulating behind the lateral malleolus, and activating the anomalously innervated lateral portion of the muscle. Lesions of the deep peroneal nerve normally cause weakness of the tibialis anterior, extensor digitorum longus, extensor hallucis longus, and extensor digitorum brevis. In the presence of the accessory deep peroneal nerve, however, the lateral portion of the extensor digitorum brevis is spared. This finding may be erroneously interpreted if the possibility of the anomaly is overlooked.[25]

# FAST VERSUS SLOW CONDUCTING FIBERS

## Temporal dispersion of the compound action potential

Although the latency measured to the onset of the muscle or nerve action potential is that of the fastest conducting fibers, the waveform of the recorded response does provide some indication as to the status of the remaining slower conducting fibers. A smaller range of conduction velocity because of loss of some nerve fibers reduces the duration of the compound action potential. Conversely, disproportionate slowing of slower conducting fibers will result in increased temporal dispersion. The greater the range is between the fastest and slowest nerve conductions, the longer is the duration of the evoked potential. In addition, temporal dispersion will be greater for proximal versus distal stimulation.[38] A method has been described for estimating the distribution of nerve fiber conduction velocities in a nerve bundle, based on a detailed model of the compound action potential as a weighted sum of asynchronous single fiber action potentials.[13, 14]

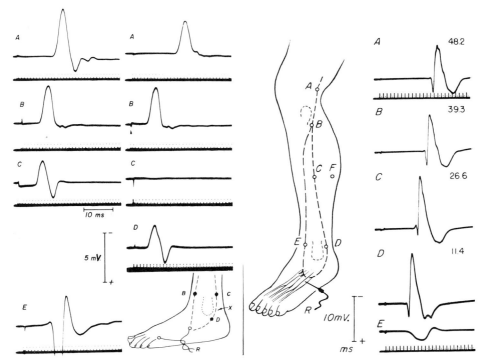

Figure 7-8

(*Left*) Compound muscle action potentials recorded from surface electrodes over the extensor digitorum brevis after a maximal stimulus to the common peroneal nerve at the knee (A), deep peroneal nerve on the dorsum of the ankle (B), accessory deep peroneal nerve posterior to the lateral malleolus (C and D), and posterior tibial nerve posterior to the medial malleolus (E) at the ankle. Left panel before and right panel after block of the accessory deep peroneal nerve with two percent lidocaine posterior to the lateral malleolus. Diagram of the foot shows the site of block (x) and the points of stimulation (B, C and D) and recording (R). (*Right*) Course of the accessory deep peroneal nerve. Action potentials recorded with coaxial needle electrode (R) in the lateral belly of the extensor digitorum brevis muscle. Stimulus applied to the common peroneal nerve at the knee (A) and just below the head of fibula (B), superficial peroneal nerve (C), accessory deep peroneal nerve posterior to the lateral malleolus (D) and deep peroneal nerve on the dorsum of the ankle (E). Note that the volume-conducted potential from the medial bellies of the extensor digitorum brevis (E) reduces amplitude of action potential of the lateral belly when both are evoked simultaneously by stimulation of the common peroneal nerve at A or B. (From Lambert,[53] with permission.)

## Block of fast or slow conducting fibers

The duration of the compound action potentials, although useful as an indirect esti-mate, is not a precise measure of slow fiber conduction. Different methods have been suggested for quantitative assessment. The principle of collision has been commonly employed.[78] The fibers with the largest diameter have the fastest conduction velocities and the lowest thresholds and are the ones initially excited with a distal stimulus of submaximal intensity. A shock of supramaximal intensity given simultaneously at a proximal site then allows selective passage of impulses in the slower fibers, because the fast fibers are blocked by antidromic activity from the distal stimulation. This assump-tion, however, is not always correct,[19] because the order of activation with threshold stimulation depends in part on the position of the stimulating electrode in relation to the different fascicles.[28, 41]

In an alternative method, paired shocks of supramaximal intensity are used.[22, 30] Without varying stimulus intensity, the proximal shock is progressively delayed after distal stimulation. When both shocks are applied simultaneously, collision occurs in all fibers. As the interval between the two stimuli is increased, the fastest fibers are the first to escape collision, while the slow fibers are still blocked. Measurement of the minimal interstimulus interval that produces a muscle action potential of normal amplitude provides an indirect assessment of the slowest conduction (Table 7-1). This method does not allow direct latency determinations of the slowest fibers. To do so, it would be necessary to block the fast conducting fibers leaving the activity in the slower fibers unaffected.

To block fast conducting fibers, nerves are activated using two sets of stimulating electrodes—one placed at the axilla and the other at the wrist. The first and third shocks, $S(A_1)$ and $S(A_2)$, respectively, are delivered through the proximal electrodes, whereas the second shock, $S(W)$, is given via the distal electrodes. The orthodromic impulse of $S(A_1)$ is blocked by the antidromic impulse of $S(W)$, so long as the distal shock is delivered before the proximal impulse reaches the distal site of stimulation. Because the motor axons are cleared of antidromic activity, the impulse of $S(A_2)$ is transmitted distally. If $S(A_1)$ precedes $S(W)$ by a time interval that allows only the fast fibers to escape collision, while the slow fibers are blocked, the motor axons are now cleared of antidromic activity in the slower fibers but not in the fast fibers. Therefore, the fast conducting fibers are blocked for the $S(A_2)$ impulse by collision with the remaining antidromic activity of $S(W)$. In this way, orthodromic impulses are selectively conducted in the slow fibers and corresponding muscle action potentials are recorded (Fig. 7-9).

This technique allows direct determination of the amplitude and latency of the slowest conducting fibers. The muscle action potential elicited by $S(A_2)$ shows progressive diminution of amplitude as an increasing number of fast conducting impulses are eliminated. The latency changes, however, are not as consistent as might be expected on theoretical grounds or on the basis of the time interval between $S(A_1)$ and $S(W)$. The exact cause of this discrepancy is not known, but it may be, at least in part, because the axons differ in length within the same nerve. If so, the fastest and slowest conducting fibers are not always the first and last to arrive at the motor end-plate, respectively. Thus, the conduction time is determined not only by the speed of the propagated impulse but also, and perhaps more importantly, by the length of fine terminal fibers innervating each muscle fiber.[64] Although the difference in length of the longest and shortest fibers is probably in the order of a few millimeters, a substantial latency difference may result, since the terminal nerve fiber is likely to conduct at a much slower rate than the more proximal segment.

## Conduction of individual motor axons

Instead of surface electrodes, needle electrodes may be used to record from different motor units within a given muscle. It is possible by this means to sample a wide range of motor fibers with different conduction characteristics. Although of theoretical interest, this technique is not as yet clinically practical and requires multiple needle insertions to isolate the slowest conducting fibers.[4, 79]

**TABLE 7-1 Range of conduction velocity in motor fibers of the ulnar nerve**

| Authors | Fastest fibers | Slowest fibers | Range |
|---|---|---|---|
| Thomas, Sears, and Gilliatt[78] | | | 15–20% |
| Poloni and Sala[65] | | | 15 m/s |
| Hopf[30] | 60.0 ± 3.2 | | 4–7 m/s |
| Hopf[31] | 60.1 ± 4.5 | 43.3 ± 2.9 | 8.7 m/s |
| Skorpil[70] | 61.1 ± 4.5 | 37.7 ± 7.1 | 22.4 m/s |

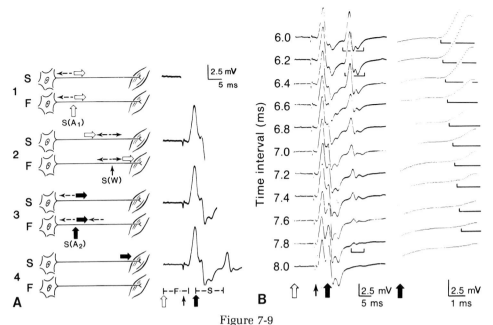

Figure 7-9

(A) Compound muscle action potential recorded by surface electrode placed over the abductor digiti minimi after stimulation of the ulnar nerve. The figures on the left are schematic diagrams showing orthodromic and antidromic impulses generated by three stimuli, S(A₁), S(W), and S(A₂) delivered at the axilla, wrist, and axilla, respectively. Note the collision between the orthodromic impulse from S(A₁) and antidromic impulse of S(W) in slow conduction fibers (S), and between the orthodromic impulse of S(A₂) and antidromic impulse of S(W) in the fast conducting fibers (F). The orthodromic impulse of S(A₂) is conducted along the slow conducting fibers and elicits the second compound muscle action potential. (B) Paired axillary shocks of supramaximal intensity were combined with a single shock at the wrist. (Compare bottom tracing in Figure 7-9A.) The first axillary stimulation, S(A₁) was followed by the wrist stimulation, S(W), given at intervals ranging from 6.0 to 8.0 ms. The second axillary shock, S(A₂) was always delivered 6.0 ms after S(W). For amplitude measurement (left half of the figure), a slow sweep was triggered by S(A₁). To determine latencies (right half), a fast sweep was triggered by S(A₂) and the response displayed after a predetermined delay of 6.0 ms.

# ASSESSMENT OF THE REFRACTORY PERIOD

## Physiologic basis

After passage of an impulse, an axon becomes totally inexcitable for a fraction of a millisecond (absolute refractory period), then gradually recovers its prestimulus excitability within the ensuing few milliseconds (relative refractory period). These two phases of decreased excitability have been extensively studied in experimental animals by direct measurement of the nerve action potentials.[1, 3, 23, 29, 77] Studies of the refractory periods in human peripheral nerves have been relatively recent and mostly limited to the sensory and mixed nerves.[2, 6, 21, 35, 36, 56, 75, 76] However, newer methods using modified paired shock techniques now enable one to study the motor fibers as well.[34, 50, 51] Although a considerable amount of data has been accumulated during the past decade for the human refractory period, the clinical value and limitations of these data have not yet been clearly delineated. This section will review various techniques and the currently available clinical data on the refractory period. A more detailed account on this subject is available elsewhere.[48]

The physiologic mechanism underlying the refractory period is based on inactivation of sodium (Na$^+$) conductance. During the absolute refractory period (0.5 to 1.0 ms), the axon is inexcitable primarily because inactivated sodium conductance at the end of the action potential cannot be immediately reactivated. During the relative refractory period (1.5 to 3.0 ms), the axon is excitable only to supramaximal stimuli, because the available sodium conductance is low. The refractory period is affected by various factors. It increases with decreasing temperature[6, 62] and with increasing age.[17] It is inversely proportional to the conduction velocity[63] and is markedly increased after experimental demyelination.[16, 54, 71, 72]

If a brief suprathreshold current is applied repetitively, conduction block occurs at the site of cathodal stimulation after one or more action potentials are generated, even if the interstimulus interval is longer than the absolute refractory period. Cathodal block, like the refractory period, is based on inactivation of sodium conductance. This type of block is relieved by a hyperpolarizing current that reduces depolarization and reactivates sodium conductance. In contrast, anodal block is due to hyperpolarization of the membrane and may be relieved by a depolarizing current that brings the transmembrane potential closer to the normal resting value.

Whereas suprathreshold current is always followed by a refractory period or conduction block, the effect of subthreshold current on the excitability of the cell membrane depends on the duration of the stimulus. A brief current usually increases the excitability by depolarizing the cell membrane. Hence, the cell may fire if a second subthreshold stimulus follows while the membrane is still partly depolarized (summation). However, a prolonged subthreshold stimulus may decrease rather than increase excitability because inactivation of sodium conductance may more than compensate for the increase in excitability due to depolarization. Thus, a slowly rising depolarizing current may inactivate sodium conductance before the depolarization reaches threshold. In this case, conduction can be blocked at the cathodal point prior to the generation of any action potentials. Reduction of nerve excitability following prolonged subthreshold stimulation is referred to as accommodation.

## Paired shock technique

To study excitability changes induced by a stimulus, a second shock may be delivered at varying time intervals after the first. This method is called the paired-shock technique or the conditioning and testing technique, because the first shock conditions the nerve, and the second impulse tests the resulting effect. If the test stimulus occurs during the refractory period induced by the conditioning stimulus, the first (conditioning) response would be normal, while the second (test) response would be absent. During the ensuing relative refractory period, the test response is reduced in amplitude and increased in latency. The paired-shock technique has been extensively used to study experimental animals.[3, 77] More recently, the sensory[6, 75, 76] and mixed fibers[21, 56] have been tested in man by measuring the nerve action potentials elicited by pairs of stimuli.

## Collision technique for study of motor fibers

To test motor fibers using the same principles, the muscle action potentials may be recorded after delivering paired stimuli to the nerve. However, the results are difficult to interpret because, with the short interstimulus interval required to study the refractory period, the muscle responses elicited by the first and second stimuli overlap. To circumvent this problem, a subtraction technique, using a signal analyzer with a memory, may be used to separate the test from the conditioning muscle response.[2, 51] The subtraction technique, which still uses successively evoked muscle responses, does not measure the nerve refractory period alone, since the size of the test response is determined by the excitability change of not only the motor axons, but also the neuromuscular junction and the muscle fibers themselves.[5] To avoid this difficulty, Hopf and Low-itzsch[34] have used paired distal stimuli at various interstimulus intervals and a single proximal stimulus to determine the refractory period of antidromic motor impulses. Alternatively, paired proximal stimuli may be combined with a single distal stimulus to block the muscle effect of the first stimulus of the pair without affecting that of the second.[45]

When paired shocks $S(A_1)$ and $S(A_2)$ at the axilla are combined with a single shock $S(W)$ at the wrist, the antidromic impulse from the wrist is eliminated by collision with the orthodromic impulse of the conditioning axillary stimulus (Fig. 7-10). Because the motor axons are now cleared of antidromic activity, the impulse of $S(A_2)$ will be transmitted distally, but only if the axons are excitable after the passage of the conditioning stimulus. Changing the $S(A_1)$–$S(W)$ interval, it is possible to adjust the point of collision and consequently the length of the nerve segment made refractory by the conditioning stimulus, before it is extinguished by the antidromic impulse. Changing the $S(A_1)$–$S(A_2)$ interval defines the range of the absolute refractory periods of different motor fibers by demonstrating the serial recovery of the test response ampli-

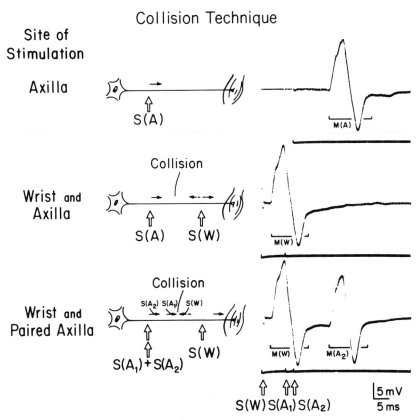

Figure 7-10

Compound muscle action potentials recorded by surface electrodes placed over the abductor digiti minimi after percutaneous stimulation of the ulnar nerve. The figures on the left are schematic diagrams showing orthodromic (solid arrows) and antidromic (dotted arrows) impulses. Axillary stimulation, S(A), was given 6.0 ms after the stimulus at the wrist, S(W), which triggered sweeps on the oscilloscope. With single stimulation at the wrist and the axilla (middle tracing), the orthodromic impulse from the axilla was extinguished by collision with the antidromic impulse from the wrist. When paired shocks were delivered at the axilla (bottom tracing), $M(A_2)$ appeared because the first axillary stimulus, $S(A_1)$, cleared the path for the orthodromic impulse of the second stimulus, $S(A_2)$. (From Kimura, Yamada, and Rodnitzky,[50] with permission.)

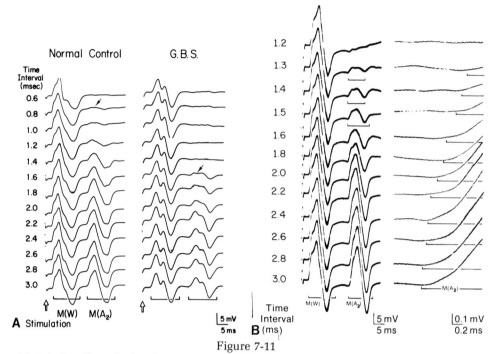

**Figure 7-11**

(A) Paired axillary shocks of just maximal intensity were combined with a single shock at the wrist. (Compare bottom tracing in Figure 7-10.) Interstimulus intervals between the two axillary stimuli ranged from 0.6 to 3.0 ms. The shock intervals were adjusted so that the second axillary shock always occurred 5.0 ms after the distal stimulus, which triggered sweeps on the oscilloscope. In the normal subject, M(A₂) first appeared (small arrow) at an interstimulus interval of 0.8 ms and recovered completely by 3.0 ms. In the patient with the Guillain-Barré syndrome, M(A₂) first appeared at the time interval of 1.6 ms and did not recover completely by 3.0 ms. (From Kimura,[45] with permission.) (B) Paired axillary shocks of just maximal intensity were combined with a single shock at the wrist. (Compare bottom tracing in Figure 7-10.) The first axillary stimulation, S(A₁), was given 6.0 ms after the shock at the wrist, S(W), so that the impulses of these two stimuli always collided 1.5 ms following the delivery of S(A₁). The second axillary shock, S(A₂), was given at intervals ranging from 1.2 to 3.0 ms after S(A₁). For amplitude measurements (left half of the figure), a slow sweep was triggered by S(W). To determine latencies (right half), a fast sweep was triggered by S(A₂) and the response displayed after a predetermined delay of 11.0 ms. (From Kimura, Yamada, and Rodnitzky,[50] with permission.)

tude (Fig. 7-11A). The duration of the relative refractory period of the most excitable fibers can be determined by changes in latency of the test response elicited at various intervals after a conditioning impulse (Fig. 7-11B). Table 7-2 summarizes the results in 20 ulnar nerves from 10 healthy subjects studied in our laboratory.[50]

## Changes in amplitude versus latency

The amplitude changes of the test response obtained with shocks of maximal intensity follow a predictable time course and are practically identical regardless of whether the shorter or longer segment is made refractory (Fig. 7-12). It is likely, therefore, that the decreased amplitude of the test response is caused by failure of nerve activation at the site of stimulation. The impulse is conducted at a slower speed than normal, if transmitted at all, during the relative refractory period (Fig. 7-13). Slowing of conduction is greatest near the absolute refractory period, followed by progressive recovery to normal

**TABLE 7-2 Interstimulus intervals of the paired shocks and conduction velocity of the test response**

(Mean ± SD)

| Length of refractory segment | Initial recovery in amplitude (test response greater than 5% of unconditioned response) | | Full recovery in amplitude (test response greater than 95% of unconditioned response) | | Full recovery in conduction velocity (test response conducts at speed greater than 95% of normal) |
|---|---|---|---|---|---|
| | Interstimulus interval between paired shocks (ms) | Conduction velocity of test impulse (% of normal) | Interstimulus interval between paired shocks (ms) | Conduction velocity of test impulse (% of normal) | Interstimulus interval between paired shocks (ms) |
| A distance normally covered in 0.5 ms | 1.16 ± 0.18 | 55.3 ± 19.2 | 2.11 ± 0.50 | 81.2 ± 17.4 | 2.65 ± 0.65 |
| A distance normally covered in 1.5 ms | 1.18 ± 0.16 | 70.3 ± 13.5 | 2.16 ± 0.52 | 87.3 ± 14.2 | 2.36 ± 0.45 |

(From Kimura, Yamada, and Rodnitzky,[50] with permission.)

as the interstimulus interval between the conditioning and test stimuli is increased. Whereas recovery in amplitude of the test response is unrelated to the length of the refractory segment, change in latency is greater with a longer refractory segment. Thus, the course of recovery in conduction time of the test response depends on the length of the refractory segment; the longer the refractory segment is, the greater is the change in latency of the test response.

The delay in latency, however, is not proportional to the length of the refractory segments. The slowing of the test impulse during the refractory period allows an increasing interval between conditioning and test impulses as they travel further distally.[77] An increasingly longer interval between the two impulses, in turn, leads to progressive recovery of the test impulse conduction velocity. Because of this regressive process, the test impulse is conducted at a relatively normal speed by the time it reaches the end of the refractory segment. This tendency is greater in the longer refractory segment than it is in the shorter segment.[45] Since change in latency per unit length

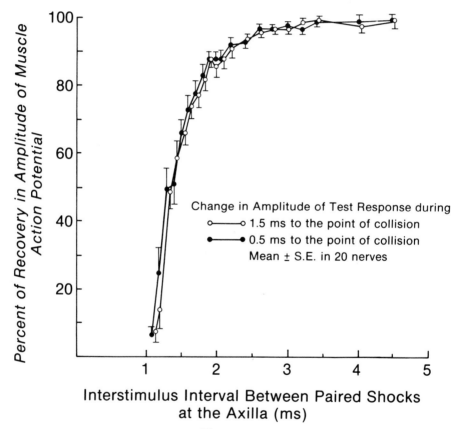

Figure 7-12

The time course of recovery in amplitude of $M(A_2)$ after the passage of a preceding impulse in 10 healthy subjects (20 responses considering right and left sides together). The response to the second shock of the pair, $M(A_2)$, was converted into a percentage of the response to a single stimulus, $M(A)$, at each interstimulus interval of paired axillary stimuli. The return of $M(A_2)$ was practically identical whether the shorter segment (normally covered in 0.5 ms) or the longer segment (normally covered in 1.5 ms) was made refractory. The gradual increase of $M(A_2)$ indicates that the absolute refractory periods of the different motor fibers vary considerably, full recovery being achieved when the least excitable fibers are no longer refractory. (From Kimura, Yamada, and Rodnitzky,[50] with permission.)

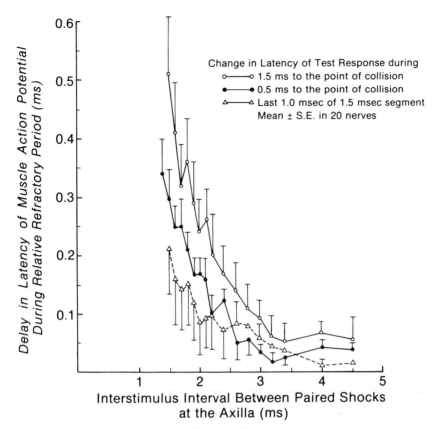

Figure 7-13

The time course of recovery in latency of M(A₂) in the same subjects as shown in Figure 7-12. The latency of M(A), the response to a single axillary shock, was subtracted from that of M(A₂), the response to the second axillary shock of the pair. The recovery was significantly slower when the longer segment normally covered in 1.5 ms was made refractory, as compared with the shorter segment normally covered in 0.5 ms. The bottom curve (triangles) was obtained by plotting the difference between the delay that occurred during the time period of 1.5 ms and that during 0.5 ms at each interstimulus interval. The values so calculated represented the delay attributable to the last two-thirds of the longer segments; that is, distance covered during the latter 1.0 ms of the 1.5 ms. (From Kimura, Yamada, and Rodnitzky,[50] with permission.)

decreases, as a longer conduction distance is studied, the average conduction velocity is faster, if the refractory segment is longer (Fig. 7-14). The same points have been illustrated in electrophysiologic studies on human sensory fibers[6] and computer simulations of conduction characteristics during the refractory period.[80]

One of the problems in studying the refractory period in human nerve is precisely measuring the amplitude and latency of the test response. This is particularly true when the signal is small and the baseline is not straight, since the onset of the evoked potential may be very gradual. Furthermore, there may be partial overlap between the test response and the preceding potential, even with the use of a collision technique. To circumvent these difficulties, Faisst and Meyer[18] have recently developed a method for the numerical quantification of the compound muscle potential in shape and latency, based on a computerized cross correlation analysis. In this technique, the height of the peak in the correlation curve gives a shape-weighted measure of the size of the test response, and the time lag of the peak indicates the delay of the test response as compared with an averaged unconditioned muscle response.

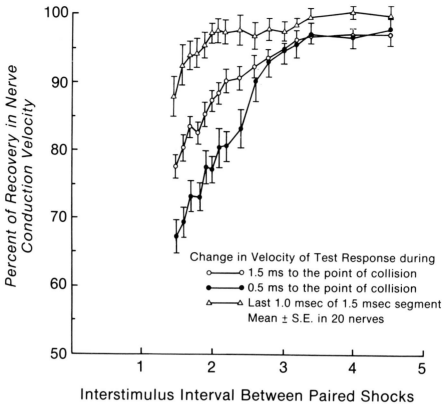

Figure 7-14

The time course of recovery in conduction velocity of M(A₂) in the same subjects shown in Figures 7-12 and 7-13. The conduction velocities were calculated assuming that the delay of M(A₂) occurred primarily in the segment proximal to the point of collision, a distance normally covered in 0.5 ms or 1.5 ms. In contrast to recovery in latency (compare Figure 7-13), the recovery in conduction velocity was significantly faster when the refractory segment was longer. The top curve (triangles) was obtained using the calculated delay of M(A₂) over the segment of nerve covered during the last 1.0 ms of the 1.5 ms. (From Kimura, Yamada, and Rodnitzky,[50] with permission.)

## Clinical value and limitations

In studies of the whole human nerve, as opposed to individual nerve fibers, it is not possible to define the absolute and relative refractory period for fibers with different conduction characteristics. Furthermore, in contrast to changes in amplitude, which follow a predictable time course, changes in latency are rather small and vary with repeated testings. Nonetheless, values of the absolute and relative refractory periods obtained in motor fibers[50] are very close to those of sensory and mixed fibers.[21] Full recovery in amplitude of the test response precedes full recovery of conduction velocity. Similar observations have been made in studying sensory and mixed human nerve fibers.[6,21,35]

Increases in the refractory period of sensory and mixed nerve fibers have been reported in diseases of the peripheral nerve.[55, 56, 75, 76] Similarly, the refractory period of median nerve sensory fibers has been shown to be increased in patients with multiple sclerosis, suggesting the possibility that peripheral nerve fibers may be affected in this disorder.[32] Conversely, the relative refractory period is known to be shortened in patients with hypokalemia of various origins.[60] Most previous studies in man have dealt with the sensory or mixed nerve fibers, but it is reasonable to assume that similar alterations may be found in the refractory characteristics of motor fibers. The clinical value and limitations of refractory period measurement have not yet been adequately evaluated. Further work is warranted to determine if such studies are of value in diagnosing diseases of the motor or sensory fibers and in elucidating their pathophysiology.

# REFERENCE SOURCES

1.  BERGMANS, J: *Physiological observations on single human nerve fibres.* In DESMEDT, JE (ED): *New Developments in Electromyography and Clinical Neurophysiology,* Vol 2. Karger, Basel, 1973, pp 89–127.

2.  BETTS, RP, JOHNSTON, DM, AND BROWN, BH: *Nerve fibre velocity and refractory period distributions in nerve trunks.* J Neurol Neurosurg Psychiatry 39:694, 1976.

3.  BISHOP, GH AND HEINBECKER, P: *Differentiation of axon types in visceral nerves by means of the potential record.* Am J Physiol 94:170, 1930.

4.  BLACKSTOCK, E, RUSHWORTH, G, AND GATH, D: *Electrophysiological studies in alcoholism.* J Neurol Neurosurg Psychiatry 35:326, 1972.

5.  BUCHTHAL, F AND ENGBAEK, L: *Refractory period and conduction velocity of the striated muscle fibre.* Acta Physiol Scand 59:199, 1963

6.  BUCHTHAL, F AND ROSENFALCK, A: *Evoked action potentials and conduction velocity in human sensory nerves.* Brain Res 3:1, 1966.

7.  BUCHTHAL, F AND ROSENFALCK, A: *Sensory potentials in polyneuropathy.* Brain 94:241, 1971.

8.  BUCHTHAL, F, ROSENFALCK, A AND TROJABORG, W: *Electrophysiological findings in entrapment of the median nerve at wrist and elbow.* J Neurol Neurosurg Psychiatry 37:340, 1974.

9.  BUNNELS, S: *Surgery of the Hand,* ed 4. JB Lippincott, Philadelphia, 1964.

10. CANNIEU, JMA: *Note sur une anastomose entre la branche profonde du cubital et le médian.* Bull Soc D'Anat Physiol Bordeaux 18:339, 1897.

11. CAVANAGH, NPC, YATES, DAH, AND SUTCLIFFE, J: *Thenar hypoplasia with associated radiologic abnormalities.* Muscle and Nerve 2:431, 1979.

12. CRUTCHFIELD, CA AND GUTMANN, L: *Hereditary aspects of accessory deep peroneal nerve.* J Neurol Neurosurg Psychiatry 36:989, 1973.

13. CUMMINS, KL, DORFMAN, LJ, AND PERKEL, DH: *Nerve fiber conduction-velocity distributions. II. Estimation based on two compound action potentials.* Electroenceph Clin Neurophysiol 46:647, 1979.

14. CUMMINS, KL, PERKEL, DH, AND DORFMAN, LJ: *Nerve fiber conduction-velocity distributions. I. Estimation based on the single-fiber and compound action potentials.* Electroenceph Clin Neurophysiol 46:634, 1979.

15. DAUBE, JR: *Percutaneous palmar median nerve stimulation for carpal tunnel syndrome.* Electroenceph Clin Neurophysiol 43:139, 1977.

16. DAVIS, FA: *Impairment of repetitive impulse conduction in experimentally demyelinated and pressure-injured nerves.* J Neurol Neurosurg Psychiatry 35:537, 1972.

17. DELBEKE, J, KOPEC, J, AND MCCOMAS, AJ: *The effects of age, temperature, and disease on the refractoriness of human nerve and muscle.* J Neurol Neurosurg Psychiatry 41:65, 1978.

18. FAISST, S AND MEYER, M: *A non-invasive computerized measurement of motor neurone refractory period and subnormal conduction in man.* Electroenceph Clin Neurophysiol, 51:548, 1981.

19. GASSEL, MM: *A study of femoral nerve conduction time.* Arch Neurol 9:607, 1963.

20. GASSEL, MM: *Sources of error in motor nerve conduction studies.* Neurology (Minneap) 14:825, 1964.

21. GILLIATT, RW AND WILLISON, RG: *The refractory and supernormal periods of the human median nerve.* J Neurol Neurosurg Psychiatry 26:136, 1963.

22. GILLIATT, RW, ET AL: *Axonal velocities of motor units in the hand and foot muscles of the baboon.* J Neurol Sci 29:249, 1976.

23. GRAHAM, HT: *The subnormal period of nerve response.* Am J Physiol 11:452, 1935.

24. GRUBER, W: *Ueber die Verbindung des Nervus medianus mit dem Nervus ulnaris am Unterarme des Menschen und der Säugethiere.* Arch Anat Physiol Med, Leipzig, 1870, pp 501–522.

25. GUTMANN, L: *Atypical deep peroneal neuropathy in presence of accessory deep peroneal nerve.* J Neurol Neurosurg Psychiatry 33:453, 1970.

26. GUTMANN, L: *Important anomalous innervations of the extremities.* American Association of Electromyography and Electrodiagnosis Meeting, 1977.

27. GUTMANN L: *Median-ulnar nerve communications and carpal tunnel syndrome.* J Neurol Neurosurg Psychiatry 40:982, 1977.

28. HODES, R, ET AL: *Low threshold associated with slow conduction velocity.* Arch Neurol 12:510, 1965.

29. HODGKIN, AL: *The Conduction of the Nervous Impulse.* The Sherrington Lectures VII, Liverpool University Press, Liverpool, 1965.

30. HOPF, HC: *Untersuchungen über die Unterschiede in der Leitgeschwindigkeit motorischer Nervenfasern beim Menschen.* Deutsche Zeitschrift Für Nervenheilkunde 183:579, 1962.

31. HOPF, HC: *Electromyographic study on so-called mononeuritis.* Arch Neurol 9:307, 1963.

32. HOPF, HC AND EYSHOLDT, M: *Impaired refractory periods of peripheral sensory nerves in multiple sclerosis.* Ann Neurol 4:499, 1978.

33. HOPF, HC AND HENSE, W: *Anomalien der motorischen Innervation an der Hand.* Z EEG-EMG 5:220, 1974.

34. HOPF, HC AND LOWITZSCH, K: *Relative refractory periods of motor nerve fibres.* In KUNZE, K AND DESMEDT, JE (EDS): *Studies on Neuromuscular Diseases.* Proceedings of the International Symposium (Giessen), Karger, Basel, 1975, pp 264–267.

35. HOPF, HC, LeQUESNE, PM, AND WILLISON, RG: *Refractory periods and lower limiting frequencies of sensory fibres of the hand.* In KUNZE, K AND DESMEDT, JE (EDS): *Studies on Neuromuscular Diseases.* Karger, Basel, 1975, pp 258–263.

36. HOPF, HC, LOWITZSCH, K, AND GALLAND, J: *Conduction velocity during the supernormal and late subnormal periods in human nerve fibres.* J Neurol 211:293, 1976.

37. INFANTE, E AND KENNEDY, WR: *Anomalous branch of the peroneal nerve detected by electromyography.* Arch Neurol 22:162, 1970.

38. ISCH, F, ET AL: *Measurement of conduction velocity of motor nerve fibres in polyneuritis and polyradiculoneuritis (abstr).* Electroenceph Clin Neurophysiol 16:416, 1964.

39. IYER, V AND FENICHEL, GM: *Normal median nerve proximal latency in carpal tunnel syndrome: A clue to coexisting Martin-Gruber anastomosis.* J Neurol Neurosurg Psychiatry 39:449, 1976.

40. JOHNSON, RK AND SHREWSBURY, MM: *Anatomical course of the thenar branch of the median nerve—Usually in a separate tunnel through the transverse carpal ligament.* J Bone Joint Surg 52A:269, 1970.

41. KADRIE, HA, ET AL: *Multiple point electrical stimulation of ulnar and median nerves.* J Neurol Neurosurg Psychiatry 39:973, 1976.

42. KAESER, HE: *Nerve conduction velocity measurements.* In VINKEN, PJ AND BRUYN, BW (EDS): *Handbook of Clinical Neurology,* Vol 7. North Holland, Amsterdam, 1970, pp 116–196.

43. KIMURA, J: *F-wave velocity in the central segment of the median and ulnar nerves. A study in normal subjects and in patients with Charcot-Marie-Tooth disease.* Neurology (Minneap) 24:539, 1974.

44. KIMURA, J: *Collision technique. Physiologic block of nerve impulses in studies of motor nerve conduction velocity.* Neurology (Minneap) 26:680, 1976.

45. KIMURA, J: *A method for estimating the refractory period of motor fibers in the human peripheral nerve.* J Neurol Sci 28:485, 1976.

46. KIMURA, J: *Electrical activity in voluntarily contracting muscle.* Arch Neurol 34:85, 1977.

47. KIMURA, J: *The carpal tunnel syndrome: Localization of conduction abnormalities within the distal segment of the median nerve.* Brain 102:619, 1979.

48. KIMURA, J: *Refractory period measurement in the clinical domain.* In WAXMAN, SA AND RITCHIE, JM (EDS): *Demyelinating Disease: Basic and Clinical Electrophysiology.* Raven Press, New York, 1981, pp 239–265.

49.  KIMURA, J, MURPHY, MJ, AND VARDA, DJ: *Electrophysiological study of anomalous innervation of intrinsic hand muscles.* Arch Neurol 33:842, 1976.

50.  KIMURA, J, YAMADA, T, AND RODNITZKY, RL: *Refractory period of human motor nerve fibres.* J Neurol Neurosurg Psychiatry 41:784, 1978.

51.  KOPEC, J, DELBEKE, J, AND McCOMAS, AJ: *Refractory period studies in a human neuromuscular preparation.* J Neurol Neurosurg Psychiatry 41:54, 1978.

52.  LAMBERT, EH: *Diagnostic value of electrical stimulation of motor nerves.* Electroenceph Clin Neurophysiol (suppl 22):9, 1962.

53.  LAMBERT, EH: *The accessory deep peroneal nerve. A common variation in innervation of extensor digitorum brevis.* Neurology (Minneap) 19:1169, 1969.

54.  LOW, PA AND McLEOD, JG: *Refractory period, conduction of trains of impulses, and effect of temperature on conduction in chronic hypertrophic neuropathy. Electrophysiological studies on the Trembler mouse.* J Neurol Neurosurg Psychiatry 40:434, 1977.

55.  LOWITZSCH, K AND HOPF, HC: *Refractory periods and propagation of repetitive mixed nerve action potentials in severe and mild neuropathy.* In HAUSMANOWA-PETRUSEWICZ, I AND JEDRZEJOWSKA, H (EDS): *Structure and Function of Normal and Diseased Muscle and Peripheral Nerve.* Proceedings of the Symposium (Kazimierz upon Vistula, Poland) Polish Medical Publisher, 1972.

56.  LOWITZSCH, K, HOPF, HC, AND SCHLEGEL, HJ: *Conduction of two or more impulses in relation to the fibre spectrum in the mixed human peripheral nerve.* In DESMEDT, JE (ED): *New Developments in Electromyography and Clinical Neurophysiology,* Vol 2. Karger, Basel, 1973, pp 272–278.

57.  MANNERFELT, L: *Studies on the hand in ulnar nerve paralysis. A clinical-experimental investigation in normal and anomalous innervation.* Acta Orthopaedica Scand (suppl 87):23, 1966.

58.  MARINACCI, AA: *Diagnosis of "all median hand."* Bull LA Neurol Soc 29:191, 1964.

59.  MARTIN, R: *Tal om Nervers allmanna Egenskapper i Manniskans Kropp.* L Salvius, Stockholm, 1763.

60.  MAURER, K, HOPF, HC, AND LOWITZSCH, K: *Hypokalemia shortens relative refractory period of peripheral sensory nerves in man.* J Neurol 216:67, 1977.

61.  NEUNDÖRFER, B AND SEIBERTH, R: *The accessory deep peroneal nerve.* J Neurol 209:125, 1975.

62.  PAINTAL, AS: *Block of conduction in mammalian myelinated nerve fibres by low temperatures.* J Physiol (Lond) 180:1, 1965.

63.  PAINTAL, AS: *Effects of temperature on conduction in single vagal and saphenous myelinated nerve fibres of the cat.* J Physiol (Lond) 180:20, 1965.

64.  PINELLI, P: *Physical, anatomical and physiological factors in the latency measurement of the M response.* Electroenceph Clin Neurophysiol 17:86, 1964.

65.  POLONI, AE AND SALA, E: *The conduction velocity of the ulnar and median nerves stimulated through a twin-needle electrode.* Electroenceph Clin Neurophysiol (suppl 22):17, 1962.

66.  RICHIE, P: *Le nerf cubital et les muscles de l'éminence thénar.* Bull Mem Soc Anat Paris 72:251, (Series 5) 1897.

67.  ROTH, G: *Vitesse de conduction motrice du nerf médian dans le canal carpien.* Ann Med Physique 13:117, 1970.

68.  SEDDON, H: *Surgical Disorders of the Peripheral Nerves,* ed 2. Churchill Livingstone, Edinburgh, 1975, pp 203–211.

69.  SIMPSON, JA: *Fact and fallacy in measurement of conduction velocity in motor nerves.* J Neurol Neurosurg Psychiatry 27:381, 1964.

70.  SKORPIL, V: *Conduction velocity of human nerve structures.* Roszpr Cesk Akad Ved 75:1, 1965.

71.  SMITH, KJ: *A sensitive method for detection and quantification of conduction deficits in nerve.* J Neurol Sci 48:191, 1980.

72.  SMITH, KJ AND HALL, SM: *Nerve conduction during peripheral demyelination and remyelination.* J Neurol Sci 48:201, 1980.

73. STREIB, EW: *Ulnar-to-median nerve anastomosis in the forearm: Electromyographic studies.* Neurology (New York) 29:1534, 1979.

74. SUNDERLAND, S: *Nerves and Nerve Injuries,* ed 2. Churchill Livingstone, Edinburgh, 1978.

75. TACKMANN, W AND LEHMANN, HJ: *Refractory period in human sensory nerve fibres.* Europ Neurol 12:277, 1974.

76. TACKMANN, W AND LEHMANN, HJ: *Relative refractory period of median nerve sensory fibres in the carpal tunnel syndrome.* Europ Neurol 12:309, 1974.

77. TASAKI, I: *Nervous Transmission.* Charles C Thomas, Springfield, Ill, 1953.

78. THOMAS, PK, SEARS, TA, AND GILLIATT, RW: *The range of conduction velocity in normal motor nerve fibres to the small muscles of the hand and foot.* J Neurol Neurosurg Psychiatry 22:175, 1959.

79. VAN DER MOST VAN SPIJK, D, HOOGLAND, RA, AND DIJKSTRA, S: *Conduction velocities compared and related to degrees of renal insufficiency.* In DESMEDT, JE (ED): *New Developments in Electromyography and Clinical Neurophysiology,* Vol 2. Karger, Basel, 1973, pp 381–389.

80. WAXMAN, SG, ET AL: *Dependence of refractory period measurements on conduction distance: A computer simulation analysis.* Electroenceph Clin Neurophysiol 47:717, 1979.

81. WIEDERHOLT, WC: *Median nerve conduction velocity in sensory fibers through carpal tunnel.* Arch Phys Med Rehabil 51:328, 1970.

82. WILBOURN, AJ AND LAMBERT, EH: *The forearm median-to-ulnar nerve communication: Electrodiagnostic aspects.* Neurology (Minneap) 26:368, 1976.

83. WINCKLER, G: *Le nerf péronier accessoire profond: Etude d'anatomie comparée.* Arch Anat Histol Embryol 18:181, 1934.

# PART 3

# ASSESSMENT OF NEUROMUSCULAR TRANSMISSION

# ANATOMY AND PHYSIOLOGY OF THE NEUROMUSCULAR JUNCTION

The neuromuscular junction is a synaptic structure that consists of the motor nerve terminal, the junctional cleft, and the muscle end-plate. Its chemical mode of transmission by release of acetylcholine (ACh) is fundamentally different from the electrical propagation of impulses that occurs in nerve and muscle. One of the important features of chemical as opposed to electrical transmission is the property of unidirectional conduction. This is achieved by the release of a transmitter substance from the axon terminal across the junctional cleft onto the muscle end-plate. The same basic principle applies to synaptic transmission in a sequence of neurons. In contrast, the nerve axons conduct an impulse in either direction, orthodromically or antidromically.

There are other physiologic characteristics common to the nerve synapse and neuromuscular junction. Analogous to synaptic delay, transmission at the muscle end-plate requires a fraction of a millisecond. Like a synapse, the neuromuscular junction fatigues when its store of immediately available neurotransmitters is depleted and its mobilization store cannot keep pace with transmitter liberation. Both synaptic and end-plate potentials are graded and nonpropagating. These local potentials are not associated with refractoriness. This is in contrast to the all-or-none response of the propagating nerve action potential, which is always followed by a refractory period. The graded response allows temporal as well as spatial summation of subliminal stimuli, thereby providing greater flexibility and adaptability.

This section will describe the physiology related to the nerve action potential at the neuromuscular junction. First, an overview of this complex event will be presented here, in preparation for a more detailed discussion on the following pages. In the presynaptic ending there are many minute vesicles, each containing up to 10,000 ACh molecules. At rest these vesicles are randomly released into the junctional cleft. When they reach the muscle end-plate, small depolarizations of the postsynaptic membrane occur. These miniature end-plate potentials (MEPP) do not attain the critical level for generation of a muscle action potential. If the motor nerve is activated and a propagating impulse reaches the nerve terminal, depolarization of the presynaptic ending triggers an influx of calcium ($Ca^{++}$) into the axon terminals, initiating the calcium-dependent release of a large number of ACh vesicles into the junctional cleft. The greatly enhanced and synchronized release of ACh gives rise to a localized nonpropagated depolarization of the postsynaptic membrane. This end-plate potential (EPP) is the result of summation of multiple MEPPs. When the EPP exceeds the excitability thresh-old of the muscle cell, an action potential is generated. Propagation of the muscle potential activates the contractile elements via excitation-contraction coupling.

# ANATOMY OF THE NEUROMUSCULAR JUNCTION

## End-plate

The name motor end-plate was originally used to describe the specialized efferent endings that terminate on a striated muscle as a whole. However, the muscle postsyn-aptic membrane alone is now commonly referred to as the end-plate. There is usually only one end-plate in each muscle fiber, and each branch of a motor axon innervates one end-plate. The myelin sheath of the motor nerve fiber is lost at the nerve terminals. Distal to the myelin sheath are Schwann cells, which separate the nerve terminals from the surrounding tissue. Thus, the neuromuscular junction consists of the motor nerve ending, Schwann cell, and muscle end-plate (Fig. 8-1). At the junctional region between the nerve ending and end-plate, Schwann cells are absent. Here, the nerve ending is found as a flattened plate lying within a surface depression of the end-plate. This

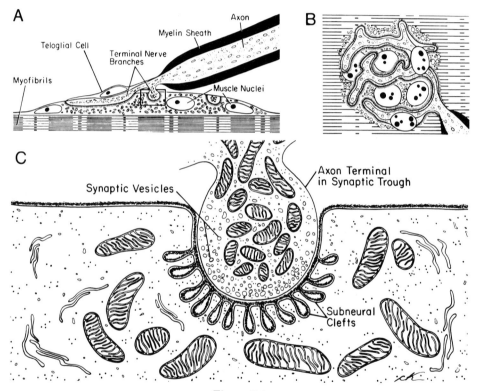

Figure 8-1
Motor end-plate as seen in histologic sections in the long axis of the muscle fiber (A) and in surface view (B) under the light microscope, and a section through the motor end-plate (an area in the rectangle on A) under the electron microscope (C). The myelin sheath ends at the junction at which the axon terminal fits into the synaptic cleft. The Schwann (teloglial) cells cover the re-maining portion without extending into the primary cleft. The plasma membrane of axon (axolem-ma) and that of muscle fiber (sarcolemma) form the presynaptic and postsynaptic membrane of the end-plate, respectively. Interdigitation of the sarcolemma gives rise to the subneural or secondary clefts. The axon terminal contains synaptic vesicles and mitochondria. (From Bloom and Fawcett,[4] with permission.)

indentation of the muscle fiber, called a synaptic gutter or a primary synaptic cleft, is about 200 to 500 angstrom deep. The postsynaptic membrane in this region is thickened and has narrow infoldings called junctional folds or secondary clefts. A large number of mitochondria, nuclei, and small granules accumulate close to the secondary clefts. Many mitochondria and synaptic vesicles also lie in the axon terminals, just proximal to the presynaptic membrane.

The ultrastructural features of the end-plates in human external intercostal muscles have been clearly delineated by Engel and Santa[20] and may be summarized as follows. Approximately 50 synaptic vesicles per $\mu m^2$ are contained in a nerve terminal that occupies an area close to 4 $\mu m^2$. The postsynaptic membrane is 10 times longer than the presynaptic membrane. The total area covered by the postsynaptic folds is about two and a half times that of the terminal itself. In diseases of neuromuscular transmission the average end-plate profile shows characteristic alterations (Fig. 8-2). In myasthenia gravis, the area occupied by the terminal is reduced, showing a simplified appearance of the postsynaptic folds. Conversely, in the myasthenic syndrome,[12] the nerve terminal area remains normal but the postsynaptic membrane is increased in length as well as in area. Marked hypertrophy of the postsynaptic membrane occurs in some end-plates. The mean synaptic vesicle diameter and mean synaptic vesicle count per unit nerve terminal area are not significantly altered in either disease. Ultrastructural changes of the motor end-plates have been observed in clinically unaffected limb muscles in patients with ocular myasthenia gravis.[53]

## Synaptic vesicles

Acetylcholine (ACh) is present inside the nerve endings, encapsulated within minute intracellular structures called synaptic vesicles. These vesicles are 300 to 500 angstrom in diameter and are usually concentrated in the presynaptic axoplasm. In addition to

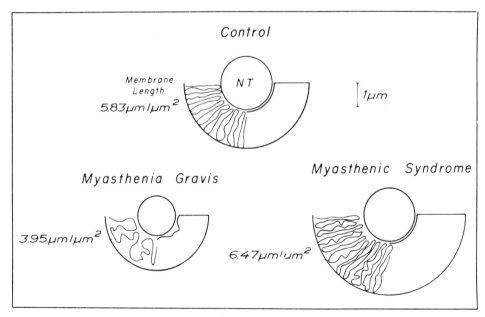

Figure 8-2
Diagrammatic representation of the motor end-plates in control, myasthenia gravis, and myasthenic syndrome drawn to the scale of the mean figure. Compared with the normal fine structure of the postsynaptic membrane there is oversimplification in myasthenia gravis and marked hypertrophy in myasthenic syndrome. (From Engel and Santa,[19] with permission.)

ACh, the nerve endings contain high concentrations of cholineacetylase which synthesizes ACh, and acetylcholinesterase which hydrolyzes ACh. The neurotransmitter and the two enzymes are also found, although to a much lesser extent, in the proximal portions of neurons, presumably because the enzymes are synthesized in the cell body before being transported to the nerve terminals.[41] It is estimated that 5000 to 10,000 molecules of ACh are contained in a vesicle.[30] This is referred to as a quantum. Some quanta (about 1000) are immediately available for release, being located adjacent to the cell membrane. Many more quanta (10,000) are contained in the mobilization store and move towards the membrane to continuously replace liberated ACh. The remaining and largest portion of quanta (300,000) forms the main store and is not directly available for release, constituting instead a reserve supply for the mobilization store.

# ELECTRICAL ACTIVITY AT THE END-PLATE

In the resting state, the interior of the muscle fibers is negatively charged, relative to the exterior, by about 90 mV. As discussed in Chapter 2, this transmembrane potential is primarily the result of an unequal distribution of inorganic ions across the membrane with a high concentration of potassium ($K^+$) intracellularly and of sodium ($Na^+$) and chloride ($Cl^-$) extracellularly. It also depends on differential permeability across the muscle membrane with a high conductance for potassium and chloride, and low conductance for sodium. The electrochemical potential equilibrium is maintained by the energy-dependent sodium-potassium pump, which compensates for a slight inward movement of sodium and outward movement of potassium at steady state (see Fig. 2-1).

## Miniature end-plate potential

The end-plates of many resting muscle fibers show a spontaneous subliminal electrical activity called miniature end-plate potential (MEPP). It represents a small depolarization of the postsynaptic membrane induced by sustained but random release of a single quantum of acetylcholine (ACh) from the nerve terminal.[25] The MEPP can be recorded with an ordinary needle electrode placed near the end-plate of the muscle fibers. For more quantitative analysis, however, a microelectrode must be inserted directly into the end-plate region to achieve a higher resolution. Each ACh quantum liberated from the nerve terminal contains a nearly equal number of ACh molecules, which is unaffected by external factors such as temperature or ionic concentration. In contrast, the frequency of the MEPP varies over a wide range. It increases with elevated temperatures and upon depolarization of the motor nerve terminals. It decreases with deficiency of calcium ($Ca^{++}$), the ion known to enhance quantal release by increasing fusion of the ACh vesicles with the membrane of the nerve terminal.

The amplitude of the MEPP, sometimes referred to as quantum size, is determined not only by the amount of ACh molecules in a vesicle but also by various other factors, such as diffusion properties of the liberated molecules, structural characteristics of the end-plate, and sensitivity of the ACh receptors. In normal human intercostal muscles, an MEPP occurs roughly every five seconds and is approximately 1 mV in amplitude when recorded intracellularly.[15] Hence, the MEPP is much below the excitability threshold of the muscle fiber and is about 1 percent of the normal end-plate potential (EPP) generated by a volley of nerve impulses. The amplitude of the MEPP is greatly reduced by a small dose of curare and is increased by neostigmine (Prostigmin).[35] The MEPPs are abolished by denervation and by nerve anesthesia. In myasthenia gravis, the average amplitude of the MEPP is reduced as a result of receptor deficiency, but the discharge frequency is normal. Conversely, the MEPP is normal in amplitude but occurs at an abnormally reduced rate in the myasthenic syndrome and in botulism, indicating defective release of ACh.

# End-plate potential

As mentioned earlier, spontaneous release of a single quantum of ACh causes MEPP that is far below the critical level necessary for generation of a muscle action potential. With the arrival of a nerve impulse, depolarization of the motor nerve ending initiates an influx of calcium into the motor axons. The increased amount of calcium accelerates fusion of the vesicle membrane with the nerve terminal membrane, thereby producing a large increase in the rate of quantal release. Massive synchronized release of ACh triggered by the arrival of a nerve action potential results in summation of many MEPPs, giving rise to a localized EPP. The amount of ACh released and the size of the EPP depend on the number of ACh quanta immediately available for the release and the concentration of calcium within the axon terminal, which in turn is determined by the level of depolarization. The mean number of quanta emitted per nerve impulse is sometimes called quantum content. It can approximately be calculated by dividing the mean amplitude of an EPP by the mean amplitude of the MEPP and is estimated to be about 100. To measure an EPP it is, of course, necessary to block muscle action potentials which otherwise would interfere with accurate recording.

Like MEPPs, EPPs are attributable to the depolarization of the motor end-plate by ACh. Under the influence of the synaptic transmitter, conductance of various diffusible ions, principally sodium and potassium, is increased. During this period, therefore, sodium and potassium ions move freely down their electrochemical gradients. The net result is depolarization of the motor end-plate. The EPP is a nonpropagated local response that declines exponentially with increasing distance from the end-plate. It may be characterized by its rise time, amplitude, and duration. It normally begins about 0.5 ms after the release of ACh, reaches its peak in about 0.8 ms, and decreases exponentially with a half decay time of about 3.0 ms. Like the excitatory postsynaptic potentials, the EPP is a graded response that can be modified by the amount of ACh quanta liberated from the nerve terminal. The degree of depolarization is also dependent upon the sensitivity of the end-plate to the depolarizing action of ACh. The important characteristic is that two or more subthreshold EPPs generated in near synchrony can summate to cause a depolarization exceeding the critical level for generation of an action potential.

# EXCITATION-CONTRACTION COUPLING

## Generation of muscle action potential

When the end-plate potential (EPP) reaches a critical level of depolarization called threshold, a muscle action potential is generated. This is an all-or-none phenomenon. A molecular change of the depolarized membrane results in the selective increase of sodium ($Na^+$) conductance followed by an increase in potassium ($K^+$) conductance. These changes are inherent to the muscle membrane, occurring irrespective of the nature of stimulus, as long as depolarization exceeds the critical value. In normal muscles, the EPP generated by a single nerve impulse is always more than adequate to excite the muscle fibers. Once the action potential is generated at the end-plate, it is propagated bidirectionally to the remaining parts of the fiber to initiate contraction. This is analogous to the propagated action potential in nerve axons, but the conduction velocity is only in the range of 3 to 5 m/s along the muscle membrane, compared with 60 m/s over the nerve.[44] A neuromuscular block results when the EPP fails to reach threshold. A subliminal EPP may be caused by insufficient liberation of ACh from the axon terminal or reduced sensitivity of the muscle end-plate. Although the generation of a muscle action potential is all-or-none for each muscle fiber, the size of the compound muscle action potential is graded, as it depends on the number of muscle fibers in which action potentials are elicited.

## Transverse and longitudinal tubules and triad

The action potential elicited at the motor end-plate in response to a nerve impulse spreads throughout the muscle fiber to activate muscle contraction. This link between electrical and mechanical activity is referred to as excitation-contraction coupling. Electrical activity of a muscle fiber can be separated temporally into two main components attributable to different structures within the fiber.[8] The first component originates at the motor end-plate and spreads along the outer surface of the muscle fiber. The second electrical component occurs within a complex tubular system that surrounds and interpenetrates the muscle fiber. This system is called the transverse tubular system, because of its transverse orientation relative to the axis of the muscle fiber. In man, tubules are found at the junctions of the A and I bands (see Fig. 11-1). This tridimensional network is structurally internal to the cell but is also continuous with extracellular fluid. Thus, the transverse tubules contain extracellular fluid and are surrounded by intracellular fluid. Consequently, the inside of the tubule is electropositive relative to the outside. Muscle action potentials are propagated along the tubules into the depth of the muscle.

Under the electron microscope, it can be seen that the myofibrils of a muscle fiber are surrounded by a second tubular system called the longitudinal tubule, or sarcoplasmic reticulum (Fig. 8-3). In contrast to the transverse tubules, these tubules are oriented longitudinally with respect to the myofibrillar axis and form a closed system devoid of continuity with either extracellular fluids or sarcoplasm. They appear as fenestrated sacs surrounding the myofibrils. The longitudinal tubules expand to form bulbous terminal cisterns on both sides of the transverse tubules where they come into close contact. The two terminal cisterns and one interposed transverse tubule form a triad in longitudinal sections of the muscle.

## Role of calcium ions

It is assumed that electromechanical coupling occurs when propagated action potentials invade the muscle fibers along the transverse tubules and come into contact with the terminal cisterns of the longitudinal tubules at the triad. Here, the action potential of the transverse tubule is coupled to the sarcoplasmic reticulum and is associated with a small electrical potential referred to as intramembranous charge movement.[7] As the action potential crosses the terminal cistern, calcium ($Ca^{++}$) is released from the longitudinal tubules into the sarcoplasm. The presence of calcium in the sarcoplasm surrounding the myofilaments initiates a chemical interaction that leads to the formation of bridges between thin and thick filaments (see Fig. 11-1). Sliding of thin filaments against thick filaments results in contraction of the myofibril, as will be further described in Chapter 11. At the end of the muscle action potential, calcium is rapidly resequestered into the longitudinal tubules, lowering the concentration of sarcoplasmic calcium. The myofibers relax as adenosine-triphosphate (ATP) breaks the existing bridges between filaments.

# POSTSYNAPTIC ABNORMALITIES

## Pathophysiology of myasthenia gravis

Intracellular recordings from the intercostal muscles have clearly delineated electrophysiologic abnormalities in myasthenia gravis.[15] At rest, miniature end-plate potentials (MEPP) occur at normal or nearly normal frequency but are significantly reduced in amplitude (i.e., quantum size is reduced). The end-plate potential (EPP) elicited by a nerve impulse is also reduced in amplitude. The number of acetylcholine (ACh) quanta liberated by a single volley remains unchanged (i.e., normal EPP quantum content is

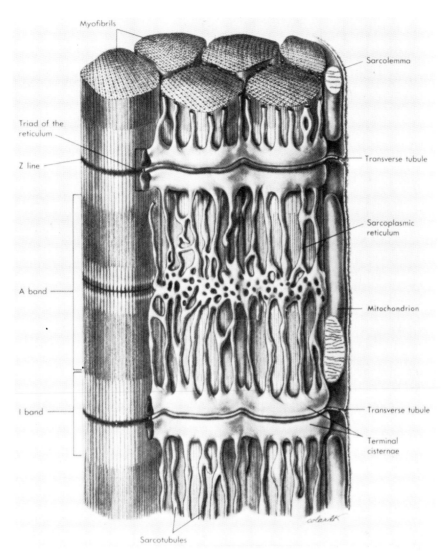

Myofibrils

Sarcolemma

Triad of the reticulum

Z line

Transverse tubule

Sarcoplasmic reticulum

A band

Mitochondrion

I band

Transverse tubule

Terminal cisternae

Sarcotubules

Figure 8-3

Anatomic relationship between the perpendicularly oriented longitudinal and transverse tubules. Electromechanical coupling is initiated at the triad of the reticulum which consists of two terminal cisterns of the longitudinal tubules and one transverse tubule between them. (From Bloom and Fawcett,[4] with permission.)

preserved). On repetitive stimulation, the number of quanta released falls gradually, as it does in a normal muscle, causing a progressive decrease in the amplitude of the EPP. With successive stimuli, progressively fewer muscle fibers generate action potentials as the EPP becomes insufficient to bring the membrane potential to the critical level. Abnormalities of neuromuscular transmission in myasthenia are more common in small motor units, perhaps because they have a lower margin of safety than the large motor units.[32, 33]

The MEPP may be reduced in amplitude because of (1) decreased numbers of ACh molecules per quantum; (2) diffusional loss of ACh within the synaptic cleft; or (3) reduced sensitivity of the ACh receptors. A presynaptic abnormality was originally thought to be present in myasthenic muscles, because postsynaptic sensitivity to carbachol and decamethonium added to the bath solution appeared to be normal.[17] This finding, however, has not been confirmed by further morphologic and electrophysiologic investigations. Indeed, microiontophoretic application of ACh at the end-plate region has since disclosed impaired postsynaptic sensitivity to ACh.[1] The observed electrophysiologic changes may also be explained on the basis of diffusional ACh loss, which can be correlated with alterations in postsynaptic membrane structure.

## Morphologic and immunologic changes

Ultrastructural histometric studies in myasthenic intercostal muscles have shown distinct deviation of the end-plate profile from normal, indicating postsynaptic membrane abnormalities.[20] More recent experiments have revealed three types of neuromuscular junctions in the surface fibers of internal and external intercostal muscles of myasthenics.[1] One group (about 25 percent) associated with mild morphologic alterations responded to the nerve stimulation with EPPs of sufficiently large amplitude to trigger an action potential. A second group, characterized histologically by a grossly altered postjunctional membrane, showed marked reduction not only in amplitude but also in frequency of the MEPP, and in amplitude of the EPP. In the last group, the end-plate was totally degenerated, showing neither MEPPs nor EPPs.

While morphologic alterations are not observed at every myasthenic end-plate, diminished MEPP amplitude can be demonstrated uniformly. It may be argued, therefore, that changes in end-plate geometry per se are not totally responsible for the physiologic defect. Using radioactively labelled alpha-bungarotoxin, a snake poison which binds to the ACh receptor, it has been shown that functional receptor sites are decreased in number in myasthenia gravis.[14, 24, 27] Further, the number of functioning ACh receptors is positively correlated with the mean amplitude of the MEPP.[31] These findings indicate the presence of an ACh receptor abnormality in myasthenia gravis. A similar physiologic defect can be produced by partially blocking the ACh receptors with curare.

Plasma exchange has been used to investigate the function of an anti-ACh receptor antibody in patients with myasthenia gravis. The inverse relationship between clinical muscle strength and antibody titers is consistent with the view that the antibody is the most important factor impairing neuromuscular transmission.[43] The exact mechanisms by which antibodies mediate obstruction of the ACh receptor is not known, but binding of antibody and complement to the receptor zone of the postsynaptic membrane has been demonstrated in myasthenic muscles.[22] Intercostal muscle biopsies show reduced number of ACh receptors in patients with myasthenia gravis.[40] In addition, antibodies are bound to many of the remaining receptors.

## Experimental models

Morphologic and physiologic abnormalities in experimental autoimmune myasthenia gravis are similar to those observed in human myasthenia gravis.[23, 46, 51] In rats with experimental autoimmune myasthenia gravis, receptor content is reduced, and receptor bound antibody is increased. These observations are consistent with the view that a reduced number of fully active receptors is primarily responsible for defective neuromuscular transmission in myasthenia gravis.[40] Disorders of the receptor protein complex in these experimental models are associated with the same electrophysiologic abnormalities as those described in the human disease. Typical histologic and electrophysiologic myasthenic features occur in mice after passive transfer of human serum fractions obtained from patients with myasthenia gravis.[52] Reduction of postsynaptic sensitivity to depolarization renders myasthenic muscles resistant to decamethonium, a neuromuscular blocking agent that causes paralysis by persistent depolarization of the end-plate region in normal muscle.[42] Antibodies to the ACh receptor do not impair the ionophore, an ion conductance modulator protein thought to control the permeability change following a reaction of ACh with ACh receptor.[49]

Intracellular recordings from muscle end-plates of immunized rabbits show reduced amplitude of MEPPs but a normal number of ACh quanta release per nerve impulse.[18] In rats with chronic experimental myasthenia, the amplitude of MEPPs is reduced, but ACh output at rest and during stimulation remains normal.[36] Following passive transfer of human myasthenia gravis to rats, reduction of MEPP amplitude does not develop immediately but occurs after the first 24 hours, reaching minimum levels by six days.[29] The delayed development of reduced MEPP amplitude indicates that a simple curarelike block of ACh receptors by IgG antibodies cannot be the sole mechanism for the defective neuromuscular transmission produced by myasthenic serum.[29]

# PRESYNAPTIC ABNORMALITIES

## Pathophysiology of myasthenic syndromes

In contrast to the receptor insensitivity of myasthenia gravis, the myasthenic syndrome[12] is characterized by defective release of acetylcholine (ACh) quanta. In this syndrome, microelectrode recordings from excised intercostal muscles reveal a normal amplitude (normal quantum size) of the miniature end-plate potentials (MEPP) and normal sensitivity of the muscle end-plate to ACh. However, since frequency of the MEPP does not increase with depolarization of the motor nerve terminal,[38] the number of ACh quanta released per single nerve impulse is much less than the normal value (small quantum content). Consequently, the end-plate potential (EPP) following a single nerve impulse is too small to trigger an action potential in some muscle fibers, leading to a reduced amplitude of the compound muscle action potential.[39]

The actual number of quanta available in the presynaptic store is probably normal, since the defect improves immediately with various maneuvers to prime the nerve terminals.[16] For example, the EPP increases progressively with repetitive stimulation of the nerve. An increase of external calcium (Ca$^{++}$) or the addition of guanidine also enhances the EPP. The low quantum number of the EPP results therefore most likely from a low probability of quantum release at the nerve terminal. Indeed, ultrastructural studies have revealed no alteration in the mean nerve terminal area or in the synaptic vesicle count per unit nerve terminal area.[20]

A new myasthenic syndrome with different types of presynaptic abnormalities has recently been described.[21] The defect is associated with deficient muscle acetylcholinesterase, decreased frequency but normal amplitude of the MEPP, decreased number of quanta liberated per nerve impulse, small nerve terminals, and focal degeneration of the postsynaptic membrane. A low number of quanta per EPP apparently results primarily from a reduced store rather than from a low probability of release, as in the case of the classic myasthenic syndrome. A congenital defect in the molecular assembly of acetylcholinesterase or its attachment to the postsynaptic membrane might represent the basic abnormality. A familial congenital myasthenic syndrome probably attributable to deficient synthesis of ACh has also been reported.[28]

## Effect of botulinum and other toxins

Defective calcium-dependent ACh release is also responsible for reduced amplitude of the EPP in a number of other conditions. In a nerve-muscle preparation blocked by botulinum toxin, the frequency of the MEPP is not affected by the addition of calcium but is significantly increased by the spider venom known to neutralize the toxin. Thus, reduced amplitude of the EPP in botulism is caused neither by blockage of calcium entry into the nerve nor by deficient storage of ACh vesicles. The toxin may interfere with the ACh release process itself, possibly by blocking exocytosis at the release sites.[34] Neuromuscular block has been produced by high concentrations of magnesium.[5,47] Experimental evidence also indicates an inhibitory effect of manganese on transmitter release at the neuromuscular junction.[2] Aminoglycoside antibiotics such as neomycin and kanamycin probably interfere with ACh release, but postsynaptic block may also play a role.[9]

# RECOVERY CYCLES OF NEUROMUSCULAR TRANSMISSION

## Release of acetylcholine molecules

The number of acetylcholine (ACh) molecules released by a nerve action potential is determined by the amount of ACh in the immediately available store and the concentration of calcium ($Ca^{++}$) at the nerve terminal. Paired or repetitive stimulation affects the release of ACh and the end-plate potential (EPP) in two opposing manners. First, there is a relative reduction in the amount of available ACh following release of a portion of the store. Thus, a smaller number of ACh quanta are released by subsequent stimuli until the mobilization store has refilled the immediately available store. On the other hand, there is a relative increase in ACh release because of accumulation of calcium in the nerve terminal. These two opposing phenomena occur in parallel but with different time courses.[11]

The recovery of the ACh store, partially depleted following the first stimulus, occurs exponentially in 5 to 10 seconds through the slow reloading of ACh ejection sites. Influx of calcium into the terminal axons takes place immediately after the nerve is depolarized, but the ion diffuses out of the axon over the next 100 to 200 ms. Accumulation of calcium, therefore, is most prominent when paired or repetitive stimulation is used with an interstimulus interval of less than 100 to 200 ms. At such fast rates of stimulation, release of ACh tends to be facilitated despite some reduction in the amount of ACh in the immediately available store. In contrast, depression of ACh release occurs with slower rates of repetition since, at such long interstimulus intervals, the negligible facilitation attributable to the electrosecretory mechanism no longer compensates for the reduction of the ACh store. Depression may also occur at high rates of stimulation, if the rate of ACh release far exceeds the rate of mobilization, leading to substantial depletion of the ACh store.

## Neuromuscular depression and facilitation

Reduction in the number of ACh quanta released by the second of two nerve impulses is referred to as neuromuscular depression. It results in a smaller EPP. The amplitude of the second compound muscle action potential decreases as EPPs no longer reach threshold in some muscle fibers. This is represented by a decrement of the muscle response to the second supramaximal stimulus. Conversely, an increase in the number of quanta released by the second nerve impulse is referred to as neuromuscular facilitation. A larger EPP as a result of facilitation must be differentiated from one caused by summation of two EPPs elicited nearly simultaneously by paired shocks with a very short interstimulus interval.[11] Both facilitation and summation result in larger compound muscle action potentials through recruitment, provided that there are additional muscle fibers to be recruited.

An increment of the muscle response through recruitment must also be differentiated from an increased amplitude without change in the number of activated muscle fibers. This phenomenon, called pseudofacilitation, simply represents better synchronization of individual muscle fiber potentials, without additional recruitment. In these instances there is no change in the total area under the waveform, which is directly proportional to the number of active muscle fibers. Whereas the total area is a more accurate indicator for the recruitment of muscle fibers, the amplitude can also be used, provided that the waveform remains relatively unchanged during repetitive stimulation.

## Normal recovery cycle

To establish the recovery cycle of neuromuscular transmission, the muscle action potentials are recorded after delivering paired stimuli to the nerve at various interstimulus intervals. The results are difficult to interpret for the first few milliseconds, since with such a short interstimulus interval, the nerve axons and muscle fibers are totally or partially inexcitable after the passage of the first impulse. Therefore, the time course of the recovery curve reflects the refractory period of the nerve and muscle in addition to the alteration of neuromuscular transmission (Fig. 8-4). With slightly longer inter-

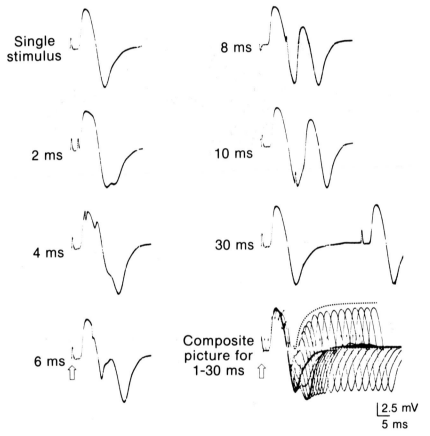

$|$ 2.5 mV

5 ms

Figure 8-4

Except for the top tracing on the left and the bottom tracing on the right, paired shocks were delivered to the median nerve at the wrist with time intervals ranging from 2 to 30 ms between conditioning (arrow) and test stimuli. The action potentials were recorded from the thenar muscles. The top tracing on the left shows a response to a single stimulus. The bottom tracing on the right is a composite picture made by superimposition of 20 paired shocks with interstimulus intervals systematically varying from 1 to 30 ms. The conditioning response of each pair appears in the same spot on the photo, superimposed exactly on top of the other. In contrast, the test responses are displaced successively according to the interstimulus interval of each pair. An imaginary line connecting the peaks of the sequential test responses represents the time course of neuromuscular excitability change following the conditioning stimulus. (From Kimura,[37] with permission.)

stimulus intervals, the effect of the refractory period is minimal, but for intervals up to 10 to 15 ms, muscle potentials cannot be measured accurately, because the first and second muscle responses overlap. With a longer interstimulus interval, the second compound muscle potential is identical in size to the first in the normal muscles. This finding, however, does not necessarily imply that the EEPs elicited by the first and second stimuli are the same.

Indeed, at interstimulus intervals up to 100 to 200 ms, the second EPP may be greater than the first reflecting a greater number of liberated quanta owing to neurosecretory potentiation. Since the EPP in response to the first stimulus exceeds the threshold of excitation in all normal muscle fibers, however, no additional recruitment is possible by the second stimulus. At a slow rate of stimulation, the number of ACh quanta released by the second stimulus is reduced even in normal muscles. Because of a large margin of safety, however, the decreased amount of ACh is still more than

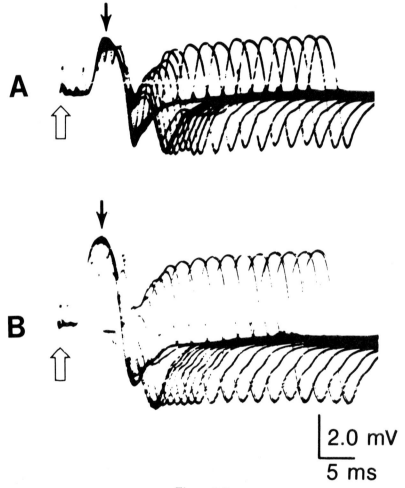

2.0 mV

5 ms

Figure 8-5

Composite pictures by superimposition of 20 paired responses from the thenar muscles. Paired stimuli were applied (open arrow) to the median nerve with interstimulus intervals ranging from 1 to 30 ms. (Compare Figure 8-4.) The conditioning response of each pair appears in the same spot of each tracing (arrows pointing down), whereas the test response is delayed according to the interstimulus interval of each pair. There is no apparent difference in the recovery curve of neuromuscular systems between a patient with myasthenia gravis (A) and a normal control (B).

adequate to cause an EPP well above the critical level of excitation in all muscle fibers. In normal muscles, therefore, the size of the compound muscle action potential remains unaltered, despite changes in the amount of ACh released in response to the second or subsequent stimuli.

## Effects of disease states

In partially curarized mammalian muscle, depression of the second muscle potential of a pair is closely related to the recovery cycle of the EPP, which reflects variations in the number of ACh quanta released by the second stimulus.[6, 10, 13] At interstimulus intervals up to 100 to 200 ms, there is calcium-dependent facilitation.[3, 10, 50] Thus, the second muscle response is equal to or greater than the first response for such short stimulus intervals. At longer intervals, the second response is smaller than the first, reflecting

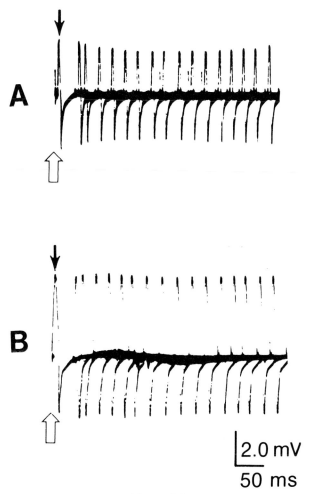

Figure 8-6
Composite pictures of 16 paired responses from the thenar muscles arranged in the same manner as in Figure 8-5. Paired shocks were delivered (open arrow) to the median nerve with interstimulus intervals ranging from 30 to 400 ms. The conditioning response of each pair appears in the same spot of each tracing (arrows pointing down), whereas the test responses are delayed successively. There was a mild but definite reduction in amplitude of the test response at the interstimulus intervals of 150 to 250 ms in the myasthenic muscle (A), but not in the normal muscle (B).

depletion of available ACh quanta in the face of a reduced margin of safety due to receptor insensitivity. The maximal depression occurs at interstimulus intervals ranging from 300 to 600 ms. This is followed by slow recovery to the control value in about 10 seconds, when ACh becomes more available through replenishment of the stores. With repetitive stimulation, the maximal depression of muscle potential occurs at the rate of about 2 to 3 per second, which is fast enough for ACh to be depleted but slow

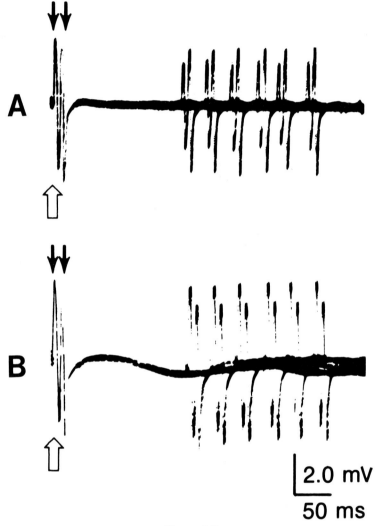

Figure 8-7

Composite pictures similar to those shown in Figures 8-5 and 8-6. Unlike the previous tracings, paired shocks with interstimulus intervals of 10 ms were used for both conditioning and test stimuli. The paired test stimuli were delivered 200 to 400 ms after the paired conditioning stimuli (open arrow). The double peaked conditioning responses appear in the same spot of each tracing (paired arrows). The second peak of the pair was slightly displaced downwards but there was no difference in amplitude of the two peaks in either myasthenia gravis (A) or in normal controls (B). In myasthenia gravis, the first peak of each test response was significantly reduced following depletion of acetylcholine (ACh) by the conditioning stimuli. The second peak of each test response, elicited 10 ms after the first, however, was considerably greater, indicating the summation of the two end-plate potentials (EPP). In the normal muscle, the first peak of the test response was of maximal size because of the margin of safety, precluding any further amplitude increase of the second peak.

enough for calcium to diffuse out of the axon. In myasthenic muscles, the neuromuscular safety margin is reduced, because the number of functional ACh receptors is small. The smaller amount of ACh, released in response to the second stimulus, then fails to activate some muscle fibers. The recovery cycle of the muscle action potential, therefore, is similar to that of curarized muscle (Figs. 8-5, 8-6, 8-7, and 8-8).

In patients with the myasthenic syndrome, the EPP elicited by a single stimulus is below activation threshold in many muscle fibers because of a defective release of ACh. If the second stimulus is given in less than a few milliseconds, the second EPP will summate with the first, activating additional muscle fibers. With the second or subsequent stimuli delivered at a longer interval, up to 100 to 200 ms, summation of the EPPs does not occur, but the second EPP still increases markedly because the electrosecretory mechanism partially overcomes the defective release of ACh (Fig. 8-8). Increased EPPs will in turn recruit some of the muscle fibers not activated by the first stimulus, leading to an increase in amplitude of the second compound muscle action potential. With paired stimuli separated by more than 100 to 200 ms, or repetitive stimuli at a slow rate, the second or subsequent EPP may be considerably less than the first, because the immediately available ACh store is reduced after the first stimulus. Diminution of the EPP, however, is not always as conspicuous as in myasthenia gravis. In some patients with the myasthenic syndrome, depletion of ACh is minimal following its limited release by the first stimulus. Consequently, decremental muscle responses, if present, may not be very prominent.

As mentioned earlier, a potentiation from summation of two EPPs at intervals less than 10 ms should be distinguished from facilitation attributable to an increased number of quanta released by the second nerve impulse.[11] True facilitation, seen at

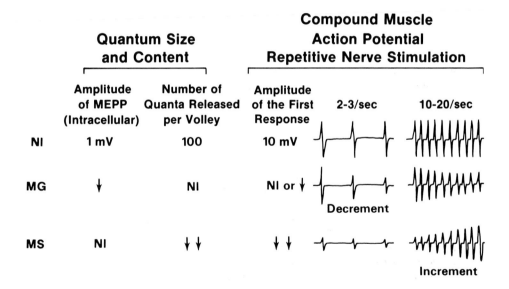

| | Quantum Size and Content | | Compound Muscle Action Potential Repetitive Nerve Stimulation | | |
|---|---|---|---|---|---|
| | Amplitude of MEPP (Intracellular) | Number of Quanta Released per Volley | Amplitude of the First Response | 2-3/sec | 10-20/sec |
| NI | 1 mV | 100 | 10 mV | | |
| MG | ↓ | NI | NI or ↓ | Decrement | |
| MS | NI | ↓↓ | ↓↓ | | Increment |

**Decrement: Reduced Quantum Content Below Safety Margin.**
**Increment: Neurosecretory Potentiation (Ca++ dependent?)**

Figure 8-8

(*Left*) Typical changes in quantum size and quantum content as determined by intracellular recordings in myasthenia gravis (MG) and myasthenic syndrome (MS). (*Right*) Decrement or increment of the compound muscle action potential to repetitive nerve stimulation. A decrease or increase in amplitude of the compound muscle potential occurs as a result of drop-out or recruitment, respectively, of individual muscle fibers according to the size of the end-plate potential (EPP).

longer interstimulus intervals up to 100 to 200 ms, is considered typical of the myasthenic syndrome. In contrast, potentiation caused by summation of the EPP is less specific as it occurs in patients with botulism or myasthenia gravis (see Fig 8-7), if the first response is less than maximal.[48] In botulism, which is characterized by the defective release of ACh, true facilitation may also be seen with paired shocks of longer intervals, although this is not as consistent as in the myasthenic syndrome.

## Post-tetanic potentiation and exhaustion

With prolonged repetitive stimulation or following a sustained voluntary muscle contraction, the immediately available store may increase as a result of a greater mobilization rate. This, coupled with the accumulation of calcium in the axon, potentiates the release of ACh and the EPP for one to two minutes (post-tetanic potentiation). Thereafter, release of ACh quanta and the EPP is reduced for up to 15 minutes, probably because of metabolic changes in the nerve terminal (post-tetanic exhaustion). This phenomenon can be experimentally elicited in muscles with a partial block by hemicholinium, which interferes with ACh synthesis, but not in those with a partial block by tubocurarine.[11] Prominent post-tetanic exhaustion also occurs in rabbits exposed to neomycin. In rat muscles, this drug causes a reduction in both the amplitude of the miniature end-plate potential (MEPP) and the number of quanta released per single nerve impulse. These findings suggest a presynaptic and postsynaptic action of neomycin.[9] The phenomenon of post-tetanic exhaustion is more marked in fast than in slow twitch muscles in the rat. Such differences in sensitivity to a blocking agent are probably postsynaptic in origin, perhaps based on the characteristics of the end-plate structure[45] or blood flow.[26]

# REFERENCE SOURCES

1.  ALBUQUERQUE, EX, ET AL: *An electrophysiological and morphological study of the neuromuscular junction in patients with myasthenia gravis.* Exper Neurol 51:536, 1976.

2.  BALNAVE, RJ AND GAGE, PW: *The inhibitory effect of manganese on transmitter release at the neuromuscular junction of the toad.* Br J Pharmacol 47:339, 1973.

3.  BETZ, WJ: *Depression of transmitter release at the neuromuscular junction of the frog.* J Physiol (Lond) 206:629, 1970.

4.  BLOOM, W AND FAWCETT, DW: *A Textbook of Histology,* ed 10. WB Saunders, Philadelphia, 1975.

5.  BRANISTEANU, DD, MIYAMOTO, MD, AND VOLLE, RL: *Effects of physiologic alterations on binomial transmitter release at magnesium-depressed neuromuscular junctions.* J Physiol (Lond) 254:19, 1976.

6.  BROOKS, VB AND THIES, RE: *Reduction of quantum content during neuromuscular transmission.* J Physiol (Lond) 162:298, 1962.

7.  CHANDLER, WK, RAKOWSKI, RF, AND SCHNEIDER, MF: *A non-linear voltage dependent charge movement in frog skeletal muscle.* J Physiol (Lond) 254:245, 1976.

8.  COSTANTIN, LL: *The role of sodium current in the radial spread of contraction in frog muscle fibers.* J Gen Physiol 55:703, 1970.

9.  DAUBE, JR AND LAMBERT, EH: *Post-activation exhaustion in rat muscle.* In DESMEDT, JE (ED): *New Developments in Electromyography and Clinical Neurophysiology,* Vol 1. Karger, Basel, 1973, pp 343–349.

10. DESMEDT, JE: *Presynaptic mechanisms in myasthenia gravis.* Ann NY Acad Sci 135:209, 1966.

11. DESMEDT, JE: *The neuromuscular disorder in myasthenia gravis. 1. Electrical and mechanical response to nerve stimulation in hand muscles.* In DESMEDT, JE (ED): *New Developments in Electromyography and Clinical Neurophysiology,* Vol 1. Karger, Basel, 1973, pp 241–304.

12. EATON, LM AND LAMBERT, E: *Electromyography and electric stimulation of nerves in diseases of motor unit. Observations on myasthenic syndrome associated with malignant tumors.* JAMA 163:1117, 1957.

13. ECCLES, JC, KATZ, B, AND KUFFLER, SW: *Nature of the "endplate potential" in curarized muscle.* J Neurophysiol 4:362, 1941.

14. ELIAS, SB AND APPEL, SH: *Acetylcholine receptor in myasthenia gravis: Increased affinity for α-bungarotoxin.* Ann Neurol 4:250, 1978.

15. ELMQVIST, D: *Neuromuscular transmission defects.* In DESMEDT, JE (ED): *New Developments in Electromyography and Clinical Neurophysiology,* Vol 1. Karger, Basel, 1973, pp 229–240.

16. ELMQVIST, D AND LAMBERT, EH: *Detailed analysis of neuromuscular transmission in a patient with the myasthenic syndrome sometimes associated with bronchogenic carcinoma.* Mayo Clin Proc 43:689, 1968.

17. ELMQVIST D, ET AL: *An electrophysiological investigation of neuromuscular transmission in myasthenia gravis.* J Physiol (Lond) 174:417, 1964.

18. ELMQVIST D, ET AL: *Acetylcholine receptor protein. Neuromuscular transmission in immunized rabbits.* Arch Neurol 34:7, 1977.

19. ENGEL, AG AND SANTA, T: *Histometric analysis of the ultrastructure of the neuromuscular junction in myasthenia gravis and in the myasthenic syndrome.* Ann NY Acad Sci 183:46, 1971.

20. ENGEL, AG AND SANTA, T: *Motor endplate fine structure.* In DESMEDT, JE (ED): *New Developments in Electromyography and Clinical Neurophysiology,* Vol 1. Karger, Basel, 1973, pp 196–228.

21. ENGEL, AG, LAMBERT, EH, AND GOMEZ, MR: *A new myasthenic syndrome with end-plate acetylcholinesterase deficiency, small nerve terminals, and reduced acetylcholine release.* Ann Neurol 1:315, 1977.

22. ENGEL, AG, LAMBERT, EH, AND HOWARD, FM, JR: *Immune complexes (IgG and C3) at the motor end-plate in myasthenia gravis.* Mayo Clin Proc 52:267, 1977.

23. ENGEL AG, ET AL: *Experimental autoimmune myasthenia gravis: A sequential and quantitative study of the neuromuscular junction ultrastructure and electrophysiologic correlations.* J Neuropath Exper Neurol 35:569, 1976.

24. FAMBROUGH, DM, DRACHMAN, DB, AND SATYAMURTI, S: *Neuromuscular junction in myasthenia gravis: Decreased acetylcholine receptors.* Science 182:293, 1973.

25. FATT, P AND KATZ, B: *Spontaneous subthreshold activity at motor nerve endings.* J Physiol (Lond) 117:109, 1952.

26. FRIESS, SL, ET AL: *Blockade in simultaneously perfused soleus and gastrocnemius muscles in the cat.* Toxicol Appl Pharmacol 18:133, 1971.

27. GREEN, DPL, ET AL: *Acetylcholine receptors.* Trans R Soc (Lond) B 270:551, 1975.

28. HART, ZH, ET AL: *A congenital familial myasthenic syndrome caused by a presynaptic defect of transmitter resynthesis or mobilization.* Neurology (New York) 29:556, 1979.

29. HOWARD, JF, JR AND SANDERS, DB: *Passive transfer of human myasthenia gravis to rats. 1. Electrophysiology of the developing neuromuscular block.* Neurology (New York) 30:760, 1980.

30. HUBBARD, JI: *Neuromuscular transmission—Presynaptic factors.* In HUBBARD, JI (ED): *The Peripheral Nervous System.* Plenum Press, New York, 1974, pp 151–180.

31. ITO, Y, ET AL: *Acetylcholine receptors and end-plate electrophysiology in myasthenia gravis.* Brain 101:345, 1978.

32. KADRIE, HA AND BROWN, WF: *Neuromuscular transmission in human single motor units.* J Neurol Neurosurg Psychiatry 41:193, 1978.

33. KADRIE, HA AND BROWN, WF: *Neuromuscular transmission in myasthenic single motor units.* J Neurol Neurosurg Psychiatry 41:205, 1978.

34. KAO, I, DRACHMAN, DB, AND PRICE, DL: *Botulinum toxin: Mechanism of presynaptic blockade.* Science 193:1256, 1976.

35. KATZ, B: *Microphysiology of the neuro-muscular junction. A physiological 'quantum of action' at the myoneural junction.* Bull Johns Hopkins Hosp 102:275, 1958.

36. KELLY, JJ, JR, LAMBERT, EH AND LENNON, VA: *Acetylcholine release in diaphragm of rats with chronic experimental autoimmune myasthenia gravis.* Ann Neurol 4:67, 1978.

37. KIMURA, J: *Electrodiagnostic study of pesticide toxicity.* In XINTARAS, C, JOHNSON, BL, AND DE GROOT, I (EDS): *Behavioral Toxicology.* U.S. Department of Health, Education and Welfare, U.S. Government Printing Office, Washington D.C., 1974, pp 174–181.

38. LAMBERT, EH AND ELMQVIST, D: *Quantal components of end-plate potentials in the myasthenic syndrome.* Ann NY Acad Sci 183:183, 1971.

39. LAMBERT, EH, OKIHIRO, M, AND ROOKE, ED: *Clinical physiology of the neuromuscular junction.* In PAUL, WM, ET AL (EDS): *Muscle.* Proceedings of the Symposium, The Faculty of Medicine, University of Alberta, Pergamon Press, London, 1965, pp 487–499.

40. LINDSTROM, JM AND LAMBERT, EH: *Content of acetylcholine receptor and antibodies bound to receptor in myasthenia gravis, experimental autoimmune myasthenia gravis, and Eaton-Lambert syndrome.* Neurology (New York) 28:130, 1978.

41. MACINTOSH, FC: *Formation, storage, and release of acetylcholine at nerve endings.* Can J Biochem Physiol 37:343, 1959.

42. MEADOWS, JC, ROSS-RUSSELL, RW, AND WISE, RP: *A re-evaluation of the decamethonium test for myasthenia gravis.* Acta Neurol Scand 50:248, 1974.

43. NEWSOM-DAVIS, J, ET AL: *Function of circulating antibody to acetylcholine receptor in myasthenia gravis: Investigation by plasma exchange.* Neurology (New York) 28:266, 1978.

44. NISHIZONO, H, SAITO, Y, AND MIYASHITA, M: *The estimation of conduction velocity in human skeletal muscle in situ with surface electrodes.* Electroenceph Clin Neurophysiol 46:659, 1979.

45. NYSTRÖM, B: *Histochemical studies of end-plate bound esterases in "slow-red" and "fast-white" cat muscles during postnatal development.* Acta Neurol Scand 44:295, 1968.

46. SATYAMURTI, S, DRACHMAN, DB, AND SLONE, F: *Blockade of acetylocholine receptors: A model of myasthenia gravis.* Science 187:955, 1975.

47. SWIFT, TR: *Weakness from magnesium-containing cathartics: Electrophysiologic studies.* Muscle and Nerve 2:295, 1979.

48. TAKAMORI, M AND GUTMANN, L: *Intermittent defect of acetylcholine release in myasthenia gravis.* Neurology (Minneap) 21:47, 1971.

49. TAKAMORI, M, IDE, Y, AND KASAI, M: *Neuromuscular defect after suppression of ion conductance.* Neurology (New York) 29:772, 1979.

50. TAKEUCHI, A: *The long-lasting depression in neuromuscular transmission of frog.* J Physiol (Japan) 8:102, 1958.

51. THORNELL, LE, ET AL: *Morphological observations on motor end-plates in rabbits with experimental myasthenia.* J Neurol Sci 29:389, 1976.

52. TOYKA, KV, ET AL: *Myasthenia gravis. Study of humoral immune mechanisms by passive transfer to mice.* N Engl J Med 296:125, 1977.

53. TSUJIHATA, M, ET AL: *Limb muscle endplates in ocular myasthenia gravis: Quantitative ultrastructural study.* Neurology (New York) 29:654, 1979.

# CHAPTER
# 9

# TECHNIQUES OF REPETITIVE STIMULATION

Nerve stimulation techniques as tests for disorders of neuromuscular transmission began with Jolly[36] who applied faradic current repeatedly at short intervals. Using a kymographic recording and visual inspection of skin displacement, he found that the size of the muscle response deteriorated rapidly in patients with myasthenia gravis during the faradization. He also noted that if the muscle was fatigued volitionally prior to the test, subsequent faradic current was less effective in eliciting a response. Conversely, faradized muscle responded poorly to subsequent volitional muscle contraction. Based on these findings Jolly concluded that the weakness in myasthenia was due to motor failure of the peripheral rather than central nervous system. The test was inadequate according to current standards in that his double coil stimulator only produced shocks of submaximal intensity, and that a mechanical rather than electrical response was recorded. His conclusion was remarkable, however, considering the limitations of his equipment.

The use of supramaximal stimulation and the recording of the muscle action potential have increased the reliability and sensitivity of nerve stimulation techniques considerably. The first to do this were Harvey and Masland,[32] who noted that in myasthenia a single muscle response was followed by a prolonged depression, during which a second maximal motor nerve stimulus excited a reduced number of muscle fibers. When the nerve was stimulated with a train of impulses, the resulting muscle action potentials showed a progressive decline in voltage. Optimal frequency of stimulation was subsequently investigated more systematically by Desmedt.[20] Various activation procedures have been designed to enhance an equivocal neuromuscular block. To maximize the accuracy of the test, attention is also directed toward the muscle temperature during recording, and to selection of appropriate muscles, as they may be differentially involved.

Except for direct microelectrode recording of end-plate potentials from muscle in vitro,[2, 26] all electrophysiologic tests offer only indirect assessments of the neuromuscular junction. However, quantitation of the motor response to paired stimuli, tetanic contraction, and repetitive stimulation at fast and slow rates provides a useful, objective measure of neuromuscular junction activity.[17, 42] These techniques have demonstrated transmission defects in a variety of disease states, including myasthenia gravis, myasthenic syndrome, botulism, amyotrophic lateral sclerosis, poliomyelitis, and multiple sclerosis. In the following discussion, the physiologic significance of decremental or incremental responses will be analyzed with reference to the differential diagnosis of clinical disorders. The characteristic electrophysiologic abnormalities for a given disease entity will be discussed later in Chapter 24.

# METHODS AND TECHNICAL FACTORS

## Belly-tendon recording

The method for stimulating the nerve and recording the muscle action potential is the same as for motor nerve conduction studies.[41] The compound muscle potential is recorded with a surface electrode ($G_1$) placed over the motor point of the tested muscle and a reference electrode ($G_2$) over the tendon (belly-tendon response). The electrical stimulus delivered to the nerve must be of supramaximal intensity to insure activation of all the motor axons innervating the muscle under study. Theoretically, any mixed or motor nerve may be tested as long as an evoked action potential can be recorded from the innervated muscle.

The initially negative potential thus recorded represents the summated electrical activity from the entire muscle fiber population, discharging relatively synchronously. The area under the negative phase is proportional to the number of muscle fibers activated, as is the amplitude, provided that the duration and waveform of the potential remain the same. In disorders of nerve conduction or neuromuscular transmission, changes in the size of the compound muscle potentials result primarily from an increase or decrease in the number of muscle fibers responding to successive stimuli. The compound muscle potential is also altered by changes in the action potentials of individual muscle fibers, as might be expected to occur in primary muscle disease.

## Movement-induced artifacts

Using repetitive stimulation particular caution is necessary to avoid a number of movement related artifacts. The action potential is, of course, significantly affected, if the recording electrodes move over the skin relative to the muscle belly in the course of repetitive stimulation. Other artifacts are less obvious. During an isotonic contraction, shortening of the muscle is associated with changes in volume conduction; that is, the spatial relationship of muscle and recording electrodes. This in turn leads to an alteration in the potential difference between the two recording electrodes, even if they are firmly attached to the skin. The stimulating electrodes may move during a train of stimulation, causing some subthreshold stimuli, even if the shock intensity is unchanged. A fallaciously small amplitude resulting from decreased numbers of nerve fibers stimulated may be mistaken for a decremental response. Use of a subcutaneous needle for stimulation is helpful in minimizing this type of artifact.

For meaningful results, therefore, it is imperative to firmly immobilize the extremity as well as the muscle under study. It is helpful to stimulate the nerve as distally as possible, since a more proximal stimulus may cause vigorous contraction of many muscles. In most instances technical problems can be identified by abrupt, irregular changes in amplitude or shape, whereas reliable responses show smooth progressive alterations. Some movement artifacts, however, may be difficult to recognize solely on the basis of changing waveforms. Thus, visual inspection of the contracting muscle is important to detect excessive movement. The most important characteristics of a reliable test are consistency and reproducibility of the change in action potential with repeated trials. Between successive trials, the muscle must be rested 30 seconds or longer, since neuromuscular transmission is subnormal for approximately 12 seconds following a single stimulus and for a greater time after repetitive impulses.

# Temperature and other factors

Some myasthenic patients notice appearance of eyelid ptosis and diplopia during exposure to warm sunlight.[4, 58] These observations can be substantiated electrophysiologically by testing weak muscles after local cooling. Four physiologic mechanisms account for the improvement of neuromuscular transmission with cooling: (1) facilitation of transmitter replacement in the presynaptic terminal;[33, 34] (2) reduction in the amount of transmitter released at the neuromuscular junction by the first of a train of impulses, leaving more quanta available for subsequent stimuli;[18] (3) decreased hydrolysis of acetylcholine (ACh) by acetylcholinesterase, allowing sustained action of the transmitter once it is released from the axon terminal;[27] and (4) increased postsynaptic receptor sensitivity to ACh.[31]

It has been shown that reduction of the intramuscular temperature from 35 to 28°C significantly increases not only the amplitude of the compound muscle action potential but also the force of the isometric twitch and tetanic contraction.[5] A distinct improvement in neuromuscular transmission has also been reported after cooling in patients with myasthenic syndrome,[55, 62] amyotrophic lateral sclerosis,[19] botulism,[63] and tick paralysis.[15] Since cooling reduces the decrement to repetitive nerve stimulation (Fig. 9-1), the control of muscle temperature is important for diagnostic application of this electrophysiologic method. If the skin temperature is below 34°C over the tested muscle, then the limb should be warmed before the test, either by immersing it in warm water or using an infrared heat lamp to avoid false negative results. Paradoxically, a decremental response may be seen during brief stimulation at high rates in normal muscles if the temperature is below 32°C.[43]

Other technical factors that must be considered include the effect of cholinesterase inhibitors. Administration of anticholinesterase drugs within a few hours before the test tends to reduce the probability of obtaining a positive result. Thus, it is advisable to discontinue the medication for several hours. A long-acting time span medication should be withheld for a longer period if clinically feasible. With an overdose of anti-

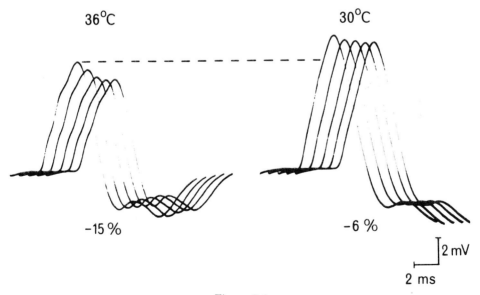

Figure 9-1
Decremental response of the hypothenar muscle with stimulation of the ulnar nerve at 2 per second in a patient with myasthenia gravis; on the left, at 36°C and on the right, following cooling of the hand to 30°C. Note the reduction in the decrement from 15 to 6 percent, and the increase in amplitude following cooling of the hand. (From Denys,[18] with permission.)

cholinesterase drugs, a single nerve impulse may cause a repetitive muscle response, and repetitive stimuli at a high rate give rise to a decremental response.

# COMMONLY USED NERVES AND MUSCLES
## Distal versus proximal muscle

In myasthenia gravis, the incidence of electrical abnormality is higher in the clinically weak proximal or facial muscles as compared with the distal muscles. In a series of experiments,[39, 40] it was shown that the decrement of electrical and mechanical responses to repetitive stimuli was two to three times as great in the platysma as in the adductor pollicis. Similarly post-tetanic facilitation was four times as great in the former as in the latter. In contrast, there was no difference between the two muscles in control subjects. The clinical features of the myasthenic syndrome may also be more prominent in the proximal muscles. In this syndrome, however, electrophysiologic abnormalities can usually be identified in any distal muscles readily accessible for recording after nerve stimulation.[9] This is in contrast to the usual absence of a decrementing response in clinically unaffected muscles of patients with myasthenia gravis. Botulism also may be associated with localized findings limited to weak muscles of the clinically affected limbs.

Theoretically any motor nerve may be tested, provided that its stimulation and recording from the innervated muscle can be accomplished. Although less sensitive, studies of the distal musculature are technically more reliable than those of more proximal limb muscles or facial muscles. Stimulation of the ulnar nerve at the elbow allows four muscles to be tested simultaneously: flexor carpi ulnaris, abductor digiti quinti, first dorsal interosseous, and adductor pollicis.[21] If the test is negative with distal muscles, the proximal muscles should be examined. Although not widely known, the spinal accessory nerve is readily accessible and a muscle action potential can be recorded selectively from the upper trapezius muscle without contamination from other muscles.[48] Selection of the nerve and muscle for study depends on the clinical problem of a given patient, but a general approach is stated below for some of the more commonly tested muscles.

## Upper limb and shoulder girdle

**HYPOTHENAR MUSCLES.** The active electrode ($G_1$) is placed over the belly of abductor digiti quinti and the reference electrode ($G_2$) on the tendon. The ulnar nerve is stimulated at the wrist in the usual fashion. The four fingers are bound together with a bandage or Velcro strap in such a way that finger abduction does not result in appreciable movement. The hand is laid flat, palm down, on an examining board and firmly, but not tightly, held by restraining metal bars which may be secured at the four corners of the board.

**THENAR MUSCLES.** The muscle potential is recorded with surface electrodes over the abductor pollicis brevis ($G_1$) and proximal phalanx of the thumb ($G_2$). The median nerve is stimulated at the wrist in the usual manner. The hand is laid flat, palm up, on the board and held from above by the restraining metal bars. The thumb is held in the adducted position so that attempted abduction results in no significant movement. The muscle is exercised by abducting the thumb against the bar.

**BICEPS.** The recording electrodes are placed over the belly ($G_1$) and tendon ($G_2$). The musculocutaneous nerve is stimulated in the axilla. The position of the arm depends on the type of restraining board available. A handlebar attached under a solid table can serve as an excellent restraint. With the patient upright in a chair, the arm is flexed approximately 45 degrees in the adducted and supinated position, with the hand holding on to the handle from below. The muscle is exercised by pulling up against the handlebar, flexing at the elbow.

**DELTOID.** The $G_1$ is placed over the belly and $G_2$, on the acromion. The brachial plexus is stimulated at Erb's point. The arm is held in the adducted position at the side, flexed at the elbow, and firmly restrained at the wrist in front of the body by the patient's opposite hand. The patient is asked to exercise by abducting the arm against his own restraint. When self-restraint is not possible because of weakness or lack of cooperation, the arm may be held adducted at the side and restrained by a Velcro strap applied firmly against the patient's trunk.

**TRAPEZIUS.** The muscle potential is recorded with surface electrodes over the upper trapezius at the angle of the neck and shoulder ($G_1$) and tendon near the acromion process ($G_2$). The spinal accessory nerve is stimulated as it descends along the posterior border of the sternocleidomastoid muscle. With the patient upright in a chair the arms are adducted and extended with the hand holding on to the bottom of the chair. Exercise is obtained by having the patient shrug the shoulders against his own restraint. In some subjects, the spinal accessory nerve is easier to stimulate with the patient in the prone position.

## Lower limb

**ANTERIOR TIBIAL.** The $G_1$ is placed over the belly and $G_2$, a few centimeters distally. The peroneal nerve is stimulated over the fibular head. With the patient sitting in a chair, the thigh is restrained firmly by Velcro straps. The foot is held on a foot board that extends from the chair so that neither the foot nor the leg moves. The muscle is exercised by dorsiflexing the foot against the restraint.

**QUADRICEPS.** The muscle potential is recorded with surface electrodes over the rectus femoris ($G_1$) and patellar tendon ($G_2$). The femoral nerve is stimulated at the groin, just lateral to the femoral artery. The thigh is fastened to the chair with Velcro straps, with the patient in the sitting position. Exercise is obtained by having the patient lift the thigh against the restraint. In some subjects, the femoral nerve is easier to stimulate in the supine position. The thigh is then bound to the bed by a Velcro strap for restraint, and the muscle is exercised by having the patient lift the foot off the bed.

## Face

**ORBICULARIS OCULI AND ORIS.** The surface electrodes are placed on the upper-outer portion of the muscle ($G_1$) and on the side of the nose ($G_2$). The facial nerve is stimulated in front of the ear. Unlike the extremities, facial muscles cannot be immobilized. Thus, the test is subject to more artifact here than elsewhere, and particular care is necessary to detect changes in amplitude induced by movement. The muscle is exercised with the patient contracting the muscle as vigorously as possible.

# PAIRED STIMULATION

## Short interstimulus intervals

As already discussed in Chapter 8, quantitative assessment of neuromuscular transmission is possible with the use of paired stimuli. In normal muscles, the first supramaximal stimulus activates the entire group of muscle fibers. The compound muscle action potential elicited by a second stimulus delivered within a few milliseconds is decreased, reflecting not only the failure at the neuromuscular junction but also the refractory period of the nerve and muscle (see Fig. 8-4). At slightly longer interstimulus intervals, the first and second potentials are essentially the same. However, at intervals less than 10 to 15 ms, the two responses are not clearly separable.

In most patients with myasthenia gravis, the maximal or near maximal muscle response is elicited by the first stimulus. At very short interstimulus intervals there is no essential difference in the time course of the recovery curve between normal and myasthenic muscles (see Fig. 8-5). In contrast, the results of paired stimuli are quite different from the normal pattern in the myasthenic syndrome with defective acetylcholine (ACh) release. At very short interstimulus intervals (up to 15 ms), there is a one and a half- to twofold increase in amplitude of the second response, if the first response is submaximal (Fig. 9-2). The increment presumably represents recruitment from summation of two EPPs in some of the fibers activated only subliminally by the first stimulus. A larger second response at short interstimulus intervals also occurs in occasional cases of myasthenia gravis and in most patients with botulism.[13]

## Longer interstimulus intervals

At interstimulus intervals longer than 15 ms, no summation of EPPs takes place. Thus, potentiation of the second response at these longer intervals represents true facilitation that results from an increased number of quanta liberated by the second stimulus. Despite a greater amount of ACh, normal muscles show no increase in the amplitude of the second muscle potential, since no additional muscle fibers can be recruited. Facilitation at this interstimulus range is also either absent or minimal in most patients with myasthenia gravis or botulism. In contrast, an increment regularly occurs at intervals ranging from 15 to 100 ms in patients with the myasthenic syndrome. Indeed, true

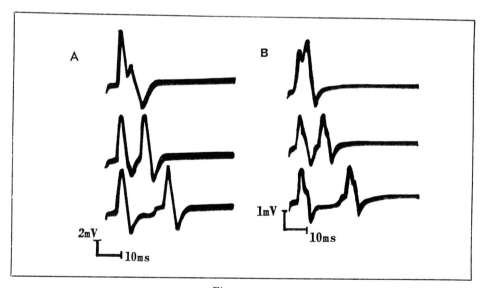

Figure 9-2
Compound muscle action potentials elicited by paired stimulation of the nerve in a normal subject (A) and in a patient with botulism (B). The paired shocks were given at interstimulus intervals of 2.5 ms (top), 15 ms (middle), and 25 ms (bottom). At the shortest interval, the test response was reduced in amplitude reflecting the refractory period in the normal subject. In contrast, the test response was greater in amplitude than the conditioning response as a result of summation of the end-plate potentials (EPP) in the patient with botulism. (From Cherington,[11] with permission.)

facilitation as defined previously is one of the essential and specific electrophysiologic features of the myasthenic syndrome.

Paired stimuli with longer interstimulus intervals are more effective in eliciting the decremental response characteristic of myasthenia gravis. Decremental response begins at intervals of about 20 ms but becomes more definite between 100 and 700 ms. It slowly returns to the baseline in about 10 seconds. The maximal depression generally occurs at an interstimulus interval of about 300 to 500 ms (see Fig. 8-6). At shorter intervals, the depression is obscured by concomitant facilitation attributable to the electrosecretory mechanism (see Fig. 8-7). The time course of the recovery curve suggests that, with repetitive stimulation, the maximum decrement also occurs at a comparable interstimulus interval. Indeed, the rate of 2 to 3 per second is generally considered the most sensitive among the slower rates of stimulation.[20]

# REPETITIVE STIMULATION AT SLOW RATES

## Method and normal values

Once the limb has been immobilized and a supramaximal stimulus determined, repetitive stimulation is delivered at a rate of 1 to 5 per second for several shocks. As discussed above, the rate generally considered most effective is 2 to 3 second, which is fast enough to cause depletion of the immediately available acetylcholine (ACh) store, but slow enough to avoid superimposed facilitation from neurosecretory mechanisms (see Fig. 8-8). Furthermore, repetitive stimulation at this rate is tolerated very well by most patients. It is least likely to result in a false positive induced by movements, since the muscle returns to its original relaxed position before the next stimulus. With a train at faster rates, change in amplitude of successive responses is more variable, because movement-related artifacts are difficult to control.

Random or irregular variations in amplitude suggest the need for a better limb restraint to minimize movement and other artifacts. Only reproducible, smooth changes in amplitude of successive potentials should be accepted for measurement. When the recording is technically satisfactory, a train of compound muscle action potentials is either stored on the oscilloscope or photographed using Polaroid film. The percentage reduction is calculated for the smallest of the first five responses, compared with the first in the same train. In normal muscles, decrement at 2 to 3 per second stimulation, if present, does not exceed 5 to 8 percent.[6, 59] In fact, the presence of any reproducible decrement is suspicious, if the extremity is firmly immobilized and the tracings are free of any technical problems, since in an optimal recording of normal muscles a train of responses is practically identical from the first to the last.

## Myasthenia gravis

In myasthenia gravis, the amount of decrement at a slow rate of stimulation is usually maximal between the first and second response, but the amplitude decreases progressively up to the fourth or fifth response (Fig. 9-3). Subsequent responses in the series then level off or, more typically, regain amplitude slightly. Occasionally, the amplitude may increase beyond the original value at rest by 10 to 20 percent after several seconds of repetitive stimulation. More characteristically, however, continued stimulation gives rise to a long slow decrement following the transient increment.[35] A reproducible decrement of 10 percent or more between the first response and the smallest of the first five responses is considered abnormal. Although changes in amplitude are considered more characteristic, progressive increase in latency may also occur in some myasthenic muscles. This is usually associated with a decremental response either at rest or during post-tetanic exhaustion. To avoid false negative tests in patients with selective involvement of localized muscles, it is necessary to sample several muscles, both proximally

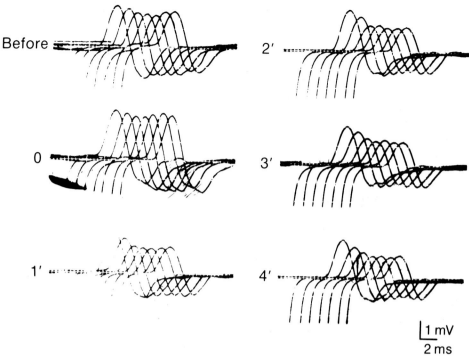

Before  2′

0  3′

1′  4′

1 mV
2 ms

Figure 9-3
Decremental responses before and after voluntary exercise in a patient with generalized myasthenia gravis. The median nerve was stimulated at the rate of 3 per second for seven shocks in each train. The compound muscle action potential was recorded from the thenar muscles. Comparing the amplitude of the fifth response with the amplitude of the first, the decrement was 25 percent at rest. It decreased to 12 percent during post-tetanic potentiation immediately after exercise and increased up to 50 percent thereafter during post-tetanic exhaustion.

and distally. Positive tests in the proximal or facial muscles are not uncommon, even when the distal limb muscles reveal no electrical abnormalities.

## Other disorders

Decrement in amplitude with a slow rate of repetitive stimulation is not exclusive to myasthenia gravis but is seen in a number of conditions with reduced margins of safety in neuromuscular transmission. These include the myasthenic syndrome (Figs. 9-4 and 9-5), botulism, multiple sclerosis,[25] motor neuron disease,[50] and regenerating nerve.[28] The response of a partially curarized muscle to a train of stimuli is very similar to that seen in myasthenic muscle in that the compound muscle action potential declines progressively during the first few impulses. In the myasthenic syndrome and in botulism, the muscle action potentials elicited by single stimuli are typically very small. Further diminution of amplitude usually occurs with a slow rate of repetitive stimulation, although the decremental tendency does not constitute an essential feature of these disorders. The administration of edrophonium (Tensilon) or neostigmine (Prostigmin) is helpful in further delineating the characteristics of defective neuromuscular transmission. These agents, which potentiate the action of ACh by blocking acetylcholinesterase, are particularly effective with postjunctional abnormalities. The diagnosis of myasthenia gravis is most likely, therefore, if the decremental tendency can be partially or completely reversed pharmacologically.

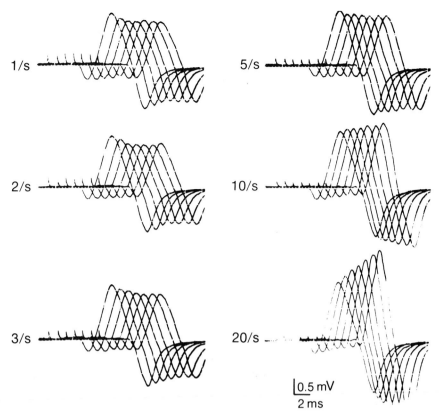

Figure 9-4

Effect of slow versus fast rates of repetitive stimulation in a patient with the myasthenic syndrome. The left median nerve was stimulated at rates of 1 through 20 per second for seven shocks in each train. The compound muscle action potential was recorded from the thenar muscles. Decremental responses occurred at slow rates of stimulation ranging from 1 to 5 per second. Incremental responses were first observed at the stimulus frequency of 10 per second and further enhanced at 20 per second.

# REPETITIVE STIMULATION AT FAST RATES

## Normal muscles

Since supramaximal stimulation of the nerve normally activates all muscle fibers, incremental responses are necessarily precluded even if increased amounts of acetylcholine (ACh) are released by subsequent stimuli. In other words, an incremental response based on recruitment of additional fibers can occur only if the first stimulus fails to activate the entire population of muscle fibers innervated by the nerve. Such is usually the case when an incremental tendency is detected in the myasthenic syndrome, in botulism, and occasionally in myasthenia gravis.

In normal muscles, the size of the potential is stable during repetitive stimulation at a rate up to 20 to 30 per second,[51] although in some healthy infants there may be progressive decline in amplitude.[14] Both decremental and incremental responses have occasionally been reported at 50 per second. However, assessment of amplitude change at such a fast rate is often rendered unreliable by inherent movement artifacts. As mentioned earlier, the amplitude of the compound muscle action potential may increase without recruitment of additional muscle fibers. This occurs commonly in nor-

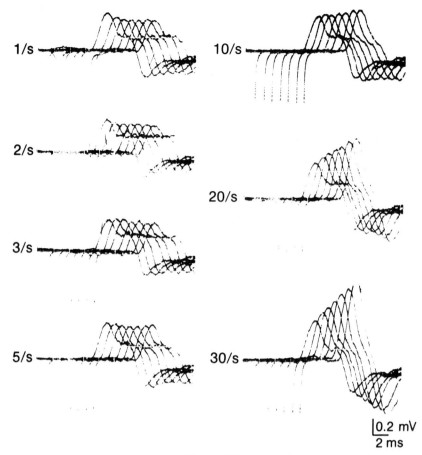

Figure 9-5

Progression of weakness in the same patient as in Figure 9-4 six weeks later. Stimulating and recording arrangements were the same. Compared with the previous study, the compound muscle action potential was smaller in amplitude, and decremental tendency was less evident at slow rates of stimulation ranging from 1 to 5 per second. Incremental responses at faster rates of stimulation were progressively more prominent as the stimulus frequency was increased from 10 to 30 per second.

mal muscles stimulated repetitively at a high rate, as a result of an increased synchrony of muscle fiber discharge. The area under the waveform, however, usually remains the same with repetitive stimulation up to 20 to 30 per second.

## Myasthenic syndrome

The most outstanding electrophysiologic finding in the myasthenic syndrome[24] is the strikingly small amplitude of the compound muscle action potential (Fig. 9-6). Indeed this diagnosis is unlikely if the response elicited by a single stimulus to any motor nerve is normal in amplitude. However, the compound muscle action potential is so variable among different subjects that an apparently low normal amplitude may in fact represent an abnormal reduction for the particular patient under consideration.

A train of stimulation at rates too rapid for demonstrating a decrementing response in myasthenia gravis may reveal significant abnormalities in the myasthenic syndrome (see Fig. 8-8). Repetitive stimulation at 10 to 50 per second is delivered for up to one minute. In the myasthenic syndrome, a remarkable increment of successive

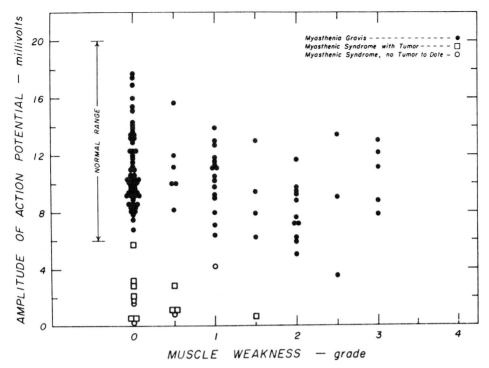

Figure 9-6

Relation of clinical estimate of weakness and the amplitude of muscle action potential in patients with myasthenia gravis and myasthenic syndrome. The ulnar nerve was stimulated by single maximal shocks and the compound muscle action potentials were recorded from the hypothenar muscles. (From Lambert, et al,[46] with permission.)

muscle action potentials occurs, leading to the normal or near normal level (see Figs. 9-4 and 9-5). The last response of a train at the end of one minute is often several times the first response in amplitude.[44] The increase is sometimes preceded by a slight initial decrement. In the myasthenic syndrome, clinical improvement with guanidine, 10 to 50 mg per kg daily, is often associated with improvement of electrophysiologic abnormalities.

## Other neuromuscular disorders

Slight potentiation (Fig. 9-7) may be seen in cases of botulism in which the amplitude of the muscle potential to a single supramaximal stimulus is also below normal. Incre-

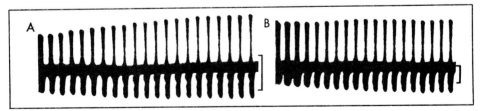

Figure 9-7

Muscle action potentials to a train of stimulation applied to the motor nerve at 50 per second in a patient with botulism. Incremental responses recorded when the patient was on a 7 mg per kg daily dose of guanidine (A) were no longer evident when the dosage was increased to 35 mg per kg (B). Vertical calibration is 2 mV. (From Cherington,[11] with permission.)

menting responses in botulism resemble those found in the myasthenic syndrome, although they are not as pronounced.[30, 52] Electrical responses may be entirely normal in early stages of botulism.[11, 12] Not infrequently, patients with myasthenia gravis also show incremental responses either during a progressive phase of the disease or during steroid therapy.[16, 49, 57, 61] An increment is more evident if the muscle action potential to a single stimulus is small. Even then, the amplitude does not usually exceed the initial value by more than 40 percent at the end of one minute. Small amplitude responses may also occur in various other disorders associated with muscle atrophy or dystrophy. However, a significant potentiation with fast rates of stimulation does not occur in the latter instances.

Similar findings may also be seen in depressed neuromuscular transmission due to antibiotic toxicity,[53] hypocalcemia or hypermagnesemia,[7, 60] or snake poisoning.[37] Thus, incrementing responses per se do not establish a diagnosis of the myasthenic syndrome. However, the degree of potentiation in this syndrome is usually considerably greater than that which may be seen in botulism, myasthenia gravis, or the other disorders noted earlier.

## Use of prolonged stimulation

A short train of several shocks usually suffices for routine evaluation of neuromuscular transmission. Prolonged stimulation at a rapid rate causes strong contraction and movement of the limb. Accordingly, artifact makes it generally unreliable as a diagnostic test. However, a longer stimulus train may be of theoretical interest to elucidate the time course of the mechanical force due to muscle contraction. The force of muscle twitch increases during prolonged stimulation in normal muscles. This phenomenon, called positive staircase, is absent or reduced in myasthenia gravis, but its diagnostic value has not yet been established.[22, 59] Whatever the purpose, repetitive stimulation should be used judiciously to avoid subjecting the patient to undue discomfort.

# EFFECT OF TETANIC CONTRACTION

Brief tetanic contraction may be achieved by repetitive electrical stimulation at 50 per second for 20 to 30 seconds or by continuous stimulation at 3 per second for a few minutes. Most subjects, however, do not tolerate prolonged electrical stimulation very well. Since a majority of patients can activate muscle potentials at rates up to 50 per second, the same effect can be accomplished simply by voluntary muscle contraction for 10 seconds to one minute. During maximal effort, inadvertent movement of recording and stimulating electrodes should be minimized by firmly immobilizing the limb. A typical postactivation cycle following voluntary or involuntary tetanic contraction of the muscle may be divided into two phases: post-tetanic potentiation[35] lasting for about two minutes, followed by post-tetanic exhaustion,[20] lasting up to 15 minutes, after which the response returns to its original level.

## Post-tetanic potentiation

Post-tetanic potentiation probably results from accumulation of calcium ($Ca^{++}$) and the increased mobilization of acetylcholine (ACh) induced by tetanic contraction. In healthy muscles, the compound muscle action potential is not appreciably affected by a larger post-tetanic end-plate potential (EPP), because pretetanic EPP already exceeds the threshold for each fiber. However, in the myasthenic syndrome post-tetanic potentiation is consistently seen (Figs. 9-8 and 9-9).

As a simple test for post-tetanic potentiation, a single shock of supramaximal intensity may be delivered to the nerve and the size of the muscle response measured before and after exercise. If defective release of ACh is responsible for the small muscle

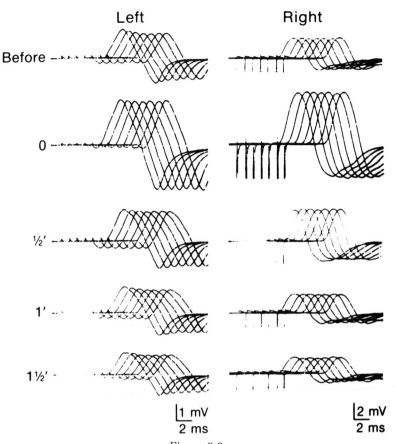

| Left | Right |
| --- | --- |

Before

0

½'

1'

1½'

| 1 mV | 2 mV |
| 2 ms | 2 ms |

Figure 9-8

Post-tetanic potentiation and exhaustion in the myasthenic syndrome. The median nerve was stimulated at the rate of 3 per second for seven shocks in each train. The compound muscle action potential was recorded from the thenar muscles. Immediately after voluntary contraction for 10 seconds the amplitude of the evoked potential increased by 70 percent on the left and 160 percent on the right, indicating a post-tetanic potentiation. One and one-half minutes later the compound muscle action potentials were smaller than the pre-exercise level on either side, representing a post-tetanic exhaustion.

response at rest, a striking increase in amplitude occurs, usually exceeding twice the baseline value.[46] Optimal duration of exercise is 10 seconds, since voluntary contraction for a longer period will result in substantial depletion of ACh and consequently lesser increases in amplitude. In general, post-tetanic potentiation greater than twice the muscle action potential at rest is suggestive of the myasthenic syndrome. A lesser degree of facilitation may occur in some patients with this syndrome as well as in occasional cases of myasthenia gravis.

Instead of a single shock, a train of 3 per second stimuli may be delivered before exercise to establish the baseline. The same train is then repeated immediately following exercise and then every 30 seconds thereafter for a few minutes. In myasthenia gravis, post-tetanic potentiation partially compensates for depletion of ACh (see Fig. 9-3). Thus, the characteristic decrementing tendency is less obvious immediately following tetanic stimulation.

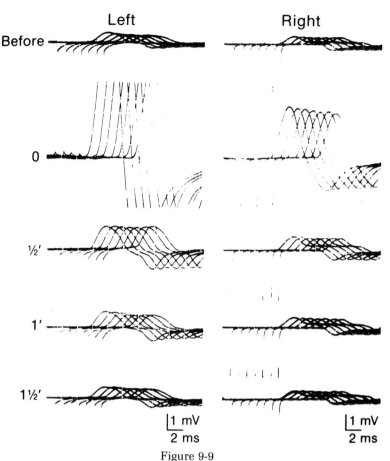

Figure 9-9

Progression of weakness in the same patient as in Figure 9-8 six weeks later. Stimulating and recording arrangements were the same. Compared with the previous study, the compound muscle action potentials were considerably smaller in amplitude on either side. Consequently, post-tetanic potentiation was more prominent and post-tetanic exhaustion less evident.

## Post-tetanic exhaustion

The post-tetanic potentiation is transient and soon followed by the post-tetanic exhaustion, which becomes apparent two to four minutes after exercise. The underlying physiologic mechanism is yet to be elucidated, but it is likely that the mobilization rate of ACh cannot keep pace with the rate of release at high stimulus repetition, thereby causing substantial depletion in the immediately available store of ACh. In normal muscles, because of a large margin of safety, the reduced amount of ACh released during post-tetanic exhaustion is still adequate to elicit a suprathreshold EPP. Neuromuscular reserve is limited in the end-plates of newborns and even less in premature infants.[38] Thus, in some normal infants, the amplitude of the compound muscle action potential progressively declines at high rates of stimulation. Post-tetanic exhaustion and relative resistance to decamethonium has also been observed in this age group.[14]

In patients with myasthenia gravis neuromuscular block worsens during post-tetanic exhaustion because of a reduced margin of safety. In some cases, an equivocal decrement at 3 per second in resting muscle may become significantly abnormal after exercise (see Fig. 9-3). In patients with the myasthenic syndrome, post-tetanic exhaustion of the EPP results in further reduction in amplitude of the originally small compound muscle action potential (Figs. 9-8 and 9-9). Thus, post-tetanic exhaustion increases the sensitivity of the nerve stimulation technique as a test of neuromuscular transmission. For observing post-tetanic exhaustion, a one minute period of voluntary contraction is optimal in order to adequately deplete the ACh store. This is in contrast to the shorter exercise period recommended for assessment of the post-tetanic potentiation.

# REPETITIVE STIMULATION IN MYOGENIC DISORDERS

Apparent decrement is also observed in patients with a number of myogenic disorders. These include myotonia, McArdle's disease, and periodic paralysis.

## Myotonia

The effect of repetitive nerve stimulation in myotonic muscles[3, 8, 45, 47] may be summarized as follows. (1) A decrementing response is common but not invariable. (2) Unlike the decremental response in myasthenia gravis, which levels off after the fourth or fifth stimulus, the decrease in amplitude is progressive for the initial few seconds. (3) This is then followed by recovery during continued stimulation for many seconds. (4) In general, the higher the rate of stimulation, the greater the change in amplitude and the shorter the latent period. (5) In patients with myotonia congenita, decrement occurs at a lower stimulation frequency than in myotonia dystrophica, and it tends to be more pronounced in the presence of clinical weakness. (6) In paramyotonia congenita, cooling potentiates both the weakness and decremental response.

The pathophysiology underlying decremental changes in myotonia is not known but may be related to the prolonged after-depolarization due to accumulation of potassium ($K^+$) in the transverse tubules.[1] The decreasing response can also be demonstrated by direct stimulation of the muscle, suggesting an abnormality of muscle rather than of the neuromuscular junction.[8] A progressive decline in amplitude of the action potential has been shown during intracellular recording of a myotonic discharge.[56] Myotonic bursts may render some of the muscle fibers refractory to subsequent stimuli. In contrast with myasthenia gravis, there is no post-tetanic potentiation or exhaustion. Indeed, the amplitude of the muscle response immediately after exercise is less than the baseline value, and the decremental tendency is greater after exercise than at rest. The resting value is restored gradually in about two to three minutes following exercise.

## McArdle's disease

In McArdle's disease, painful muscle contracture develops on exertion. The stiff muscle is electrically silent. With rapid repetitive stimulation of a motor nerve, there is a progressive decrease in amplitude of the compound muscle action potential coinciding with the development of contracture.[23, 54]

## Periodic paralysis

In periodic paralysis, the amplitude of the muscle action potential elicited by a single stimulus is reduced during a paralytic episode. The amplitude may progressively increase with repetitive stimulation of the motor nerve at high rates[29] or during intermittent repetitive stimulation,[10] although it falls again during rest.

# REFERENCE SOURCES

1. ADRIAN, RH AND BRYANT, SH: *On the repetitive discharge in myotonic muscle fibres.* J Physiol (Lond) 240:505, 1974.

2. ALBUQUERQUE, EX, ET AL: *An electrophysiological and morphological study of the neuromuscular junction in patients with myasthenia gravis.* Exp Neurol 51:536, 1976.

3. AMINOFF, MJ, ET AL: *The declining electrical response of muscle to repetitive nerve stimulation in myotonia.* Neurology (Minneap) 27:812, 1977.

4. BORENSTEIN, S AND DESMEDT, JE: *Temperature and weather correlates of myasthenic fatigue.* Lancet 2:63, 1974.

5. BORENSTEIN, S AND DESMEDT, JE: *Local cooling in myasthenia. Improvement of neuromuscular failure.* Arch Neurol 32:152, 1975.

6. BOTELHO, SY, ET AL: *Evaluation of the electromyogram of patients with myasthenia gravis.* Arch Neurol Psychiatry 67:441, 1952.

7. BRANISTEANU, DD, MIYAMOTO, MD, AND VOLLE, RL: *Effects of physiologic alterations on binomial transmitter release at magnesium-depressed neuromuscular junctions.* J Physiol (Lond) 254:19, 1976.

8. BROWN, JC: *Muscle weakness after rest in myotonic disorders: An electrophysiological study.* J Neurol Neurosurg Psychiatry 37:1336, 1974.

9. BROWN, JC AND JOHNS, RJ: *Diagnostic difficulties encountered in the myasthenic syndrome sometimes associated with carcinoma.* J Neurol Neurosurg Psychiatry 37:1214, 1974.

10. CAMPA, JF AND SANDERS, DB: *Familial hypokalemic periodic paralysis. Local recovery after nerve stimulation.* Arch Neurol 31:110, 1974.

11. CHERINGTON, M: *Botulism: Electrophysiologic and therapeutic observations.* In DESMEDT, JE (ED): *New Developments in Electromyography and Clinical Neurophysiology,* Vol 1. Karger, Basel, 1973, pp 375–379.

12. CHERINGTON, M: *Botulism. Ten-year experience.* Arch Neurol 30:432, 1974.

13. CHERINGTON, M AND GINSBERG, S: *Type B botulism: Neurophysiologic studies.* Neurology (Minneap) 21:43, 1971.

14. CHURCHILL-DAVIDSON, HC AND WISE, RP: *Neuromuscular transmission in the newborn infant.* Anesthesiology 24:271, 1963.

15. COOPER, BJ AND SPENCE, I: *Temperature-dependent inhibition of evoked acetylcholine release in tick paralysis.* Nature 263:693, 1976.

16. DAHL, DS AND SATO, S: *Unusual myasthenic state in a teen-age boy.* Neurology (Minneap) 24:897, 1974.

17. DAUBE, JR: *Electrophysiologic testing for disorders of the neuromuscular junction.* American Association of Electromyography and Electrodiagnosis, August, 1978.

18. DENYS, EH: *Minimonograph #14: The role of temperature in electromyography.* American Association of Electromyography and Electrodiagnosis, 1980.

19. DENYS, EH AND NORRIS, FH, JR: *Amyotrophic lateral sclerosis—Impairment of neuromuscular transmission.* Arch Neurol 36:202, 1979.

20. DESMEDT, JE: *The neuromuscular disorder in myasthenia gravis. 1. Electrical and mechanical response to nerve stimulation in hand muscles.* In DESMEDT, JE (ED): *New Developments in Electromyography and Clinical Neurophysiology,* Vol 1. Karger, Basel, 1973, pp 241–304.

21. DESMEDT, JE AND BORENSTEIN, S: *Diagnosis of myasthenia gravis by nerve stimulation.* Ann NY Acad Sci 274:174, 1976.

22. DESMEDT, JE, ET AL: *Muscular dystrophy and myasthenia gravis. Muscle contraction properties studied by the staircase phenomenon.* In DESMEDT, JE (ED): *New Developments in Electromyography and Clinical Neurophysiology,* Vol 1. Karger, Basel, 1973, pp 380–399.

23. DYKEN, ML, SMITH, DM, AND PEAKE, RL: *An electromyographic diagnostic screening test in McArdle's disease and a case report.* Neurology (Minneap) 17:45, 1967.

24. EATON, LM AND LAMBERT, EH: *Electromyography and electric stimulation of nerves in diseases of motor unit. Observations on myasthenic syndrome associated with malignant tumors.* JAMA 163:1117, 1957.

25. EISEN, A, ET AL: *Reduced neuromuscular transmission safety factor in multiple sclerosis.* Neurology (New York) 28:598, 1978.

26. ELMQVIST, D: *Neuromuscular transmission defects.* In DESMEDT, JE (ED): *New Developments in Electromyography and Clinical Neurophysiology,* Vol 1. Karger, Basel, 1973, pp 229–240.

27. FOLDES, FF, ET AL: *The influence of temperature on neuromuscular performance.* J Neural Transm 43:27, 1978.

28. GILLIATT, RW: *Nerve conduction in human and experimental neuropathies.* Proc R Soc Med (Lond) 59:989, 1966.

29. GROB, D, JOHNS, RJ, AND LILJESTRAND, Ä: *Potassium movement in patients with familial periodic paralysis. Relationship to the defect in muscle function.* Am J Med 23:356, 1957.

30. GUTMANN, L AND PRATT, L: *Pathophysiologic aspects of human botulism.* Arch Neurol 33:175, 1976.

31. HARRIS, JB AND LEACH, GDH: *The effect of temperature on end-plate depolarization of the rat diaphragm produced by suxamethonium and acetylcholine.* J Pharm Pharmacol 20:194, 1968.

32. HARVEY, AM AND MASLAND, RL: *The electromyogram in myasthenia gravis.* Bull Johns Hopkins Hosp 48:1, 1941.

33. HOFMANN, WW, PARSONS, RL, AND FEIGEN, GA: *Effects of temperature and drugs on mammalian motor nerve terminals.* Am J Physiol 211:135, 1966.

34. HUBBARD, JI, JONES, SF, AND LANDAU, EM: *The effect of temperature change upon transmitter release, facilitation and post-tetanic potentiation.* J Physiol (Lond) 216:591, 1971.

35. JOHNS, RJ, GROB, D, AND HARVEY, AM: *Studies in neuromuscular function. 2. Effects of nerve stimulation in normal subjects and in patients with myasthenia gravis.* Bull Johns Hopkins Hosp 99:125, 1956.

36. JOLLY, F: *Myasthenia gravis pseudoparalytica.* Berliner Klinische Wochenschrift 32:33, 1895.

37. KAMENSKAYA, MA AND THESLEFF, S: *The neuromuscular blocking action of an isolated toxin from the elapid (oxyuranus scutellactus).* Acta Physiol Scand 90:716, 1974.

38. KOENIGSBERGER, MR, PATTEN, B, AND LOVELACE, RE: *Studies of neuromuscular function in the newborn: 1. A comparison of myoneural function in the full term and the premature infant.* Neuropädriatrie 4:350, 1973.

39. KRARUP, C: *Electrical and mechanical responses in the platysma and in the adductor pollicis muscle: In patients with myasthenia gravis.* J Neurol Neurosurg Psychiatry 40:241, 1977.

40. KRARUP, C: *Electrical and mechanical responses in the platysma and in the adductor pollicis muscle: In normal subjects.* J Neurol Neurosurg Psychiatry 40:234, 1977.

41. LAMBERT, EH: *Electromyography and electric stimulation of peripheral nerves and muscle.* In *Clinical Examinations in Neurology,* ed 4. Departments of Neurology, Physiology, and Biophysics, Mayo Clinic and Mayo Foundation, WB Saunders, Philadelphia, 1976, pp 298–329.

42. LAMBERT, EH: *Electromyographic responses to repetitive stimulation of nerve.* American Academy of Neurology, Special Course #16, April 23–28, 1979.

43. LAMBERT, EH: *Neuromuscular transmission studies.* American Association of Electromyography and Electrodiagnosis, Third Annual Continuing Education Course, September 25, 1980.

44. LAMBERT, EH AND ROOKE, ED: *Myasthenic state and lung cancer.* In BRAIN, WR AND NORRIS, FH, JR (EDS): *Contemporary Neurology Symposia,* Vol 1. *The Remote Effects of Cancer on the Nervous System.* Grune & Stratton, New York, 1965, pp 67–80.

45. LAMBERT, EH, MILLIKAN, CH, AND EATON, LM: *Stage of neuromuscular paralysis in myotonia.* Am J Physiol 171:741, 1952.

46. LAMBERT, EH, ET AL: *Myasthenic syndrome occasionally associated with bronchial neoplasm: Neurophysiologic studies.* In VIETS, HR (ED): *Myasthenia Gravis. The Second International Symposium Proceedings,* Charles C Thomas, Springfield, Ill, 1961, pp 362–410.

47. LUNDBERG, PO, STÅLBERG, E, AND THIELE, B: *Paralysis periodica paramyotonica. A clinical and neurophysiological study.* J Neurol Sci 21:309, 1974.

TECHNIQUES OF REPETITIVE STIMULATION

48. MA, DM, WASSERMAN, EJL, AND GIEBFRIED, J: *Repetitive stimulation of the trapezius muscle: Its value in myasthenic testing.* Muscle and Nerve 3:439, 1980.

49. MAYER, RF AND WILLIAMS, IR: *Incrementing responses in myasthenia gravis.* Arch Neurol 31:24, 1974.

50. MULDER, DW, LAMBERT, EH, AND EATON, LM: *Myasthenic syndrome in patients with amyotrophic lateral sclerosis.* Neurology (Minneap) 9:627, 1959.

51. ÖZDEMIR, C AND YOUNG, RR: *The results to be expected from electrical testing in the diagnosis of myasthenia gravis.* Ann NY Acad Sci 274:203, 1976.

52. PICKETT, J, ET AL: *Syndrome of botulism in infancy: Clinical and electrophysiological study.* N Engl J Med 295:770, 1976.

53. PITTINGER, C AND ADAMSON, R: *Antibiotic blockade of neuromuscular function.* Ann Rev Pharmacol 12:169, 1972.

54. RICKER, K AND MERTENS, HG: *Myasthenic reaction in primary muscle fibre disease.* Electroenceph Clin Neurophysiol 25:413, 1968.

55. RICKER, K, HERTEL, G, AND STODIECK, S: *The influence of local cooling on neuromuscular transmission in the myasthenic syndrome of Eaton and Lambert.* J Neurol 217:95, 1977.

56. RÜDEL, R AND KELLER, M: *Intracellular recording of myotonic runs in dantrolene-blocked myotonic muscle fibres.* In BRADLEY, WG, GARDNER-MEDWIN, D, AND WALTON, JN (EDS): *Recent Advances in Myology.* Proceedings of the Third International Congress on Muscle Diseases, Excerpta Medica, Amsterdam, 1975, pp 441–445.

57. SCHWARTZ, MS AND STÅLBERG, E: *Myasthenia gravis with features of the myasthenic syndrome. An investigation with electrophysiologic methods including single-fiber electromyography.* Neurology (Minneap) 25:80, 1975.

58. SIMPSON, JA: *Myasthenia gravis: A new hypothesis.* Scott Med J 5:419, 1960.

59. SLOMIĆ, A, ROSENFALCK, A, AND BUCHTHAL, F: *Electrical and mechanical responses of normal and myasthenic muscle with particular reference to the staircase phenomenon.* Brain Res 10:1, 1968.

60. SWIFT, TR: *Weakness from magnesium-containing cathartics: Electrophysiologic studies.* Muscle and Nerve 2:295, 1979.

61. TAKAMORI, M AND GUTMANN, L: *Intermittent defect of acetylcholine release in myasthenia gravis.* Neurology (Minneap) 21:47, 1971.

62. WARD, CD AND MURRAY, NMF: *Effect of temperature on neuromuscular transmission in the Eaton-Lambert syndrome.* J Neurol Neurosurg Psychiatry 42:247, 1979.

63. WRIGHT, GP: *The neurotoxins of clostridium botulinum and clostridium tetani.* Pharmacol Rev 7:413, 1955.

# CHAPTER
# 10

# ACTIVATION PROCEDURES AND OTHER METHODS

Not all muscles are significantly affected in patients with diseases of the neuromuscular junction. Thus, the conventional nerve stimulation technique does not always uncover electrophysiologic abnormalities to substantiate the clinical diagnosis. The sensitivity of this technique can be further increased by imposing a metabolic stress on the muscles, thereby reducing the safety factor for neuromuscular transmission. Various tests have been introduced to improve the diagnostic sensitivity of the nerve stimulation technique, while avoiding false-positive results. Commonly employed activation methods include the ischemic test[10] and the regional curare test.[20] Both procedures are well tolerated in normal muscles but lead to a transmission defect in occult as well as overtly myasthenic muscles.

When testing neuromuscular transmission by means of paired or repetitive electrical stimuli applied to the peripheral nerve, electrical activity of the contracting muscle is ordinarily recorded to demonstrate decremental responses. The fatigability of the muscle force can also be measured simultaneously, but an accurate recording of mechanical activity is possible in only a few muscles. In addition to the nerve stimulation technique, analysis of motor unit potentials in conventional electromyography is of value in evaluating disorders of neuromuscular transmission. In particular, assessment of the extraocular muscles by a needle electrode provides useful information in patients with ocular myasthenia. More recently, single fiber electromyography has been added to the list of electrophysiologic methods. Calculation of jitter is a very sensitive measure of neuromuscular transmission and has proven to be one of the most useful. The in vitro analysis of miniature end-plate potentials of intercostal muscles is another physiologic means that allows a direct quantitative measure of neuromuscular transmission,[11] although the technique is not feasible as a routine clinical study.

There are a number of other laboratory methods for objectifying the diagnosis of myasthenia gravis. These include tonography and infrared optokinetic nystagmography for patients with ocular myasthenia[38, 42] and the stapedius reflex for patients with weakness of the facial muscles.[2] In addition, the effects of edrophonium (Tensilon) or neostigmine (Prostigmin) are studied in connection with the electrophysiologic methods mentioned earlier for quantitative assessments. Based on the immunologic abnormalities, measurement of serum antibodies against the muscle end-plate has been used successfully as a diagnostic test.[1, 24, 25] As a part of clinical evaluation, pulmonary function tests also provide useful objective criteria in documenting neuromuscular fatigue.[16, 29]

# ISCHEMIC TEST

A double-step test has been introduced to increase the diagnostic sensitivity of nerve stimulation techniques in patients with mild, generalized myasthenia gravis or ocular myasthenia gravis.[4, 9] The first step consists of continuous supramaximal stimulation of the ulnar nerve at a rate of 3 per second for four minutes and recording the compound muscle action potential from the ulnar-innervated intrinsic hand muscles or the flexor carpi ulnaris in the forearm. The muscles are then tested several times at 30 second intervals by a train of 3 per second stimulation for several shocks and the amount of decrement within each 3 per second trial determined. If the first step produces a negative or equivocal result, ischemia is induced by a cuff inflated above arterial pressure proximal to the stimulation site. The same procedure is then repeated.

## Normal response

In normal subjects, the amplitude of the compound muscle action potential may be stable or become progressively smaller after two or three minutes of continuous 3 per second stimulation under ischemia. In the series by Desmedt and Borenstein,[10] the amplitude of the last response in a four minute stimulation ranged from 50 to 110 percent of the first. Even if the size of the muscle response is reduced during ischemic exercise, the subsequent 3 per second tests elicit no decrementing response within each train in the intrinsic hand muscles. Such reduction in amplitude without significant decrement may be caused by conduction block of the nerve during ischemia. The amplitude returns to normal in about three minutes if the cuff is released. Decrements in the 3 per second series occur in the intrinsic hand muscles of normals only after a more prolonged period of ischemic exercise lasting 7 to 15 minutes. The flexor carpi ulnaris is, for unknown reasons, more sensitive to this procedure and normal subjects may show decremental responses in the 3 per second series following four minutes of ischemic exercise.

## Myasthenic response

In myasthenic hand muscles, the ischemic exercise at 3 per second stimulation for four minutes generally elicits marked exhaustion. The amplitude of the muscle response decreases markedly two to three minutes after the beginning of the continuous 3 per second stimulation. A train of 3 per second stimulation following ischemic exercise shows increased block in the overtly myasthenic muscle. More importantly, subclinical involvement may be uncovered when there is no clear abnormality of neuromuscular transmission before ischemic exercise. A similar period of ischemia with only one 3 per second test every two minutes and no continuous exercise does not significantly affect the neuromuscular block. Thus, muscles with subclinical myasthenia develop decrement only when sensitized by both ischemia and sustained exercise. If ischemic muscles are cooled 1 to 2°C, neuromuscular transmission will improve.[5] Therefore, it is important to avoid such a temperature drop to minimize the incidence of false-negative results.

Supramaximal stimuli at 2 to 3 per second are optimal for demonstrating the decrement in myasthenic muscles as discussed earlier. The duration of the ischemic exercise should be at least two minutes to unmask the reduced safety factor, but it should not exceed five minutes to avoid the decrementing response seen in normal muscles. Thus, Desmedt and Borenstein[10] recommend 3 per second stimulation for four minutes before and four minutes during ischemia. This procedure excludes false-positive results in the hand muscles, yet is adequate to reveal significant decrements in subclinical myasthenic muscles. Various muscles are affected to different degrees in the same patient with myasthenia gravis. Neuromuscular block may be apparent in the resting state in some muscles, whereas it occurs only with exercise in others. Still other muscles are without demonstrable neuromuscular failure even after considerable stress is placed on the system. The double step test of Desmedt and Borenstein[10] has been helpful in elucidating different degrees of myasthenic involvement in the same patient. How much additional help this procedure provides in the early diagnosis of myasthenia gravis remains to be further investigated.[31]

# REGIONAL CURARE TEST

The amount of acetylcholine (ACh) released with each nerve impulse normally produces an end-plate potential (EPP) that substantially exceeds the critical level for excitation of all the muscle fibers. Because of this margin of safety, a latent deficit of neuromuscular transmission may remain undetected clinically or electrophysiologically. The functional reserve may be reduced or eliminated by the administration of curare, which causes a nondepolarizing block by competing with ACh for the end-plate receptors. Sensitivity to curare may be used to assess the defect of neuromuscular transmission. The smaller the margin of safety, the less curare is required to eliminate the reserve.

## Principles and procedures

The systemic administration of curare, however, has not been widely used because of its potential hazard. Instead, a reduced dose of curare may be regionally injected at the wrist with a pressure tourniquet occluding the forearm circulation. Muscular strength in the limb may be studied by changes in grip strength[13] or in force of evoked muscle contraction.[12] However, the effect of curare is best analyzed by changes in amplitude of the compound muscle action potentials elicited by a train of stimulation to the nerve in the upper limb rendered ischemic.[6, 19, 20, 21, 22]

The neuromuscular block restricted to one forearm and hand may be achieved by regional intravenous administration of about one twentieth of the usual curarizing dose. The following steps are recommended.[18] A blood pressure cuff is applied to the forearm. A scalp vein needle, pointing distally, is inserted into a superficial forearm vein. The arm is then elevated for one minute to drain venous circulation. With the arm in that position, the cuff is inflated to about 250 mm Hg, at least 100 mm Hg above systolic pressure. The arm is lowered and a solution of 0.2 mg d-tubocurarine in 20 cc of 0.9 percent sodium chloride is rapidly injected. The cuff remains inflated for six and a half minutes after the start of the injection. Repetitive stimulation at 3 per second is applied five minutes and again six minutes after the start of the injection, with the arm still ischemic. The cuff is then deflated allowing blood to circulate before the next trains of 3 per second are given at eight minutes and again at nine minutes after injection. If decrements of greater than 10 percent are obtained, stimulation is repeated at 10 minutes for confirmation. If the decrement is equivocal, post-tetanic exhaustion is evaluated with 3 per second stimulus trains at one-minute intervals for 10 minutes following a tetanus.

## Clinical value and limitations

The regional curare test is considered safe in equivocal or mildly myasthenic patients. Therefore, an anesthetist need not be present under ordinary circumstances. Nonetheless, the procedure should be avoided in patients with established myasthenia gravis. The exposure of severely myasthenic patients should be rare, if the regional curare test is reserved as a measure of last resort and performed only when the conventional nerve stimulation techniques fail to reveal abnormalities in suspected cases. Horowitz and Sivak[20] reported a series of 600 patients referred for evaluation of possible myasthenia gravis. The diagnosis was verified electrophysiologically in 320 (53 percent), using conventional repetitive stimulation at the wrist and shoulder. Of the remaining 280 patients, the regional curare test was abnormal in 72 (26 percent), including 52 (74 percent) of 70 patients with definite generalized myasthenia gravis, 13 (10 percent) of 136 patients with possible generalized myasthenia gravis, and 7 (14 percent) of 49 ocular myasthenics.

The concentration of curare that reaches the muscles depends on diffusion through the volume of tissue, which is probably quite variable from one case to the next. Thus, normal and pathologic responses cannot always be clearly delineated using different dosages of curare.[17] Nonetheless, the regional curare test appears to be useful in establishing the defect of neuromuscular transmission in the hand muscles, especially in patients with ocular myasthenia. Some investigators feel, however, that the use of curare or other provocative techniques are unnecessary in the diagnosis of 95 percent of patients with myasthenia gravis.[31] It is important to remember that undue sensitivity to curare has been reported not only in myasthenia gravis,[35] but also in amyotrophic lateral sclerosis[28] and muscular weakness after administration of antibiotics.[33] Therefore, the decrementing response of muscle potentials demonstrated by the regional curare test must be interpreted in the light of the clinical context, since it may not necessarily be indicative of myasthenia gravis.

# ELECTROMYOGRAPHY

In normal muscles, a given motor unit potential firing repetitively under voluntary control is identical in shape and amplitude every time it discharges, as long as the needle electrode remains in the same location relative to the motor unit. In myasthenic muscles, the end-plate potentials of some individual muscle fibers may not reach the critical level in response to each nerve impulse because of a reduced margin of safety. Consequently, not all the individual muscle fibers, although innervated by the same axon, discharge when the motor unit is activated repetitively, resulting in amplitude variability of motor unit potentials. This in turn is responsible, at least in part, for diminished mean amplitude and duration of motor unit potentials in weak muscles of myasthenic patients.[30]

## Varying motor unit potentials

The needle is slowly advanced or retracted until single motor unit potentials are isolated and then maintained in the same location. A defect in neuromuscular transmission is often suggested by the variability in the sound of an isolated motor unit potential over the loudspeaker during minimal contraction of the muscle. To document changing amplitude and shape of the unit, repetitive motor unit discharges may be stored on the oscilloscope or photographed. Accurate quantitative assessment of neuromuscular transmission cannot be achieved by this method. Unlike the nerve stimulation technique, however, the needle examination is not restricted to the limited number of muscles innervated by a readily accessible nerve. Further, the muscle does not have to be immobilized for this purpose. Thus, the method is useful in testing muscles that cannot be properly evaluated with repetitive stimulation of the nerve. Extraocular muscles are such examples, and these can be tested by ocular electromyography as described in Chapter 14. Ocular electromyography shows a progressive decrease in amplitude and frequency during a prolonged period of voluntary contraction in patients with ocular myasthenia gravis.[36] This can be partially reversed by administration of edrophonium (Tensilon) intravenously.[23]

The effect of edrophonium on motor unit potentials has been studied in patients with myasthenia gravis. It is characterized by reversal of the diminished amplitude and duration that is observed during weak contraction, and reversal of the reduction in amplitude seen during maximal effort. In a series of 12 patients studied by Pinelli[32] using computer averaging, the mean amplitude of motor unit potentials in the extensor digitorum communis increased 30 to 130 percent in nine patients, and the mean duration increased 10 to 25 percent in seven patients, following intravenous injection of edrophonium. In three other patients, the amplitude of motor unit potentials increased in a facial or extraocular muscle, but not in the extensor digitorum communis. In four patients, there were significant changes in the motor unit potentials, even though repetitive nerve stimulation failed to uncover a decremental response in the opponens pollicis muscle. Thus, careful assessment of motor unit potentials before and after administration of edrophonium appears to be a sensitive test for early detection of defects in neuromuscular transmission.

## Jitter and blocking

The single fiber recording is another electromyographic procedure that has proven useful in early detection of neuromuscular disturbances. It allows assessment of single fiber neuromuscular transmission and provides an important new method in the evaluation of myasthenia gravis.[39, 40] The technique is described in detail later in Chapter 15, but essential points will be discussed briefly here. If a pair of single fiber potentials are recorded simultaneously, fluctuation of the neuromuscular transmission can be determined by the stability of the second response of the pair. Neuromuscular disturbances are characterized by either blocking or by increased jitter as follows.

When a motor unit is voluntarily activated, the end-plate potentials (EPP) normally reach threshold in all single muscle fibers belonging to the unit. If the EPP is subthreshold owing to reduced safety margin, then blocking occurs and the single muscle fiber potential drops out. This is seen on standard needle recordings as a reduction in the size of the motor unit potential. If an EPP barely reaches the necessary level, its rate of rise tends to be slow and the action potential is delayed, although not blocked. If a pair of single fiber potentials is recorded simultaneously, a delay of the action potential in either fiber is seen as an increased interpotential interval or increased jitter. It is probably the first sign of neuromuscular instability. Since it usually precedes blocking of single potential, increase in the jitter value is seen without variation of motor unit potentials or decrementing response to repetitive stimulation of the nerve. Single fiber electromyography is technically more demanding than the conventional method, but with additional training, it can now be performed using commercially available recording units. It has proven to be the most sensitive of many electrophysiologic techniques currently available for the assessment of neuromuscular transmission.

# OTHER TECHNIQUES

## Microelectrode recording

Microelectrode recordings from single intercostal muscles enable one to quantitatively measure the size of the acetylcholine (ACh) quantum and the number of ACh quanta released per volley of the nerve impulse. These determinations in turn allow precise definition of an abnormality of neuromuscular transmission. At present it is the only method capable of distinguishing myasthenia gravis, myasthenic syndrome, and other disorders involving the neuromuscular junction, with certainty. The method has been important in defining the underlying pathophysiology of disordered neuromuscular transmission. The technique is essential in quantitative assessment of the production and mobilization of ACh as well as the sensitivity of motor end-plate. This method, however, cannot be used as a routine clinical test, since it requires biopsy of the intercostal muscles.

# Tonography

Other techniques not ordinarily used in an electromyographic laboratory include edrophonium (Tensilon) tonography. This is a standardized method for a measurement of the intraocular pressure that results in part from contraction of the extraocular muscles.[23] An electronic tonometer is used to measure the pressure before and after administration of edrophonium.[14, 15] Muscle action potentials may be recorded simultaneously with needle electrodes placed in the extraocular muscles. In normal subjects, intraocular pressure may fall on the average 1.6 to 1.8 mm Hg over a one-minute period, after an intravenous injection of edrophonium up to 10 mg.[8] Ocular electromyography is not significantly affected.

Intraocular pressure may be reduced in patients with decreased extraocular tone, as in ocular myasthenia. In patients with decreased extraocular tone, edrophonium produces changes in tonography coincident with a moderate increase in electrical activity in the extraocular muscles. Rise in intraocular pressure by a mean of 1.6 mm Hg occurs within 35 seconds of injection of edrophonium, as a result of a sudden increase in extraocular muscle tone. This phenomenon, however, is not specific to ocular myasthenia, having been reported in ocular myositis without other features of myasthenia gravis.[42] Intraocular pressure may also rise with Valsalva maneuver, resulting in a false-positive edrophonium tonography. A control injection of saline is often administered first to identify this phenomenon.

# Stapedius reflex

Bilateral contraction of the stapedius muscles occurs in response to unilateral sound stimulation. This in turn induces changes in the acoustic impedance of the middle ear, and prevents hyperacusis. Thus, the function of the stapedius muscle can be measured by impedance audiometry. In normal subjects, the stapedius reflex occurs with a sound stimulus 70 dB to 100 dB above the hearing threshold. There is no decay in the sustained contraction with stimulus durations up to one minute for frequencies of 250 to 1000 Hz.

In patients with myasthenia gravis, weakened stapedius muscles result in hyperacusis due to enhanced transmission of sound in the 1 to 4 KHz range. This is associated with weakness of the acoustic reflex, which is thus induced only by high sound intensity.[27] In addition, reflex contraction of the stapedius muscle shows a rapid decrement, indicating an increased neuromuscular fatigability.[2] This is analogous to the decremental response to repetitive electrical stimulation in myasthenic muscles elsewhere. After administration of edrophonium, hyperacusis diminishes, reflecting a stronger acoustic reflex, and the decay of the stapedius reflex to repetitive sound stimulation is improved. As a diagnostic test of myasthenia gravis, the stapedius reflex may provide the only electrophysiologic abnormality.[41]

# Tests for oculomotor function

Electronystagmography is considered useful in patients with ocular myasthenia, since it measures fatigue of extraocular movements. Amplitude, velocity, and frequency of optokinetic nystagmus are recorded. The technique is used to demonstrate oculomotor improvement following administration of edrophonium. In patients with ocular myasthenia, edrophonium induces an increase in previously reduced amplitude and velocity of the fast component of optokinetic nystagmus.[3] Neuromuscular fatigue with subsequent beneficial response to edrophonium is seen in 50 percent of myasthenic patients.[8] However, the amplitude and rate of nystagmus is quite variable when recorded by electrooculography. The optokinetic nystagmus may also be recorded with an infrared reflection technique, which improves the sensitivity of the test.[38] In this method, neuropharmacologic effect can be graded by numerical criteria rather than visual inspection to make the evaluation of edrophonium response simple and objective.[37]

Lancaster red-green test is another technique used to detect oculomotor improvement following administration of edrophonium.[34] In patients with myasthenia gravis, there is a definite change in the pattern of ocular deviations as measured with the red-green test. The amplitude and frequency are restored after rest or with administration of edrophonium. Velocity of saccadic ocular movements can be measured by the infrared recording technique or by electrooculography.[26] In myasthenic patients, ocular velocities increase following administration of edrophonium.

# REFERENCE SOURCES

1. ALMON, RR, ANDREW, CG, AND APPEL, SH: Serum globulin in myasthenia gravis: Inhibition of α-bungarotoxin binding to acetylcholine receptors. Science 186:55, 1974.

2. BLOM, S AND ZAKRISSON, JE: The stapedius reflex in the diagnosis of myasthenia gravis. J Neurol Sci 21:71, 1974.

3. BLOMBERG, LH AND PERSSON, T: A new test for myasthenia gravis. Preliminary report. Acta Neurol Scand 41(suppl 13):363, 1965.

4. BORENSTEIN, S AND DESMEDT, JE: New diagnostic procedures in myasthenia gravis. In DESMEDT, JE (ED): New Developments in Electromyography and Clinical Neurophysiology, Vol 1. Karger, Basel, 1973, pp 350–374.

5. BORENSTEIN, S AND DESMEDT, JE: Local cooling in myasthenia: Improvement of neuromuscular failure. Arch Neurol 32:152, 1975.

6. BROWN, JC AND CHARLTON, JE: A study of sensitivity to curare in myasthenic disorders using a regional technique. J Neurol Neurosurg Psychiatry 38:27, 1975.

7. BROWN, JC, CHARLTON, JE, AND WHITE, DJK: A regional technique for the study of sensitivity to curare in human muscle. J Neurol Neurosurg Psychiatry 38:18, 1975.

8. CAMPBELL, MJ, ET AL: Ocular myasthenia: Evaluation of Tensilon tonography and electronystagmography as diagnostic tests. J Neurol Neurosurg Psychiatry 33:639, 1970.

9. DESMEDT, JE: The neuromuscular disorder in myasthenia gravis. 1. Electrical and mechanical response to nerve stimulation in hand muscles. In DESMEDT, JE (ED): New Developments in Electromyography and Clinical Neurophysiology, Vol 1. Karger, Basel, 1973, pp 241–304.

10. DESMEDT, JE AND BORENSTEIN, S: Double-step nerve stimulation test for myasthenic block: Sensitization of postactivation exhaustion by ischemia. Ann Neurol 1:55, 1977.

11. ELMQVIST, D: Neuromuscular transmission defects. In DESMEDT, JE (ED): New Developments in Electromyography and Clinical Neurophysiology, Vol 1. Karger, Basel, 1973, pp 229–240.

12. FELDMAN, SA AND TYRRELL, MF: A new theory of the termination of action of the muscle relaxants. Proc R Soc Med 63:692, 1970.

13. FOLDES, FF, ET AL: A new curare test for the diagnosis of myasthenia gravis. JAMA 203:649, 1968.

14. GLASER, JS: Tensilon tonography in the diagnosis of myasthenia gravis. Invest Ophthalmol 6:135, 1967.

15. GLASER, JS, MILLER, GR, AND GASS, JDM: The edrophonium tonogram test in myasthenia gravis. Arch Ophthalmol 76:368, 1966.

16. GRIGGS, RC, ET AL: Evaluation of pulmonary function in neuromuscular disease. Arch Neurol 38:9, 1981.

17. HERTEL, G, RICKER, K, AND HIRSCH, A: The regional curare test in myasthenia gravis. J Neurol 214:257, 1977.

18. HOROWITZ, SH: The regional curare test and electrophysiologic diagnosis of myasthenia gravis. Am Acad Neurol, Special Course #16, April 23–28, 1979.

19. HOROWITZ, SH AND KRARUP, C: A new regional curare test of the elbow flexors in myasthenia gravis. Muscle and Nerve 2:478, 1979.

20. HOROWITZ, SH AND SIVAK, M: The regional curare test and electrophysiologic diagnosis of myasthenia gravis: Further studies. Muscle and Nerve 1:432, 1978.

21. HOROWITZ, SH, ET AL: *Regional curare test in evaluation of ocular myasthenia.* Arch Neurol 32:84, 1975.

22. HOROWITZ, SH, ET AL: *Electrophysiologic diagnosis of myasthenia gravis and the regional curare test.* Neurology (Minneap) 26:410, 1976.

23. KORNBLUETH, W, ET AL: *Contraction of the oculorotary muscles and intraocular pressure. A tonographic and electromyographic study of the effect of edrophonium chloride (Tensilon) and succinylcholine (Anectine) on the intraocular pressure.* Am J Ophthalmol 49:1381, 1960.

24. LEFVERT, AK, ET AL: *Determination of acetylcholine receptor antibody in myasthenia gravis: Clinical usefulness and pathogenetic implications.* J Neurol Neurosurg Psychiatry 41:394, 1978.

25. LINDSTROM, JM, ET AL: *Experimental autoimmune myasthenia gravis and myasthenia gravis: Biochemical and immunochemical aspects.* Ann NY Acad Sci 274:254, 1976.

26. METZ, HS, SCOTT, AB, AND O'MEARA, DM: *Saccadic eye movements in myasthenia gravis.* Arch Ophthalmol 88:9, 1972.

27. MORIOKA, WT, ET AL: *Audiotympanometric findings in myasthenia gravis.* Arch Otolaryngol 102:211, 1976.

28. MULDER, DW, LAMBERT, EH, AND EATON, LM: *Myasthenic syndrome in patients with amyotrophic lateral sclerosis.* Neurology (Minneap) 9:627, 1959.

29. O'DONOHUE, WJ, ET AL: *Respiratory failure in neuromuscular disease. Management in a respiratory intensive care unit.* JAMA 235:733, 1976.

30. OOSTERHUIS, HJGH, ET AL: *The mean duration of motor unit action potentials in patients with myasthenia gravis.* Electroenceph Clin Neurophysiol 32:697, 1972.

31. ÖZDEMIR, C AND YOUNG, RR: *The results to be expected from electrical testing in the diagnosis of myasthenia gravis.* Ann NY Acad Sci 274:203, 1976.

32. PINELLI, P: *The effect of anticholinesterases on motor unit potentials in myasthenia gravis.* Muscle and Nerve 1:438, 1978.

33. PITTINGER, C AND ADAMSON, R: *Antibiotic blockade of neuromuscular function.* Ann Rev Pharmacol 12:169, 1972.

34. RETZLAFF, JA, ET AL: *Lancaster red-green test in evaluation of edrophonium effect in myasthenia gravis.* Am J Ophthalmol 67:13, 1969.

35. ROWLAND, LP, ARANOW, H, JR, AND HOEFER, PFA: *Observations on the curare test in the differential diagnosis of myasthenia gravis.* In VIETS, HR (ED): Myasthenia Gravis. The Second International Symposium Proceedings, Charles C Thomas, Springfield, Ill, 1961, pp 411–434.

36. SEARS, ML, WALSH, FB, AND TEASDALL, RD: *The electromyogram from ocular muscles in myasthenia gravis.* Arch Ophthalmol 63:791, 1960.

37. SPECTOR, RH AND DAROFF, RB: *Edrophonium infrared optokinetic nystagmography in the diagnosis of myasthenia gravis.* Ann NY Acad Sci 274:642, 1976.

38. SPECTOR, RH, DAROFF, RB, AND BIRKETT, JE: *Edrophonium infrared optokinetic nystagmography in the diagnosis of myasthenia gravis.* Neurology (Minneap) 25:317, 1975.

39. STÅLBERG, E, EKSTEDT, J, AND BROMAN, A: *Neuromuscular transmission in myasthenia gravis studied with single fibre electromyography.* J Neurol Neurosurg Psychiatry 37:540, 1974.

40. STÅLBERG, E, TRONTELJ, JV, AND SCHWARTZ, MS: *Single-muscle-fiber recording of the jitter phenomenon in patients with myasthenia gravis and in members of their families.* Ann NY Acad Sci 274:189, 1976.

41. WARREN, WR, ET AL: *Stapedius reflex decay in myasthenia gravis.* Arch Neurol 34:496, 1977.

42. WRAY, SH AND PAVAN-LANGSTON, D: *A reevaluation of edrophonium chloride (Tensilon) tonography in the diagnosis of myasthenia gravis. With observations on some other defects of neuromuscular transmission.* Neurology (Minneap) 21:586, 1971.

PART

# 4

# ELECTROMYOGRAPHY

# CHAPTER
# 11

# ANATOMY
# AND PHYSIOLOGY
# OF SKELETAL MUSCLE

The skeletal muscles contain extrafusal and intrafusal fibers that are distinct anatomically as well as physiologically. The extrafusal fibers are contractile elements innervated by alpha motor neurons and occupy the bulk of muscle mass. The intrafusal fibers, known as muscle spindles, are stretch sensitive receptors found in parallel with the extrafusal fibers. They are innervated by gamma motor neurons. The Golgi tendon organs also respond to stretch, but they are aligned in series with the tendon of the extrafusal fibers. The muscle spindles and Golgi tendon organ continuously monitor and regulate the tonus of reflexively or volitionally contracting extrafusal fibers. The smallest unit of muscle contraction is the motor unit, which consists of a single motor neuron and all the muscle fibers innervated by its axon.

Electromechanical coupling which precedes the muscle contraction has already been described in conjunction with neuromuscular transmission in Chapter 8. The initial event of a muscle contraction is the depolarization of the end-plate region by acetylcholine (ACh) released at the neuromuscular junction in response to a nerve impulse. Once the action potential is generated, it is propagated along the muscle membrane. Ionized calcium ($Ca^{++}$) is released into the sarcoplasm. Chemical interaction of the ionized calcium with thin filaments leads to the formation of bridges between the thin and thick filaments. The sliding of thin filaments between the thick filaments results in a shortening of the muscle fibers.

This section will present an anatomic description of the contractile elements, the mechanism underlying the shortening of the muscle fibers, and the anatomy and physiology of motor units.

## FUNCTIONAL ANATOMY

### Gross anatomy of muscle

A connective tissue called epimysium surrounds the surface of each muscle (Fig. 11-1). Each muscle consists of many fascicles bound by the coarse sleeves of the connective tissue, called perimysium. Each fascicle contains many muscle fibers which are surrounded by a delicate network of fine connective tissue, called endomysium. A muscle fiber is the smallest anatomic unit capable of contraction. Its average diameter ranges

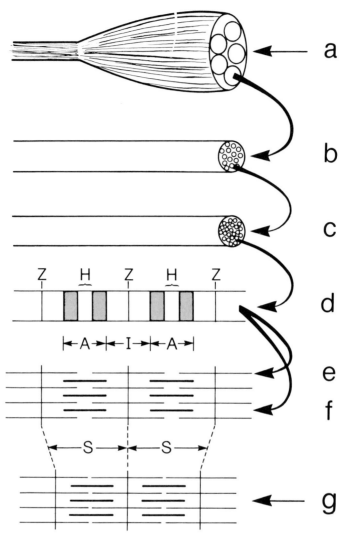

Figure 11-1

Anatomic composition of the skeletal muscle. The epimysium surrounds the entire muscle (a) which is subdivided into many fascicles and bound by perimysium (b). Individual muscle fibers (c) in the fascicle are covered by endomysium. Each muscle fiber contains many bundles of myofibers (d) which in turn consist of thin (e) and thick (f) myofilaments. Thin actin filaments slide relative to thick myosin filaments during muscle contraction (g).

from 10 $\mu$m in the newborn to 50 $\mu$m in an adult.[20] Individual muscle fibers range from 2 to 12 cm in length, some extending the entire length of the muscle and others only through a short segment of the total length.

The surface membrane of a muscle fiber is a thin sheath called sarcolemma and contains multiple nuclei distributed beneath. The membrane is similar to that of an axon with regard to its functional properties of excitability and conductivity. The conduction velocity of muscle fibers, however, is considerably slower than that of nerve axons and is estimated to be 4 to 5 m/s.[20, 44, 87] The intracellular content of a muscle fiber is semifluid plasma called sarcoplasm. Within the sarcoplasm are many bundles of cylindrical myofibrils, which are a thin, threadlike substance with light and dark bands of striations.

# Myofibrils and myofilaments

Under the electron miscroscope myofibrils are seen to consist of two types of myofilaments which are the basic substrates for the contraction of muscle fibers. The transverse striations seen by light microscopy are due to specific arrangements between these two types of myofilaments. The structural subunit extending between two adjacent Z-lines is called the sarcomere. The center of the sarcomere contains longitudinally oriented thick myosin myofilaments. Thin actin filaments extend from either side of the Z-line into the two adjacent sarcomeres and interdigitate with the myosin filaments. The thick filaments consist of only myosin molecules which are assembled to form parallel elongated rods. The thin filaments contain not only actin molecules but also two other proteins, troponin and tropomyosin, which are intimately bound to actin molecules. The globular shaped troponins are attached to each end of the long and thin tropomyosin molecules, which in turn are continuously interwoven along the length of actin molecules (Fig. 11-2). During muscle fiber contraction, individual filaments do not shorten, but actin filaments slide relative to the myosin filaments, thereby bringing the adjacent Z-lines closer together. Consequently, the sarcomere shortens.[16]

# Mechanism of contraction

The exact mechanism of the sliding is not yet known, but it is postulated that calcium($Ca^{++}$)-dependent bridges link the actin and myosin filaments. At rest, tropomyosin blocks the formation of bridges between myosin and actin. The propagated action potential, spreading into the sarcoplasmic reticulum via the transverse tubules, releases calcium from the terminal cistern of the longitudinal tubules. The free calcium binds to troponin, the only calcium-receptive protein in the contractile system. This interaction shifts the position of tropomyosin relative to the actin molecule, allowing the globular heads of myosin to gain access to actin molecules. Myosin-actin cross-bridges are formed, pulling the actin filaments past the myosin filaments. The tension developed by a sarcomere is likely to be related to the number of cross-bridges formed by this chemical interaction. Old bridges are shorn following the dissociation of adenosine triphosphate (ATP) of actin and myosin.

Without a sustained muscle action potential, calcium is sequestered into the sarcoplasmic reticulum through ATP-dependent active transport. The removal of calcium from troponin allows tropomyosin to return to the resting position, and the muscle relaxes.[43, 107] In McArdle's disease, characterized by deficiency of muscle phosphorylase, this initial step of muscle relaxation does not occur, presumably because of insufficient ATP. Failure of relaxation results in persistent shortening of the muscle in the absence of ongoing muscle action potentials. This condition, called contracture, is best seen following exercise under ischemic conditions (Fig. 11-3).

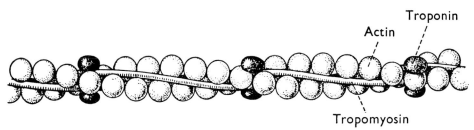

Figure 11-2
Fine structure of the thin actin filament. Actin molecules are attached to globular-shaped troponin and rod-shaped tropomyosin in an orderly arrangement. (From Ebashi, Endo, and Ohtsuki[43] with permission.)

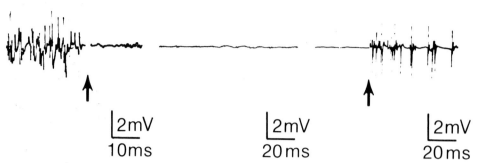

Figure 11-3

Contracture during ischemic exercise in a 66-year-old man with McArdle's disease. The forearm was made ischemic with an inflated pressure tourniquet placed around the arm, while the patient exercised the forearm flexors. The muscle action potential was recorded continuously with a concentric needle electrode inserted in the flexor digitorum profundus. Contracture began 45 seconds after the start of ischemic exercise (arrow in a), and persisted (b). Electrical activity returned 15 minutes after the cuff was released (arrow in c). (Courtesy of E. Peter Bosch, M.D., Department of Neurology, University of Iowa Hospitals and Clinics.)

## TYPES OF MUSCLE FIBERS

Muscle fibers may be subdivided based on their histologic and physiologic profiles. Important differentiating characteristics include enzymatic properties demonstrated by histochemical reactions, rate of rise in twitch tension (which determines the speed of contraction), degree of fatigability, and the nature of motor innervation. As summarized in Table 11-1, the muscle fibers are commonly designated as Type I or Type II, according to histochemical reactions;[13, 42, 48] as slow (S), fast resistant (FR), or fast fatiguing (FF), based on twitch and fatigue characteristics;[30] and as slow oxidative (SO), fast oxidative glycolytic (FOG), or fast glycolytic (FG), based on twitch and enzymatic properties.[92]

### Type I and Type II fibers

Based on histochemical reactions (Fig. 11-4), human muscle fibers may be subdivided into two types. Type I fibers react strongly to oxidative enzymes such as nicotinamide adenine dinucleotide dehydrogenase (NADH) and reduced diphosphopyridine nucleotide (DPNH), and weakly to both phosphorylase and myofibrillar adenosine triphosphatase (ATPase). Type II fibers show the reverse reactivity.[42] There are three subtypes of Type II fibers: IIA, IIB, and IIC, which can be defined by their ATPase reactions (Table 11-1) following preincubation at different pH values.[12, 13, 48] Type IIC fibers are fetal precursor cells and are rarely seen in adult muscles. The speed of contraction is usually directly related to the myosine ATPase content.[4] Thus, in general, it is possible to correlate the fiber types with physiologic data in that the slow and fast twitch fibers are histochemically Type I and II, respectively.[28, 68] However, this association is not necessarily one to one. For example, all the muscle fibers are fast in the histochemically mixed extensor digitorum longus of the rat,[34] and the myosine ATPase activity is greater in slow soleus muscle than in fast gastrocnemius muscle in cats. Thus, the intensity of histochemical ATPase reaction cannot be used as a sole criterion in distinguishing fast and slow twitch fibers.[31]

**TABLE 11-1 Types of muscle fibers**

| 1. Commonly used designations | | | |
|---|---|---|---|
| Fiber types[13] | Type I | Type IIA | Type IIB |
| Twitch and fatigue characteristics[30] | slow (S) | fast resistant (FR) | fast fatigue (FF) |
| Twitch and enzymatic properties[92] | slow oxidative (SO) | fast oxidative-glycolytic (FOG) | fast glycolytic (FG) |
| **2. Properties of muscle fibers** | | | |
| Resistance to fatigue | high | high | low |
| Oxidative enzymes | high | high | low |
| Phosphorylase (glycolytic) | low | high | high |
| Adenosine triphosphate | low | high | high |
| Twitch speed | low | high | high |
| Twitch tension | low | high | high |
| **3. Characteristics of motor units** | | | |
| Size of cell body | small | large | large |
| Size of motor unit | small | large | large |
| Diameter of axons | small | large | large |
| Conduction velocity | low | high | high |
| Threshold for recruitment | low | high | high |
| Firing frequency | low | high | high |
| Frequency of miniature end-plate potentials (MEPP) | low | high | high |

## Fast and slow twitch fibers

Muscle fibers may be divided into fast versus slow groups on the basis of their contraction time, defined as the time interval between the beginning of contraction and the development of peak tension in response to a single stimulus.[92] In addition, force-velocity curves and the rates of decay are also distinguishing. Slow fibers (S) have high oxidative properties (SO) and are resistant to fatigue. Fast fibers may be further divided into two subgroups: the fast resistant (FR) fibers have high oxidative and glycolytic properties (FOG) and are resistant to fatigue. The fast fatigue (FF) fibers are high in glycolytic activity but low in oxidative enzyme (FG) and are easily fatigable.[30] These findings suggest that glycolytic capacity is generally related to twitch characteristics, whereas oxidative capability is related to fatigability.

## Fast and slow muscles

When a muscle consists mainly of one muscle fiber type, the muscle itself may be designated as either slow or fast. Slow muscles are usually, but not always, deeper red in color. This probably reflects a higher myoglobin content. Fast muscles tend to be whitish in color. Functionally, slow muscles usually subserve a tonic postural role (e.g., the soleus in the cat), whereas fast muscles are used in phasic, willed movements (e.g., the wing muscles of a chicken). This distinction, however, is not clear in man because slow and fast twitch motor units are not segregated but are mixed in most limb muscles.[25] The percentage of the slow twitch fibers may be only very grossly estimated, using the oxidative reaction. High oxidative fibers comprise 90 percent of the human triceps surae and tibialis anterior, 60 percent of the biceps, and 50 percent of the triceps muscles. The fibers with contraction times longer than 60 ms predominate in the soleus and gastrocnemius, whereas they constitute one half, one third, and only a few percent of the tibialis anterior, biceps, and triceps, respectively.[18] Slow oxidative fibers have

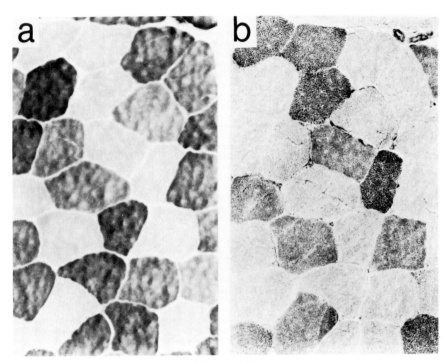

Figure 11-4
Cross-section of a normal skeletal muscle. The same preparation was stained with adenosine triphosphatase at pH of 9.4 (ATPase) and nicotinamide adenine dinucleotide dehydrogenase (NADH) in a and b, respectively. The darker fibers are Type II in a and Type I in b. (Courtesy of Linda Ansbacher, M.D. and Michael N. Hart, M.D., Department of Pathology, University of Iowa Hospitals and Clinics.)

been found in 38, 44, 47, and 61 percent of the superficial and deep areas of the vastus lateralis and of the vastus medialis, respectively.[62]

## Effect of innervation

If the nerve normally innervating a fast fiber is transplanted to a slow fiber, the originally slow muscle fiber will acquire the properties of a fast muscle fiber.[26, 63, 94, 110] Thus, the mechanical characteristics of muscle fibers are apparently determined by the type of innervation.[23] The exact physiologic mechanisms are not known, but this regulation probably takes place partly because of different motor neuron activity and partly by the axoplasmic transport of trophic substances from the nerve to muscle. Although the characteristics of the spike potential are the same, after-hyperpolarization is significantly shorter in motor neurons innervating fast twitch muscles than those supplying slow twitch muscles.[45]

The results of animal experiments seem to indicate that fast and slow rates of stimulation are responsible for producing fast and slow contractility of muscle fibers, respectively.[70, 93] In man, a greater number of slow fibers are found in athletes engaged in endurance training,[52] whereas fast fibers are more prominent in weight lifters.[104] In patients with chronic neuromuscular diseases, characteristic muscle fiber histochemistry is preserved only as long as motor neuron differentiation remains. Alterations in histochemical properties correlate with changes in the firing properties and the axonal conduction velocity of the motor neurons.[8] However, there has been no success in changing basic muscle contractility in man by exercise training alone.[2, 52, 104] Thus, motor neuron activity does not seem sufficient in itself to alter the distribution of fast and slow fibers in a muscle. The findings in favor of additional important neurotrophic influences from nerve upon muscle[55] include trophic effects of neurons on muscle in tissue cultures[111] and the inverse relationship of nerve length on the time interval before the development of muscle membrane changes after nerve section.[32]

# STRETCH SENSITIVE RECEPTORS

## Anatomy of muscle spindles

Muscle spindles consist of small specialized muscle fibers that are sensitive to muscle tension and are encapsulated by connective tissue. The intrafusal fibers of the muscle spindles are shorter in length (4 to 10 mm) and smaller in diameter (0.2 to 0.35 mm) than the extrafusal fibers of striated muscle.[64] The connective tissue capsule surrounding the intrafusal fiber is attached through the sarcolemma of the extrafusal fibers to the origin and insertion of the muscle. Thus, the muscle spindles are situated in parallel with the striated muscle fibers. Two distinct types of intrafusal fibers, nuclear bag and nuclear chain,[9] can be distinguished on the basis of the nuclear arrangement in their equatorial regions (Fig. 11-5). Nuclear bag fibers are expanded about their midpoint over a short length of about 100 $\mu$m by a collection of some 50 nuclei. Nuclear chain fibers contain a linear array of nuclei along the center of the fiber. Bag fibers are usually, but not always, longer and thicker than the chain fibers.

The afferent and efferent nerves that supply muscle spindles each have two different kinds of endings: primary (annulospiral) and secondary (flower-spray) sensory endings; and plate (single, discrete) and trail (multiple, diffuse) motor endings, respectively. The primary sensory ending spirals around the center of both bag and chain fibers, whereas the secondary ending terminates more peripherally and chiefly on nuclear chain fibers. Primary endings give rise to group IA afferent nerve fibers. These large diameter fast conducting sensory fibers subserve the monosynaptic stretch reflex. In contrast, the secondary ending gives rise to group II afferent nerve fibers that termi-

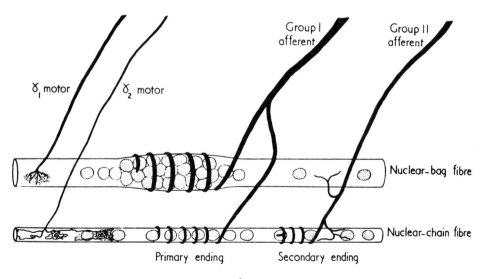

(after Boyd)

Figure 11-5

Simplified diagram of the central region (about 1 mm) of the nuclear bag fiber (top) and nuclear chain fiber (bottom). There are two types of motor endings, two types of afferent fibers, and two types of gamma motor neurons. (From Matthews,[71] with permission.)

nate on spinal interneurons. While both kinds of motor endings can innervate either type of intrafusal fiber, plate and trail endings occur preferentially on nuclear bag and chain fibers, respectively.

## Function of muscle spindles

Muscle spindles may be characterized by their dynamic and static states. A dynamic afferent response occurs during active stretching of the spindles (velocity), whereas a static response is maintained as long as the sensory endings are stretched (length). The primary ending is sensitive to velocity of muscle stretch as well as its length, but the secondary ending mainly responds to length (Fig. 11-6). The fusimotor system may influence either the dynamic or static muscle spindle response.[24, 71] The trail endings mediate static changes. The role of fibers terminating in plate endings remains to be determined but may be dynamic in type. It is likely that the bag and chain fibers receive a sufficiently distinctive motor innervation to preferentially subserve dynamic versus static fusimotor effects.[73]

The very complex functioning of muscle spindles may be simplified as follows (Table 11-2). There are two types of intrafusal fibers, nuclear bag and nuclear chain; two types of sensory receptor endings, primary and secondary, giving rise to group IA and group II afferent fibers, respectively; and two types of fusimotor endings, plate and

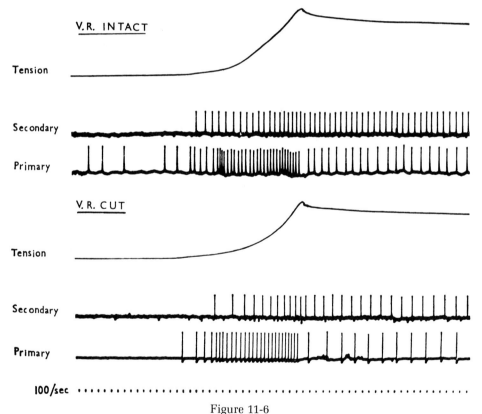

Figure 11-6

Responses of primary and secondary endings to a rapidly applied stretch before (top) and after (bottom) cutting the ventral root. A steady intrafusal contraction was maintained by spontaneous fusimotor discharge in the decerebrate cat. The primary endings are much more sensitive to stretch than the secondary endings, but both types are equally sensitive to changes in muscle length. (From Matthews,[72] with permission.)

## TABLE 11-2 Sensory endings of muscle spindles

| | Primary sensory ending | Secondary sensory ending |
|---|---|---|
| Location | Both bag and chain fibers | Mainly chain fibers |
| Sensitivity | Both length and velocity | Mainly length |
| Fusimotor system | Both dynamic and static | Mainly static |
| Form of ending | Half rings and annulospirals | Spirals and flower-sprays |
| Length of ending | About 300 $\mu$m | About 400 $\mu$m |
| Type of afferent fiber | Group IA | Group II |
| Diameter of afferent fiber | 12–20 $\mu$m | 6–12 $\mu$m |

trail, which are preferentially dynamic and static in function. Nuclear chain fibers are innervated mainly by fusimotor fibers with trail endings and by both types of sensory afferents. Overall they seem best suited to regulate static muscle length. On the other hand, nuclear bag fibers are preferentially innervated by fusimotor fibers with plate endings and by primary sensory endings. They would seem best equipped to modulate dynamic muscle function.

## The Golgi tendon organ

In contrast to muscle spindles, the Golgi tendon organ is arranged in series with extra-fusal striated muscle fibers. It discharges during active muscle contraction as well as during passive stretch. These endings give rise to group IB afferent fibers that partici-pate in disynaptic inhibition of motor neurons innervating the parent muscle. The Golgi tendon organ was once believed to provide a safety function by reflexively inhibiting the motor neurons when the magnitude of their firing reached a level that would cause excessive muscle tension. More recently, however, it has become clear that the thresh-old tension required to excite the tendon organ is much less than previously believed, especially if the tension is developed by contraction rather than passive stretch.[61] Thus it is likely that tendon organs, being excited during mild tension, continuously monitor and adjust the magnitude of muscle contraction.

# ANATOMY OF THE MOTOR UNIT

By definition[69] the motor unit consists of a single motor neuron and the few hundred muscle fibers that it innervates. Under normal conditions, contraction of a motor unit is an all-or-none phenomenon; that is, all motor unit fibers contract simultaneously. Thus, even though the smallest contractile element of the muscle may be a myofibril, the functional unit of the motor system is the motor unit.[97]

## Motor unit count

In 1971, McComas and his associates[76] introduced a new method to estimate the num-ber of motor units in human limb muscles.[14, 77, 96] The technique consists of delivering graded electrical stimulation to a whole nerve and comparing peak-to-peak amplitude of successively activated compound muscle action potentials. It is assumed that each increment in amplitude of the evoked potentials occurs by the addition of one single motor unit and that the units initially excited are representative for the muscle under study. These assumptions are, however, not widely accepted. The thresholds of two or more axons frequently overlap. At threshold stimulus intensity, therefore, the number of motor units recruited fluctuates unreliably. Moreover, the motor units initially acti-vated may not be associated with average evoked potential amplitude.[15] Thus, even with modified techniques using an averager, larger motor units are still excluded from computation.[15] Despite the shortcomings outlined above, there is currently no other noninvasive method to evaluate the number of functional motor units in man. The mean number of motor units estimated by this technique is about 200 for extensor digitorum brevis[3, 76] and 250 to 340 for the thenar muscles.[14, 74] Subnormal numbers of functioning motor units have been found in several disorders, including Duchenne muscular dystrophy.[75]

## Innervation ratio

The average size of a motor unit may be estimated by dividing the total number of extrafusal fibers by the number of innervating motor axons. This so-called innervation ratio varies greatly, depending on muscle function. A ratio as small as 3:1 may be found in extrinsic eye muscles that require fine gradations of movement. The ratio may be as high as 30:1 to 120:1 in some limb muscles subserving only coarse movement.[103] Table 11-3 summarizes the results of an innervation study.[49] The territory of a particular motor unit can be estimated histologically[35] or electrically as shown in Table 11-4.[19]

## Distribution of muscle fibers

Since muscle fibers belonging to a given motor unit have identical histologic characteristics, the apparent random distribution of different histologic fiber types seen in muscle cross-sections indicates considerable overlap in the territories of adjacent motor units.[62] The scattering of muscle fibers belonging to a given motor unit has also been demonstrated using single fiber electromyography.[47, 99, 100]

Motor unit overlap is substantiated by another mapping technique.[11, 41, 46] A single ventral root nerve fiber is isolated and stimulated repetitively. The muscle is excised immediately after tetanic stimulation, and a frozen section is stained for glycogen. Muscle fibers belonging to the motor unit of the stimulated axon remain unstained because their glycogen has been exhausted. This method not only confirms the histochemical uniformity of a given motor unit but also the territorial overlapping of adjacent motor units. Indeed, it is rare to see a muscle fiber of a single motor unit in direct contact with other fibers of the same unit.

### TABLE 11-3 Summary of innervation study

| 1. Material | 2. Muscle | 3. No. of large nerve fibers | 4. No. of muscle fibers | 5. Calculated no. of motor units | 6. Mean no. of fibers per motor unit | 7. Mean diam. of muscle fibers (μm) | 8. Cross sectional area of motor units (mm²) |
|---|---|---|---|---|---|---|---|
| ♂ 22 | Platysma | 1,826 | 27,100 | 1,096 | 25 | 20 | 0.008 |
| ♂ 40 | Brachioradialis | right 525 | > 129,200 | 315 | > 410 | 34 | |
| | | left 584 | | 350 | | | |
| ♂ 22 | First dorsal interosseus | 199 | 40,500 | 119 | 340 | 26 | 0.18 |
| ♂ 54 | First | 155 | 10,038 | 93 | 108 | 19 | 0.031 |
| ♀ 29 | lumbrical | 164 | 10,500 | 98 | 107 | 21 | 0.037 |
| ♂ 40 | Anterior | 742 | 250,200 | 445 | 562 | | |
| ♂ 22 | tibial | | 292,500 | | 657 | 57 | 1.7 |
| ♂ 28 | Gastrocnemius | 965 | 1,120,000 | 579 | 1,934 | | |
| ♂ 22 | medial head | | 946,000 | | 1,634 | 54 | 3.4 |

(From Feinstein, et al, [49] with permission.)

**TABLE 11-4 Mean values of motor unit territory and maximum voltage in normal muscles**

| Muscle | Number of muscles | Number of motor units | Spike level (μV) | Territory at spike level (mm) | Standard deviation (mm) | Maximum voltage (μV) | Standard deviation (μV) |
|---|---|---|---|---|---|---|---|
| Biceps brachii .......... | 24 | 129 | 100 | 5.1 ± 0.2 | 2.4 | 370 ± 17 | 190 |
| Deltoideus.......... | 7 | 52 | 100 | 6.7 ± 0.4 | 3.0 | 450 ± 27 | 190 |
| Extensor digitorum communis ... | 11 | 43 | 100 | 5.5 ± 0.3 | 2.1 | 800 ± 59 | 390 |
| Opponens pollicis.......... | 10 | 34 | 150 | 7.4 ± 0.4 | 2.6 | 1,000 ± 83 | 500 |
| Rectus femoris.......... | 9 | 65 | 100 | 10.0 ± 0.6 | 4.6 | 550 ± 38 | 300 |
| Biceps femoris.......... | 5 | 35 | 150 | 8.8 ± 0.7 | 4.1 | 900 ± 67 | 400 |
| Tibialis anterior .......... | 8 | 47 | 100 | 7.0 ± 0.4 | 3.0 | 620 ± 43 | 300 |
| Extensor digitorum brevis ........ | 5 | 25 | 200 | 11.3 ± 0.8 | 4.1 | 3,000 ± 300 | 1,500 |

(From Buchthal, Erminio, and Rosenfalck,[19] with permission.)

A more recent study suggests that the arrangement of mammalian muscle fibers is not in fact random but is ordered at certain stages of development to minimize adjacencies of individual muscle fibers belonging to the same motor unit.[108] Such arrangement may have the functional advantage of maximizing muscle action potential dispersal for smooth muscle contraction and in compensating for lost motor units.

Based on histologic findings in partially denervated muscle, Buchthal, Guld, and Rosenfalck[21, 22] once proposed that the fibers of each motor unit might be divided into subunits, each containing an average of 10 to 30 fibers. According to this theory, the motor unit potential recorded during routine electromyography represents the completely synchronized firing of all fibers belonging to a subunit. This concept, however, was not substantiated by electrophysiologic studies in rat phrenic-hemidiaphragm preparation[67] or in rat peroneus longus muscle.[88] Histochemical studies showed that there were no groupings of fibers within the motor unit in rat or cat muscle.[10, 41, 46] Moreover, it has been shown that high amplitude spikes could be derived from a single muscle fiber in human muscles.[47, 95] Using the single fiber needle, Stålberg[98] found no evidence of muscle fiber grouping within a motor unit in normal extensor digitorum communis or biceps brachii muscles. From these findings, it seems reasonable to abandon the concept of the subunit in normal human muscle.[17]

# PHYSIOLOGY OF THE MOTOR UNIT

Types of muscle fibers were described earlier in this chapter and summarized in Table 11-1. Different types of motor units can be characterized using the same criteria, since all the muscle fibers of a given motor unit have identical histologic and physiologic properties. Pertinent animal and human data will be briefly reviewed, as they pertain to the understanding of motor unit potentials in clinical electromyography.

## Animal experiments

Series of animal experiments have clearly established that the fundamental physiologic properties of motor units are closely related to the size of the motor neuron (see Table 11-1). Larger motor neurons supply a greater number of muscle fibers (i.e., have larger innervation ratios).[58, 79, 109] Their axons, also of relatively large diameter, have higher conduction velocities.[65, 78] Large motor units develop higher twitch tensions and faster twitch contractions but fatigue more quickly compared with small motor units.[29, 31, 59, 60] Finally motor neurons are recruited, not at random but in an orderly manner: In response to central stimulation small motor neurons are preferentially activated before large neurons (size principle).[58, 65, 66]

In brief, the larger the cell body is: the greater the conduction velocity, the stronger the twitch tension, the faster the twitch contraction, and, in general, the greater the tendency to fatigue. Smaller motor neurons, innervating smaller motor units, discharge initially with minimal effort, and larger motor neurons discharge only with a greater effort of contraction.

## Recruitment

Most of the above findings in animals are also applicable to man (see Table 11-1). In the first dorsal interosseous muscle of the human, the motor units recruited early at low threshold have lower twitch tensions and slower twitch contractions, compared with those units recruited at higher levels of activation.[27, 83, 84, 85] Activation threshold is correlated with axon diameter,[51] axon conduction velocity,[7, 50, 57] and motor unit size.[83, 84, 85] High and low threshold motor units also differ histochemically.[106] Attempts have been made to distinguish tonic and phasic motor units on the basis of their firing pattern and the order of recruitment.[105] More recent studies, however, have shown a relatively continuous rather than distinctly bimodal pattern of recruitment.[50, 56, 84, 85, 89]

Exceptions in the recruitment order of motor units have been reported under some experimental circumstances.[5, 53, 54] However, the size principle of Henneman generally applies to any voluntary activation of motor units, including rapid ramp or ballistic contractions.[37, 39, 90, 91] Desmedt and Godaux[38] have recently extended the size principle to the order of presynaptic inhibition after activation of IA afferent fibers by tonic vibration. The recruitment order is preserved in patients with neuropathy and motor neuron disease, but a random pattern of recruitment has been reported in patients with previous transection of the ulnar nerve.[82]

## Twitch characteristics

Fast and slow units have been identified in different human muscles whose twitch contraction approximates the contraction time of the whole muscle.[96] The muscle twitch attributable to a single motor unit may be recorded and analyzed if an averager is triggered by impulses of that unit.[83, 84, 85, 86, 101] Twitch tensions range from 0.1 to 1.0 g, whereas contraction times vary between 20 and 100 ms.

As in animals, the twitch tension generated by a motor unit is proportional to its action potential amplitude and the voluntary force required for its activation. The units recruited with slight contraction have smaller twitch tensions and slower contraction times. They are also fatigue-resistant compared with the units recruited with stronger contraction.[101] Partially denervated muscles have prolonged contraction times and reduced twitch tension as a whole.[80] It is not clear, however, whether the twitch tension of individual motor units becomes larger[77] or smaller,[82] following denervation.

## Rate coding

It has long been debated whether increasing force occurs because of recruitment of previously inactive motor neurons or because of the increased firing of already active units. In early studies, discharge frequency appeared to stabilize over a wide range of forces, although the firing rate ranged from several to 30 impulses per second.[6, 33, 36, 102] Therefore, it was suggested by some that rate coding was mostly related to fine control at the beginning of contraction and during maximal effort. More recent work in humans,[85, 86] however, has emphasized the importance of rate coding for increasing force, as originally suggested by Adrian and Bronk.[1]

Recruitment must be responsible for increasing force at low levels of contraction, since all units begin firing at about the same rate ranging from 5 to 15 impulses per second.[37, 50, 85] When most units have been recruited, additional increases in force must result from faster firing of individual motor units. In strong or ballistic contractions, instantaneous firing rates of 60 to 120 impulses per second have been recorded at the onset.[37] Firing rates are in general higher in myopathy and lower in neuropathy compared with controls,[40] although the difference may be significant only in severely weak muscles.[81]

# REFERENCE SOURCES

1. ADRIAN, ED AND BRONK, DW: *The discharge of impulses in motor nerve fibres. Part II. The frequency of discharge in reflex and voluntary contractions.* J Physiol (Lond) 67:119, 1929.

2. ANDERSEN, P AND HENRIKSSON, J: *Capillary supply of the quadriceps femoris muscle of man: Adaptive response to exercise.* J Physiol (Lond) 270:677, 1977.

3. BALLANTYNE, JP AND HANSEN, S: *New method for the estimation of the number of motor units in a muscle. 2. Duchenne, limb-girdle and facioscapulohumeral, and myotonic muscular dystrophies.* J Neurol Neurosurg Psychiatry 37:1195, 1974.

4. BÁRÁNY, M AND CLOSE, RI: *The transformation of myosin in cross-innervated rat muscles.* J Physiol (Lond) 213:455, 1971.

5. BASMAJIAN, JV: *Control and training of individual motor units.* Science 141:440, 1963.

6. BIGLAND, B AND LIPPOLD, OCJ: *Motor unit activity in the voluntary contraction of human muscle.* J Physiol (Lond) 125:322, 1954.

7. BORG, J, GRIMBY, L, AND HANNERZ, J: *Axonal conduction velocity and voluntary discharge properties of individual short toe extensor motor units in man.* J Physiol (Lond) 277:143, 1978.

8. BORG, J, GRIMBY, L, AND HANNERZ, J: *Motor neuron firing range, axonal conduction velocity, and muscle fiber histochemistry in neuromuscular diseases.* Muscle and Nerve 2:423, 1979.

9. BOYD, IA: *The structure and innervation of the nuclear bag muscle fibre system and the nuclear chain muscle fibre system in mammalian muscle spindles.* Philos Trans R Soc (Lond) 245:81, 1962.

10. BRANDSTATER, ME AND LAMBERT, EH: *A histological study of the spatial arrangement of muscle fibers in single motor units within rat tibialis anterior muscle.* Bull American Association of Electromyography and Electrodiagnosis 16:82, 1969.

11. BRANDSTATER, ME AND LAMBERT, EH: *Motor unit anatomy.* In DESMEDT, JE (ED): *New Developments in Electromyography and Clinical Neurophysiology,* Vol 1. Karger, Basel, 1973, pp 14–22.

12. BROOKE, MH AND KAISER, KK: *The use and abuse of muscle histochemistry.* Ann NY Acad Sci 228:121, 1974.

13. BROOKE, MH, WILLIAMSON, E, AND KAISER, KK: *The behavior of four fiber types in developing and reinnervated muscle.* Arch Neurol 25:360, 1971.

14. BROWN, WF: *A method for estimating the number of motor units in thenar muscles and the changes in motor unit count with ageing.* J Neurol Neurosurg Psychiatry 35:845, 1972.

15. BROWN, WF AND MILNER-BROWN, HS: *Some electrical properties of motor units and their effects on the methods of estimating motor unit numbers.* J Neurol Neurosurg Psychiatry 39:249, 1976.

16. BUCHTHAL, F AND KAISER, E: *The rheology of the cross striated muscle fibre with particular reference to isotonic conditions.* Dan Biol Medd (No 7) 21:1, 1951.

17. BUCHTHAL, F AND ROSENFALCK, P: *On the structure of motor units.* In DESMEDT, JE (ED): *New Developments in Electromyography and Clinical Neurophysiology,* Vol 1. Karger, Basel, 1973, pp 71–85.

18. BUCHTHAL, F AND SCHMALBRUCH, H: *Contraction time and fibre types in intact human muscle.* Acta Physiol Scand 79:435, 1970.

19. BUCHTHAL, F, ERMINIO, F, AND ROSENFALCK, P: *Motor unit territory in different human muscles.* Acta Physiol Scand 45:72, 1959.

20. BUCHTHAL, F, GULD, C, AND ROSENFALCK, P: *Propagation velocity in electrically activated muscle fibres in man.* Acta Physiol Scand 34:75, 1955.

21. BUCHTHAL, F, GULD, C, AND ROSENFALCK, P: *Volume conduction of the spike of the motor unit potential investigated with a new type of multielectrode.* Acta Physiol Scand 38:331, 1957.

22. BUCHTHAL, F, GULD, C, AND ROSENFALCK, P: *Multielectrode study of the territory of a motor unit.* Acta Physiol Scand 39:83, 1957.

23. BUCHTHAL, F, SCHMALBRUCH, H, AND KAMIENIECKA, Z: *Contraction times and fiber types in neurogenic paresis.* Neurology (Minneap) 21:58, 1971.

24. BULLER, AJ: *The motor unit in reflex action.* In CREESE, R (ED): *Recent Advance in Physiology,* ed 8. J & A Churchill, London, 1963.

25. BULLER, AJ: *The physiology of the motor unit.* In WALTON, JN (ED): *Disorders of Voluntary Muscle,* ed 3. Churchill Livingstone, London, 1974.

26. BULLER, AJ, ECCLES, JC, AND ECCLES, RM: *Interactions between motoneurons and muscles in respect of the characteristic speeds of their responses.* J Physiol (Lond) 150:417, 1960.

27. BURKE, D, SKUSE, NF, AND LETHLEAN, AK: *Isometric contraction of the abductor digiti minimi muscle in man.* J Neurol Neurosurg Psychiatry 37:825, 1974.

28. BURKE, RE AND TSAIRIS, P: *The correlation of physiological properties with histochemical characteristics in single muscle units.* Ann NY Acad Sci 228:145, 1974.

29. BURKE, RE, ET AL: *Physiological types and histochemical profiles in motor units of the cat gastrocnemius.* J Physiol (Lond) 234:723, 1973.

30. BURKE, RE, ET AL: *Mammalian motor units: Physiological-histochemical correlation in three types in cat gastrocnemius.* Science 174:709, 1971.

31. BURKE, RE, ET AL: *Direct correlation of physiological and histochemical characteristics in motor units of cat triceps surae muscle.* In DESMEDT, JE (ED): *New Developments in Electromyography and Clinical Neurophysiology,* Vol 1. Karger, Basel, 1973, pp 23–30.

32. CARD, DJ: *Denervation: Sequence of neuromuscular degenerative changes in rats and the effect of stimulation.* Exp Neurol 54:251, 1977.

33. CLAMANN, HP: *Activity of single motor units during isometric tension.* Neurology (Minneap) 20:254, 1970.

34. CLOSE, R: *Properties of motor units in fast and slow skeletal muscles of the rat.* J Physiol (Lond) 193:45, 1967.

35. COËRS, C AND WOOLF, AL: *The Innervation of Muscle. A Biopsy Study.* Charles C Thomas, Springfield, Ill, 1959.

36. DASGUPTA, A AND SIMPSON, JA: *Relation between firing frequency of motor units and muscle tension in the human.* Electromyography 2:117, 1962.

37. DESMEDT, JE AND GODAUX, E: *Fast motor units are not preferentially activated in rapid voluntary contractions in man.* Nature 267:717, 1977.

38. DESMEDT, JE AND GODAUX, E: *Mechanism of the vibration paradox: Excitatory and inhibitory effects of tendon vibration on single soleus muscle motor units in man.* J Physiol (Lond) 285:197, 1978.

39. DESMEDT, JE AND GODAUX, E: *Voluntary motor commands in human ballistic movements.* Ann Neurol 5:415, 1979.

40. DIETZ, V, ET AL: *Discharge characteristics of single motor fibres of hand muscles in lower motoneurone diseases and myopathies.* In KUNZE, K AND DESMEDT, JE (EDS): *Studies on Neuromuscular Diseases.* Proc Int Symp Giessen, Karger, Basel, 1975, pp 122–127.

41. DOYLE, AM AND MAYER, RF: *Studies of the motor unit in the cat. A preliminary report.* Bull School Med Univ Maryland 54:11, 1969.

42. DUBOWITZ, V: *Histochemical aspects of muscle disease.* In WALTON, JN (ED): *Disorders of Voluntary Muscle,* ed 3. Churchill Livingstone, London, 1974,

43. EBASHI, S, ENDO, M, AND OHTSUKI, I: *Control of muscle contraction.* Q Rev Biophys 2:351, 1969.

44. EBERSTEIN, A AND GOODGOLD, J: *Slow and fast twitch fibers in human skeletal muscle.* Am J Physiol 215:535, 1968.

45. ECCLES, JC: *Specificity or neural influence on speed of muscle contraction.* In GUTMANN, E AND HNIK, P (EDS): *The Effect of Use and Disuse on Neuromuscular Functions.* Elsevier, Amsterdam, 1963 pp 111–128.

46. EDSTRÖM, L AND KUGELBERG, E: *Histochemical composition, distribution of fibres and fatiguability of single motor units.* J Neurol Neurosurg Psychiatry 31:424, 1968.

47. EKSTEDT, J: *Human single muscle fiber action potentials.* Acta Physiol Scand 61(suppl 226):1, 1964.

48. ENGEL, WK: *Selective and nonselective susceptibility of muscle fiber types.* Arch Neurol 22:97, 1970.

49. FEINSTEIN, B, ET AL: *Morphologic studies of motor units in normal human muscles.* Acta Anat (Basel) 23:127, 1955.

50. FREUND, HJ, BÜDINGEN, HJ, AND DIETZ, V: *Activity of single motor units from human forearm muscles during voluntary isometric contractions.* J Neurophysiol 38:933, 1975.

51. FREUND, HJ, ET AL: *Discharge characteristics of single motor units in normal subjects and patients with supraspinal motor disturbances.* In DESMEDT, JE (ED): *New Developments in Electromyography and Clinical Neurophysiology,* Vol 3. Karger, Basel, 1973 pp 242–250.

52. GOLLNICK, PD, ET AL: *Effect of training on enzyme activity and fiber composition of human skeletal muscle.* J Appl Physiol 34:107, 1973.

53. GRIMBY, L AND HANNERZ, J: *Recruitment order of motor units on voluntary contraction: Changes induced by proprioceptive afferent activity.* J Neurol Neurosurg Psychiatry 31:565, 1968.

54. GRIMBY, L AND HANNERZ, J: *Disturbances in voluntary recruitment order of low and high frequency motor units on blockades of proprioceptive afferent activity.* Acta Physiol Scand 96:207, 1976.

55. GUTMANN, E: *Considerations of neurotrophic relations in the central and peripheral nervous system.* Acta Neurobiol Exp 35:841, 1975.

56. HANNERZ, J: *Discharge properties of motor units in relation to recruitment order in voluntary contraction.* Acta Physiol Scand 91:374, 1974.

57. HANNERZ, J AND GRIMBY, L: *The afferent influence on the voluntary firing range of individual motor units in man.* Muscle and Nerve 2:414, 1979.

58. HENNEMAN, E: *Relation between size of neurons and their susceptibility to discharge.* Science 126:1345, 1957.

59. HENNEMAN, E, SOMJEN, G, AND CARPENTER, DO: *Functional significance of cell size in spinal motoneurons.* J Neurophysiol 28:560, 1965.

60. HENNEMAN, E, SOMJEN, G, AND CARPENTER, DO: *Excitability and inhibitibility of motoneurons of different sizes.* J Neurophysiol 28:599, 1965.

61. HOUK, J AND HENNEMAN, E: *Responses of Golgi tendon organs to active contractions of the soleus muscle of the cat.* J Neurophysiol 30:466, 1967.

62. JOHNSON, MA, ET AL: *Data on the distribution of fibre types in thirty-six human muscles. An autopsy study.* J Neurol Sci 18:111, 1973.

63. KARPATI, G AND ENGEL, WK: *"Type grouping" in skeletal muscles after experimental reinnervation.* Neurology (Minneap) 18:447, 1968.

64. KENNEDY, WR: *Innervation of normal human muscle spindles.* Neurology (Minneap) 20:463, 1970.

65. KERNELL, D: *Input resistance, electrical excitability, and size of ventral horn cells in cat spinal cord.* Science 152:1637, 1966.

66. KERNELL, D AND SJÖHOLM, H: *Recruitment and firing rate modulation of motor unit tension in a small muscle of the cat's foot.* Brain Res 98:57, 1975.

67. KRNJEVIĆ, K AND MILEDI, R: *Motor units in the rat diaphragm.* J Physiol (Lond) 140:427, 1958.

68. KUGELBERG, E: *Properties of the rat hind-limb motor units.* In DESMEDT, JE (ED): *New Developments in Electromyography and Clinical Neurophysiology,* Vol 1. Karger, Basel, 1973, pp 2–13.

69. LIDDELL, EGT AND SHERRINGTON, CS: *Recruitment and some other features of reflex inhibition.* Proc R Soc Lond B 97:488, 1925.

70. LØMO, T, WESTGAARD, RH, AND DAHL, HA: *Contractile properties of muscle: Control by pattern of muscle activity in the rat.* Proc R Soc Lond B 187:99, 1974.

71. MATTHEWS, PBC: *Muscle spindles and their motor control.* Physiol Rev 44:219, 1964.

72. MATTHEWS, PBC: *Mammalian Muscle Receptors and Their Central Actions.* Edward Arnold, Ltd, London, 1972.

73. MATTHEWS, PBC: *The advances of the last decade of animal experimentation upon muscle spindles.* In DESMEDT, JE (ED): *New Developments in Electromyography and Clinical Neurophysiology,* Vol 3. Karger, Basel, 1973, pp 95–125.

74. McCOMAS, AJ: *Neuromuscular Function and Disorders.* Butterworth and Co., London, 1977.

75. McCOMAS, AJ, SICA, REP, AND BRANDSTATER, ME: *Further motor unit studies in Duchenne muscular dystrophy.* J Neurol Neurosurg Psychiatry 40:1147, 1977.

76. McCOMAS, AJ, ET AL: *Electrophysiological estimation of the number of motor units within a human muscle.* J Neurol Neurosurg Psychiatry 34:121, 1971.

77. McCOMAS, AJ, ET AL: *Functional compensation in partially denervated muscles.* J Neurol Neurosurg Psychiatry 34:453, 1971.

78. McLEOD, JG AND WRAY, SH: *Conduction velocity and fibre diameter of the median and ulnar nerves of the baboon.* J Neurol Neurosurg Psychiatry 30:240, 1967.

79. McPhedran, AM, Wuerker, RB, and Henneman, E: *Properties of motor units in a homogenous red muscle (soleus) of the cat.* J Neurophysiol 28:71, 1965.

80. Miller, RG: *Dynamic properties of partially denervated muscle.* Ann Neurol 6:51, 1979.

81. Miller, RG and Sherratt, M: *Firing rates of human motor units in partially denervated muscle.* Neurology (New York) 28:1241, 1978.

82. Milner-Brown, HS, Stein, RB, and Lee, RG: *Contractile and electrical properties of human motor units in neuropathies and motor neurone disease.* J Neurol Neurosurg Psychiatry 37:670, 1974.

83. Milner-Brown, HS, Stein, RB, and Yemm, R: *The contractile properties of human motor units during voluntary isometric contractions.* J Physiol (Lond) 228:285, 1973.

84. Milner-Brown, HS, Stein, RB, and Yemm, R: *The orderly recruitment of human motor units during voluntary isometric contractions.* J Physiol (Lond) 230:359, 1973.

85. Milner-Brown, HS, Stein, RB, and Yemm, R: *Changes in firing rate of human motor units during linearly changing voluntary contractions.* J Physiol (Lond) 230:371, 1973.

86. Monster, AW and Chan, H: *Isometric force production by motor units of extensor digitorum communis muscle in man.* J Neurophysiol 40:1432, 1977.

87. Nishizono, H, Saito, Y, and Miyashita, M: *The estimation of conduction velocity in human skeletal muscle in situ with surface electrodes.* Electroenceph Clin Neurophysiol 46:659, 1979.

88. Norris, FH, Jr, and Irwin. RL: *Motor unit area in a rat muscle.* Am J Physiol 200:944, 1961.

89. Person, RS and Kudina, LP: *Discharge frequency and discharge pattern of human motor units during voluntary contraction of muscle.* Electroenceph Clin Neurophysiol 32:471, 1972.

90. Petajan, JH: *Clinical electromyographic studies of diseases of the motor unit.* Electroenceph Clin Neurophysiol 36:395, 1974.

91. Petajan, JH and Philip, BA: *Frequency control of motor unit action potentials.* Electroenceph Clin Neurophysiol 27:66, 1969.

92. Peter, JB, et al: *Metabolic profiles of three fiber types of skeletal muscle in guinea pigs and rabbits.* Biochemistry 11:2627, 1972.

93. Pette, D, et al: *Effects of long-term electrical stimulation on some contractile and metabolic characteristics of fast rabbit muscles.* Pflügers Arch 338:257, 1973.

94. Romanul, FCA and Van der Meulen, JP: *Slow and fast muscles after cross innervation. Enzymatic and physiological changes.* Arch Neurol 17:387, 1967.

95. Rosenfalck, P: *Intra- and extracellular potential fields of active nerve and muscle fibres.* Acta Physiol Scand (Suppl 321):1, 1969.

96. Sica, REP, et al: *Motor unit estimations in small muscles of the hand.* J Neurol Neurosurg Psychiatry 37:55, 1974.

97. Sissons, HA: *Anatomy of the motor unit.* In Walton, JN (ed): *Disorders of Voluntary Muscle,* ed 3. Churchill Livingstone, London, 1974.

98. Stalberg, E: *Single fibre electromyography for motor unit study in man.* In Shahani, M (ed): *The Motor System: Neurophysiology and Muscle Mechanisms.* Elsevier, Amsterdam, 1976.

99. Stålberg, E and Ekstedt, J: *Single fibre EMG and microphysiology of the motor unit in normal and diseased human muscle.* In Desmedt, JE (ed): *New Developments in Electromyography and Clinical Neurophysiology,* Vol 1. Karger, Basel, 1973, pp 113–129.

100. Stålberg, E, Schiller, HH, and Schwartz, MS: *Safety factor in single human motor endplates studied in vivo with single fibre electromyography.* J Neurol Neurosurg Psychiatry 38:799, 1975.

101. Stephens, JA and Usherwood, TP: *The mechanical properties of human motor units with special reference to their fatiguability and recruitment threshold.* Brain Res 125:91, 1977.

102. Tanji, J and Kato, M: *Recruitment of motor units in voluntary contraction of a finger muscle in man.* Exp Neurol 40:759, 1973.

103. Tergast, P: *Ueber das Verhältniss von Nerve und Muskel.* Arch Mikr Anat 9:36, 1873.

104. Thorstensson, A: *Muscle strength, fibre types and enzyme activities in man.* Acta Physiol Scand (Suppl 433):8, 1976.

ACTIVATION PROCEDURES AND OTHER METHODS

**233**

105. TOKIZANE, T AND SHIMAZU, H: *Functional Differentiation of Human Skeletal Muscle.* Charles C Thomas, Springfield, Ill, 1964.

106. WARMOLTS, JR AND ENGEL, WK: *Open-biopsy electromyography. I. Correlation of motor unit behavior with histochemical muscle fiber type in human limb muscle.* Arch Neurol 27:512, 1972.

107. WEBER, A AND MURRAY, JM: *Molecular control mechanisms in muscle contraction.* Physiol Rev 53:612, 1973.

108. WILLISON, RG: *Arrangement of muscle fibers of a single motor unit in mammalian muscles (letter to the editor).* Muscle and Nerve 3:360, 1980.

109. WUERKER, RB, McPHEDRAN, AM AND HENNEMAN, E: *Properties of motor units in a heterogeneous pale muscle (m. gastrocnemius) of the cat.* J Neurophysiol 28:85, 1965.

110. YELLIN, H: *Neural regulation of enzymes in muscle fibers of red and white muscle.* Exp Neurol 19:92, 1967.

111. YOUNKIN, SG, ET AL: *Substances moved by axonal transport and released by nerve stimulation have an innervation-like effect on muscles.* Science 200:1292, 1978.

# 12

# TECHNIQUES AND NORMAL FINDINGS

Electromyography tests the integrity of the entire motor system, which consists of upper and lower motor neurons, the neuromuscular junction, and muscle. With further subdivisions in each category, there are seven possible sites of involvement that may cause muscle weakness (Fig. 12-1). The knowledge of physiologic mechanisms underlying normal muscle contraction is a prerequisite for understanding the electrophysiologic abnormalities found in various disorders of the motor system. Electromyographers must also be thoroughly familiar with multiple factors that can significantly affect the outcome of recordings. These include not only the variables related to the age of patients and the particular muscle under study, but also those variables inherent in the electrical characteristics of the needle electrodes and recording apparatus, as discussed earlier.

Electromyography is best considered an extension of the physical examination rather than simply a laboratory procedure. Different muscle groups must be selected for examination according to the clinical symptoms and signs of the patient. Each muscle must be sampled many times not only at rest, but also during different degrees of muscle contraction. Depending upon the findings of initially tested muscles, the examiner must decide the course of subsequent exploration. Thus, no rigid protocol can be recommended for a routine electromyographic examination. Certain guidelines will be presented, but a flexible approach is essential to fulfill the needs of individual patients.

## PRINCIPLES OF ELECTROMYOGRAPHY

### External recording of muscle potential

The electrical property of the muscle discussed in Chapter 2 related to the muscle fiber action potentials recorded with intracellular microelectrodes. In clinical electromyography, muscle action potentials are recorded with extracellular electrodes. Because internal and external recordings are opposite in polarity, an internally positive action potential is recorded as a negative spike. A triphasic waveform is generated as the impulse approaches, reaches, and leaves a recording electrode through a volume conductor. If the muscle fiber is damaged by the needle, however, a negative spike cannot

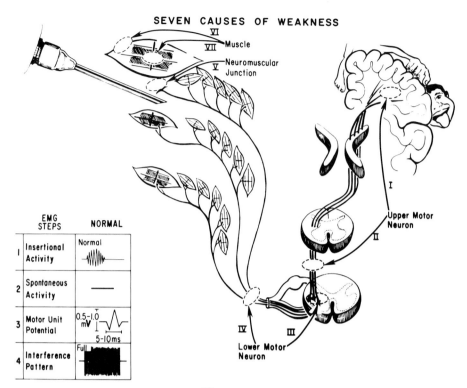

**SEVEN CAUSES OF WEAKNESS**

| EMG STEPS | NORMAL |
|---|---|
| 1 Insertional Activity | Normal |
| 2 Spontaneous Activity | — |
| 3 Motor Unit Potential | 0.5–1.0 mV / 5–10ms |
| 4 Interference Pattern | Full |

Figure 12-1

Schematic illustration of the motor system showing seven anatomic levels that may be affected by a lesion causing muscle weakness. They include (1) upper motor neuron from the cortex to the spinal cord; (2) lower motor neuron consisting of the anterior horn cell and nerve axon; (3) neuromuscular junction; and (4) muscle membrane and contractile substrate. The four steps of performing electromyography are also shown diagrammatically together with normal findings. The figure of cortical representation is adapted from Netter.[53]

be generated at the site of recording. The action potential will then consist of a large positivity initially followed by low amplitude, long duration negativity.

The action potential is constant in amplitude, duration, and waveform every time it fires, but the externally recorded potential varies depending on its spatial relationship to the recording electrode. Indeed, the amplitude of an action potential falls off to less than 10 percent at a distance of 1 mm from the generator source. In normal muscles, action potentials are generated only in response to neural impulses. Thus, all muscle fibers belonging to a motor unit fire simultaneously, producing a motor unit potential. Denervated muscle fibers become unstable, as they are no longer under neural control. Individual muscle fibers will then fire with a regular rhythm in the absence of apparent external stimuli. These single fiber potentials are recorded as spontaneous activity in electromyography.

## Contraindications for electromyography

Two groups of patients require special attention before electromyographic examination: those with bleeding tendencies and those unusually susceptible to recurrent systemic infections. It is important that the electromyographer routinely inquire about these possibilities, since patients usually fail to provide the information unless specifically asked. If potential problems exist, the referring physician must be consulted and a decision made weighing the possible benefits against the risks. Patients receiving anticoagulants should have bleeding and prothrombin times tested before being subjected to needle examination. The same applies to any coagulopathy in general. Routine electromyographic examination is contraindicated in patients with hemophilia[61] or severe thrombocytopenia. In the latter, if the platelet count is more than 20,000 per mm³, the bleeding tendency may be minimal and hemostasis can be accomplished simply by local pressure. Transient bacteremia as the result of needle examination could cause endocarditis in patients with valvular disease or with prosthetic valves. Although prophylactic administration of antibiotics is not generally recommended,[63] unnecessary needle examinations should be avoided in these patients.

When dealing with neuromuscular disorders, clinical features are supplemented not only by electrophysiologic but also by biochemical and histologic findings. Serum creatine kinase (CK) is high in certain muscle diseases such as muscular dystrophy and polymyositis.[31] The level may also be elevated significantly by the combination of electromyography, diurnal variation, and prolonged exercise,[4, 12, 48, 54] although needle examination by itself should not induce misleadingly high creatine kinase levels in normal persons. In one study,[13] no significant changes in creatine kinase levels occurred within two hours after electromyographic studies. It reached a peak value (one and one-half times baseline) in six hours and returned to baseline 48 hours after the examination. To avoid potential confusion, it is advisable to test serum enzymes prior to needle examination. However, elevated serum creatine kinase activities should be considered abnormal, even if the serum is drawn after electromyographic examination.

To establish a clinical diagnosis, it is often necessary to obtain a muscle biopsy. Muscle fibers are repeatedly traumatized during insertion and movement of the needle electrode. In addition to well-known findings of localized inflammation, focal myopathic changes may be produced by prior insertion of electromyographic or hypodermic needles. Thus, if a muscle biopsy is contemplated, it is best to avoid needle examination of the muscle under consideration.

## Recording technique

Electromyographic examination of skeletal muscle is usually performed in four steps:

1. A needle electrode is placed in the muscle and electrical activity associated with its insertion is evaluated (insertional activity).

2. The muscle is evaluated at rest, that is, with the needle stationary in a relaxed muscle (spontaneous activity).

3. Muscle potentials evoked by isolated discharges of motor neurons are recorded with mild voluntary contraction of the muscle (motor unit potentials).

4. The change in electrical potential is assessed as the level of muscle contraction gradually increases and eventually reaches a maximum (recruitment and interference pattern).

The needle electrode registers muscle action potentials from a limited area in the muscle. Therefore, for an adequate survey of the muscle under study, it is necessary to sample many different areas by frequently repositioning the needle. This is done by manually advancing or withdrawing the needle in very small steps and maintaining the needle in each new position with a firm grip. It is recommended that needle examinations be done at least in four directions from a single puncture site to minimize discomfort. Additional needle punctures may be required when dealing with larger muscles so that proximal, central, and distal portions are sampled. We use an oscilloscope sweep speed of 5 to 10 ms per cm and whatever gain is necessary to maximize the recorded potentials without truncating the peaks. The optimal range is usually between 50 to 100 μV per cm when studying insertional and spontaneous activities and between 100 μV to 1 mV per cm for assessment of motor unit potentials. Obviously, a lower gain suffices for study of high amplitude potentials. In our laboratory, the low and high frequency filters are usually set at 20 Hz and 10 KHz, respectively, but a low frequency filter of 10

Hz or less may be desirable when determining the duration of motor unit potentials.

# INSERTIONAL ACTIVITY

## Origin and characteristics

As an electrode is inserted into muscle, brief bursts of electrical activity are normally seen.[38, 70] The same discharges are also observed whenever the needle is repositioned within the muscle. The insertional activity is of short duration, averaging a few hundred milliseconds, and lasts little longer than the movement of the needle (Fig. 12-2). It appears as repetitive high frequency spikes in a cluster that normally has large positive deflection.[73] This is accompanied by a crisp static sound over the loudspeaker. The same activity is also referred to as the injury potential, since it is felt to represent discharges from muscle fibers injured or mechanically stimulated as the skeletal muscle is penetrated.

## Clinical significance

Based on the wave forms seen on the oscilloscope and perhaps more importantly by the sound over the loudspeaker, the insertional activity can be somewhat loosely categorized as normal, decreased, or increased. Quantitative analysis, however, is difficult, since the level of response depends, among other things, on the magnitude and speed of needle movement. It is nonetheless considered an important measure of muscle excitability and may be abnormally reduced in fibrotic muscles or exaggerated in denervating or inflammatory processes. The insertional activity often gives the first clue to the presence and nature of a muscle abnormality and directs the electromyographer toward the proper course of subsequent examination. As mentioned earlier, each muscle should be sampled in several locations by shifting the electrode from one point to another within the muscle. Otherwise, patchy areas of hyperexcitability, if present, may remain undetected.

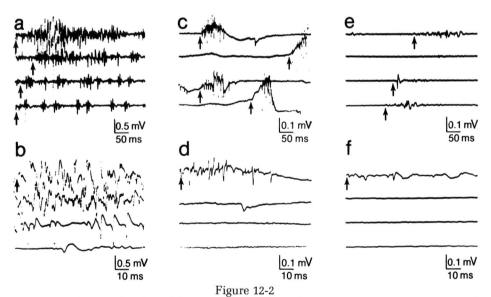

Figure 12-2

Increased (a, b) normal (c, d), and decreased (e, f) insertional potentials induced by movements of the needle (arrows). The tracings were obtained from the first dorsal interosseus in a patient with tardy ulnar palsy (a, b), tibialis anterior in a control subject (c, d), and fibrotic deltoid of a patient with severe dermatomyositis (e, f).

In denervated muscles, insertion of the exploring needle may provoke fibrillation potentials[70] and positive sharp waves.[71] These early abnormalities of denervation are sometimes difficult to distinguish from a normal insertional activity which may also take the form of positive sharp potentials. Using a mechanical electrode inserter to allow quantitative analysis of the electrical activity, Wiechers[72] found that one or two isolated positive waves could appear in normal muscles at the end of the insertional activity. However, none of these positive potentials fired repetitively or in trains, and none were reproducible with further insertions. Their audio characteristics were also different from those of positive sharp waves associated with denervation. These findings suggest that, when examining the muscle for evidence of early denervation, isolated positive waves induced by insertion must be considered nonspecific, unless they are reproducible in trains and associated with characteristic audio displays reminiscent of the spontaneous discharge.

## END-PLATE ACTIVITIES

If the needle is stationary and the muscle at rest, no electrical activity is detected in normal subjects, except when the needle is in the end-plate region irritating the small intramuscular nerve terminals. End-plate activities are of two types: low amplitude, undulating end-plate noise (Fig. 12-3) and high amplitude intermittent spikes (Fig. 12-4). These two types of end-plate potentials occur conjointly or independently and are

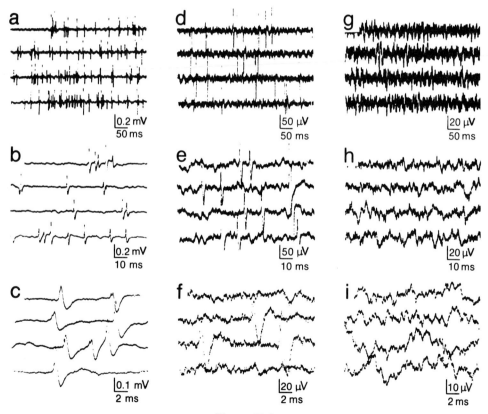

Figure 12-3

End-plate activities recorded from the tibialis anterior in a healthy subject. Two types of potentials are shown: the initially negative end-plate spikes and low amplitude end-plate noise. The spikes (a, b, c) and end-plate noise (g, h, i) may appear separately, although they are more commonly observed together (d, e, f). The spike activity is much larger in amplitude than the end-plate noise which is usually seen only with high gain.

usually associated with a dull pain, which is relieved by changing the position of the needle slightly. Although both types of end-plate activity are considered physiologic, they are often excessive when encountered in denervated muscles.

## End-plate noise

Background activity in the end-plate region consists of frequently recurring small, short, negative potentials, 10 to 50 $\mu$V in amplitude and 1 to 2 ms in duration. They

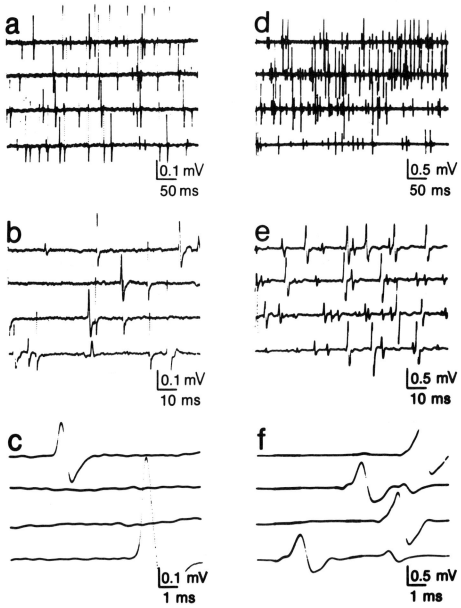

Figure 12-4

End-plate spikes recorded from the abductor pollicis brevis in a normal subject (a, b, c) and in a patient with the carpal tunnel syndrome (d, e, f). End-plate activities are sometimes unusually prominent in denervated muscle, but their quantitative assessment is difficult. Fibrillation potentials, if recorded at the end-plate, also appear as initially negative discharges.

occur irregularly, giving rise to a characteristic sound that is much like a sea shell held to the ear. Buchthal and Rosenfalck[7] have suggested that these discharges probably represent extracellularly recorded miniature end-plate potentials (MEPP). Wiederholt[74] has presented histologic evidence that end-plate noise indeed represents MEPPs. As discussed in Chapter 8, the MEPPs are nonpropagating depolarizations of the end-plate caused by spontaneous release of acetylcholine (ACh) quanta, which, if recorded in vivo with intracellular microelectrodes, are seen as monophasic, positive potentials, about 1 mV in amplitude.[21] When recorded with extracellular electrodes these potentials are opposite in sign and much reduced in amplitude.

## End-plate spikes

Intermittent spikes are 100 to 200 $\mu$V in amplitude, 3 to 4 ms in duration, and fire at an irregular frequency of 5 to 50 impulses per second.[7] They are always initially negative and should not be confused with fibrillation potentials, which are initially positive unless recorded at the end-plate region. Although often referred to as nerve potentials, the spikes probably represent discharges of single muscle fibers excited by intramuscular nerve terminals irritated by the needle.[7]

Small irregularly occurring positive potentials may be recorded in the end-plate region with the use of a concentric needle electrode. These positive discharges have been shown to represent cannula-recorded end-plate spikes which are reversed in polarity and reduced in amplitude.[57] These potentials are not observed by monopolar recordings. They are smaller, shorter, and more irregular than the positive waves seen in denervation and tend to occur in small distal muscles, possibly reflecting higher innervation ratios.[58] These positive potentials have no clinical significance but must be distinguished on the basis of their irregularity and shorter duration from the positive sharp waves of denervated muscles.

# MOTOR UNIT POTENTIALS

Under normal circumstances, the smallest functional unit of muscle contraction is the motor unit, which consists of a group of muscle fibers innervated by a single motor neuron (Fig. 12-5). Isolated discharges recorded during mild voluntary muscle contraction represent the sum of a number of single muscle fiber potentials belonging to the same unit. Within a single motor unit, individual muscle fibers discharge nearly synchronously. The configuration of the motor unit potential is related to the anatomic features of the motor unit in general and to the spatial and temporal relationships of individual muscle fiber potentials in particular.[6, 8, 9, 10]

## Factors determining motor unit profiles

Specific factors include the number of muscle fibers innervated by the motor neuron (innervation ratio), the number of muscle fibers per given cross-sectional area (fiber density), the propagation velocity in the terminal axon twigs, and the integrity of neuromuscular transmission. These factors vary with age and between different muscle groups. The motor units activated by minimal voluntary contraction also differ physiologically from those recruited with maximal contraction. With decreasing intramuscular temperature from 37 to 30°C, the mean motor unit duration increases by 10 to 30 percent and the mean amplitude decreases by 2 to 5 percent per °C. The number of polyphasic potentials increases as much as tenfold with a 10°C decrease.[11] The amplitude of a motor unit potential does not increase despite the local facilitatory effect of cooling on the muscle membrane, presumably because lower temperatures also increase differential slowing and desynchronization.

Other important variables include the spatial relationship of the recording electrode to the discharging muscle fibers and the physiologic characteristics (e.g., resist-

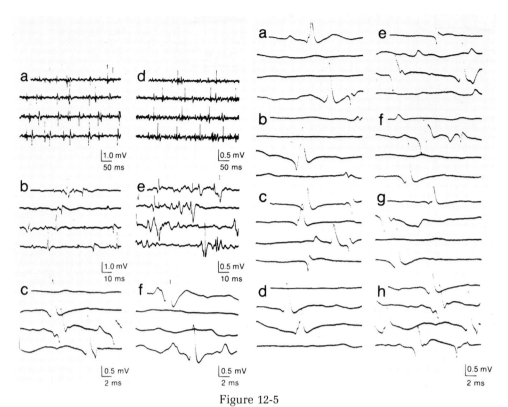

Figure 12-5

*(Left)* Normal motor unit potentials from minimally contracted biceps in a 40-year-old healthy man (a, b, c) and maximally contracted tibialis anterior in a 31-year-old woman with hysterical weakness (d, e, f). The amplitude, duration, and waveform are normal in both, but the firing frequency is inappropriately low for the presumed maximal effort in the latter. *(Right)* Normal variations of motor unit potentials from the biceps in the same healthy subject as shown at left. Tracings a through h represent eight different sites of recording.

ance and capacitance) of the intervening tissue. A motor unit potential may be described by its amplitude, rise time, duration, and number of phases.[16] These characteristics remain unchanged as long as the electrode maintains the same relative position within the motor unit. With slight positional shifts of the electrode, however, new motor unit profiles will appear, reflecting a new spatial relationship between the needle and the motor unit. Finally, there are a number of nonphysiologic factors that significantly influence the recorded potentials. These include the type of needle electrode, size of the recording surface (i.e., lead-off area), electrical characteristics of the amplifier, choice of oscilloscope gain, sweep or filters, and the methods of storage and replay.

## Amplitude

Although all the individual muscle fibers in a motor unit discharge in near synchrony, the amplitude of a motor unit potential is primarily determined by a limited number of muscle fibers—those that are located near the tip of the recording needle (Fig. 12-6). This is because the amplitude of single muscle fiber potentials falls off to less than 50 percent at a distance of 200 to 300 $\mu$m from the muscle fiber and to less than 1 percent a few millimeters away.[9, 10, 20, 44] Thiele and Böhle[66] found that fewer than 20 muscle fibers lying within a 1 mm radius of the electrode tip contribute to the high voltage spike of the motor unit potential. Therefore, in order to precisely determine the ampli-

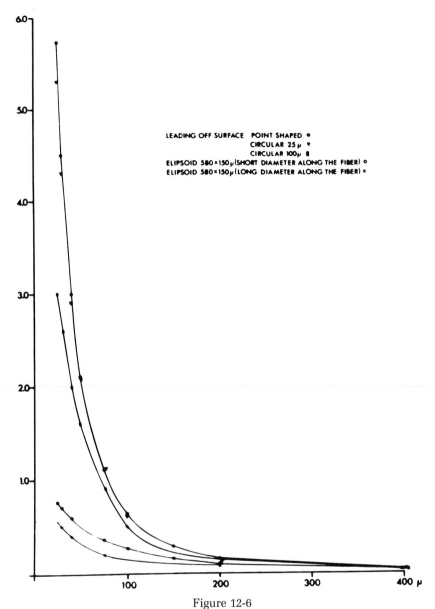

Figure 12-6

Reduction in amplitude of recorded response as the electrode is moved away from the source. With a large leading-off surface, the amplitude is low even near the spike generator and changes relatively little as the distance between the electrode and the source increases. Amplitude change per unit distance is much steeper with a smaller leading-off surface. See Figure 15-1 for further explanation. (From Ekstedt and Stålberg,[20] with permission.)

tude characteristics of a motor unit, it is necessary to explore the same motor unit at different recording sites. The amplitude normally ranges from several hundred microvolts to a few millivolts with a concentric needle, or nearly twice as great with a monopolar needle with its smaller lead-off surface.

## Rise time

The rise time of a motor unit potential is measured from the initial positive peak to the subsequent negative peak (see Fig. 2-6). It is an indicator of the distance between the recording tip of the electrode and the discharging muscle fibers; the shorter the rise time is, the closer the unit, because a potential is attenuated by the resistance and capacitance of the intervening tissue which acts as a high frequency filter. Rise time should be less than 500 $\mu$s, and preferably 100 to 200 $\mu$s, before a unit is accepted for measurement. A motor unit with a short rise time produces a sharp, crisp sound over the loudspeaker. Thus, sound characteristics can provide an important clue to the proximity of the unit to the electrode. If the discharge is associated with a dull sound, the electrode should be repositioned until crisp sounds are detected. The rise time is then measured to determine if the potential is acceptable for assessing its amplitude and duration.

## Duration

The duration of a motor unit potential is measured from the initial take-off until the return to baseline (Table 12-1). It is a function of synchrony in the firing of many individual muscle fibers belonging to a common motor unit. Synchrony in turn is determined by the variability in length and conduction velocity of the axon terminals and muscle fibers. Although the spike amplitude of a motor unit potential is primarily determined by muscle fibers near the electrode, its duration is significantly affected by distant muscle fibers. Fibers at a distance of more than 1 mm are responsible for the initial and terminal phases of low amplitude potentials. Total duration normally ranges from 2 to 10 ms but is significantly increased by age. Buchthal[5] found that the mean durations of motor units at the ages of three and 75 were 7.3 ms and 12.8 ms in biceps brachii, 9.2 ms and 15.9 ms in tibialis anterior, and 4.3 and 7.5 ms in the facial muscles, respectively.

## Phases

A phase is defined as that portion of a wave between the departure from and return to baseline. The number of phases is determined by counting the number of negative and positive peaks to and from the baseline and is equal to the number of baseline crossings plus one. Normally, motor units have four phases or less. Polyphasic motor unit potentials with more than four phases are occasionally seen, but do not exceed 5 to 15 percent of the total population in a healthy muscle if recorded with a concentric needle electrode. Polyphasic activities are generally higher with the use of a monopolar needle but the exact incidence is not known. Some action potentials show several directional changes (turns) without crossing the baseline. They are called serrated action potentials or, less appropriately, complex or pseudopolyphasic potentials. Both polyphasic and serrated potentials are measures of fiber synchrony.

# QUANTITATIVE MEASUREMENTS

## Conventional assessment

In clinical electromyography, motor unit parameters are assessed by simple observation of oscilloscope displays and listening to audio characteristics. By these simple means, an experienced examiner can detect abnormalities with reasonable certainty. Although subjective assessment may be satisfactory for the detection of unequivocal abnormalities, it is often inadequate for demonstrating less obvious deviations or for assessing mixed patterns of abnormalities. In these circumstances, quantitative measurements of motor unit potentials are helpful. If a standardized method is used, quantitative descriptions also allow meaningful comparison of test results sequentially or from one laboratory to another.

## TABLE 12-1 Mean action potential duration (ms) in various muscles at different ages[1] (Concentric electrodes)

| Age in years | Arm muscles | | | | | | Leg muscles | | | | | Facial musc. | Age in years |
| --- | --- | --- | --- | --- | --- | --- | --- | --- | --- | --- | --- | --- | --- |
| | Deltoideus | Biceps brachii | Triceps brachii | Extensor digitorum communis | Opponens pollicis; interosseus | Abductor digiti quinti | Biceps femoris; quadriceps | Gastrocnemius | Tibialis anterior | Peroneus longus | Extensor digitorum brevis | Orbicularis oris superior; triangularis; frontalis | |
| 0 | 8.8 | 7.1 | 8.1 | 6.6 | 7.9 | 9.2 | 8.0 | 7.1 | 8.9 | 6.5 | 7.0 | 4.2 | 0 |
| 3 | 9.0 | 7.3 | 8.3 | 6.8 | 8.1 | 9.5 | 8.2 | 7.3 | 9.2 | 6.7 | 7.2 | 4.3 | 3 |
| 5 | 9.2 | 7.5 | 8.5 | 6.9 | 8.3 | 9.7 | 8.4 | 7.5 | 9.4 | 6.8 | 7.4 | 4.4 | 5 |
| 8 | 9.4 | 7.7 | 8.6 | 7.1 | 8.5 | 9.9 | 8.6 | 7.7 | 9.6 | 6.9 | 7.6 | 4.5 | 8 |
| 10 | 9.6 | 7.8 | 8.7 | 7.2 | 8.6 | 10.0 | 8.7 | 7.8 | 9.7 | 7.0 | 7.7 | 4.6 | 10 |
| 13 | 9.9 | 8.0 | 9.0 | 7.4 | 8.9 | 10.3 | 9.0 | 8.0 | 10.0 | 7.2 | 7.9 | 4.7 | 13 |
| 15 | 10.1 | 8.2 | 9.2 | 7.5 | 9.1 | 10.5 | 9.2 | 8.2 | 10.2 | 7.4 | 8.1 | 4.8 | 15 |
| 18 | 10.4 | 8.5 | 9.6 | 7.8 | 9.4 | 10.9 | 9.5 | 8.5 | 10.5 | 7.6 | 8.4 | 5.0 | 18 |
| 20 | 10.7 | 8.7 | 9.9 | 8.1 | 9.7 | 11.2 | 9.8 | 8.7 | 10.8 | 7.8 | 8.6 | 5.1 | 20 |
| 25 | 11.4 | 9.2 | 10.4 | 8.5 | 10.2 | 11.9 | 10.3 | 9.2 | 11.5 | 8.3 | 9.1 | 5.4 | 25 |
| 30 | 12.2 | 9.9 | 11.2 | 9.2 | 11.0 | 12.8 | 11.1 | 9.9 | 12.3 | 8.9 | 9.8 | 5.8 | 30 |
| 35 | 13.0 | 10.6 | 12.0 | 9.8 | 11.7 | 13.6 | 11.8 | 10.6 | 13.2 | 9.5 | 10.5 | 6.2 | 35 |
| 40 | 13.4 | 10.9 | 12.4 | 10.1 | 12.1 | 14.1 | 12.2 | 10.9 | 13.6 | 9.8 | 10.8 | 6.4 | 40 |
| 45 | 13.8 | 11.2 | 12.7 | 10.3 | 12.5 | 14.5 | 12.5 | 11.2 | 13.9 | 10.1 | 11.1 | 6.6 | 45 |
| 50 | 14.3 | 11.6 | 13.2 | 10.7 | 12.9 | 15.0 | 13.0 | 11.6 | 14.4 | 10.5 | 11.5 | 6.8 | 50 |
| 55 | 14.8 | 12.0 | 13.6 | 11.1 | 13.3 | 15.5 | 13.4 | 12.0 | 14.9 | 10.8 | 11.9 | 7.0 | 55 |
| 60 | 15.1 | 12.3 | 13.9 | 11.3 | 13.6 | 15.8 | 13.7 | 12.3 | 15.2 | 11.0 | 12.2 | 7.1 | 60 |
| 65 | 15.3 | 12.5 | 14.1 | 11.5 | 13.9 | 16.1 | 14.0 | 12.5 | 15.5 | 11.2 | 12.4 | 7.3 | 65 |
| 70 | 15.5 | 12.6 | 14.3 | 11.6 | 14.0 | 16.3 | 14.1 | 12.6 | 15.7 | 11.4 | 12.5 | 7.4 | 70 |
| 75 | 15.7 | 12.8 | 14.4 | 11.8 | 14.2 | 16.5 | 14.3 | 12.8 | 15.9 | 11.5 | 12.7 | 7.5 | 75 |

[1] The values given in the table are mean values from different subjects without evidence of neuromuscular disease. The standard deviation of each value is 15 percent (20 potentials for each muscle). Therefore, deviations up to 20 percent are considered within the normal range when comparing measurements in a given muscle with the values of the table.
(From Buchthal,[5] with permission.)

# Selection and analysis

For quantitative analysis, the standard concentric needle electrode with a lead-off surface of about 0.07 mm² is commonly used. The amplifier frequency response is set to cover the 10 Hz to 10 KHz range and the standard gain is set at 100 to 500 $\mu$V per cm. Skin temperature should be greater than 34°C to maintain the muscle temperature at about 37°C.[18] In normal subjects single motor units may be readily isolated during mild to moderate contraction by moving or rotating the needle gently until crisp discharges are heard. It is essential that the motor unit potentials selected for quantitative assessment have rise times less than 500 $\mu$s. A storage oscilloscope with a delay line offers a distinct advantage for the identification and quantification of motor unit potentials. There is considerable variability of recorded potentials from one motor unit to another and within the same motor unit depending upon the relative position of the needle tip to the source of discharge. Thus it is recommended that at least 20 different motor unit potentials be recorded and measured in each muscle to determine the average value.[5] This procedure usually requires multiple needle insertions.

Useful criteria for various aspects of motor unit potentials have been established by Buchthal.[5] Table 12-1 summarizes his normal values for motor unit duration in different muscles and age groups. In this study, duration was measured from the point of take-off to the return to baseline. A late or satellite component,[43] seen as a separate peak after return to baseline, was excluded from the duration measurement. The range of normal values, however, cannot be applied indiscriminately because of its dependence on many factors other than just the parameter of the motor unit potential itself as discussed earlier in this chapter. For meaningful quantitative studies, each laboratory should construct its own table of normal values.

# Automated methods

Different investigators have explored the possibility of automatically analyzing motor unit potentials using analog[52] or digital techniques.[59] Motor unit potentials from a needle electrode are amplified, converted to a digital equivalent, and analyzed with a digital computer. Some of the parameters measured are duration, amplitude, polarity, number of phases, and integrated area under the waveform.[40] One of the inherent difficulties with computer analysis centers on the selection of motor units. In one early method[59] motor units were selected by visual inspection using a monitor scope, before being processed for automated analysis. With another technique[35] motor units were automatically accepted if their peak-to-peak amplitudes exceeded 100 $\mu$V. In this system, the duration of motor units was measured at 20 $\mu$V above the baseline and the number of phases having a deflection exceeding 40 $\mu$V were counted.

Different investigators have shown no major discrepancy between the results of the conventional time-consuming methods and those quickly analyzed by computers.[34, 36, 37, 39, 45] Indeed, computer analysis may be more accurate and efficient[30] in discriminating clearly abnormal electromyographic patterns and distinguishing between typical neuropathic and myopathic changes.[62] It remains to be seen, however, if these techniques are helpful in resolving borderline cases in which conventional methods fail to provide useful information.

# Frequency spectrum

Muscle action potentials may be considered as a summation of many sine waves of different frequencies. Thus, its frequency spectrum provides another objective means to characterize motor unit potentials. This is particularly convenient in evaluating the duration of motor units; the shorter the duration, the greater the high frequency compo-

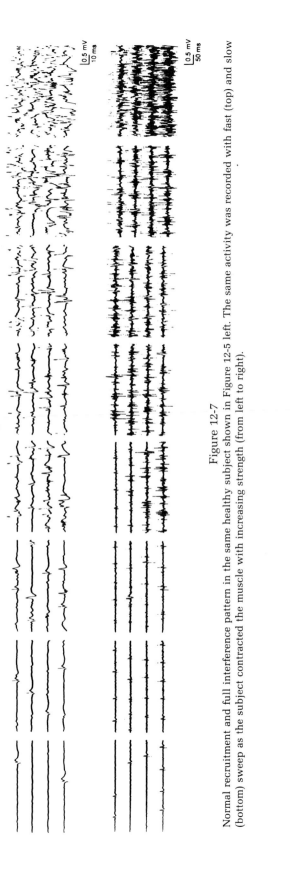

Figure 12-7

Normal recruitment and full interference pattern in the same healthy subject shown in Figure 12-5 left. The same activity was recorded with fast (top) and slow (bottom) sweep as the subject contracted the muscle with increasing strength (from left to right).

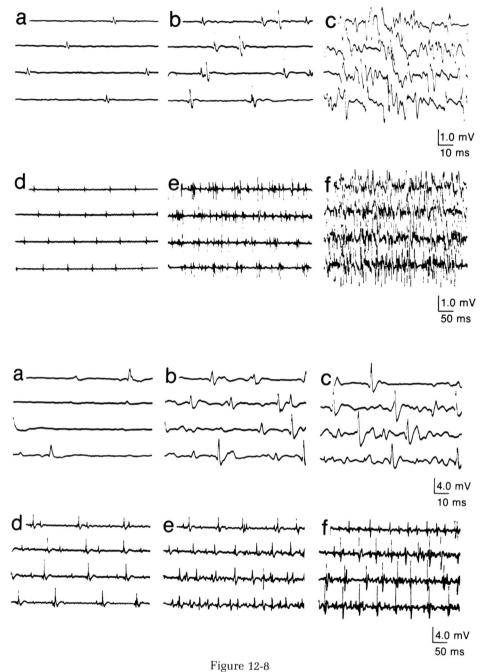

Figure 12-8

(*Top*) Normal recruitment of the triceps in a 44-year-old healthy man. The same activity was recorded with fast (top) and slow sweep (bottom) during minimal (a, d), moderate (b, e), and maximal contraction (c, f). (*Bottom*) Reduced recruitment of the tibialis anterior in a 44-year-old man with amyotrophic lateral sclerosis. A single motor unit discharged rapidly during strong contraction.

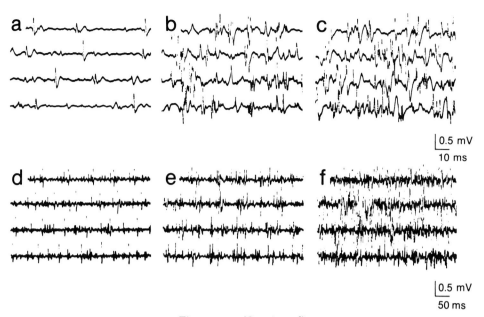

0.5 mV
10 ms

0.5 mV
50 ms

Figure 12-8 (Continued)

(Above) Early recruitment and full interference pattern of the quadriceps in a 20-year-old patient with limb-girdle dystrophy. An excessive number of motor units discharged for the amount of muscle force exerted during weak contraction.

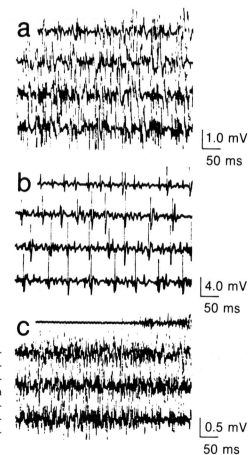

1.0 mV
50 ms

4.0 mV
50 ms

0.5 mV
50 ms

Figure 12-9

Interference patterns of the triceps in a 44-year-old healthy man (a); of the tibialis anterior in a 52-year-old man with amyotrophic lateral sclerosis (b); and of the quadriceps in a 20-year-old patient with limb-girdle dystrophy (c). Note discrete single motor unit discharge in (b) and abundant motor unit potentials with reduced amplitude in (c).

TECHNIQUES AND NORMAL FINDINGS

nents. Frequency analysis can be performed either with electronic filters or by a digital computer. The results are usually presented as a histogram of amplitude against frequency. Different authors have studied frequency spectra in normal and diseased muscles.[32] In normal muscles, peak amplitude was found to be between 100 and 200 Hz during maximal contraction.[68] There was a shift of the peak amplitude to a higher frequency in myopathy[60] and to a lower frequency in anterior horn cell lesions.[22] Despite the clear difference between myopathy and neuropathy, the clinical value of frequency analysis is limited by its variability. Indeed, frequency spectra change significantly depending upon needle position and level of muscle contraction.[15]

# DISCHARGE PATTERN OF MOTOR UNIT

## Recruitment

The physiologic principles underlying the orderly activation of motor units have already been discussed in Chapter 11. Mild voluntary contraction causes isolated low frequency (1 to 2 impulses per second) discharges of one or a few motor units. Effort to increase muscle force is associated with two separate but related changes in the pattern of motor unit discharge: (1) recruitment of previously inactive units; and (2) more rapid firing of already active units (Fig. 12-7). Which of the two plays a greater role is not known, but both mechanisms operate simultaneously. Assessment of the recruitment pattern during routine electromyography depends on knowing how many motor units should normally be firing for the force being exerted. The recruitment pattern is normal if the number of motor units is appropriate for the effort (Fig. 12-8 Top, left), reduced if there are fewer discharging units than expected (Fig. 12-8 Bottom, left), and increased if too many units are recruited for minimal effort of contraction (Fig. 12-8 Top, right).

A healthy subject should be able to voluntarily activate only one or two motor units initially. As discussed in Chapter 11, normal recruitment occurs in a fixed order according to the size principle.[29] Thus, the motor units activated early are relatively small, probably representing Type I muscle fibers. Those recruited later are considerably larger, reflecting participation of Type II units.[69] A measure of firing pattern used in clinical electromyography is the recruitment frequency; that is, the firing frequency of a motor unit when an additional unit in the vicinity begins to fire. Normally, the recruitment frequency is 5 to 20 impulses per second during mild contraction, but this varies for different types of motor units.[14, 56] Another measure of recruitment is the ratio of the average motor unit firing rate to the number of active units. Normally this ratio is less than 5 with, for example, three units firing less than 15 impulses per second each.[17] If 2 units are firing over 20 impulses per second, the ratio is more than 10, indicating a loss of motor units.

## Interference pattern

With greater contraction, many motor units begin to fire very rapidly (Fig. 12-9). Simultaneous activation of different units no longer allows recognition of individual motor unit potentials. Hence, this summated response is usually referred to as the interference pattern. It is a measure of the density or number of spikes and the average amplitude of all the available motor unit potentials. It depends on the descending input to the motor neuron pool, the number of motor neurons capable of discharging, and the configuration and firing frequency of each motor unit potential. Analyzing the interference pattern is important to determine not only how many motor units are discharging at maximal effort but also whether the number of firing units is appropriate for the muscle force exerted.

# Automatic analysis

Parameters of individual motor unit potentials are best assessed at low levels of voluntary contraction which tend to activate only low-threshold motor neurons. Quantitative analysis of a wider range of motor neurons can be accomplished by studying the recruitment pattern during moderate or strong muscle contraction. Willison[75] described an automated technique that takes into account the pattern of recruitment. The number of directional changes of a waveform that exceeds a minimum excursion without necessarily crossing the baseline is designated as the number of turns. This characteristic, rather than the number of individual spikes, is measured along with amplitude during a fixed period of time from a number of different sites (Fig. 12-10). The amplitude is measured from a point of change in direction to the next, not from baseline to peak. Only potentials greater than 100 $\mu$V are selected to avoid contamination by noise.[26, 27] This analysis is not limited to low levels of muscle contraction but depends on constant patient effort while recording from multiple sites.

A special purpose digital computer has been developed for automatic analysis and display of the total number of reversals, histograms of the intervals between potential reversals, and cumulative amplitude of all potentials during a certain time period.[19] One study[22] showed a 10 to 25 percent reproducibility for the number of turns and mean amplitude tested during repeated trials. Less intersubject difference was encountered when a relative rather than an absolute force was required for each individual. Reproducibility was best at 30 percent of the maximum force.

Quantitative measurements of single motor units and recruitment pattern are complementary. Analysis of individual potentials allows precise comparison between normal and abnormal motor units and provides a measure of their temporal stability. In

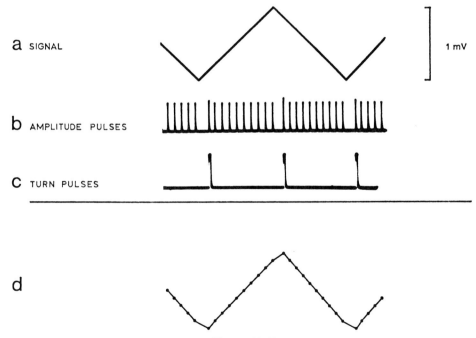

Figure 12-10
Conversion of calibration waveform (a) into two serial pulse trains: amplitude (b) and turns (c). The outputs of these two pulse generators characterize the original input accurately, as evidenced by graphical reconstruction of the waveform (d) by plotting from b and c. (From Hayward and Willison,[27] with permission.)

contrast, the latter method is best used for assessing overall muscle performance by demonstrating the number and pattern of motor unit recruitment. These methods are not widely used at this time but seem promising as a supplement to routine electromyography.[2, 24, 25, 28, 49]

# ELECTRICAL POTENTIAL AND MUSCLE FORCE

During maximal effort, single motor units will discharge at frequencies ranging from 25 to 50 impulses per second. Despite the intermittent electrical activation of individual motor units, the mechanical response fuses at high discharge frequencies and relatively even tension develops. With a high degree of fusion, a summated contraction produces more than twice the tension of a single twitch. Contraction of the whole muscle is very smooth not only because the responses of individual motor units fuse, but also because different motor units fire asynchronously. The maximal mechanical response is called tetanic contraction.

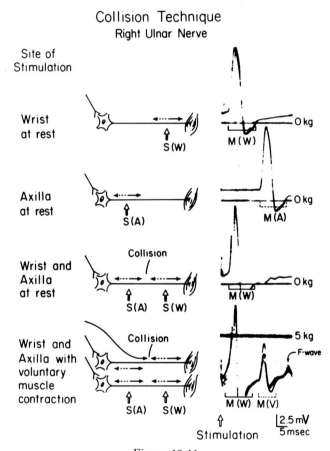

Figure 12-11

Compound muscle action potentials, M(W) and M(A), from the first dorsal interosseous and muscle force (straight line). With stimulation at the wrist and axilla at rest, the orthodromic impulse from the axilla was extinguished by collision. When the same shocks were delivered with voluntary effort (bottom tracing), M(V) appeared in proportion to the number of axons in which a voluntary impulse first collided with an antidromic impulse from the wrist. (From Kimura,[33] with permission.)

# Rectification and integration

Waveform integration has been used to correlate muscle force and electrical activity. To determine the total area under a waveform, the polarity of all negative peaks is reversed, a process called full-wave rectification. The rectified potential consists of only positive deflections and the area between the waveform and baseline can now be determined electrically.[1] The integral of a waveform is directly proportional to the amplitude, frequency, and duration of the original potential. A linear relationship between the integrated electromyogram and the isometric tension produced by the submaximally contracting muscle has been demonstrated.[3, 41, 42, 46, 47, 50, 64, 67]

# Collision technique

The collision technique has been used to determine the relationship between the electrical potential and force produced by voluntary contraction of the first dorsal interosseous muscle. Shocks of supramaximal intensity, delivered at either the wrist or axilla, elicit nearly identical compound muscle action potentials, M(W) or M(A) (Fig. 12-11). If shocks are applied simultaneously at the wrist and axilla with the subject at rest, M(W) but not M(A) is elicited because the orthodromic impulse from the axilla is extinguished by collision with the antidromic impulse from the wrist. However, M(A) is not completely blocked if the same paired shocks are delivered while the muscle is voluntarily contracted. In this situation some antidromic impulses from the wrist first collide with voluntary impulses and, therefore, cannot interfere with the impulse evoked by

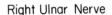

Right Ulnar Nerve

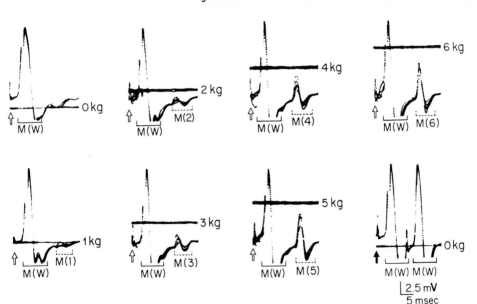

Figure 12-12

Correlation between muscle force and electrical activity, right ulnar nerve. Stimulation (open arrow) and recording as for bottom tracing in Figure 12-11 in the same subject. Muscle force ranged from 0 to 6.0 kg (straight line). In the last tracing, paired stimuli (closed arrow) were delivered at the wrist to allow the second M(W) to appear with the same time delay as M(V). First and second M(W) were nearly identical, indicating that alteration in neuromuscular excitability was negligible. (From Kimura,[33] with permission.)

axillary stimulation. The fraction of M(A) so recorded is termed M(V), as it represents the magnitude of the voluntary impulse. This technique produces in effect a synchronized equivalent to the asynchronous motor neuron activity associated with voluntary contraction.[33] The amplitude of the compound muscle action potential M(V) thus recorded relates directly and linearly to the force of contraction under isometric conditions (Fig. 12-12).

The recruitment and discharge pattern of single motor units can best be studied by direct recording of firing units with a needle electrode during weak voluntary contraction.[51, 55, 56, 65] However, the identification of single motor units by this means becomes difficult during strong muscle contraction because of the presence of a large shower of spikes from many different units. Moreover, the few motor units that may be selected for observation do not necessarily reveal the behavior of the total population of motor neurons. The collision technique provides a direct means to relate a measurement of the discharge pattern of the motor neuron pool to muscle force over a wide range of voluntary contraction.

# REFERENCE SOURCES

1. BAK, MJ AND LOEB, GE: *A pulsed integrator for EMG analysis.* Electroenceph Clin Neurophysiol 47:738, 1979.

2. BERGMANS, J: *Clinical applications. Applications to EMG.* In RÉMOND, A (ED): *EEG Informatics. A Didactic Review of Methods and Applications of EEG Data Processing.* Elsevier, Amsterdam, 1977.

3. BOUISSET, S: *EMG and muscle force in normal motor activities.* In DESMEDT, JE (ED): *New Developments in Electromyography and Clinical Neurophysiology,* Vol 1. Karger, Basel, 1973 pp 547, 583.

4. BROOKE, MH, ET AL: *The prolonged exercise test.* Neurology (New York) 29:636, 1979.

5. BUCHTHAL, F: *An Introduction to Electromyography.* Scandinavian University Books, Copenhagen, 1957.

6. BUCHTHAL, F: *The general concept of the motor unit.* In ADAMS, RD, EATON, LM, AND SHY, GM (EDS): *Neuromuscular Disorders.* Williams & Wilkins, Baltimore, 1960.

7. BUCHTHAL, F AND ROSENFALCK, P: *Spontaneous electrical activity of human muscle.* Electroenceph Clin Neurophysiol 20:321, 1966.

8. BUCHTHAL, F, GULD, C, AND ROSENFALCK, P: *Action potential parameters in normal human muscle and their dependence on physical variables.* Acta Physiol Scand 32:200, 1954.

9. BUCHTHAL, F, GULD, C, AND ROSENFALCK, P: *Volume conduction of the spike of the motor unit potential investigated with a new type of multielectrode.* Acta Physiol Scand 38:331, 1957.

10. BUCHTHAL, F, GULD, C, AND ROSENFALCK, P: *Multielectrode study of the territory of a motor unit.* Acta Physiol Scand 39:83, 1957.

11. BUCHTHAL, F, PINELLI, P, AND ROSENFALCK, P: *Action potential parameters in normal human muscle and their physiological determinants.* Acta Physiol Scand 32:219, 1954.

12. CHERINGTON, M, LEWIN, E, AND MCCRIMMON, A: *Serum creatine phosphokinase changes following needle electromyographic studies.* Neurology (Minneap) 18:271, 1968.

13. CHRISSIAN, SA, STOLOV, WC, AND HONGLADAROM, T: *Needle electromyography: Its effect on serum creatine phosphokinase activity.* Arch Phys Med Rehabil 57:114, 1976.

14. CLAMANN, HP: *Activity of single motor units during isometric tension.* Neurology (Minneap) 20:254, 1970.

15. COSI, V AND MAZZELLA, GL: *Frequency analysis in clinical electromyography: A preliminary report.* Electroenceph Clin Neurophysiol 27:100, 1969.

16. DAUBE, JR: *The description of motor unit potentials in electromyography.* Neurology (New York) 28:623, 1978.

17. DAUBE, JR: *Needle Examination in Electromyography.* American Association of Electromyography and Electrodiagnosis, Mayo Clinic, Rochester, Minnesota, 1979.

18. DESMEDT, JE: *The neuromuscular disorder in myasthenia gravis. 1. Electrical and mechanical response to nerve stimulation in hand muscles.* In DESMEDT, JE (ED): *New Developments in Electromyography and Clinical Neurophysiology,* Vol 1. Karger, Basel, 1973.

19. DOWLING, MH, FITCH, P, AND WILLISON, RG: *A special purpose digital computer (Biomac 500) used in the analysis of the human electromyogram.* Electroenceph Clin Neurophysiol 25:570, 1968.

20. EKSTEDT, J AND STÅLBERG, E: *How the size of the needle electrode leading-off surface influences the shape of the single muscle fibre action potential in electromyography.* Computer Prog Biomed 3:204, 1973.

21. FATT, P AND KATZ, B: *An analysis of the end-plate potential recorded with an intra-cellular electrode.* J Physiol (Lond) 115:320, 1951.

22. FEX, J AND KRAKAU, CET: *Some experiences with Walton's frequency analysis of the electromyogram.* J Neurol Neurosurg Psychiatry 20:178, 1957.

23. FUGLSANG-FREDERIKSEN, A AND MÅNSSON, A: *Analysis of electrical activity of normal muscle in man at different degrees of voluntary effort.* J Neurol Neurosurg Psychiatry 38:683, 1975.

24. FUGLSANG-FREDERIKSEN, A, SCHEEL, U, AND BUCHTHAL, F: *Diagnostic yield of analysis of the pattern of electrical activity and of individual motor unit potentials in myopathy.* J Neurol Neurosurg Psychiatry 39:742, 1976.

25. FUGLSANG-FREDERIKSEN, A, SCHEEL, U, AND BUCHTHAL, F: *Diagnostic yield of the analysis of the pattern of electrical activity of muscle and of individual motor unit potentials in neurogenic involvement.* J Neurol Neurosurg Psychiatry 40:544, 1977.

26. HAYWARD, M: *Automatic analysis of the electromyogram in healthy subjects of different ages.* J Neurol Sci 33:397, 1977.

27. HAYWARD, M AND WILLISON, RG: *The recognition of myogenic and neurogenic lesions by quantitative EMG.* In DESMEDT, JE (ED): *New Developments in Electromyography and Clinical Neurophysiology,* Vol 2. Karger, Basel, 1973 pp 448–453.

28. HAYWARD, M AND WILLISON, RG: *Automatic analysis of the electromyogram in patients with chronic partial denervation.* J Neurol Sci 33:415, 1977.

29. HENNEMAN, E: *Relation between size of neurons and their susceptibility to discharge.* Science 126:1345, 1957.

30. HIROSE, K, UONO, M, AND SOBUE, I: *Quantitative electromyography comparison between manual values and computer ones on normal subjects.* Electromyogr Clin Neurophysiol 14:315, 1974.

31. HUGHES, RC, ET AL: *Serum creatine kinase studies in the detection of carriers of Duchenne dystrophy.* J Neurol Neurosurg Psychiatry 34:527, 1971.

32. KAISER, E AND PETERSÉN, I: *Muscle action potentials studied by frequency analysis and duration measurement.* Acta Neurol Scand 41(suppl 13):213, 1965.

33. KIMURA, J: *Electrical activity in voluntarily contracting muscle.* Arch Neurol 34:85, 1977.

34. KOPEC, J AND HAUSMANOWA-PETRUSEWICZ, I: *Histogram of muscle potentials recorded automatically with the aid of the averaging computer "ANOPS".* Electromyography 9:371, 1969.

35. KOPEC, J AND HAUSMANOWA-PETRUSEWICZ, I: *Application of automatic analysis of electromyograms in clinical diagnosis.* Electroenceph Clin Neurophysiol 36:575, 1974.

36. KOPEC, J AND HAUSMANOWA-PETRUSEWICZ, I: *On-line computer application in clinical quantitative electromyography.* Electromyogr Clin Neurophysiol 16:49, 1976.

37. KOPEC, J, ET AL: *Automatic analysis in electromyography.* In DESMEDT, JE (ED): *New Developments in Electromyography and Clinical Neurophysiology,* Vol 2. Karger, Basel, 1973.

38. KUGELBERG, E AND PETERSÉN, I: *"Insertion activity" in electromyography. With notes on denervated muscle response to constant current.* J Neurol Neurosurg Psychiatry 12:268, 1949.

39. KUNZE, K: *Quantitative EMG analysis in myogenic and neurogenic muscle diseases.* In DESMEDT, JE (ED): *New Developments in Electromyography and Clinical Neurophysiology,* Vol 2. Karger, Basel, 1973 pp 469–476.

**ACTIVATION PROCEDURES AND OTHER METHODS**

40. KUNZE, K AND ERBSLÖH, F: *Automatic EMG analysis, a new approach.* Electroenceph Clin Neurophysiol 25:402, 1968.

41. KURODA, E, KLISSOURAS, V, AND MILSUM, JH: *Electrical and metabolic activities and fatigue in human isometric contraction.* J Appl Physiol 29:358, 1970.

42. LAM, HS, MORGAN, DL, AND LAMPARD, DG: *Derivation of reliable electromyograms and their relation to tension in mammalian skeletal muscles during synchronous stimulation.* Electroenceph Clin Neurophysiol 46:72, 1979.

43. LANG, AH AND PARTANEN, VSJ: *"Satellite potentials" and the duration of motor unit potentials in normal, neuropathic and myopathic muscles.* J Neurol Sci 27:513, 1976.

44. LANG, AH AND TUOMOLA, H: *The time parameters of motor unit potentials recorded with multi-electrodes and the summation technique.* Electromyogr Clin Neurophysiol 14:513, 1974.

45. LEE, RG AND WHITE, DG: *Computer analysis of motor unit action potentials in routine clinical electromyography.* In DESMEDT, JE (ED): *New Developments in Electromyography and Clinical Neurophysiology,* Vol 2. Karger, Basel, 1973 454–461.

46. LENMAN, JAR: *A clinical and experimental study of the effects of exercise on motor weakness in neurological disease.* J Neurol Neurosurg Psychiatry 22:182, 1959.

47. LIPPOLD, OCJ: *The relation between integrated action potentials in a human muscle and its isometric tension.* J Physiol (Lond) 117:492, 1952.

48. MAEYENS, E, JR AND PITNER, SE: *Effect of electromyography on CPK and aldolase levels.* Arch Neurol 19:538, 1968.

49. McCOMAS, AJ AND SICA, REP: *Automatic quantitative analysis of the electromyogram in partially denervated distal muscles: Comparison with motor unit counting.* Le J Canadien des Sciences Neurol 5:377, 1978.

50. MILNER-BROWN, HS AND STEIN, RB: *The relation between the surface electromyogram and muscular force.* J Physiol (Lond) 246:549, 1975.

51. MILNER-BROWN, HS, STEIN, RB, AND YEMM, R: *Changes in firing rate of human motor units during linearly changing voluntary contractions.* J Physiol (Lond) 230:371, 1973.

52. MOOSA, A AND BROWN, BH: *Quantitative electromyography: A new analogue technique for detecting changes in action potential duration.* J Neurol Neurosurg Psychiatry 35:216, 1972.

53. NETTER, FH: *The Ciba Collection of Medical Illustrations.* Vol 1. *A compilation of paintings on the normal and pathologic anatomy of the nervous system with a supplement on the hypothalamus.* Ciba Pharmaceutical Co., New York, 1962.

54. PEDINOFF, S AND SANDHU, RS: *Electromyographic effect on serum creatine phosphokinase in normal individuals.* Arch Phys Med Rehabil 59:27, 1978.

55. PERSON, RS: *Rhythmic activity of a group of human motoneurones during voluntary contraction of a muscle.* Electroenceph Clin Neurophysiol 36:585, 1974.

56. PETAJAN, JH: *Clinical electromyographic studies of diseases of the motor unit.* Electroenceph Clin Neurophysiol 36:395, 1974.

57. PICKETT, JB: *Small sputtering positive waves—Cannula recorded "nerve" potentials.* Electroenceph Clin Neurophysiol 45:178, 1978.

58. PICKETT, JB AND SCHMIDLEY, JW: *Sputtering positive potentials in the EMG: An artifact resembling positive waves.* Neurology (New York) 30:215, 1980.

59. RATHJEN, R, SIMONS, DG, AND PETERSON, CR: *Computer analysis of the duration of motor-unit potentials.* Arch Phys Med Rehabil 49:524, 1968.

60. RICHARDSON, AT: *Electromyography in myasthenia gravis and the other myopathies.* Am J Phys Med 38:118, 1959.

61. SCRANTON, PE, HASIBA, U, AND GORENC, TJ: *Intramuscular hemorrhage in hemophiliacs with inhibitors.* JAMA 241:2028, 1979.

62. SICA, REP, McCOMAS, AJ, AND FERREIRA, JCD: *Evaluation of an automated method for analysing the electromyogram.* Le J Canadien des Sciences Neurol 5:275, 1978.

63. SKAGGS, H, ET AL: *Guidelines in EMG.* Professional Standards Committee, American Association of Electromyography and Electrodiagnosis, 1979.

64. STEPHENS, JA AND TAYLOR, A: *The relationship between integrated electrical activity and force in normal and fatiguing human voluntary muscle contractions.* In DESMEDT, JE (ED): *New Developments in Electromyography and Clinical Neurophysiology,* Vol 1. Karger, Basel, 1973 pp 623–627.

65. TANJI, J AND KATO, M: *Recruitment of motor units in voluntary contractions of a finger muscle in man.* Exp Neurol 40:759, 1973.

66. THIELE, B AND BÖHLE, A: *Number of spike-components contributing to the motor unit potential.* Z EEG-EMG 9:125, 1978.

67. VREDENBREGT, J AND RAU, G: *Surface electromyography in relation to force, muscle length and endurance.* In DESMEDT, JE (ED) *New Developments in Electromyography and Clinical Neurophysiology,* Vol 1. Karger, Basel, 1973 pp 607–622.

68. WALTON, JN: *The electromyogram in myopathy: Analysis with the audio-frequency spectrometer.* J Neurol Neurosurg Psychiatry 15:219, 1952.

69. WARMOLTS, JR AND ENGEL, WK: *Open-biopsy electromyography. I. Correlation of motor unit behavior with histochemical muscle fiber type in human limb muscle.* Arch Neurol 27:512, 1972.

70. WEDDELL, G, FEINSTEIN, B, AND PATTLE, RE: *The electrical activity of voluntary muscle in man under normal and pathological conditions.* Brain 67:178, 1944.

71. WIECHERS, DO: *Mechanically provoked insertional activity before and after nerve section in rats.* Arch Phys Med Rehabil 58:402, 1977.

72. WIECHERS, DO: *Electromyographic insertional activity in normal limb muscles.* Arch Phys Med Rehabil 60:359, 1979.

73. WIECHERS, DO, STOW, R, AND JOHNSON, EW: *Electromyographic insertional activity mechanically provoked in biceps brachii.* Arch Phys Med Rehabil 58:573, 1977.

74. WIEDERHOLT, WC: *"End-plate noise" in electromyography.* Neurology (Minneap) 20:214, 1970.

75. WILLISON, RG: *Analysis of electrical activity in healthy and dystrophic muscle in man.* J Neurol Neurosurg Psychiatry 27:386, 1964.

# 13
# TYPES OF ABNORMALITY

As discussed in Chapter 12, electrical signals registered during electromyography are extracellular recordings of propagating muscle action potentials. Except for end-plate noise and the brief insertional activity coincident with needle placement there are normally no electrical discharges in a relaxed muscle. Several types of spontaneous discharges occur in some diseases of the nerve and muscle, although they do not necessarily carry the same clinical significance. Fibrillation potentials and positive sharp waves are derived from single spontaneous discharges of individual motor units. Complex repetitive discharges are of unknown origin but probably represent high frequency discharges from single or multiple muscle fibers.

Under normal circumstances, the smallest unit of volitional contraction is a motor unit. Hence, a motor unit potential is the smallest volitionally generated electrical activity that can be recorded by the conventional needle electromyography. In diseases of the nerve and muscle, the motor unit may be affected structurally or functionally, leading to alterations in waveform and discharge patterns of muscle action potentials. Because certain patterns of electrical abnormalities may be associated with a particular pathologic process, the study of muscle action potentials provides information regarding the nature of the disease.

Electromyography is useful as a clinical tool only if the findings are interpreted in light of the patient's history, physical examination, and other diagnostic studies. However, based solely on the four steps of electromyography described in Chapter 12 (see Fig. 12-1), motor dysfunction may be divided into upper and lower motor neuron disorders, and myogenic lesions. Types of abnormalities will be detailed below in each of the four steps. Typical electromyographic findings associated with each disease category are shown diagrammatically in Figures 13-1 through 13-3 and summarized in Figure 13-4. As a means of introduction, the illustrations emphasize the basic principles at the risk of oversimplification. These points will be amplified and certain variations will be clarified in the text to complement the diagrams.

## INSERTIONAL ACTIVITY
### Decreased versus increased activity

A marked diminution or absence of insertional activity usually indicates a reduced number of healthy muscle fibers as, for example, in fibrotic or severely atrophied mus-

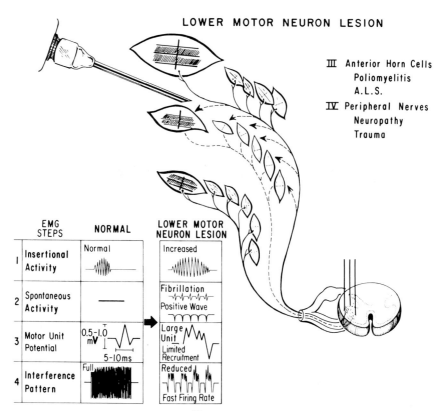

LOWER MOTOR NEURON LESION

III Anterior Horn Cells
Poliomyelitis
A.L.S.

IV Peripheral Nerves
Neuropathy
Trauma

| EMG STEPS | | NORMAL | LOWER MOTOR NEURON LESION |
|---|---|---|---|
| 1 | Insertional Activity | Normal | Increased |
| 2 | Spontaneous Activity | | Fibrillation / Positive Wave |
| 3 | Motor Unit Potential | 0.5–1.0 mV / 5–10ms | Large Unit / Limited Recruitment |
| 4 | Interference Pattern | Full | Reduced / Fast Firing Rate |

Figure 13-1

Typical findings in lower motor neuron lesions. They include (1) increased insertional activity; (2) spontaneous activities in the form of fibrillation potentials and positive sharp waves, (3) large amplitude, long duration polyphasic motor unit potentials; and (4) discrete single unit activity firing rapidly during maximal effort of contraction. The diagram illustrates denervation and reinnervation of a group of muscle fibers supplied by a diseased axon. (Compare Figure 12-1.)

cles (see Fig. 12-2). The insertional activity may also be absent when muscle fibers are functionally inexcitable, as is known to occur during attacks of familial periodic paralysis. The absence of insertional activity may also occur because of a faulty needle or because the needle is not moving through the muscle (as assumed by the examiner). An abnormal increase in insertional activity outlasting the cessation of needle movement is often associated with irritability of the muscle or, more specifically, instability of the muscle membrane (see Fig. 12-2). This is usually associated with frank denervation, although it may also occur in myotonic disorders and certain other myogenic disorders, including myositis.[42] In addition, some apparently normal individuals may show a variant of normal insertional activity associated with one or two isolated positive potentials at the end of the discharge.[79, 80] This must be distinguished from insertional positive waves, which are more sustained, rhythmic, and reproducible as described below.

## Insertional positive waves

After cessation of the needle movement, insertional activity may be followed by a briefly sustained run of positive waves lasting several seconds to minutes. Less frequently, a train of negative spikes with or without initial positivity may be seen instead of positive sharp waves. They discharge at a slow frequency, ranging 1 to 30 impulses per second, and are indistinguishable in waveform from the spontaneous discharges recorded from frankly denervated muscles at rest. Abnormal insertional activity of this

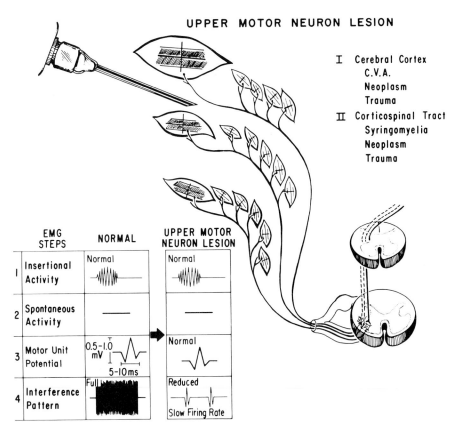

## UPPER MOTOR NEURON LESION

I Cerebral Cortex
C.V.A.
Neoplasm
Trauma

II Corticospinal Tract
Syringomyelia
Neoplasm
Trauma

| EMG STEPS | | NORMAL | UPPER MOTOR NEURON LESION |
|---|---|---|---|
| 1 | Insertional Activity | Normal | Normal |
| 2 | Spontaneous Activity | | |
| 3 | Motor Unit Potential | 0.5–1.0 mV / 5–10ms | Normal |
| 4 | Interference Pattern | Full | Reduced / Slow Firing Rate |

Figure 13-2

Typical findings in upper motor neuron lesions. They include (1) normal insertional activity; (2) no spontaneous activity; (3) normal motor unit potential if detected in an incomplete paralysis; and (4) reduced interference pattern with slow rates of firing of individual motor unit potentials. The diagram illustrates degeneration of the corticospinal tract resulting in a reduced number of descending impulses reaching the anterior horn cells and consequently to the muscle fibers supplied by those axons.

type appears in the early stages of denervation, 10 days to 2 weeks after nerve injury, before the appearance of spontaneous activity, but similar insertional discharges are also seen in some patients with mild forms of myotonic disorders. It may also occur in chronically denervated muscles or in association with rapidly progressive degeneration of muscle fibers in acute polymyositis. In these cases, positive sharp waves also appear spontaneously—not initiated by needle movement (Fig. 13-5). By definition, however, insertional activity is evoked by the mechanical stimulus of the needle, even if it continues after cessation of needle movement; whereas true spontaneous activities occur without apparent triggering mechanisms. Differentiation may be somewhat arbitrary in some cases, since spontaneous activity is often enhanced by needle movement.

Because of its resemblance to myotonic discharges in waveform and sound, insertional positive waves or negative spikes seen in denervated muscles are sometimes called pseudomyotonia, although a more descriptive term is preferable. The insertional positive waves associated with early denervation are briefer than those seen in myotonic disorders and usually lack the waxing and waning quality, showing abrupt onset and termination. However, distinction between the two can be difficult and may be a source of error. Insertional positive waves of denervation may occur in the absence of spontaneous activity. A few positive waves in the first seconds after insertion of the needle

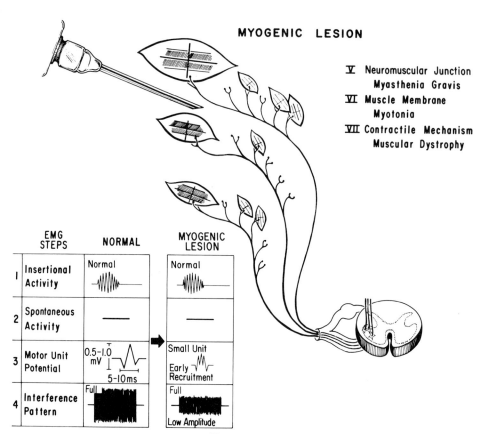

**MYOGENIC LESION**

V Neuromuscular Junction
  Myasthenia Gravis
VI Muscle Membrane
  Myotonia
VII Contractile Mechanism
  Muscular Dystrophy

| EMG STEPS | | NORMAL | MYOGENIC LESION |
|---|---|---|---|
| 1 | Insertional Activity | Normal | Normal |
| 2 | Spontaneous Activity | — | — |
| 3 | Motor Unit Potential | 0.5-1.0 mV 5-10ms | Small Unit Early Recruitment |
| 4 | Interference Pattern | Full | Full Low Amplitude |

Figure 13-3

Typical findings in myogenic lesions. They include (1) normal insertional activity; (2) no spontaneous activity, although there are some notable exceptions; (3) low amplitude, short duration, polyphasic motor unit potentials; and (4) early recruitment leading to low amplitude, full interference pattern at less than maximal effort of contraction. The diagram illustrates random loss of individual muscle fibers resulting in reduced number of fibers per motor unit.

may then mimic a mild form of myotonic discharge. On the other hand, insertional positive waves associated with an abortive form of myotonic discharge, when very brief, resemble those of early denervation. Recognition of the myotonic phenomenon is especially difficult immediately after prolonged exercise, which tends to diminish the after-discharge electrically as well as clinically. Insertional positive waves have been described in otherwise normal subjects, possibly representing a form fruste of myotonia congenita.[80]

# MYOTONIC DISCHARGE

Myotonia is a sustained contraction of the muscle following voluntary movement or after electrical or mechanical stimulation. It is a clinical phenomenon commonly seen in a variety of disorders, including myotonia congenita, myotonia dystrophica, chondrodystrophic myotonia, paramyotonia congenita, and hyperkalemic periodic paralysis.[16, 50] The electromyographic correlates of clinical myotonia consist of rhythmic discharges. Triggered by insertion of the needle electrode, they last for long periods after the external source of excitation has come to rest. Myotonic discharges are usually found in conjunction with clinical myotonia in the disorders listed above. Infrequently, similar discharges occur in polymyositis, Type II glycogen storage disease (acid maltase

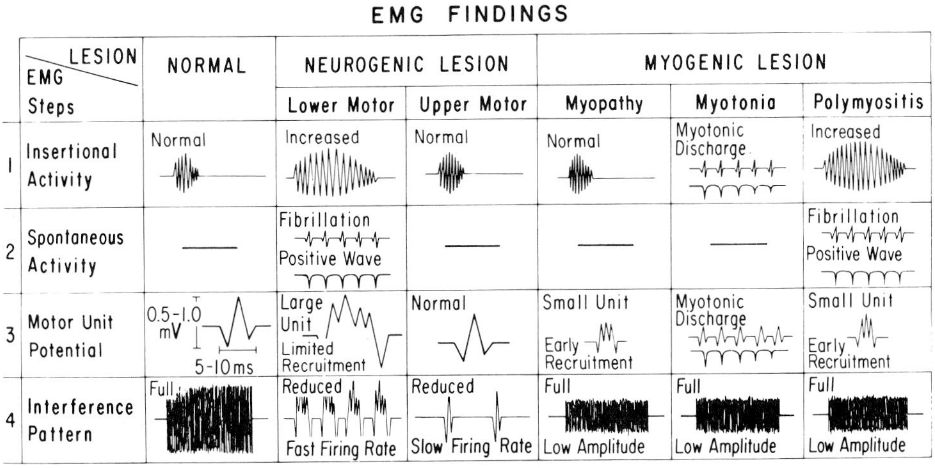

EMG FINDINGS

| LESION / EMG Steps | NORMAL | NEUROGENIC LESION | | MYOGENIC LESION | | |
|---|---|---|---|---|---|---|
| | | Lower Motor | Upper Motor | Myopathy | Myotonia | Polymyositis |
| 1 Insertional Activity | Normal | Increased | Normal | Normal | Myotonic Discharge | Increased |
| 2 Spontaneous Activity | | Fibrillation / Positive Wave | | | | Fibrillation / Positive Wave |
| 3 Motor Unit Potential | 0.5-1.0 mV / 5-10ms | Large Unit / Limited Recruitment | Normal | Small Unit / Early Recruitment | Myotonic Discharge | Small Unit / Early Recruitment |
| 4 Interference Pattern | Full | Reduced / Fast Firing Rate | Reduced / Slow Firing Rate | Full / Low Amplitude | Full / Low Amplitude | Full / Low Amplitude |

Figure 13-4

Typical findings in lower and upper motor neuron disorders and myogenic lesions as shown in Figures 13-1 through 13-3. Myotonia shares many features common to myopathy in general but is additionally characterized by myotonic discharges triggered by insertion of the needle and with voluntary effort to contract the muscle. Polymyositis shows combined features of myopathy and neuropathy, including (1) increased insertional activity; (2) abundant spontaneous discharges; (3) small amplitude, short duration, polyphasic motor unit potentials; and (4) early recruitment leading to low amplitude, full interference pattern.

deficiency),[34] and other disorders with chronic denervation that are not typically associated with clinical myotonia.

## Positive versus negative discharge

Myotonic discharges take two forms, probably depending on the spatial relationship between the recording surface of the needle and the discharging muscle fibers. One type of myotonic discharge occurs as a sustained run of positive waves ranging from 10 $\mu$V to 1 mV in amplitude (Fig. 13-6). The initial sharp positivity is followed by a slow negative component of a much longer duration. These positive sharp waves, like those of denervation, probably represent action potentials recorded from an injured area of the muscle fiber. A second type of myotonic discharge consists of a sustained run of negative spikes with a small initial positivity (Fig. 13-6). They also range from 10 $\mu$V to 1 mV in amplitude and resemble fibrillation potentials seen in denervation. In contrast to the positive sharp waves usually initiated by needle insertion, the negative spikes tend to occur at the beginning of slight volitional contraction. Both positive waves and negative spikes typically wax and wane in amplitude over the range of 10 $\mu$V to 1 mV, varying inversely to the rate of firing. Their frequency may increase or decrease within the range of 50 to 100 impulses per second, giving rise to a characteristic noise over the loudspeaker. It is reminiscent of the sound generated by an accelerating or decelerating motorcycle or chain saw. It has also been likened to the sound of a dive-bomber, although this analogy is not a very good one in my personal experience (with dive-bombers).

## Pathophysiology

The pathophysiology of the myotonic discharge has not been clearly established in man. It is known, however, that a decrease in resting chloride ($Cl^-$) conductance results in repetitive electrical activity in isolated frog[26] and mammalian skeletal muscle.[47] The electrophysiologic abnormality of hereditary myotonia in goats can also be explained

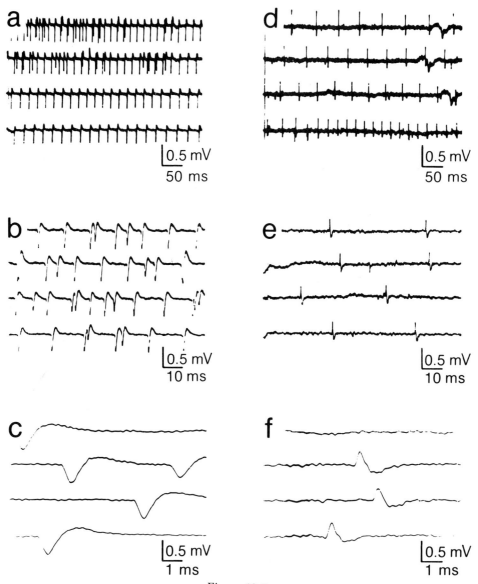

Figure 13-5

Spontaneous discharge from the right paraspinal muscle in a 62-year-old woman with polymyositis. Two types of discharges are shown: trains of positive sharp waves (a, b, c) and negative spikes (d, e, f) initiated by insertion of the needle electrode. The lack of initial positivity indicates that the negative spikes were recorded near the end-plate region, although they do not represent physiologic end-plate spikes. Note the absence of waxing and waning quality typically associated with myotonic potentials. (Compare Figure 13-6.)

by decreased chloride conductance.[46] In normal fibers the presence of chloride conductance stabilizes the membrane potential by shunting the depolarizing current and dampening its effect.[36] Conversely, the absence of chloride conductance in effect raises the resistance of the membrane. Since the depolarization for generation of an action potential is calculated as $E = IR$, where I and R are current and resistance, respectively, increased resistance will reduce the amount of current necessary to achieve the required voltage.[26]

As the critical level of depolarization is reached, a rapid change in sodium ($Na^+$) conductance occurs and initiates an action potential. The action potential falls with

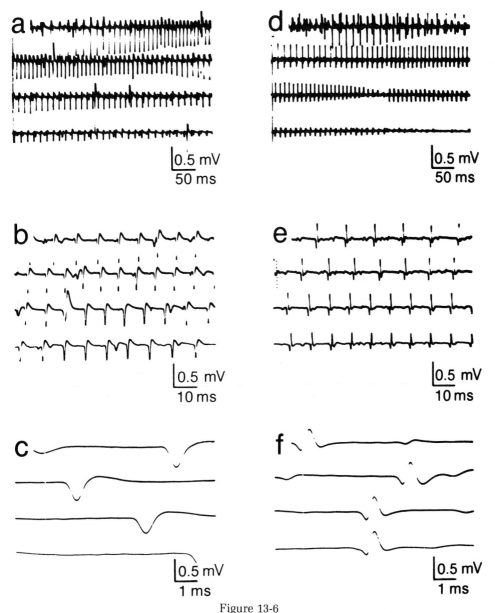

Figure 13-6

Myotonic discharge from the right anterior tibialis in a 39-year-old man with myotonic dystrophy. Two types of discharges are shown: trains of positive sharp waves (a, b, c) and negative spikes with initial positivity (d, e, f). Waxing and waning quality of these discharges are apparent in a and d.

inactivation of sodium conductance and delayed activation of potassium ($K^+$) conductance which tends to hyperpolarize the membrane. As potassium conductance slowly returns to its resting value, the cell becomes slightly depolarized relative to the previous hyperpolarized state. In an unstable membrane with increased resistance as a result of lowered chloride conductance, this slow change in potassium conductance is sufficient to trigger another action potential, and the cycle repeats itself.[8] Thus, the process of depolarization begins as soon as repolarization ends, leading to a series of repetitive action potentials. It remains to be seen whether the explanation of myotonic phenomena based on low chloride conductance can be extended to human disorders.[43]

# SPONTANEOUS ACTIVITY
## Origin and clinical significance

In the first two weeks after denervation, the sensitivity of a muscle fiber to acetylcholine (ACh) increases by as much as 100-fold.[6, 48, 70] This phenomenon is known as denervation hypersensitivity. It has been postulated that spontaneous discharges of denervated muscle fibers may represent hypersensitive responses to small quantities of circulating ACh.[20] The role of some circulating substance is supported by the absence of fibrillation potentials following artificially induced ischemia[33] and in isolated muscle fibers.[69] In rats, fibrillation potentials have been silenced by application of α-bungarotoxin or atropine sulfate.[7] Thus, the receptor molecules for these agents are essential for the production of fibrillations.

Some observations and experimental data have been marshalled against the ACh-hypersensitivity hypothesis. The amount of circulating ACh reaching the endplate is limited, since acetylcholinesterase concentrated in this region continuously catalyzes the hydrolysis of ACh to choline and acetate. Denervation hypersensitivity reflects the development of many highly sensitive sites over the entire muscle fiber, rather than a specific increase in end-plate sensitivity itself.[1] Spontaneous activity, however, seems to originate only in the end-plate zone and not elsewhere in nonjunctional membrane.[2] Further, these discharges continue to occur after the infusion of curare.[69] Denervation of frog muscle may cause increased sensitivity to ACh but produces no spontaneous activity.[49] These findings suggest that denervation hypersensitivity is not the sole explanation for the generation of spontaneous activity. One alternative hypothesis invokes slowly changing membrane potentials of metabolic origin which may periodically reach the critical level and evoke propagated spikes.[45]

Spontaneous activity, if reproducible in at least two muscle sites, is an unequivocal sign of abnormality and one of the most useful findings in clinical electromyography. It is usually seen in denervated muscle but may also occur in certain primary muscle diseases discussed later in the section on fibrillation potential. However, spontaneous activity may not appear until two to three weeks after nerve injury. Thus, the absence of spontaneous activity does not preclude denervation during the early weeks of presumed nerve injury. When found in disorders of the lower motor neuron, the distribution of spontaneous potentials can aid in the localization of lesions affecting the spinal cord, root, plexus, or peripheral nerve.

As a rule, spontaneous activity is not found in paretic limbs of patients with upper motor neuron disorders or disuse atrophy. Positive waves and fibrillation potentials in hemiplegic patients have been reported[39] but not always confirmed.[18] Some argue that spontaneous activity seen in these patients is, at least in part, caused by secondary disease of the lower motor neurons, since entrapment and traction causing subclinical or clinical neuropathy or radiculopathy may be present. Although an increasing number of electromyographers have now become convinced that fibrillation potentials and positive sharp waves can be seen unilaterally in individuals with acute upper motor neuron lesions, this observation is at present still controversial. Further studies are necessary to elucidate the true incidence and the possible etiology of this type of discharge. Spontaneous activity may also be found in the paraspinous muscles, following myelography in patients with previously normal electromyographic studies. These abnormalities develop by the first day after the procedure and resolve by the fourth day.[77]

There are four basic types of spontaneous activity: fibrillation potentials, positive sharp waves, fasciculation potentials, and complex repetitive discharges. Fibrillation potentials are discharges from single muscle fibers. Positive sharp waves are considered by some to be a special form of fibrillation potential.[19] They probably represent single fiber potentials recorded from an injured area of the fiber in which, because of the standing depolarization of the damaged tissue, the propagating action potential approaches but fails to generate a negative spike. Fasciculation potentials are spontaneous discharges from groups of muscle fibers and are analogous to motor unit potentials. Complex repetitive discharges probably result from the rapid firing of many muscle fibers that are activated ephaptically at a point of lateral contact by a spontaneously activated single fiber, which serves as a pacemaker.[22, 67] The frequency and pattern of discharge may be determined by two different, usually independent, mechanisms: rhythmic depolarization of denervated muscle fibers and circus movements of currents between muscle fibers.[37]

The spontaneous potentials arising from single muscle fibers are not accompanied by visible muscle movement. Isolated muscle twitches over a localized area may be seen with fasciculations and complex repetitive discharges. In contrast, spontaneous muscle discharges seen in myokymia and the other cramp syndromes are associated with sustained muscle contraction. These entities will be dealt with in Chapter 26.

Fibrillation potentials and positive sharp waves may be graded as follows:

(+1) Transient runs of positive discharges that occur only after moving the needle electrode. Strictly speaking, this is an insertional rather than spontaneous activity (i.e., insertional positive waves).

(+2) Occasional spontaneous potentials at rest in more than two different sites.

(+3) Resting activities present at rest, regardless of the position of the needle electrode.

(+4) Abundant spontaneous potentials nearly filling the screen of the oscilloscope.

## Fibrillation potentials

This term refers to spontaneous discharges that are 1 to 5 ms in duration and 20 to 200 μV in amplitude when recorded with a concentric needle electrode.[14, 59] They are initially positive, unless recorded from the end-plate, and diphasic or triphasic in waveform (Fig. 13-7). When the needle electrode is within the end-plate zone, fibrillation potentials are diphasic with initial negativity and may be difficult to differentiate from physiologic end-plate spikes, which are also initially negative. Thus, spontaneous activity must be recorded away from the end-plate region to be considered clinically significant. Fibrillation potentials typically fire in a regular pattern at a rate of 1 to 30 impulses per second with an average frequency of 13 impulses per second.[14] An irregular firing pattern has also been seen infrequently. Over the loudspeaker, the fibrillation potential produces a crisp, clicking noise reminiscent of the sound caused by wrinkling tissue paper. Fibrillation potentials tend to be facilitated by warming the muscle or by the administration of cholinesterase inhibitors, such as edrophonium (Tensilon) or neostigmine (Prostigmin). In contrast, moderate cooling of the muscle or hypoxia tends to suppress fibrillation potentials. It is sometimes necessary to warm the muscle under study for an adequate assessment of the spontaneous activity.

Fibrillation potentials and voluntarily activated single fiber potentials have the same shape and amplitude distribution when studied with single fiber electromyography (SFEMG).[66] When the potentials appear in a train there is no change in shape between the first and the last potentials. These findings indicate that fibrillation potentials originate from single muscle fibers, a view consistent with the observation that they are the smallest potentials recorded by the needle electrode.[20, 38] The earlier belief[14, 17] that they may be generated by a subunit consisting of 10 to 30 muscle fibers is no longer held, since the concept of the subunit itself has been abandoned.[15]

This potential, although usually regarded as pathognomonic of denervation, may occasionally be found in otherwise healthy muscles. The isolated appearance of fibrillation potentials, therefore, cannot be considered as absolute evidence of abnormality, unless they are detected in at least two different areas of the muscle. The presence of fibrillation potentials is highly suggestive of lower motor neuron disorders, which in-

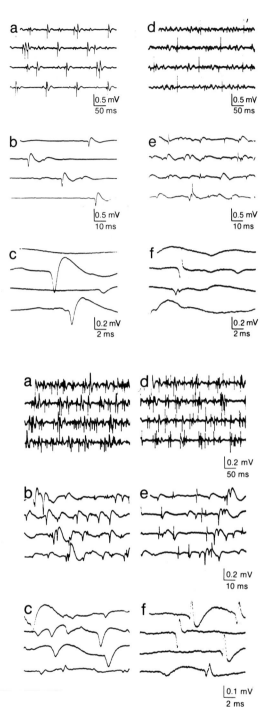

Figure 13-7

(*Top*) Spontaneous activity of the anterior tibialis in a 68-year-old woman with amyotrophic lateral sclerosis. Two types of discharges shown are positive sharp waves (a, b, c) and fibrillation potentials (d, e, f). (*Bottom*) Spontaneous activity of the paraspinal muscle in a 40-year-old man with radiculopathy. Two types of discharges shown are positive sharp waves (a, b, c) and fibrillation potentials (d, e, f).

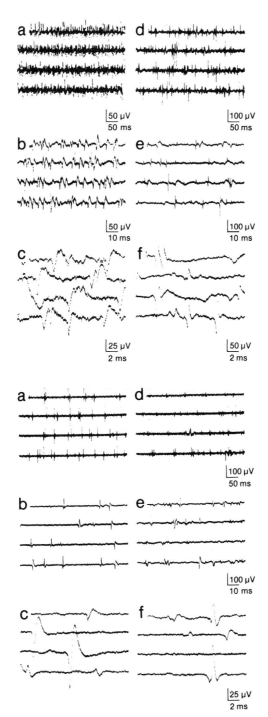

Figure 13-7 (*Continued*)

(*Top*) Spontaneous activity of the deltoid (a, b, c) and tibialis anterior (d, e, f) in a 9-year-old boy with a 6-week history of dermatomyositis. Two types of discharges shown are positive sharp waves (a, b, c) and fibrillation potentials (d, e, f). (*Bottom*) Spontaneous activity of the tibialis anterior in a 7-year-old boy with Duchenne dystrophy. Two types of discharges shown are positive sharp waves (a, b, c) and fibrillation potentials (d, e, f).

clude diseases of the anterior horn cells, radiculopathies, plexopathies, and mono- and polyneuropathies with axonal degeneration. However, spontaneous discharges by no means preclude a myopathic process or a disease of neuromuscular junction. They are commonly seen in muscular dystrophy, dermatomyositis, and polymyositis, and less frequently in myasthenia gravis and botulism.[28, 54] The spontaneous discharges are also found, although not consistently, in facioscapulohumeral dystrophy, limb girdle dystrophy, oculopharyngeal dystrophy,[31] myotubular (centronuclear) myopathy,[65] and trichinosis.[75, 76]

Buchthal and Rosenfalck[14] found fibrillation potentials in 20 of 76 patients with progressive muscular dystrophy. Fibrillation potentials observed in this disease are at least in part produced by denervation of muscle fibers secondary to muscle necrosis.[21] Spontaneous activity in polymyositis has been ascribed to increased membrane irritability,[4] inflammation of intramuscular nerve fibers,[58] or focal degeneration separating a part of the muscle fiber from the end-plate region.[63] In any case, muscle fibers are likely to be functionally denervated in this condition, since SFEMG and histochemical techniques have revealed changes in the terminal innervation pattern indicative of reinnervation.[32]

## Positive sharp waves

These discharges consist of an initial positive spike followed by a slow negative potential much lower in amplitude but longer in duration than the positive deflection, forming the characteristic waveform resembling a saw-tooth. They are often associated with insertion of the needle but also occur spontaneously, firing rhythmically at regular intervals (Fig. 13-7). The origin of positive sharp waves has not been clearly established, but the absence of a negative spike may be attributable to electrode positioning near a damaged part of the muscle fiber. It has been postulated that positive sharp waves represent single fiber discharges recorded from an injured area of the fiber. If so, they have the same significance as fibrillation potentials, which they frequently accompany. However, for some undetermined reasons, positive sharp waves tend to appear before the fibrillation potentials following nerve section.[79]

Like fibrillation potentials, positive sharp waves occur rarely, if at all, in a healthy muscle. They are regularly encountered in denervated muscles but also occur in a variety of myositic conditions, including polymyositis, dermatomyositis, trichinosis, ischemic myositis, and dystrophic muscles, particularly in muscular dystrophy. As discussed earlier, positive sharp waves may be present only as part of insertional activity in the early stage of denervation, although distinction between spontaneous and insertional activity is somewhat arbitrary. As mentioned previously the positive potentials that form the major component of myotonic discharges are nearly identical in waveform to positive sharp waves associated with denervation. However, myotonic discharges are always triggered by insertion of the needle or by mild voluntary contraction, and characteristically wax and wane.

## Fasciculation potentials

Visible twitching of muscle bundles was once referred to as fibrillation, a term now reserved for the electromyographic description of spontaneously firing single muscle fibers. To avoid confusion, Denny-Brown and Pennybacker[20] proposed the term fasciculation to represent spontaneous contraction of motor units. Fasciculation potentials are now defined as spontaneous discharges of a group of muscle fibers representing either a whole or possibly part of a motor unit (Fig. 13-8). When fasciculations occur in the depth of the muscle, they are not necessarily accompanied by visible twitches. In these instances, electromyography allows detection of fasciculation that would otherwise remain unrecognized. The generator source for fasciculations has not yet been

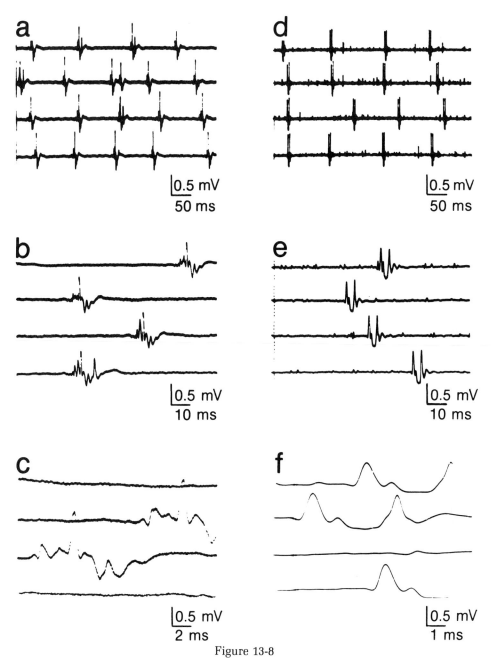

Figure 13-8

Fasciculation potentials in two patients with polyneuropathy. Recordings were obtained from the tibialis anterior in both, one showing a very polyphasic potential of long duration (a, b, c) and the other a double-peaked complex discharge suggesting a doublet (d, e, f). Fasciculation potentials are not always abnormal in waveform as shown here and are usually indistinguishable in shape from voluntarily activated motor unit potentials.

completely elucidated, but the existing evidence suggests that the neural discharge may originate in the spinal cord or anywhere along the length of the peripheral nerve.[78] Fasciculation potentials may sometimes persist after distal nerve block. If the nerve supply to a fasciculating muscle is totally removed, however, fasciculations remain for about four days, and then disappear.[27]

Fasciculation potentials commonly represent isolated discharges of one motor unit and are referred to as single fasciculation potentials. There are occasionally more complex bursts consisting of grouped or repetitive discharges.[64] The latter must be distinguished from voluntary motor unit discharges which may have the same grouped pattern. In differentiating volitional motor units from fasciculations, it is helpful to determine whether the discharges are under voluntary control. Various maneuvers, including voluntary contraction of antagonistic muscles, may be of value. Attempts to volitionally increase or decrease the firing rate should not influence the discharge pattern of fasciculation. Vermicular movement of skin, called myokymia, may be associated with grouped fasciculation potentials but can also be caused by a large number of single fasciculation potentials. This pattern will be discussed further in Chapter 26, but they usually occur in bursts at regular intervals of 0.1 to 10 seconds, with 2 to 10 spikes firing at 30 to 40 impulses per second in each burst (Fig. 13-9).

Fasciculation potentials are commonly but not exclusively found in diseases of anterior horn cells. They also occur in irritative lesions of the root and peripheral nerves, such as radiculopathy and entrapment neuropathy, in which they may be limited to the myotomes of the affected root or nerve. Additionally, they have been observed in the muscular pain-fasciculation syndrome[35] and in occasional patients with polyradicular neuropathies such as Charcot-Marie-Tooth disease and the Guillian-Barré syndrome. In a number of patients with cervical spondylotic myelopathy, fasciculations have been noted in the lower extremities.[40, 41] Since these spontaneous activities often disappear following surgical decompression for cervical spondylosis, it is postulated that loss of inhibition caused by myelopathy results in fasciculations in the leg. Other possible mechanisms include vascular insufficiency, cord traction, and denervation, but there is no anatomic or physiologic evidence to support these hypotheses. Fasciculation potentials are also seen in metabolic derangements such as tetany, thyrotoxicosis, and overdose of anticholinesterase medication.[19] Grouped fasciculation potentials sometimes have an ominous significance because of their frequent association with either amyotrophic lateral sclerosis or progressive spinal muscular atrophy. They also occur in other degenerative diseases of the anterior horn cells, including poliomyelitis and syringomyelia.

Either single or grouped spontaneous discharges may occur in otherwise normal muscle and are sometimes, but not always, associated with cramps.[57] Data obtained from a questionnaire survey of a group of 539 healthy medical personnel indicate that 70 percent have experienced some type of muscle twitches.[56] Because of the serious implications, it is important to differentiate this form of fasciculation from those asso-

---

Figure 13-9

(*Top*) Myokymic discharges in a 21-year-old woman with multiple sclerosis. The patient had visible undulating movement of the facial muscles on the right. Characteristic bursts of spontaneous activity were recorded from the orbicularis oris (a, b, c, d) as well as orbicularis oculi (e, f, g, h). In d, each sweep was triggered by a recurring spontaneous potential to show a repetitive pattern of the waveform. (*Bottom*) Myokymic discharges in a 57-year-old man with a 2-week history of the Guillian Barré syndrome and a nearly complete peripheral facial palsy. Despite the absence of visible undulating movement, rhythmically recurring spontaneous discharges appeared in the upper (a, b, c), and lower (d, e, f) portions of the left orbicularis oris. In c and f, each sweep was triggered by a recurring spontaneous potential to show the repetitive pattern.

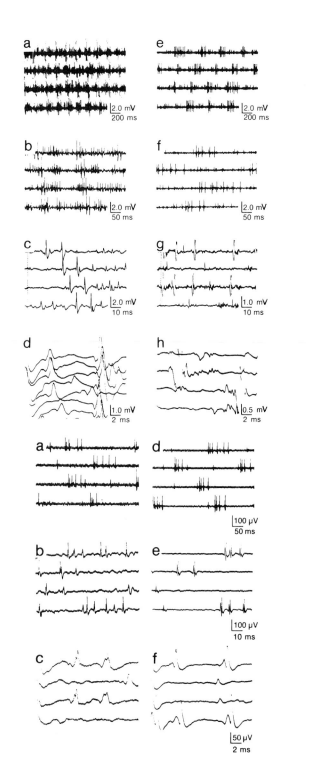

ciated with motor neuron disease, but thus far no reliable single method is available to distinguish one from the other on the basis of their action potentials. Although attempts have been made to characterize waveforms of these two forms of fasciculations,[57] there is nothing distinctive in the appearance of either potential.[71] The frequency of discharge, however, may possibly separate the two types, since fasciculations in motor neuron disease occur with an average interval of 3.5 seconds, compared with 0.8 second for the other type.[71]

In conclusion, fasciculations by themselves cannot be regarded as pathologic unless either fibrillation potentials or positive sharp waves are simultaneously demonstrated. Excluding those seen in healthy subjects, the presence of fasciculation tends to suggest disease of the lower motor neuron. Since it can originate at any level from the anterior horn cells to axon terminals, its significance must be determined in the context of other electrophysiologic and clinical findings. Fasciculations seen in otherwise normal muscle are referred to by some as benign, as opposed to malignant, when associated with motor neuron disease;[57] but the dichotomy is not generally accepted, because there is no reliable method for distinguishing the two. Instead, fasciculation potentials should be characterized by their waveform, amplitude, duration, and frequency of occurrence.

## Complex repetitive discharges

These potentials are sometimes called bizarre high frequency discharges, although the use of the term is now discouraged. They are also referred to, even less appropriately, as pseudomyotonia, because of their superficial resemblance to myotonic discharges, although they characteristically lack the waxing and waning quality. These potentials are 50 µV to 1 mV in amplitude and up to 50 to 100 ms in duration, representing a group of muscle fibers firing in near synchrony (Figs. 13-10 and 13-11). They discharge repetitively at slow or fast rates, usually ranging from 5 to 100 impulses per second. The waveform, which is typically polyphasic and complex, remains uniform from one discharge to another, although a sudden change in shape may also occur. These discharges typically begin abruptly and maintain a constant rate of firing for a short period. Their cessation is as abrupt as their onset. Over the loudspeaker, they resemble the sound of a machine gun.

When recorded using a single fiber electrode,[67] complex repetitive discharges contain up to 10 or more distinct single fiber action potentials separated by intervals ranging from less than 0.5 ms to as much as 100 to 200 ms. The individual spikes within the complex fire in the same order, as the discharge recurs repetitively. The burst is initiated by one fiber in the complex serving as a pacemaker for one or several other fibers that are driven ephaptically.[67] In successive cycles the principal pacemaker is re-excited by one of the remaining fibers that was activated late in the previous cycle, and the whole cycle is repeated, until the pacemaker fibers become subnormally excitable and block. Spikes in complex repetitive discharges are often high amplitude compared with fibrillation potentials. Thus, their stronger electrical field may be more effective in ephaptically activating neighboring muscle fibers.

This discharge is seen in a wide variety of myopathic and lower motor neuron disorders. These include muscular dystrophy, polymyositis, and chronic denervation such as motor neuron disease, long-standing radiculopathy, or chronic polyneuropathy. It is also seen in myxedema and Schwarz-Jampel syndrome. In a large series studied by Emeryk, Hausmanowa-Petrusewicz, and Nowak,[22] the discharge occurred most commonly in Duchenne dystrophy, spinal muscular atrophy, and Charcot-Marie-Tooth disease. The same complex repetitive discharges are occasionally seen in apparently healthy subjects, especially in the iliopsoas muscles, in which they probably represent a clinically silent irritative process. Complex repetitive discharges must be distinguished from similar discharges seen in myokymia, neuromyotonia, and cramp syn-

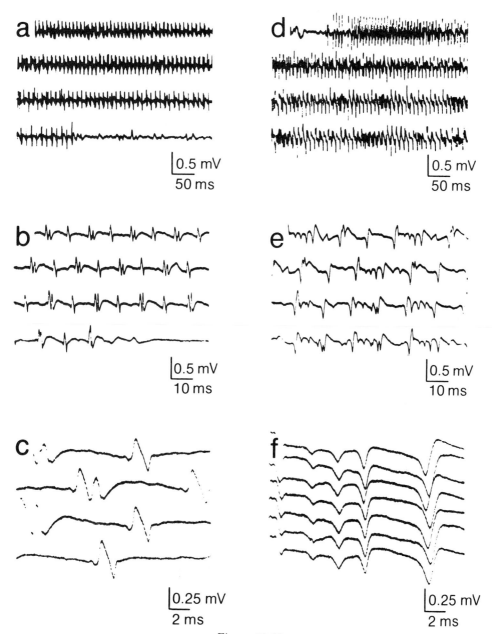

Figure 13-10

Complex repetitive discharges of the left quadriceps in a 58-year-old man with herniated lumbar disc. Two types of discharges shown are trains of single- or double-peaked negative spikes (a, b, c) and complex positive sharp waves (d, e, f). In f, each sweep was triggered by a recurring motor unit potential to show remarkable reproducibility of the waveform within a given train.

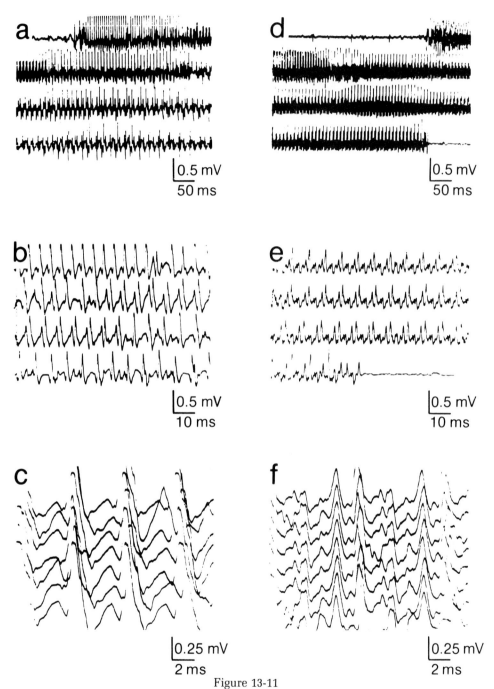

Figure 13-11

Complex repetitive discharges with trains of negative spikes from the same muscle shown in Figure 13-10. Note gradual decline of discharge frequency in one train (a, b, c) but not in the other (d, e, f). Abrupt onset and cessation are characteristic (a, d, e). In c and f, each sweep was triggered by a recurring motor unit potential to show detailed patterns of the waveform.

dromes, by their characteristic waveform and firing pattern as will be described in Chapter 26.

# MOTOR UNIT POTENTIALS

A motor unit potential is defined by its amplitude, rise time, duration, phases, stability, and territory. In a wide range of neuromuscular disorders, these parameters may be affected in various combinations. Abnormalities of motor unit potentials per se do not establish a specific diagnosis. However, the general distinction between myopathic and lower motor neuron disorders is usually possible. In myopathies, motor unit potentials are smaller in size as a result of random loss of muscle fibers. In neuropathy or anterior horn cell disease, motor unit potentials are normal or larger than normal in size, but reduced in number, reflecting functional or structural loss of axons. Thus, taken together with abnormalities of insertional and spontaneous activities, changes in the size and recruitment pattern of the motor unit potential play an essential role in the classification of weakness in diseases of the nerve and muscle.[29]

## Abnormalities of motor unit potentials

In the following discussion, abnormalities of each parameter of the motor unit potential will be described and emphasis given to contrasting alterations commonly seen in myopathic versus lower motor neuron disorders. For each type of abnormality, a number of associated disease categories will be mentioned. However, the clinical and electromyographic features of each disease entity will be dealt with in greater detail in Chapters 20 through 26.

The amplitude of the motor unit potential varies greatly with the position of the needle electrode relative to the discharging unit. Even if the rise time of the motor unit potential is less than 500 $\mu$s, indicating that the recording surface is close enough to the unit under study, there is no way of determining the exact number of single muscle fibers contributing to the spike amplitude. In general, the amplitude of a motor unit potential does not aid in determining the size of the motor unit territory, although it may be taken as an indicator of muscle fiber density within the motor unit: the higher the amplitude is, the closer together are the muscle fibers near the recording surface. The duration of the motor unit potential is a better index of the motor unit territory. Distant units, while not contributing to the amplitude of the negative spike, significantly add to the motor unit duration, increasing the time of the initial and terminal positivity. For meaningful assessment, the duration of motor unit potentials must be compared with the normal range for the same muscle in the same age group.[9]

A majority of motor unit potentials are diphasic or triphasic in normal muscles, although 5 to 15 percent may be polyphasic, having four or more phases. An increased number of polyphasic units is nonspecific and can be seen either in myopathy, neuropathy, or motor neuron disease (Fig. 13-12). Polyphasia simply indicates increased temporal dispersion of muscle fiber potentials within a motor unit. Excessive temporal dispersion, in turn, may be the result of difference in conduction time along the terminal branch of the nerve or over the muscle fiber membrane. In partially paretic muscles during neurapraxia or an acute stage of axonotomesis, motor unit potentials, if recorded at all, are normal in waveform, since the motor units innervated by the surviving axons remain unchanged (Fig. 13-13).

Motor units normally discharge semirhythmically, and successive motor unit potentials are nearly identical in configuration. During muscle fatigue, the discharge rate of the motor unit decreases and the rhythm may become irregular, but the shape of the motor unit potential remains the same. In the presence of defective neuromuscular transmission, the amplitude of a motor unit potential, firing repetitively during sustained muscle contraction, may fluctuate or progressively diminish. This is expected if

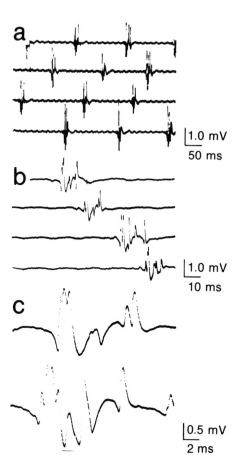

Figure 13-12
Polyphasic motor unit potentials from the anterior tibialis in a 52-year-old man with amyotrophic lateral sclerosis. The repetitively discharging single motor unit showed temporal variability in waveform, suggesting intermittent blocking of some axon terminals.

some of the muscle fibers of the unit drop out intermittently as the store of immediately available acetylcholine (ACh) is depleted during repetitive discharges (see Fig. 13-12). The fatigue of the motor unit potential is seen not only in myasthenia gravis, myasthenic syndrome, and botulism, but also occasionally in motor neuron disease, poliomyelitis, syringomyelia, and during the early stages of reinnervation. As mentioned in Chapter 10, waveform variability of a repetitively firing motor unit potential can be used as a test of neuromuscular transmission, especially in those muscles not accessible by conventional nerve stimulation techniques. In myotonia congenita, a characteristic decline in amplitude of the motor unit potentials typically recovers during continued contraction.

Another abnormal discharge pattern is the doublet or triplet (see Fig. 13-8). In this condition, the motor unit discharges regularly during voluntary contraction, but each potential consists of two to three isolated spikes, representing repetitive firing of the motor unit at very short intervals. This should be distinguished from polyphasic motor units which are not repetitive discharges. In doublet or double discharges, two action potentials occur consistently in the same relationship to one another at intervals of 2 to 20 ms. If they occur at a longer interval, ranging from 20 to 80 ms, they are referred to as paired discharges. In triplets, the interval between the first two is usually shorter than that between the last two but both are in the range of 2 to 20 ms. These multiple discharges are often seen in latent tetani, in other metabolic disease, or during hyperventilation, and probably represent hyperexcitability of the motor neuron pool.[61] Other disorders commonly associated with this type of discharge include poliomyelitis,[72] motor neuron disease,[68] the Guillain-Barré syndrome,[60] other neuropathies, radiculopathy,

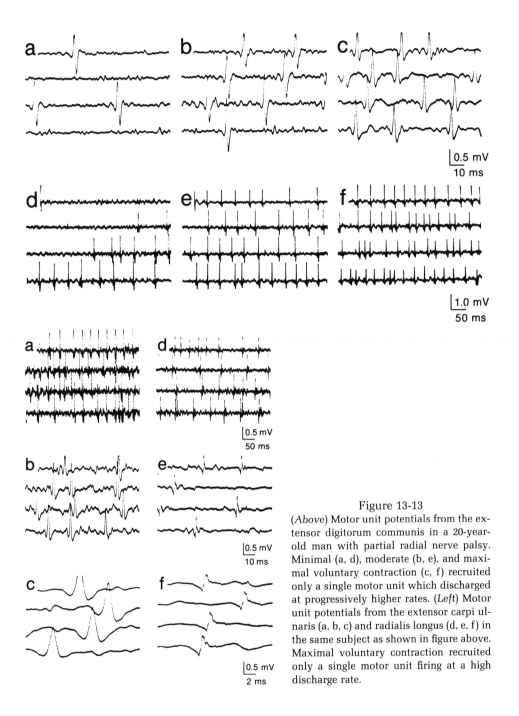

Figure 13-13

(*Above*) Motor unit potentials from the extensor digitorum communis in a 20-year-old man with partial radial nerve palsy. Minimal (a, d), moderate (b, e), and maximal voluntary contraction (c, f) recruited only a single motor unit which discharged at progressively higher rates. (*Left*) Motor unit potentials from the extensor carpi ulnaris (a, b, c) and radialis longus (d, e, f) in the same subject as shown in figure above. Maximal voluntary contraction recruited only a single motor unit firing at a high discharge rate.

and myotonic dystrophy.[51] Doublets may also occur physiologically at the beginning and termination of muscular contraction but are otherwise not seen in normal muscles.[53] The exact origin and clinical significance of multiple discharges remain to be elucidated. No correlation has been found between spontaneous fasciculations and the double discharges of voluntarily activated motor unit potentials.[52]

## Lower motor neuron versus myopathic disorders

The motor unit potential is frequently increased in amplitude as well as in duration (Fig. 13-14) with diseases of the lower motor neuron, such as motor neuron disease, poliomyelitis, and syringomyelia, and in diseases of the peripheral nerve, such as chronic neuropathy and reinnervation after nerve injury. In these disorders, the functional motor unit territory is increased, indicating either abnormal synchronization of two or more motor units at the cord level or anatomic reorganization of denervated muscle fibers into a more cohesive motor unit by means of axon sprouting. Large functional units are associated with increased duration of the motor unit potential, reflecting greater variability in length and conduction time along the axon terminals within the unit. The amplitude of the motor unit potential is also increased, not because of the enlarged territory, but as a result of increased fiber density.

Borenstein and Desmedt[5] have studied motor unit potentials during reinnervation after traumatic nerve lesions. Their findings may be summarized as follows. After complete nerve transection, motor unit potentials become increasingly more polyphasic as additional muscle fibers are incorporated. Temporal instability of a motor unit potential results from marked latency variability of regenerating motor axons and intermittent segmental conduction block. After a partial nerve lesion, there is extensive collateral reinnervation of the dennervated muscle fibers by healthy motor axons. Late components linked to the main unit will then be added to the original motor unit potentials. These long latency components may be overlooked in free running modes but can readily be appreciated if the sweep is triggered by a recurring motor unit potential itself and the potential is displayed in its entirety with the use of a delay line.

In general, reduction in amplitude and duration of the motor unit potential (Fig. 13-15) occurs in primary myopathic disorders, such as muscular dystrophy, congenital or other myopathies, periodic paralysis, myositis, and disorders of neuromuscular transmission, including myasthenia gravis, myasthenic syndrome, and botulism. All these entities have in common the random loss of functional muscle fibers from each motor unit. This may be caused by muscle degeneration, inflammation, metabolic changes, or failure of neuromuscular activation. In extreme cases, only a single muscle fiber of a motor unit can be activated voluntarily, and the motor unit potential becomes indistinguishable from a fibrillation potential. The short 1 to 2 ms duration spikes produce a high frequency sound over the loudspeaker, reminiscent of spontaneously discharging fibrillation potentials. Unlike the electrophysiologic changes in some inherited myopathies, those in metabolic or toxic myopathies are often reversible.[10] Mild metabolic and endocrine myopathies characteristically show little or no alteration in duration or amplitude of the motor unit potential.

Contrasting changes in amplitude and duration of the motor unit potential generally differentiate myopathic from lower motor neuron disorders.[11, 12, 13, 30] The overall concordance of electromyography and histochemical findings from muscle biopsies has been reported to be around 90 percent or greater.[3, 11, 12, 29] However, unequivocal distinction cannot always be made.[23] Sick axon terminals in distal neuropathy, for example, may result in random loss of muscle fibers within a motor unit. Similarly, during early reinnervation, immature motor units consist of only a few muscle fibers. Motor unit potentials may then be polyphasic and of low amplitude and short duration. In both instances a neuropathic process will produce changes in the motor unit potential that are classically associated with myopathy.

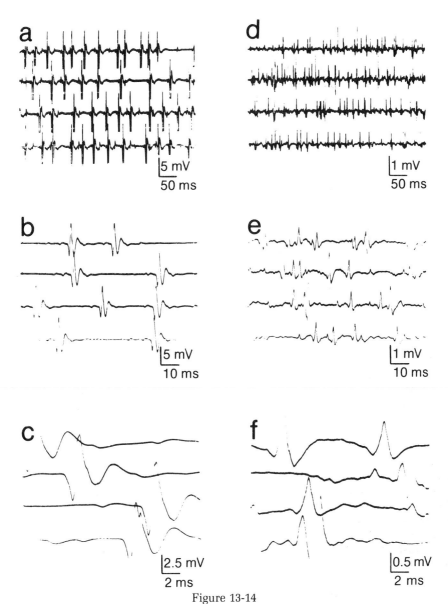

Figure 13-14

Large amplitude, long duration motor unit potentials from the first dorsal interosseus (a, b, c) compared with relatively normal motor unit potentials from orbicularis oculi (d, e, f) in a patient with polyneuropathy. Note discrete single unit interference pattern during maximal voluntary contraction.

Conversely, in some myopathic disorders, motor unit potentials may have a very long duration and may be confused with neuropathic change.[21, 44, 55] Long latency potentials are particularly common in myopathies with regenerating muscle fibers. These potentials commonly appear quite distinct from the main unit, thus giving rise to the terms satellite and parasite potentials, now discarded in favor of the more descriptive name, late component. If fiber density is increased by regeneration, then amplitude may also be much greater than ordinarily expected in myopathy.

Thus, when interpreting abnormalities of motor unit potentials and correlating them with clinical diagnoses, the oversimplified dichotomy between myopathy and

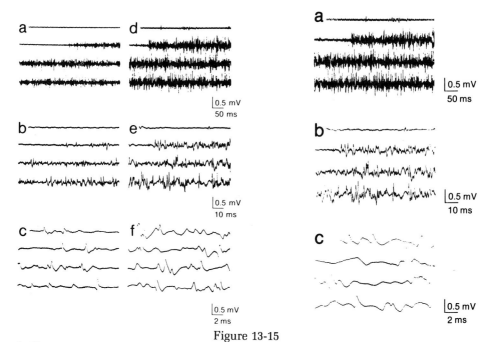

Figure 13-15

(*Left*) Low amplitude, short duration motor unit potentials from the biceps (a, b, c) and tibialis anterior (d, e, f) in a 7-year-old boy with Duchenne dystrophy. (Compare Figure 13-7 bottom right.) Minimal voluntary contraction recruited an excessive number of motor units in both muscles. (*Right*) Low amplitude, short duration motor unit potentials from the biceps in a 50-year-old woman with polymyositis. A high number of discharging motor units during minimal muscle contraction indicates very early recruitment.

lower motor neuron disorder is not always appropriate.[24, 25, 73, 74] Findings are not necessarily the same among the different muscles in a patient or even from one part to another in the same muscle. Thus, one must examine many muscles, sampling each muscle in several areas. In a given disease state, muscles with minimal dysfunction may show no abnormality, whereas very severely diseased muscles may reveal only nonspecific end-stage change. Optimal muscles to examine are those moderately affected but not totally destroyed by the disease process. Despite some uncertainties, the electromyographic division between myopathies and lower motor neuron disorders is usually possible in most patients with definite weakness.

# RECRUITMENT PATTERN

## Lower and upper motor neuron disorders

The recruitment pattern of the motor unit potential is primarily determined by the number of functional motor neurons and the average size of the motor unit. If the excitable motor neurons are reduced in number, as is usually the case with motor neuron disease and disorders of the root and peripheral nerve, a limited number of motor units discharge and the recruitment is said to be reduced or limited. To maintain a certain force, these excitable motor neurons must fire at an inappropriately rapid rate to compensate. In extreme instances, a single motor unit produces the discrete or so-called picket fence interference pattern at maximal effort (Fig. 13-16).

When decreased recruitment results from failure of descending impulses, motor units discharge more slowly than expected for normal maximal contraction (Fig. 13-17). Thus, a lower motor neuron lesion with a rapid rate of discharge can be distinguished

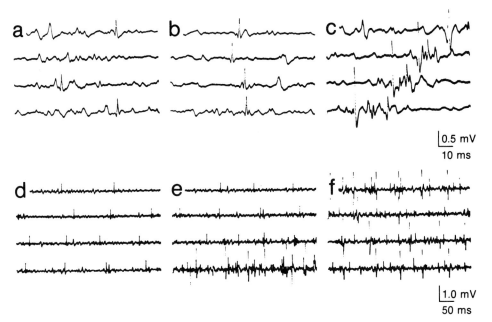

Figure 13-16
Reduced recruitment and incomplete interference pattern of the mildly paretic extensor carpi radialis in a 20-year-old man with partial radial nerve palsy. The rate of firing rather than the number of discharging motor units increased during minimal (a, d), moderate (b, e), and maximal voluntary contraction (c, f). (Compare Figure 13-13.)

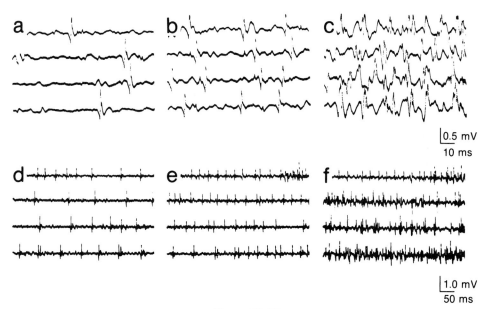

Figure 13-17
Reduced recruitment and incomplete interference pattern of the tibialis anterior in a 31-year-old woman with hysterical weakness. Minimal (a, d), moderate (b, e), and maximal (c, f) effort to contract the muscle altered neither the rate of firing nor the number of discharging motor units appreciably.

from an upper motor neuron lesion or hysterical paralysis with a slow rate of discharge, even though the interference pattern may be reduced in either case. In addition, hysterical weakness or poor cooperation is associated with irregular firing of motor units, not seen in patients with a genuine paresis.

## Myopathy

When motor unit potentials are low in amplitude and short in duration early recruitment is expected. This may be regarded as functional compensation, since the smaller the motor unit is, the greater is the number of units required to maintain a given force. With slight voluntary effort, many units begin to fire almost instantaneously (Fig. 13-

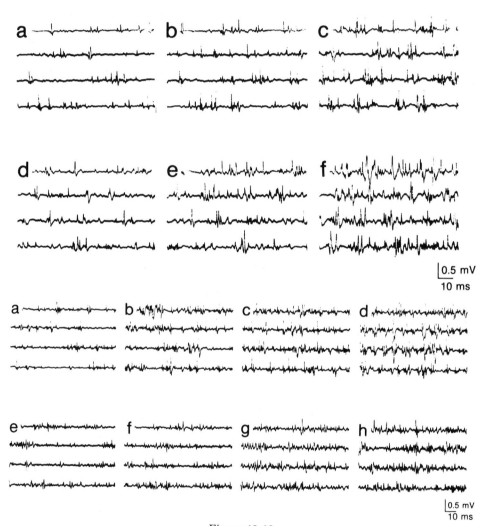

0.5 mV
10 ms

0.5 mV
10 ms

Figure 13-18

(*Top*) Early recruitment of the deltoid (a, b, c) and tibialis anterior (d, e, f) in a 9-year-old boy with a 6-week history of dermatomyositis. (Compare Figure 13-7 top right.) Note abundant motor units discharging with minimal (a, d), mild (b, e), and moderate contraction (c, f). (*Bottom*) Early recruitment of the biceps (a, b, c, d) and tibialis anterior (e, f, g, h) in a 7-year-old boy with Duchenne dystrophy. (Compare Figure 13-7 bottom right.) An excessive number of motor unit potentials appeared during minimal (a, e), mild (b, f), moderate (c, g), and maximal contraction (d, h).

18). With increasing force, a full interference pattern develops at less than maximal contraction, although its amplitude may be substantially reduced, reflecting the decreased fiber density of individual motor units. However, the interference pattern may be incomplete in advanced myogenic disorders in which there is loss of whole motor units rather than individual muscle fibers. Whereas early recruitment is considered characteristic of a myopathic process, it also occurs in diseases of neuromuscular transmission.

## Involuntary movement

Movement disorders with involuntary motor symptoms may be associated with electromyographic findings resembling changes seen in lower motor neuron disease. Tremor is characterized by bursts of motor unit potentials firing at a fairly constant rate. Although many motor units fire in a group during each burst, there is no fixed temporal or spatial relationship among them. Thus, successive bursts are variable in amplitude, duration, waveform, and number of motor unit potentials. When tremor is not clinically obvious, a tremor burst could be mistaken for a polyphasic long duration motor unit potential, unless the varying appearance and rhythmic pattern are recognized. Different types of tremor can be characterized by electromyographic recordings of their rate, rhythm, and distribution.[62]

In most other involuntary movement disorders, individual motor unit potentials are normal, but their recruitment is not under voluntary control. These include stiffman syndrome, common cramps, tetanus, tetani, and hemifacial spasm. Synkinesis seen in hemifacial spasm or following aberrant regeneration is associated with unintended activation of motor units in the muscle not being voluntarily contracted (see Fig. 14-1). Simultaneous recording from multiple muscles confirms the presence of synkinesis by demonstrating time-locked discharge of aberrant motor unit potentials. This is particularly important in differentiating spontaneous activity from synkinetic discharges. These entities will be described in Chapter 26.

# REFERENCE SOURCES

1.   AXELSSON, J AND THESLEFF, S: *A study of supersensitivity of denervated mammalian skeletal muscle.* J Physiol (Lond) 149:178, 1957.

2.   BELMAR, J AND EYZAGUIRRE, C: *Pacemaker site of fibrillation potentials in denervated mammalian muscle.* J Neurophysiol 29:425, 1966.

3.   BLACK, JT, ET AL: *Diagnostic accuracy of clinical data, quantitative electromyography and histochemistry in neuromuscular disease. A study of 105 cases.* J Neurol Sci 21:59, 1974.

4.   BOHAN, A AND PETER, JB: *Polymyositis and dermatomyositis.* N Engl J Med 292:344, 1975.

5.   BORENSTEIN, S AND DESMEDT, JE: *Range of variations in motor unit potentials during reinnervation after traumatic nerve lesions in humans.* Ann Neurol 8:460, 1980.

6.   BROWN, GL: *The actions of acetylcholine on denervated mammalian and frog's muscle.* J Physiol (Lond) 89:438, 1937.

7.   BRUMBACK, RA, ET AL: *The effect of pharmacologic acetylcholine receptor on fibrillation and myotonia in rat skeletal muscle.* Arch Neurol 35:8, 1978.

8.   BRYANT, SH: *The electrophysiology of myotonia, with a review of congenital myotonia of goats.* In DESMEDT, JE (ED): *New Developments in Electromyography and Clinical Neurophysiology,* Vol 1. Karger, Basel, 1973 pp 420–450.

9.   BUCHTHAL, F: *An Introduction to Electromyography.* Scandinavian University Books, Copenhagen, 1957.

10.   BUCHTHAL, F: *Electrophysiologic abnormalities in metabolic myopathies and neuropathies.* Acta Neurol Scand (suppl 43)46:129, 1970.

11.   BUCHTHAL, F: *Diagnostic significance of the myopathic EMG.* In ROWLAND, LP (ED): *Pathogenesis of Human Muscular Dystrophies.* Proceedings of the Fifth International Scientific

Conference of the Muscular Dystrophy Association, Durango, Colorado, June, 1976, Excerpta Medica, Amsterdam, 1977.

12. BUCHTHAL, F: *Electrophysiological signs of myopathy as related with muscle biopsy.* Acta Neurol (Napoli) 32:1, 1977.

13. BUCHTHAL, F AND ROSENFALCK, P: *Electrophysiological aspects of myopathy with particular reference to progressive muscular dystrophy.* In BOURNE, GH AND GOLARZ, MN (EDS): *Muscular Dystrophy in Man and Animals.* Hafner Publishing Company, New York, 1963.

14. BUCHTHAL, F AND ROSENFALCK, P: *Spontaneous electrical activity of human muscle.* Electroenceph Clin Neurophysiol 20:321, 1966.

15. BUCHTHAL, F AND ROSENFALCK, P: *On the structure of motor units.* In DESMEDT JE (ED): *New Developments in Electromyography and Clinical Neurophysiology,* Vol 1. Karger, Basel, 1973 pp 71–85.

16. BUCHTHAL, F, ENGBAEK, L, AND GAMSTORP, I: *Paresis and hyperexcitability in adynamia episodica hereditaria.* Neurology (Minneap) 8:347, 1958.

17. BUCHTHAL, F, GULD, C, AND ROSENFALCK, P: *Multielectrode study of the territory of a motor unit.* Acta Physiol Scand 39:83, 1957.

18. CHOKROVERTY, S AND MEDINA, J: *Electrophysiological study of hemiplegia.* Arch Neurol 35:360, 1978.

19. DAUBE, JR: *Needle Examination in Electromyography.* American Association of Electromyography and Electrodiagnosis, Minimonograph #11, Rochester, Minnesota, 1979.

20. DENNY-BROWN, D AND PENNYBACKER, JB: *Fibrillation and fasciculation in voluntary muscle.* Brain 61:311, 1938.

21. DESMEDT, JE AND BORENSTEIN, S: *Regeneration in Duchenne muscular dystrophy. Electromyographic evidence.* Arch Neurol 33:642, 1976.

22. EMERYK, B, HAUSMANOWA-PETRUSEWICZ, I, AND NOWAK, T: *Spontaneous volleys of bizarre high frequency potentials (b.h.f.p.) in neuro-muscular diseases. Part I. Occurrence of spontaneous volleys of b.h.f.p. in neuro-muscular diseases. Part II. An analysis of the morphology of spontaneous volleys of b.h.f.p. in neuromuscular diseases.* Electromyogr Clin Neurophysiol (Part I) 14:303, 1974. (Part II) 14:339, 1974.

23. ENGEL, WK: *Brief, small, abundant motor-unit action potentials. A further critique of electromyographic interpretation.* Neurology (Minneap) 25:173, 1975.

24. ENGEL, WK AND WARMOLTS, JR: *Multiplicity of muscle changes postulated from motoneuron abnormalities.* In CASSENS, RG (ED): *Muscle Biology.* Marcel Dekker, New York, 1972.

25. ENGEL, WK AND WARMOLTS, JR: *The motor unit. Diseases affecting it in toto or in portio.* In DESMEDT, JE (ED): *New Developments in Electromyography and Clinical Neurophysiology,* Vol 1. Karger, Basel, 1973 pp 141–177.

26. FALK, G AND LANDA, JF: *Effects of potassium on frog skeletal muscle in a chloride-deficient medium.* Am J Physiol 198:1225, 1960.

27. FORSTER, FM, BORKOWSKI, WJ, AND ALPERS, BJ: *Effects of denervation on fasciculations in human muscle. Relation of fibrillations to fasciculations.* Arch Neurol Psychiatry 56:276, 1946.

28. FUSFELD, RD: *Electromyographic abnormalities in a case of botulism.* Bulletin of the Los Angeles Neurological Societies 35:164, 1970.

29. HAUSMANOWA-PETRUSEWICZ, I, AND JEDRZEJOWSKA, H: *Correlation between electromyographic findings and muscle biopsy in cases of neuromuscular disease.* J Neurol Sci 13:85, 1971.

30. HAUSMANOWA-PETRUSEWICZ, I, ET AL: *Electromyography in neuro-muscular diagnostics.* Electromyography 7:203, 1967.

31. HEFFERNAN, LP, REWCASTLE, NB, AND HUMPHREY, JG: *The spectrum of rod myopathies.* Arch Neurol 18:529, 1968.

32. HENRIKSSON, KG AND STÅLBERG, E: *The terminal innervation pattern in polymyositis: A histochemical and SFEMG study.* Muscle and Nerve 1:3, 1978.

33. HNÍK, P AND ŠKORPIL, V: *Fibrillation activity in denervated muscle.* In GUTMANN, E (ED): *The Denervated Muscle.* Czech Acad Sci, Prague, 1962 pp 135–150.

34. HUDGSON, P, ET AL: *Adult myopathy from glycogen storage disease due to acid maltase deficiency.* Brain 91:435, 1968.

35. HUDSON, AJ, BROWN, WF, AND GILBERT, JJ: *The muscular pain-fasciculation syndrome.* Neurology (New York) 28:1105, 1978.

36. HUTTER, OF AND NOBLE, D: *The chloride conductance of frog skeletal muscle.* J Physiol (Lond) 151:89, 1960.

37. JABLECKI, C AND KNOLL, D: *Fibrillation potentials and complex repetitive discharges* (abst). Electroenceph Clin Neurophysiol 50:242P, 1980.

38. JASPER, H AND BALLEM, G: *Unipolar electromyograms of normal and denervated human muscle.* J Neurophysiol 12:231, 1949.

39. JOHNSON, EW, DENNY, ST, AND KELLEY, JP: *Sequence of electromyographic abnormalities in stroke syndrome.* Arch Phys Med Rehabil 56:468, 1975.

40. KASDON, DL: *Cervical spondylotic myelopathy with reversible fasciculations in the lower extremities.* Arch Neurol 34:774, 1977.

41. KING, RB AND STOOPS, WL: *Cervical myelopathy with fasciculations in the lower extremities.* J Neurosurg 20:948, 1963.

42. KUGELBERG, E AND PETERSÉN, I: *"Insertion activity" in electromyography. With notes on denervated muscle response to constant current.* J Neurol Neurosurg Psychiatry 12:268, 1949.

43. KUHN, E: *Myotonia. The clinical evidence.* In DESMEDT, JE (ED): *New Developments in Electromyography and Clinical Neurophysiology,* Vol 1. Karger, Basel, 1973.

44. LANG, AH AND PARTANEN, VSJ: *"Satellite potentials" and the duration of motor unit potentials in normal, neuropathic and myopathic muscles.* J Neurol Sci 27:513, 1976.

45. LI, CL, SHY, GM, AND WELLS, J: *Some properties of mammalian skeletal muscle fibres with particular reference to fibrillation potentials.* J Physiol (Lond) 135:522, 1957.

46. LIPICKY, RJ AND BRYANT, SH: *A biophysical study of the human myotonias.* In DESMEDT, JE (ED): *New Developments in Electromyography and Clinical Neurophysiology,* Vol 1. Karger, Basel, 1973 pp 451–463.

47. LÜLLMANN, H: *Das Verhalten normaler und denervierter Skelemuskulatur in chloridfreiem Medium (Methylsulfat-Tyrodelösung).* Naunyn-Schmiedeberg's Arch exp Path u Pharmak 240:351, 1961.

48. MAILLIS, AG AND JOHNSTONE, BM: *Observations on the development of muscle hypersensitivity following chronic nerve conduction blockage and recovery.* J Neurol Sci 38:145, 1978.

49. MILEDI, R: *The acetylcholine sensitivity of frog muscle fibres after complete or partial denervation.* J Physiol (Lond) 151:1, 1960.

50. MORRISON, JB: *The electromyographic changes in hyperkalaemic familial periodic paralysis.* Ann Phys Med 5:153, 1960.

51. PARTANEN, VSJ: *Double discharges in neuromuscular diseases.* J Neurol Sci 36:377, 1978.

52. PARTANEN, VSJ: *Lack of correlation between spontaneous fasciculations and double discharges of voluntarily activated motor units.* J Neurol Sci 42:261, 1979.

53. PARTANEN, VSJ AND LANG, AH: *An analysis of double discharges in the human electromyogram.* J Neurol Sci 36:363, 1978.

54. PETERSÉN, I AND BROMAN, AM: *Elektromyografiska fynd från ett fall av botulism.* Nordisk Med 65:259, 1961.

55. PICKETT, JB: *Late components of motor unit potentials in a patient with myoglobinuria.* Ann Neurol 3:461, 1978.

56. REED, DM AND KURLAND, LT: *Muscle fasciculations in a healthy population.* Arch Neurol 9:363, 1963.

57. RICHARDSON, AT: *Muscle fasciculation.* Arch Phys Med Rehabil 35:281, 1954.

58. RICHARDSON, AT: *Clinical and electromyographic aspects of polymyositis.* Proc R Soc Med 49:111, 1956.

59. ROSENFALCK, P AND BUCHTHAL, F: *Studies on fibrillation potentials of denervated human muscle.* Electroenceph Clin Neurophysiol (suppl 22):130, 1962.

60. ROTH, G: *Réflexe d'axone moteur.* Arch Suisses Neurol Neurochir Psychiatr 109:73, 1971.

**TYPES OF ABNORMALITY**

**287**

61. SCHERRER, J AND METRAL, S: *Electromyography.* In VINKEN, PJ AND BRUYN, GW (EDS): *Handbook of Clinical Neurology,* Vol 1. *Disturbances of Nervous Function.* North-Holland, Amsterdam, 1969.

62. SHAHANI, BT AND YOUNG, RR: *The blink, H, and tendon vibration reflexes.* In GOODGOLD, J AND EBERSTEIN, A (EDS): *Electrodiagnosis of Neuromuscular Diseases,* ed 2. Williams & Wilkins, Baltimore, 1977 pp 245–263.

63. SIMPSON, JA: *Handbook of Electromyography and Clinical Neurophysiology.* Vol 16. *Neuromuscular Diseases.* Elsevier, Amsterdam, 1973.

64. SINDERMANN, F, ET AL: *Unusual properties of repetitive fasciculations.* Electroenceph Clin Neurophysiol 35:173, 1973.

65. SPIRO, AJ, SHY, GM, AND GONATAS, NK: *Myotubular myopathy. Persistence of fetal muscle in an adolescent boy.* Arch Neurol 14:1, 1966.

66. STÅLBERG, E AND EKSTEDT, J: *Single fibre EMG and microphysiology of the motor unit in normal and diseased human muscle.* In DESMEDT, JE (ED): *New Developments in Electromyography and Clinical Neurophysiology,* Vol 1. Karger, Basel, 1973.

67. STÅLBERG, E AND TRONTELJ, JV: *Single Fiber Electromyography.* The Mirvalle Press Limited, Old Woking, Surrey U.K., 1979.

68. TARASCHI, G AND LANZI, G: *Décharges multiples d'une unité motrice, durant l'activité volontaire dans un cas de sclérose latérale amyotrophique.* Electroenceph Clin Neurophysiol (suppl 22):146, 1962.

69. THESLEFF, S: *Spontaneous electrical activity in denervated rat skeletal muscle.* In GUTMANN, E (ED): *Proceedings of the Symposium on Effect of Use and Disuse on Neuromuscular Functions.* Czech Acad Sci, Prague, 1963.

70. TROJABORG, W: *Early electrophysiologic changes in conduction block.* Muscle and Nerve, 1:400, 1978.

71. TROJABORG, W AND BUCHTHAL, F: *Malignant and benign fasciculations.* Acta Neurol Scand (suppl 13)41:251, 1965.

72. VALLE, M: *Décharges multiples dans la poliomyélite par mécanismes fonctionnels non-reconductibles à cryptotetanie.* Electroenceph Clin Neurophysiol (suppl 22):144, 1962.

73. WARMOLTS, JR AND ENGEL, WK: *Open-biopsy electromyography. I. Correlation of motor unit behavior with histochemical muscle fiber type in human limb muscle.* Arch Neurol 27:512, 1972.

74. WARMOLTS, JR AND MENDELL, JR: *Open-biopsy electromyography. Direct correlation of a pattern of excessively recruited, pathologically small motor unit potentials with histologic evidence of neuropathy.* Arch Neurol 36:406, 1979.

75. WAYLONIS, GW AND JOHNSON, EW: *The electromyogram in acute trichinosis: Report of four cases.* Arch Phys Med Rehabil 45:177, 1964.

76. WAYLONIS, GW AND JOHNSON, EW: *Electromyographic findings in induced trichinosis.* Arch Phys Med Rehabil 46:615, 1965.

77. WEBER, RJ AND WEINGARDEN, SI: *Electromyographic abnormalities following myelography.* Arch Neurol 36:588, 1979.

78. WETTSTEIN, A: *The origin of fasciculations in motoneuron disease.* Ann Neurol 5:295, 1979.

79. WIECHERS, DO: *Mechanically provoked insertional activity before and after nerve section in rats.* Arch Phys Med Rehabil 58:402, 1977.

80. WIECHERS, DO AND JOHNSON, EW: *Diffuse abnormal electromyographic insertional activity: A preliminary report.* Arch Phys Med Rehabil 60:419, 1979.

# 14

# EXAMINATION OF NON-LIMB MUSCLES

The muscles of mastication—face, soft palate, and tongue—are as readily accessible to the needle electrode as the skeletal muscles in the limbs. Electromyographic evaluation of laryngeal muscles requires the assistance of an otolaryngologist for proper placement of the needle electrode. Extraocular muscles are also difficult to approach although their physiologic and pharmacologic properties are not different from those of the peripheral skeletal muscles.[18] Because of the special skill and knowledge required in safely placing the electrode in the intended muscles, electromyography of the extraocular muscles is best undertaken with the help of an ophthalmologist.

The truncal musculature can be studied as easily as the muscles of the extremities, using the same technique. The examination of the abdominal and paraspinal muscles is important in the assessment of the intercostal nerves and posterior rami of the spinal nerves, respectively. The external anal sphincter can also be adequately tested in an ordinary electromyographic laboratory. The paraurethral muscles, however, are preferably studied in conjunction with cystometry and other urodynamic evaluations, which are beyond the scope of this book.[15, 25, 37, 50, 59]

## MUSCLES OF THE FACE, LARYNX, AND NECK

Voluntary muscles innervated by the cranial nerves are studied using the same technique as for the skeletal muscles of the limbs. The laryngeal and extraocular muscles are exceptions, as will be discussed below. The most commonly tested muscles are the masseter, temporalis, orbicularis oculi, orbicularis oris, tongue, trapezius, and sternocleidomastoid. Insertion of a needle electrode is best accomplished if the muscle is immobilized by holding its belly between the index finger and thumb of the examiner.

### Facial muscles

Because of anatomic proximity, the needle electrode placed in the orbicularis oris or oculi may detect distant potentials generated in the masseter or temporalis muscle. This should be avoided by having the patient open the mouth slightly when testing motor unit potentials of the mimetic muscles of the face. Motor unit potentials are generally of short duration in the facial muscles although a wide variety of values has been reported, ranging from 2.28 ± 0.3 ms (mean ± SD) by Petersén and Kugelberg[47] to 5 to 6 ms by Buchthal and Rosenfalck.[24] The orbicularis oris contains some muscle fibers crossing from one side to the other. In case of unilateral denervation, therefore, activity of muscle fibers innervated by the normal facial nerve on the unaffected side may be recorded on the affected side. Anesthetic block of the normal facial nerve may then be necessary to establish a complete loss of innervation on the side of the lesion.[22]

After nerve injury, fibrillation potentials tend to appear slightly earlier in the facial than in the limb muscles. Detection of spontaneous activity is important in differentiating structural damage to the axon from functional block of the facial nerve in patients with peripheral facial palsy. The brevity and small amplitude of normal motor unit potentials makes it difficult to distinguish them from spontaneous fibrillation potentials in waveform (Fig. 14-1). For an accurate assessment of fibrillation potentials therefore, it is essential that the facial muscle under study be completely relaxed. As in the skeletal muscles elsewhere, the electrical evidence of reinnervation in the form of nascent units may occur before the return of voluntary movement. Aberrant regeneration is the rule rather than the exception, once the nerve is degenerated from the

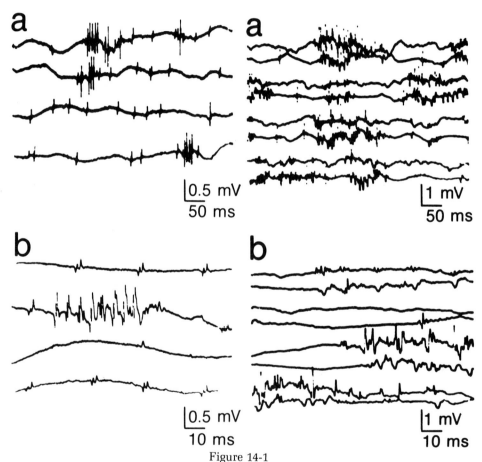

Figure 14-1

Motor unit potentials recorded in a 54-year-old woman with hemifacial spasm. (*Left*) Recurrent spontaneous bursts of high frequency discharges are shown at a slow (a) and fast sweep (b) during continuous recording from the orbicularis oris with the patient at rest. (*Right*) Simultaneous recording from the orbicularis oculi (top tracing in each pair) and oris (bottom). The patient was asked to blink quickly several times. Synkinesis demonstrated in this figure is characteristic of hemifacial spasm.

proximal trunk (see Fig. 16-9).[41] Random regeneration may occur between two branches of the facial nerve, or between two distinct but anatomically close nerves, such as the facial and trigeminal nerves.[56] In these cases, electromyographic studies with simultaneous recording from the affected muscles substantiate the presence of synkinesis (Fig. 14-1).

## Laryngeal and nuchal muscles

The motor functions of the glossopharyngeal and vagal nerves are similar, since both innervate the larynx, the latter by recurrent branches. Paralytic involvement of the vocal cord, palate, and pharyngeal and laryngeal muscles is not usually tested in an ordinary electromyographic laboratory. A flexible wire electrode is suitable for studies of these anatomic structures. The insertion of the electrode is best carried out with the help of an otolaryngologist. Examination of the tongue is simpler. The conventional needle electrode is usually placed in the lateral portion of the tongue with only mild discomfort. To study spontaneous activity, the tongue should be relaxed on the floor of the mouth with the electrode in place. Motor unit potentials are recorded when the tongue is deviated away from the needle. Conversely, muscle potentials are inhibited with deviation towards the needle. When the tongue is protruded in the midline, both sides are contracting simultaneously. In this position, the tongue is often restless and tremulous, and it may be difficult to evaluate electromyographically. The exact innervation ratio of these muscles is not known, but the value probably falls between those of the extraocular and limb muscles.

The spinal accessory nerve supplies the sternocleidomastoid and the upper portion of the trapezius. The sternocleidomastoid is unique because of its primarily ipsilateral supranuclear control, as opposed to most other movements which are controlled by the contralateral cerebral hemisphere.[5] Unilateral activation of the sternocleidomastoid turns the head away from the contracting muscle. The muscle on the opposite side is reciprocally inhibited in healthy subjects but not in patients with torticollis (Fig. 14-2). Bilateral contraction of this muscle flexes the head forward. The trapezius is activated when the patient shrugs the shoulders upwards towards the ears. Both muscles can be tested with ease using a regular electromyographic needle.

# EXTRAOCULAR MUSCLES

Electromyography of the extraocular muscles was introduced by Björk[7] and Björk and Kugelberg.[9,10] The technique was refined by Breinin[18] who also provided detailed descriptions of the methods and normal findings. More recent reviews on this subject are available.[20,42,52] The test is most useful in differentiating causes of paralytic squint, such as denervation, ocular myopathy, and myasthenia gravis. Ocular electromyography may also be valuable in detecting abnormalities of eye movements attributable to mechanical limitations. These include squint secondary to dislocation of the globe, anomalies in tendon attachment, presence of fascial bands connecting one muscle with another, and fibrous tissue partly replacing the extraocular muscles. Assessment of electrical activity of the extraocular muscles reveals no abnormality in most patients with mechanical strabismus. Electromyographic activity is not affected by passive movement of the eyes.

## Recording technique

Monopolar needle electrodes currently in use are similar to those developed by Björk and Kugelberg.[9,10] These needle electrodes are about 0.25 mm in diameter and are insulated along the length of the shaft, except for the tip, which is bare. The indifferent electrode is placed on the tip of the nose or a blepharostat attached to the eyelid. A fine

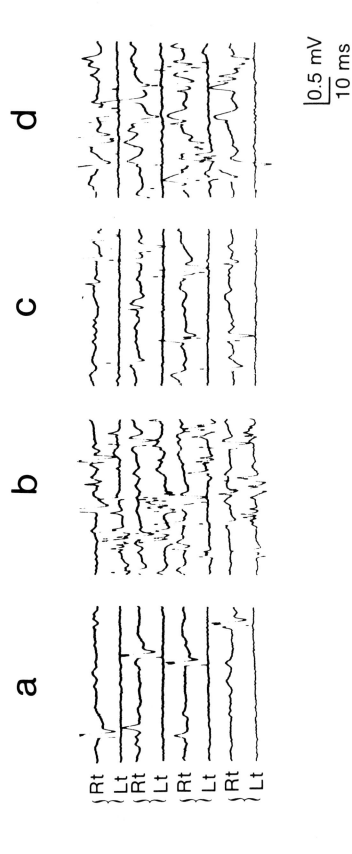

Figure 14-2

Torticollis on the right in a 30-year-old woman. Muscle action potentials were registered simultaneously from right (upper tracing of each pair) and left (lower tracing) sternocleidomastoid. Sequential recordings were obtained with the patient either facing straight ahead (a and c) or turning the head to the right (b) or left (d). The muscle on the right continuously discharged regardless of the head position, whereas the muscle on the left was electrically silent; except when turning the head to the opposite direction (b).

0.5 mV

10 ms

concentric electrode, 1 to 1½ inches long and similar to a 30-gauge hypodermic needle in diameter, is more convenient for study of the extraocular muscles. The concentric needle recommended by Breinin[18] is 0.25 mm in external diameter with a leading-off surface diameter of 0.08 mm. Another concentric electrode with an external diameter of 0.5 mm and leading-area of 0.015 mm² has also been used.[30] A second needle electrode may be simultaneously placed in an agonist or antagonist muscle to study synergistic actions or reciprocal inhibition.

Ocular electromyography is done with the patient supine on the examining table. Placement of the needle electrodes through the skin of the lid is properly done by an ophthalmologist, who is familiar with the anatomy of the eye and the extraocular muscles. The inferior oblique is the most easily reached, but any of the remaining extraocular muscles can be explored. The superior oblique is least accessible, requiring a needle considerably longer than the ordinary electrode. A topical anesthetic is applied to the eye before the needle is inserted subconjunctivally into the belly of a muscle along its long axis. The electrode position is adjusted by monitoring the waveform and sound of motor unit discharges.

The procedure is generally well tolerated with minimal discomfort, although it is difficult, if not impossible, to perform in an uncooperative patient. To evaluate voluntary eye movements, the subject must be awake during the examination. This requirement precludes the use of any form of general anesthesia when performing ocular electromyography as a diagnostic test. Electrical activity decreases during general, retrobulbar, or local anesthesia as the level deepens, leading to complete electrical silence with the eyes assuming a position of divergence.[16, 17, 18] Rare complications include ecchymoses of the conjunctiva, subcapsular hemorrhage, and exposure keratitis, all of which clear without sequelae.[9, 18, 44] Inadvertent perforation of the globe is a more serious complication that can occur, especially in the presence of undetected glaucoma.

## Unique properties of extraocular muscles

The eyes move rapidly and accurately. This precisely controlled movement of a constant load is achieved by complex coactivation of synergistic muscles and relaxation of the antagonists. Sherrington first described this principle of reciprocal inhibition based on studies done on the extraocular muscles. The eye muscles are capable of discharging at a rate of up to 200 impulses per second[9] in contrast to the usual rates of firing of less than 50 impulses per second in the skeletal muscles of the limbs. Compared with the limb muscles, extraocular muscle fibers are very thin, ranging from 10 to 50 μm in diameter.[19] The muscle fiber content of ocular motor units is small, varying from 6 to 12[14, 55] to 23.[29] These values are considerably less than the innervation ratio in the limb muscles, which has been estimated to be 100 to 2000.[21, 32, 51] The low innervation ratio and other physiologic characteristics of the extraocular muscles permit rapid and very finely graded eye movements. The existence of both slow and fast twitch fibers has recently been documented in the extraocular muscles.[19] The role of the slow fibers is not clearly delineated, but the long-lasting contraction of an extraocular muscle to the application of acetylcholine (ACh) or succinylcholine has been attributed to the slow fiber system. The characteristic monophasic, low amplitude potential of a slow fiber can often be obtained by sampling the surface layer of the extraocular muscle.[20]

Ocular electromyography is generally quite similar to that of the peripheral skeletal muscles, but there are certain electrophysiologic characteristics peculiar to the extraocular muscles. As in the muscles of the extremities, a brief insertional activity is recorded with placement of the needle electrode, presumably representing an injury potential. Unlike the limb musculature, however, extraocular muscles are not electrically silent following the cessation of needle movement. Continuous electrical discharges result from the tonic activity of the muscles required to maintain the eyes in the primary position during the alert state. With ocular movement, motor unit discharge increases in the contracting muscles and decreases in the antagonists (Fig. 14-3). Complete electrical silence of the antagonist is accomplished only with the reciprocal inhibition associated with rapid contraction of the active muscle in fast eye movements.[10]

Reflecting the small diameter of the muscle fiber and low innervation ratio, motor unit potentials in the extraocular muscles are smaller in size than those in the limb muscles. Björk and Kugelberg[9] found an amplitude of $108 \pm 9.2$ µV (mean $\pm$ SD) and a duration of $1.60 \pm 0.06$ ms, whereas Faurschou Jensen[30] reported a slightly longer duration with a mean value of $2.8 \pm 0.1$ ms. Breinin[20] considers the normal amplitude to range from 20 to 600 µV averaging 200 µV in the primary position, and the normal duration from 1 to 2 ms with an average of 1.5 ms. As in the limb muscles, individual potentials are usually triphasic in waveform and rarely polyphasic. With maximal effort of contraction they discharge at a rate of up to 200 impulses per second.[9]

## Neurogenic extraocular palsy

Electromyographic findings of a neurogenic extraocular palsy caused by lesions of the third, fourth, or sixth nerve are in principle the same as those in denervated limb muscles. Denervation potentials are harder to evaluate in the extraocular muscles, however, in view of the tonic discharge normally present with the eyes in the primary position. The problem is compounded by the brevity of the normal motor unit potentials, which resemble fibrillation potentials.[23] However, denervation potentials can be recognized with certainty if they occur independently of any attempted contraction in

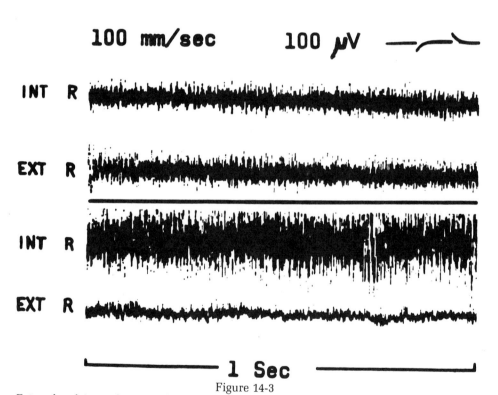

Figure 14-3

External and internal rectus of the left eye in a normal subject, recorded simultaneously for comparison. Upper tracing shows essentially equal and constant activity of normal amplitude in both muscles. Lower tracing was taken when eye was turned strongly into field of action of internal rectus. Note increased motor unit activity of this muscle and corresponding reciprocal decrease in activity of external rectus. (From Van Allen and Blodi,[57] with permission.)

a totally paretic muscle.[8] After reinnervation, polyphasic potentials are not as conspicuous in the extraocular muscles as they are in skeletal muscles elsewhere, although the amplitude and duration of motor unit potentials may be increased. Large motor unit potentials are frequently noted in aberrant regeneration of oculomotor nerves.[20]

Neurogenic weakness of the extraocular muscles is suspected with slow recruitment of motor units during voluntary contraction. The interference pattern is reduced approximately in proportion to the degree of paresis. In a totally paretic muscle no motor units can be activated with attempted maximal contraction. However, complete electrical silence is rare, even in severe palsies. The interference pattern may consist of repetitive discharges from a single motor unit in severe, but incomplete, paralysis. Mild palsies without definite limitations of rotation are associated with abundant electrical activity in the remaining normal units. They are, therefore, difficult to distinguish from ordinary strabismus, which is characteristically associated with a normal motor unit discharge on attempted rotation into the field of action.

## Myopathy and myasthenia gravis

In contrast to a neurogenic paralysis, ocular myopathy is typically associated with the absence of denervation potentials and the preservation of a normal interference pattern.[11, 45] This is consistent with a random loss of individual muscle fibers without significant change in the number of functional motor units. Motor unit potentials may be of reduced amplitude and short duration in ocular myopathies.[31] Such findings have been demonstrated in progressive external ophthalmoplegia, thyroid ophthalmopathy, and pseudotumor of the orbit.[20] Except in advanced cases, however, the reduction in fiber content expected to occur in myopathy is often difficult to substantiate electromyographically. This is because the diameter of the muscle fiber is small and the innervation ratio is low in normal extraocular muscles. A higher mean firing frequency has been shown to occur in ocular myopathy, when automatic frequency analysis is used, but this is of limited clinical value in detecting abnormalities in individual patients.[18]

The ocular muscles are commonly affected early in myasthenia gravis, causing diplopia associated with abnormal fatigue of eye movements. Thus, electromyography of the extraocular muscles may help to establish the diagnosis, even if extremity muscles are normal clinically and electrically. In myasthenia gravis the amplitude of a motor unit potential typically fluctuates or progressively declines when the same unit is repetitively activated, and sustained maximal contraction may cause a progressive decrease in the number of discharging motor units. The interference is often reduced and of low amplitude. The diagnosis of myasthenia gravis may be established if the interference pattern returns to normal immediately following administration of edrophonium (Tensilon).[16] When ptosis is the presenting sign, the levator palpebrae may be tested, but this muscle is extremely difficult to localize. In patients receiving anticholinesterase therapy, over-medication may result in clinical and electrical abnormalities induced by cholinergic block. Ocular myasthenia may be associated with myopathic changes of the extraocular muscle that do not respond to the administration of anticholinesterase.[45]

## Other types of gaze palsy

Musculofacial anomalies generally result in limitation of gaze in one direction, either vertically or horizontally. If an apparent paralysis is purely mechanical, the electrical activity of the contracting muscle remains physiologic, showing normal motor unit potentials and a complete interference pattern disproportionate to the failure of rotation. In a blow-out fracture of the orbit, the globe may be prevented from normal rotation by incarceration of the extraocular muscle in the fracture line. In such a case, ocular electromyography establishes the presence of normally innervated muscle by demonstrating abundant activity which follows the effort to rotate the eye. This is not the case if the limitation of rotation is the result of a direct injury to the nerve or muscle.

Duane's syndrome is a congenital deficiency of ocular motility presumably secondary to fibrosis of individual extraocular muscles. The syndrome typically consists of impaired abduction of one eye, and retraction and ptosis on attempted adduction of the same eye. It has been postulated that a fibrotic lateral rectus neither contracts on abduction nor relaxes on adduction. Electromyographic findings are compatible with this view, in that the lateral rectus shows a reduced number of motor unit potentials when activated, and fails to produce electrical silence when reciprocally inhibited.[17, 49] Furthermore, a central supranuclear lesion may disrupt normal reciprocal inhibition (Fig. 14-4) and contribute to the ophthalmoplegia in this condition.[12]

Limitation of eye movements may occur on a central basis as in internuclear ophthalmoplegia.[3, 43] In this syndrome caused by a lesion of the medial longitudinal fasciculus, the eye on the side of the lesion fails to adduct, despite the integrity of the peripheral motor system. Supranuclear disturbances can be demonstrated in ocular electromyography by the altered pattern of innervation. The medial rectus has normal electrical discharges with the eyes in the primary position but shows neither an increase in activity on attempted adduction nor reciprocal inhibition on attempted abduction.

The Möbius syndrome consists of facial diplegia and restriction of horizontal eye movements. Electromyographic studies show synchronous bursts of activity from the medial and lateral rectus rather than the normally expected reciprocal pattern of innervation (Fig. 14-5). Although this syndrome has been referred to as congenital paralysis or nuclear agenesis of the sixth or seventh nerves, these findings would suggest that a supranuclear lesion is in part responsible for the abnormal ocular motility in these patients.

Nystagmus can be demonstrated using a pair of electrodes inserted into the extraocular muscles.[20] A reciprocal relationship between orbicularis oculi and levator palpebrae has also been described using electromyographic techniques.[58]

# TRUNCAL MUSCULATURE

## Abdominal muscles

Muscles of the upper and lower extremities are supplied by the anterior rami of the cervical and lumbosacral spinal nerves, respectively. Analogous to this anatomic arrangement, intercostal and abdominal muscles are innervated by 12 pairs of intercostal nerves derived from the anterior rami of the thoracic spinal nerves. Involvement of the intercostal nerve results in segmental paralysis of respiration. Weakness of the abdominal muscles causes protrusion of the abdomen on coughing and deviation of the umbilicus to the unaffected side by unopposed action of the normal muscle. The study of the abdominal muscles may be helpful in detecting the presence of a lesion at the thoracic levels, which do not have appendicular representation in the extremities. Exact localization of the involved cord level, however, is often difficult because of the considerable overlap in segmental representation. Each segmental level is supplied by at least two adjoining intercostal nerves in both thoracic and abdominal regions.

The abdominal musculature can be tested by needle examination just as easily as the muscles of the four extremities. The external oblique is tested at the anterior axillary line 5 to 10 cm above the anterior superior spine of the iliac crest. The needle must be inserted obliquely along the course of the muscle fibers, which run medially and downward. If the needle is placed too deep it will be in the internal oblique or transverse abdominis (or the abdominal cavity). Even with the patient completely relaxed, volume-conducted potentials may be registered from the intercostal muscles firing

## Left Eye

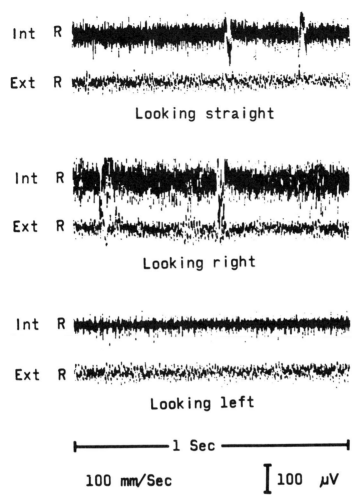

Int R

Ext R

Looking straight

Int R

Ext R

Looking right

Int R

Ext R

Looking left

|——————— 1 Sec ———————|

100 mm/Sec          ⌶ 100 μV

Figure 14-4

External and internal rectus of the left eye, recorded simultaneously in a patient with Duane's syndrome. Innervation pattern of the internal rectus is normal. There is no increment nor decrement of the external rectus on attempted gaze to the left or to the right, although the electrical activity of this muscle is normal in the primary position. (From Blodi, Van Allen and Yarbrough,[12] with permission.)

rhythmically with respiration. This activity must be distinguished from spontaneous discharges, which are unrelated to the breathing cycle. To study motor unit potentials, the patient is asked to contract the muscle by bending the upper trunk forward. The abdominal rectus is tested between the linea alba, connecting the xiphoid and umbilicus in the midline, and the linea semilunaris, which form the lateral margin of the rectus. The needle is inserted into the muscle so as to avoid the three transverse tendinous bands located at the xiphoid, umbilicus, and halfway in between.[34] The muscle is activated for the assessment of motor unit potentials by asking the patient to bend forward against a resistance.

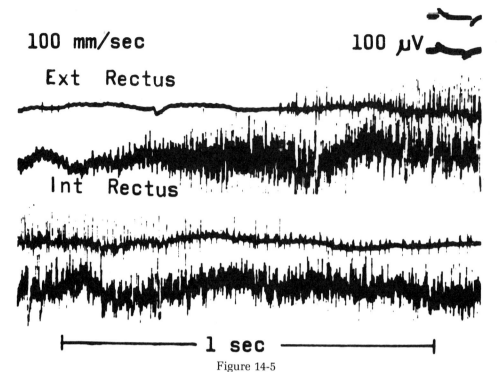

Figure 14-5

External and internal rectus of the left eye, recorded simultaneously in a patient with the Möbius syndrome. Record is continuous. Note spontaneous volley in external rectus, with simultaneous waxing of activity in internal rectus. There is no evidence of normal reciprocal innervation. (From Van Allen and Blodi,[57] with permission.)

## Paraspinal muscles

In contrast to the muscles of the extremities and abdominal musculature, the paraspinal muscles are supplied by the posterior ramus of the spinal nerves at respective segmental levels. Documentation of electromyographic abnormalities in this region is quite important to identify a radicular lesion that affects the spinal nerve at a point proximal to its bifurcation into the posterior and anterior rami (see Fig. 13-7 bottom left). With a more distally located lesion at the level of the plexus or the peripheral nerve, the paraspinal muscles are entirely spared, since the posterior rami are not affected. Examination of paraspinal muscle is of critical value in the investigation of cervical or lumbar disc herniation.[35, 38, 39] In fact, within one to two weeks after the onset of radiculopathy, electrical abnormalities may be limited to this region. Some systemic disorders, most notably polymyositis, may affect the paraspinal muscles preferentially.[1, 53]

There are two portions of paraspinal muscles—short spinal muscles, also called multifidus, and long spinal muscles, known as longissimus dorsi. The short spinal muscles are the deeper of the two and are located immediately posterior to the transverse process. They are innervated fairly discretely by the corresponding posterior rami. To study this portion of the paraspinal muscle, the needle must be inserted deep, just lateral to the spinal process, toward the transverse process. The long spinal muscles are more superficial, extending several centimeters to either side of the spinous process and ligamentum nuchae.[34] There is considerable overlap of innervation extending at least one to two segments caudally and rostrally. This portion of the muscle can be reached quite superficially if the needle is inserted 2 to 3 cm lateral to the spinous process either at the cervical or lumbar level.

Complete relaxation of the paraspinal muscles is sometimes difficult to achieve. The subjects should lie in a lateral decubitus or prone position with pillows under the neck or abdomen for cervical and lumbar studies, respectively. To relax cervical paraspinal muscles, we find it best to ask the patient to bend the head forward, pressing the forehead against the table. For lumbar examination, we ask the patient to slightly raise the hips toward the ceiling. Motor unit potentials are normally of low amplitude and short duration, especially in the cervical region. Thus, they may be easily mistaken for fibrillation potentials, unless complete relaxation is attained.

# ANAL SPHINCTER

The anal sphincter is innervated by the anal pudendal nerve, which derives from the anterior division of S-2, S-3, and S-4 spinal nerves. The anal sphincter is normally under volitional control and shares similar physiologic properties with the skeletal muscles of the limbs. Since the initial attempt by Beck,[6] electromyography has long been used for kinesiologic studies of the normal anal sphincter at rest and during defecation. Floyd and Walls[33] recorded electrical potentials from this muscle with surface electrodes during waking and sleeping. They found that sphincter activity was increased by coughing, speaking, and body movements of the trunk, and decreased greatly during sleep. Other electrodes used include dental needles with a 25 $\mu$m wire in the center[40] for kinesiologic studies and steel needle[54] for recording electrical discharges associated with reflex contraction upon digital stretching of the sphincter. For routine clinical electromyography of the anal sphincter, the conventional concentric or monopolar needle electrodes are quite adequate.

Electromyographic studies objectively quantitate sphincter dysfunction in neurologic disorders.[60] They help establish or rule out the possibility of agenesis of the striate sphincter in the preoperative assessment of the newborn with an imperforate anus. Electrical studies not only localize the sphincter precisely, if it is present, but also determine its functional capacity.[2] The anal sphincter may be injured during parturition, prostatectomy, or rectal surgery, including repair of an anal fistula or prolapse. Electromyography may be used to determine the extent of damage in such cases. It is also valuable in confirming the integrity of the anal sphincter for possible ilioconduit surgery in patients with prominent urologic dysfunction, since anal and external urethral sphincters share a common segmental derivation. Electromyography of the urethral sphincter is best performed in a laboratory equipped for urodynamic investigations.

Chantraine[25] and Jesel, Isch-Treussard, and Isch[37] have reviewed methods for studying the anal sphincter. The patient may assume the lateral decubitus, knee-chest, or modified lithotomy position. Of these, the lateral decubitus position may be preferred in adults and older children and modified lithotomy position in infants. Sphincter tone is tested first by digital examination. With a gloved finger still placed in the anus, the needle is inserted through the perianal skin adjacent to the mucocutaneous junction. The tip of the electrode should be located close to the anal orifice, 0.5 to 1 cm from the ring. The ring of the anal orifice may be divided into four parts. Anterior and posterior quadrants should be examined on both sides. The anal sphincter is tested at rest and while contracted voluntarily or reflexively.

## Resting and voluntary activities

Unlike peripheral skeletal muscles, the anal sphincter maintains a certain tonus even when the muscle is not volitionally contracted. With the subject at rest, isolated motor unit potentials fire at a low rate. This activity varies considerably with changes in subject position. The activity continues during sleep, although the discharge rate is much less than during wakefulness. Complete absence of sphincter activity is obtained only during attempted defecation. Conversely, volitional contraction of the anal sphincter inhibits rectal motility based on reciprocal innervation between the rectal musculature and the striated muscle of the anal sphincter. Because of physiologic tonic activity at rest, detection of abnormal spontaneous potentials is difficult in the partially denervated muscle. Thus, fibrillation potentials and positive sharp waves can be identified with certainty only when sphincter tone is absent or markedly reduced.

To test voluntary activity, the patient is asked to contract the sphincter as though attempting to hold a bowel movement. The average size of the motor unit potentials has been reported to be 5.5 to 7.5 ms in duration and 0.2 to 0.5 μV in amplitude.[25, 46] Reflex activity is elicited simply by digital examination of the anal sphincter, but coughing and crying also activate the muscle.[33, 54] The interference pattern should normally be complete whether induced volutarily or reflexively. A system of grading the interference pattern has been developed,[4, 60] but, as in the skeletal muscles of the limb, its reliability depends on patient cooperation. Some patients are unable to relax or contract the sphincter under pretense, in response to requests of the examiner. In these patients, electromyographic appraisal of sphincteric tone is particularly difficult, and

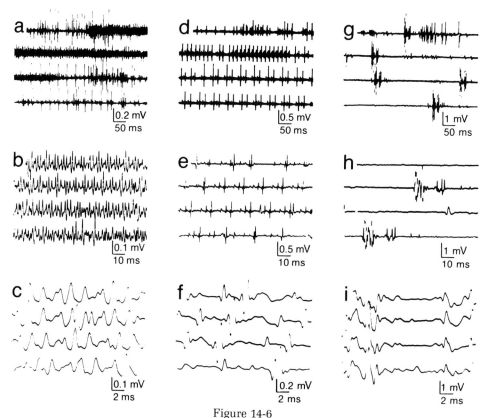

Figure 14-6

Recording from anal sphincter in a 16-year-old girl with incontinence. Tracings include continuous discharge at high frequency, resembling very prominent end-plate noise (a, b, c), complex repetitive potentials (d, e, f), and very polyphasic fasciculation potential (g, h, i), all recorded in a localized small area of the sphincter while the patient was completely relaxed. In i, each sweep was triggered by a recurring fasciculation potential to show consistent late components which follow the major discharge.

care must be taken not to misinterpret this as a central lesion. With some experience, however, it is usually possible to correlate electrical activity and sphincter tone with reasonable accuracy.

## Central versus peripheral paralysis

Paralysis of the striated sphincter may result from a pure central lesion, pure peripheral lesion, or a mixed central and peripheral lesion. In central paralysis, voluntary activity is reduced or absent, although the muscle can be activated reflexively. Reduced voluntary activity produces an incomplete interference pattern that consists of motor unit potentials of normal amplitude discharging at low frequency. If voluntary activity is entirely lost, the low frequency discharge normally seen at rest continues during maximal effort to contract the muscle.

Peripheral paralysis of the anal sphincter is usually caused by lesions in the cauda equina, or in the sacral or pudendal plexus. When paralysis is incomplete, a few motor units can be volitionally activated. In contrast to central paralysis, the surviving units show polyphasic potentials of a long duration. They discharge at a high frequency. In an acute cauda equina syndrome, the initial paralysis may be secondary to a functional block. If axonal degeneration occurs, fibrillation potentials or positive sharp waves appear. Complex repetitive discharges may also be seen (Fig. 14-6). The sphincter muscle, however, is not conspicuously denervated in amyotrophic lateral sclerosis.[48]

A mixture of central and peripheral paresis may be seen in congenital malformations, vascular disease, or traumatic injury of the conus medullaris.[13, 27, 36] Spina bifida with meningomyelocele is perhaps one of the most common spinal cord lesions affecting both upper and lower motor neurons.[26] Electromyography of the anal sphincter in these cases shows absent or markedly reduced voluntary activity. Reflex activity, if present, is also significantly reduced, showing isolated high frequency discharges of a few motor units. With complete damage to the sacral segment of the conus medullaris, no sphincter activity can be induced either voluntarily or reflexively. Spontaneous denervation potentials are, however, usually recorded in these cases.[28]

# REFERENCE SOURCES

1. ALBERS, JW, ET AL: *Spontaneous electrical activity and muscle biopsy abnormalities in polymyositis and dermatomyositis.* Muscle and Nerve 2:503, 1979.

2. ARCHIBALD, KC AND GOLDSMITH, EI: *Sphincteric electromyography.* Arch Phys Med Rehabil 48:387, 1967.

3. BACH-Y-RITA, P AND COLLINS, CC (EDS): *The Control of Eye Movements.* Academic Press, New York, 1971.

4. BAILEY, JA, POWERS, JJ, AND WAYLONIS, GW: *A clinical evaluation of electromyography of the anal sphincter.* Arch Phys Med Rehabil 51:403, 1970.

5. BALAGURA, S AND KATZ, RG: *Undecussated innervation to the sternocleidomastoid muscle: A reinstatement.* Ann Neurol 7:84, 1980.

6. BECK, A: *Elektromyographische Untersuchungen Sphincter ani.* Arch Physiol 224:278, 1930.

7. BJÖRK, Å: *Electrical activity of human extrinsic eye muscles.* Experientia 8:226, 1952.

8. BJÖRK, Å: *Electromyographic study of conditions involving limited mobility of the eye, chiefly due to neurogenic pareses.* Br J Ophthalmol 38:528, 1954.

9. BJÖRK, Å AND KUGELBERG, E: *Motor unit activity in the human extraocular muscles.* Electroenceph Clin Neurophysiol 5:271, 1953.

10. BJÖRK, Å AND KUGELBERG, E: *The electrical activity of the muscles of the eye and eyelids in various positions and during movement.* Electroenceph Clin Neurophysiol 5:595, 1953.

11. BLODI, FC AND VAN ALLEN, MW: *Electromyographic studies in some neuro-ophthalmologic disorders.* XVIII Concilium Ophthalmologicum, Vol 2, (Belgica), 1958, p 1621.

12. BLODI, FC, VAN ALLEN, MW, AND YARBROUGH, JC: *Duane's syndrome: A brain stem lesion.* Arch Ophthalmol 72:171, 1964.

13. BONNAL, J, STEVENAERT, A, AND CHANTRAINE, A: *Bilan électromyographique pré et postopératoire du spina bifida avec troubles neurologiques.* Neuro-Chir (Paris) 15:299, 1969.

14. BORS, E: *Über das Zahlenverhältnis zwischen Nerven- und Muskelfasern.* Anat Anz 60:415, 1926.

15. BRADLEY, WE, ET AL: *Detrusor and urethral electromyography.* J Urol 114:891, 1975.

16. BREININ, GM: *Electromyography—A tool in ocular and neurologic diagnosis. I. Myasthenia gravis.* Arch Ophthalmol 57:161, 1957.

17. BREININ, GM: *Electromyography—A tool in ocular and neurologic diagnosis. II. Muscle palsies.* Arch Ophthalmol 57:165, 1957.

18. BREININ, GM: *The Electrophysiology of Extraocular Muscle with Special Reference to Electromyography.* University of Toronto Press, Toronto, 1962.

19. BREININ, GM: *The structure and function of extraocular muscle—An appraisal of the duality concept.* Am J Ophthalmol 72:1, 1971.

20. BREININ, GM: *Ocular electromyography.* In GOODGOLD, J AND EBERSTEIN, A (EDS): *Electrodiagnosis of Neuromuscular Diseases,* ed 2. Williams & Wilkins, Baltimore, 1977.

21. BUCHTHAL, F: *The general concept of the motor unit.* In ADAMS, R, EATON, L, AND SHY, GM (EDS): *Neuromuscular Disorders,* Vol 38. Williams & Wilkins, Baltimore, 1960.

22. BUCHTHAL, F: *Electromyography in paralysis of the facial nerve.* Arch Otolaryngol (Stockh) 81:463, 1965.

23. BUCHTHAL, F: *Electrophysiological abnormalities in metabolic myopathies and neuropathies.* Acta Neurol Scand (suppl 43)46:129, 1970.

24. BUCHTHAL, F AND ROSENFALCK, P: *Action potential parameters in different human muscles.* Acta Psychiatr Neurol Scand 30:125, 1955.

25. CHANTRAINE, A: *EMG examination of the anal and urethral sphincters.* In DESMEDT, JE (ED): *New Developments in Electromyography and Clinical Neurophysiology,* Vol 2. Karger, Basel, 1973, pp 421–432.

26. CHANTRAINE, A, LLOYD, K, AND SWINYARD, CA: *The sphincter ani externus in spina bifida and myelomeningocele.* J Urol (Baltimore) 95:250, 1966.

27. CHANTRAINE, A, STEVENAERT, A, AND TIMMERMANS, L: *Electromyographic study before and after operation in spina bifida with myelomeningocele: A preliminary report.* Dev Med Child Neurol (suppl 13):136, 1967.

28. CHANTRAINE, A, ET AL: *Evolution électromyographique du bilan pré- et postopératoire du spina bifida avec troubles neurologiques.* Acta Paediat Belg 22:127, 1968.

29. CHRISTENSEN, E: *Topography of terminal motor innervation in striated muscles from stillborn infants.* Am J Phys Med 38:65, 1959.

30. FAURSCHOU JENSEN, S: *The normal electromyogram from the external ocular muscles.* Acta Ophthalmol 49:615, 1971.

31. FAURSCHOU JENSEN, S: *Endocrine ophthalmoplegia. Is it due to myopathy or to mechanical immobilization?* Acta Ophthalmol 49:679, 1971.

32. FEINSTEIN, B, ET AL: *Morphologic studies of motor units in normal human muscles.* Acta Anat 23:127, 1955.

33. FLOYD, WF AND WALLS, EW: *Electromyography of the sphincter ani externus in man.* J Physiol (Lond) 122:599, 1953.

34. GOODGOLD, J: *Anatomical Correlates of Clinical Electromyography.* Williams & Wilkins, Baltimore, 1974.

35. GOUGH, JG AND KOEPKE, GH: *Electromyographic determination of motor root levels in erector spinae muscles.* Arch Phys Med Rehabil 47:9, 1966.

36. INGBERG, HO AND JOHNSON, EW: *Electromyographic evaluation of infants with lumbar meningomyelocele.* Arch Phys Med Rehabil 44:86, 1963.

37. JESEL, M, ISCH-TREUSSARD, C, AND ISCH, F: *Electromyography of striated muscle of anal and urethral sphincters.* In DESMEDT, JE (ED): *New Developments in Electromyography and Clinical Neurophysiology,* Vol 2. Karger, Basel, 1973.

38. JOHNSON, EW AND MELVIN, JL: *The value of electromyography in the management of lumbar radiculopathy.* Arch Phys Med Rehabil 50:720, 1969.

39. JONSSON, B: *Morphology, innervation, and electromyographic study of the erector spinae.* Arch Phys Med Rehabil 50:638, 1969.

40. KAWAKAMI, M: *Electro-myographic investigation on the human external sphincter muscle of anus.* Jpn J Physiol 4:196, 1954.

41. KIMURA, J, RODNITZKY, RL, AND OKAWARA, S: *Electrophysiologic analysis of aberrant regeneration after facial nerve paralysis.* Neurology (Minneap) 25:989, 1975.

42. LENMAN, JAR AND RITCHIE, AE: *Clinical Electromyography,* ed 2. J.B. Lippincott, Philadelphia, 1977.

43. LOEFFLER, JD, HOYT, WF, AND SLATT, B: *Motor excitation and inhibition in internuclear palsy.* Arch Neurol 15:664, 1966.

44. MARG, E, JAMPOLSKY, A, AND TAMLER, E: *Elements of human extraocular electromyography.* Arch Ophthalmol 61:258, 1959.

45. PAPST, W, ESSLEN, E, AND MERTENS, HG: *Klinische Erfahrungen mit der Elektromyographie bei oculären Myopathien.* Zusamm Deutsch Ophth Ges, 1957.

46. PETERSÉN, I AND FRANKSSON, C: *Electromyographic study of the striated muscles of the male urethra.* Br J Urol 27:148, 1955.

47. PETERSÉN, I AND KUGELBERG, E: *Duration and form of action potential in the normal human muscle.* J Neurol Neurosurg Psychiatry 12:124, 1949.

48. SAKUTA, M, NAKANISHI, T, AND TOYOKURA, Y: *Anal muscle electromyograms differ in amyotrophic lateral sclerosis and Shy-Drager syndrome.* Neurology (New York) 28:1289, 1978.

49. SATO, S: *Electromyographic study on retraction syndrome.* Jpn J Ophthalmol 4:57, 1960.

50. SCOTT, FB, QUESADA, EM, AND CARDUS, D: *The use of combined uroflowimetry, cystometry and electromyography in evaluation of neurogenic bladder dysfunction.* In BOYARSKY, S (ED): *Neurogenic Bladder.* Williams & Wilkins, Baltimore, 1967, pp 106–114.

51. SISSONS, HA: *Anatomy of the motor unit.* In WALTON, JN (ED): *Disorders of Voluntary Muscle,* ed 3. Churchill-Livingstone, London, 1974.

52. STRACHAN, IM: *Clinical electromyography of the extra-ocular muscles.* Br Orthopt J 26:60, 1969.

53. STREIB, EW, WILBOURN, AJ, AND MITSUMOTO, H: *Spontaneous electrical muscle fiber activity in polymyositis and dermatomyositis.* Muscle and Nerve 2:14, 1979.

54. TAVERNER, D AND SMIDDY, FG: *An electromyographic study of the normal function of the external anal sphincter and pelvic diaphragm.* Dis Colon Rectum 2:153, 1959.

55. TORRE, M: *Nombre et dimensions des unités motrices dans les muscles extrinsèques de l'oeil et, en général, dans les muscles squélettiques reliés à des organes de sens.* Arch Suisses Neurol Psychiatr 72:362, 1953.

56. TROJABORG, W AND SIEMSSEN, SO: *Reinnervation after resection of the facial nerve.* Arch Neurol 26:17, 1972.

57. VAN ALLEN, MW AND BLODI, FC: *Neurologic aspects of the Möbius syndrome. A case study with electromyography of the extraocular and facial muscles.* Neurology (Minneap) 10:252, 1960.

58. VAN ALLEN, MW AND BLODI, FC: *Electromyographic study of reciprocal innervation in blinking.* Neurology (Minneap) 12:371, 1962.

59. VEREECKEN, RL AND VERDUYN, H: *The electrical activity of the paraurethral and perineal muscles in normal and pathological conditions.* Br J Urol 42:457, 1970.

60. WAYLONIS, GW AND KRUEGER, KC: *Anal sphincter electromyography in adults.* Arch Phys Med Rehabil 51:409, 1970.

# SINGLE FIBER ELECTROMYOGRAPHY

The motor unit is the smallest component of muscle contraction that can be activated individually. Single motor unit potentials can easily be recorded with the coaxial needle electrode of Adrian and Bronk,[1] bipolar concentric needle, or monopolar needle (see Fig. 3-1). These electrodes, however, do not discriminate between potentials from different muscle fibers within a motor unit, all of which fire more or less synchronously. A variety of recording methods have been used to study muscle fiber physiology within the motor unit in more detail than is possible with conventional electromyography. These methods include the multi-electrode needle of Buchthal, Guld, and Rosenfalck,[3] introduced primarily to measure the territory of a motor unit, and the single fiber needle of Ekstedt and Stålberg.[7]

The smaller recording surface of the single fiber needle allows extracellular recording of single muscle fiber action potentials in voluntarily contracting human muscles. The method is termed single fiber electromyography (SFEMG). A number of papers have appeared describing different uses of this technique for the study of normal and disordered motor units. Of these applications, two are most useful as supplements to conventional electromyography: (1) measurement of fiber density—the number of single fiber action potentials within the recording radius of the electrode; and (2) determination of electromyographic jitter—the variability of the interpotential interval between two or more single muscle fibers belonging to the same motor unit. These and other findings of SFEMG in various neurologic disorders have been summarized by Stålberg and Trontelj.[34]

## RECORDING APPARATUS

### Electrode characteristics

The single fiber needle electrode has a much smaller leading-off surface and is therefore close to fewer muscle fibers than the conventional needle.[12] In addition, distortions of the electrical field induced by shunting effect of the metallic surface is much reduced (Fig. 15-1). This is advantageous for selective recording from single muscle fibers, since without shunting, the amplitude of the action potential decreases almost exponentially as the recording electrode is moved away from the source.[17] Thus, the slope of the line

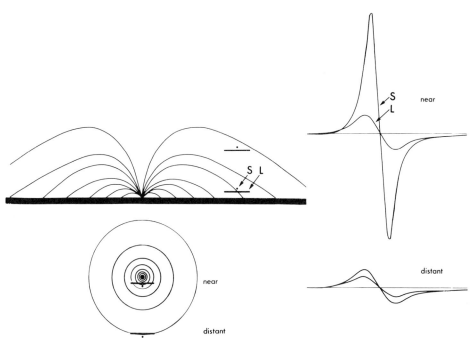

Figure 15-1

Electrical field around a muscle fiber recorded with a small (S) and a large (L) leading-off surface. When placed very close to the generator source, a large recording area shunts the high density isopotential lines more than a small recording area. Thus, the recorded potential is less in amplitude with a larger leading-off surface than with a smaller leading-off surface. See Figure 12-6 for relationship between the amplitude recorded and the electrode distance from the source. (From Stålberg and Trontelj,[34] with permission.)

describing the relationship between the recorded amplitude and the distance of the electrode from the generator is very steep (see Fig. 12-6). This in turn results in sharp discrimination of single fiber potentials as interference from action potentials of neighboring muscle fibers is minimal. An electrode diameter of 25 to 30 $\mu$m has been shown to be optimal for this purpose.[9]

In comparison, the conventional needle electrode has a leading-off surface of about 150 $\times$ 600 $\mu$m (see Fig. 3-1). With this larger leading-off surface, shunting is prominent and, more importantly, disproportionately greater near the source owing to the higher density of isopotential lines (Fig. 15-1). Thus, amplitude is comparatively less near the potential generator. Farther from the source the shunting effect is not very pronounced with either type of electrode, reflecting the larger radius of the isopotential lines and lower gradient of the electrical field. With large leading-off surfaces, therefore, the action potential does not decrease exponentially with increasing recording distance, as might be theoretically expected.[15] Consequently, there is relatively little difference between potentials derived from near and distant fibers with the conventional needle electrode.

Single fiber potentials can be further selectively increased by bipolar recordings in which two small wires are separated by a short interelectrode distance, as opposed to a monopolar arrangement with a reference electrode outside the muscle (see Fig. 3-1). The suggested interelectrode distance is 200 $\mu$m, long enough to avoid substantial decrease of the recorded action potential, while still not recording from two independent sources.[34]

## Amplifier settings

Because of the small leading-off surface, the electrical impedance of a single fiber electrode is much higher than that of a conventional monopolar or concentric needle. It is on the order of 100 Kohms at 1 KHz for platinum, although the value varies for different metals. To maintain a high signal-to-noise ratio, therefore, the amplifier must have a very high input impedance on the order of 100 megohms. With the electrode and the amplifier connected, the common mode rejection ratio or differential amplification between the signal and the interference potential should be better than 200.[34] The amplifier gain is initially set at 0.2 to 1 mV per cm with a sweep speed of 0.2 to 1 ms per cm. For detailed analysis of jitter and waveforms, a faster sweep speed is recommended.

Single fiber action potentials recorded near the potential generator are of short duration and high amplitude and thus consist mainly of high frequency components. When recorded at a distance, however, volume-conducted potentials are distorted by muscle tissue, which tends to filter high frequency components and have a larger proportion of low frequency discharges. Thus, distant potentials are selectively attenuated by a low-frequency cut-off of 500 Hz, for example. Volume-conducted background activity is then substantially reduced, whereas the action potential from fibers close to the electrode decreases by less than 10 percent.[16, 17] This slight change in shape of the single fiber potential is acceptable for measurements of propagation velocity, fiber density, and jitter. However, the high-pass (low-frequency) filter setting should be lowered considerably to 2 to 10 Hz for studying waveforms. A high-frequency cut-off of 35 KHz is ideal, but in practice the low-pass (high-frequency) filter may be lowered to 20 KHz without substantially altering the amplitude or shape of the single fiber action potential.

# SINGLE FIBER POTENTIAL

The potential generated by a single fiber is a biphasic spike with a rise time of 75 to 200 $\mu$s and total duration of about 1 ms, when recorded with an optimally placed single-fiber electrode.[6] The peak-to-peak amplitude is usually between 1 to 7 mV, but the value may be as low as 200 $\mu$V or as high as 15 to 20 mV. The recording site is decisive for amplitude, which attenuates exponentially with distance from the discharging muscle fiber as mentioned earlier.[17] Using a time resolution of 5 to 10 $\mu$s, the shape of the potential remains constant with successive discharges. The frequency spectrum ranges from 100 Hz to 10 KHz with a peak at 1.61 $\pm$ 0.30 KHz.[15]

## Recording procedures

Electrical stimulation or voluntary contraction can be used to generate motor unit potentials for single fiber electromyography (SFEMG). Cutaneous stimulation tends to activate many motor units simultaneously and makes single fiber recording difficult. In contrast, stimulation of an end-plate zone with a bipolar needle electrode can activate only a few terminal twigs of a motor neuron. The excited terminal twigs in the region conduct the action potential antidromically to the remaining nerve twigs and activate the whole motor unit.[26, 33] This allows recording of the SFEMG from a single motor unit firing in response to electrical stimulation. Although this technique reliably generates isolated motor unit potentials, slight steady voluntary muscle contraction usually produces a technically similar response and is the preferred method of studying SFEMG.

Ekstedt and Stålberg[10] recommend the following recording procedures during slight voluntary activation of the muscle: With the subject comfortably lying or seated, the needle is inserted into the slightly contracting muscle. The amplifier gain is set at 1 mV per cm on the oscilloscope screen. The needle is slowly advanced until the clear, high-pitched sound of a single fiber action potential is audible over the loudspeaker. The needle is then carefully rotated, advanced, or retracted to maximize the potential on the oscilloscope. The trigger level is set on the initial positive deflection of the action potential, and the consecutive discharges are superimposed on Polaroid film or a storage scope screen. If the action potentials are derived from a single muscle fiber, the waveform of the successive discharge is constant. Varying waveforms indicate a composite action potential that must be discarded from the analysis.

## Recommended criteria

In general, a potential may be accepted as generated by a single muscle fiber if the peak-to-peak amplitude exceeds 200 $\mu$V, the rise time from the positive to negative peak is less than 300 $\mu$s, and the waveform of successive discharges is constant when assessed with a time resolution of 10 $\mu$s or better. The same criteria are applicable in recording single fiber potentials with a commercially available SFEMG system. Accuracy in recording, however, is to a great degree dependent on the time resolution of the amplifier and other particulars of the recording system. Like any normative data, therefore, the ideal is for each laboratory to establish its own normal values.

Occasionally, it is possible to record single muscle fiber action potentials with conventional needle electrodes if a high-pass filter is used to eliminate low-frequency responses below 500 Hz to 1 KHz, which are mainly volume conducted from distant muscle fibers.[2] With this type of recording, it is difficult to accurately distinguish single fiber responses from summated potentials of more than one fiber, although it sometimes reveals abnormal complexity and instability of the motor unit not otherwise appreciated. Recording with low-frequency attenuation of the motor unit potential may bridge the gap between the SFEMG and conventional electromyography.[22]

# FIBER DENSITY

## Definition and clinical significance

If the single-fiber electrode is inserted into a slightly contracting normal muscle, randomly recorded activity generally derives from only one muscle fiber. However, occasionally the electrode may be placed close to two or more muscle fibers of the same motor unit. The recorded activity then consists of multiple single-fiber potentials discharging synchronously within the recording radius of the single fiber electrode (Fig. 15-2). The electromyographic fiber density is defined as the mean number of associated single-fiber potentials that fire almost synchronously with the initially identified potential at each random insertion of the single-fiber electrode.[32] In the normal adult muscle the average uptake radius is about 250 to 300 $\mu$m, using a monopolar derivation.[34] Thus, the motor unit fiber density defined above indicates the average number of single muscle fibers belonging to the same motor unit within this radius.

Fiber density is a measure of muscle fiber clustering rather than the total number of muscle fibers within a motor unit. Random loss of muscle fibers within the motor unit is generally not well detected by this technique, since by definition the lowest possible value is 1.0. However, a local concentration of action potentials is detected as an increase in fiber density, which usually indicates the presence of collateral sprouting.[37] Fiber density is said to be more sensitive than histochemical fiber grouping in identifying rearrangements within the motor unit.[34] Normally, fiber density is slightly higher in the frontalis and lower in the biceps brachii. In general, it is slightly higher under the age of 10 years and over the age of 60 (Table 15-1). Fiber density increases slowly during life with faster progression after the age of 70 years, perhaps indicating degeneration of motor neurons with aging, compensated for by reinnervation.[32]

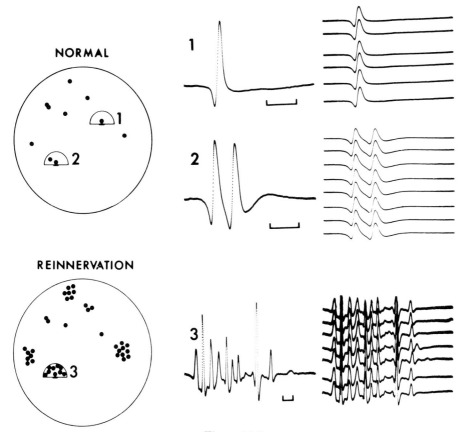

Figure 15-2

Fiber density in normal and reinnervated muscles. All muscle fibers belonging to one motor unit (small closed circles) discharge synchronously, but the recording radius of the single fiber electrode (half circle) normally contains only one (1) or two (2) muscle fibers. Following reinnervation, however, a large number of fibers (3) are clustered within the same radius, reflecting an increase in fiber density. Time calibration is 1 ms. (From Stålberg and Trontelj,[34] with permission.)

## Determination of fiber density

To determine the fiber density, the needle is slowly advanced so that a single-fiber potential is recorded with the leading-off surface of the electrode optimally positioned close to the identified fiber. In practice this is achieved by moving the needle tip back and forth and rotating it until the maximal amplitude of the identified potential is obtained. When the first action potential is maximized, the number of simultaneously firing single muscle fibers is counted for a time interval of at least 5 ms after the triggering spike. The needle is then further advanced until another single muscle fiber potential is recorded. To be included, an action potential must have an amplitude exceeding 200 $\mu$V and a rise time shorter than 300 $\mu$s with a high-pass filter of 500 Hz. The trigger level of the oscilloscope is set at 200 $\mu$V, otherwise small potentials fulfilling the criteria would remain undetected.

This procedure is repeated at 20 to 30 different sites in the muscle, and the fiber density is calculated as the average number of simultaneously firing single muscle fibers within the recording radius of the single fiber electrode. For example, if isolated discharges of a single muscle fiber occur in 15 different insertions and two fibers dis-

TABLE 15-1 Fiber density in normal subjects

| Muscles | AGES 10–25 years<br>m SD n | 26–50 years<br>m SD n | 51–75 years<br>m SD n | above 75 years<br>m SD n |
|---|---|---|---|---|
| Frontalis | 1.61 0.21 (11) | 1.72 0.21 (15) | | |
| Deltoid | 1.36 0.16 (20) | 1.40 0.11 (10) | | |
| Biceps | 1.25 0.09 (20) | 1.33 0.07 (17) | | |
| Extensor digitorum communis | 1.47 0.16 (61) | 1.49 0.16 (98) | 1.57 0.17 (59) | 2.13 0.41 (21) |
| 1st dorsal interosseus | 1.33 0.13 (14) | 1.45 0.12 (6) | | |
| Rectus femoris | 1.43 0.18 (11) | 1.57 0.23 (14) | | |
| Tibialis anterior | 1.57 0.22 (18) | 1.56 0.22 (21) | 1.77 0.12 (4) | 3.8 (1) |
| Extensor digitorum brevis | 2.07 0.42 (16) | 2.62 0.30 (11) | | |

Table 5. Fibre density in different muscles of normal subjects arranged in four age groups. Number of subjects (n) in parenthesis.

(From Stålberg and Trontelj,[34] with permission.)

charge in 15 other insertions, the average fiber density would be 1.5.[32] In some disease states, single muscle fiber potentials form such a complex pattern that the number of associated discharges may be difficult to count. Therefore, instead of fiber density, it is sometimes convenient to report the percentage of needle insertions that encounter only one single fiber potential without associated discharges. Isolated potentials of one single fiber occur in 65 to 70 percent of random insertions in the normal extensor digitorum communis. Only two fibers discharge in the remaining 30 to 35 percent, and triple potentials occur in 5 percent or less.[32]

## Duration and mean interspike intervals

During the fiber density search, the duration of the action potential complex can also be determined within the recording radius of the needle electrode. This value is defined as the time difference between the first and last single fiber potentials of the same motor unit recorded at each random insertion. It is a measure of the difference in nerve terminal conduction, neuromuscular transmission, and muscle fiber conduction times within the recording radius of the needle. In practice, this is measured from the point of baseline intersection of the first potential, which is greater than 200 $\mu$V in amplitude and less than 300 $\mu$s in rise time, to the corresponding point of the last potential fulfilling the same criteria. At least 20 such measurements are made and the average value obtained. The duration is less than 4 ms in over 95 percent of all multiple potential recordings in the extensor digitorum communis. In contrast, values as high as 40 to 50 ms may be seen in some pathologic conditions.

Another parameter, mean interspike interval (MISI), is calculated by dividing the total duration by the number of intervals (number of spikes minus one). The normal range of MISI in the extensor digitorum communis is 0.3 to 0.7 ms. This value is increased in muscular dystrophy, polymyositis, and early reinnervation.[34]

# JITTER

## Definition and clinical significance

If single fiber potentials are recorded from a muscle after repetitive stimulation of its nerve, the latencies of the elicited response are almost, but not exactly, the same with each stimulus.[6] This latency variability, on the order of tens of microseconds, is referred to as electromyographic jitter, the term previously used in the engineering literature to denote instability of a time-base generator.[8] The motor end-plate is considered to be the main source of jitter in normal muscles.[6] A slight change in the rising slope of the end-plate potential (Fig. 15-3) and fluctuation in the critical level of depolarization necessary for generation of an action potential probably account for most of the variability in transmission time at the neuromuscular junction. Jitter may also reflect the variability in the conduction of impulses along the nerve and muscle fibers, but these factors are considered negligible as discussed later. The stimulation technique may be used in patients who are in coma, and others who are unable to voluntarily activate muscle.

In cooperative patients, however, jitter measurements can best be made in a voluntarily contracting muscle. For this purpose, single fiber potentials are simultaneously recorded from two muscle fibers innervated by adjacent terminal branches of the same axon (Fig. 15-4). The interpotential interval then represents the difference in conduction time from the common branching point to the recording electrode along separate axon terminals and muscle fibers within the same motor unit. Electromyographic jitter is expressed as the degree of variability in the interpotential interval. Sometimes, following increases in the interpotential interval, the second potential fails to appear. This phenomenon, referred to as blocking, is more commonly seen in pathologic conductions such as myasthenia gravis, although it may also occasionally be seen in normal subjects over age 50.[11]

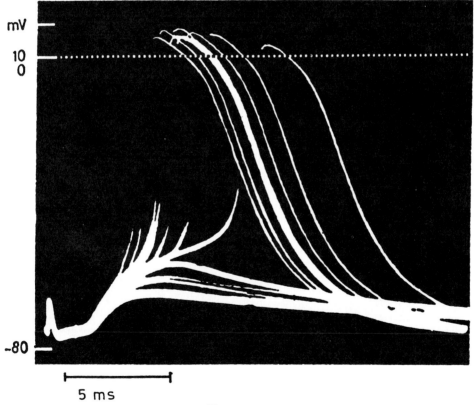

Figure 15-3
End-plate potentials (EPP) and action potentials recorded intracellularly from the end-plate region of a human muscle fiber. Variation in amplitude and slope of EPP is considered one of the main factors contributing to the variability of neuromuscular transmission time (jitter). (From Elmqvist, et al,[14] with permission.)

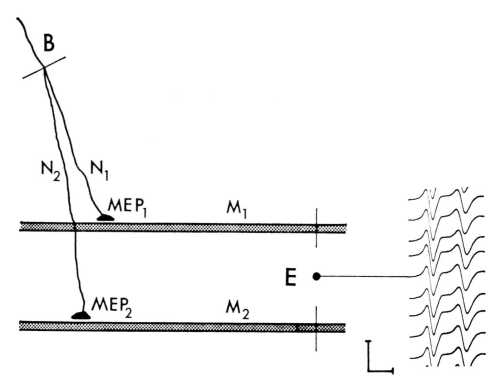

Figure 15-4

Determination of jitter by simultaneous recording from two muscle fibers, $M_1$ and $M_2$, within the same motor unit. The potential from $M_1$ that triggers the sweep is displayed from the onset with the use of a delay line. The potential from $M_2$ appears after a short interpotential interval determined by the difference in conduction time from the common branching point (B) to the recording electrode (E). The variability of the interpotential interval (jitter) mainly occurs at the motor endplates, but changes in propagation time along the terminal axons and muscle fibers also contribute. Calibration in the strip recording: 2mV and 500μs. (From Dahlbäck, Ekstedt, and Stålberg,[4] with permission.)

Propagation of a second impulse along the nerve and muscle is slowed during the refractory period following a preceding impulse. This delay may differentially affect the activation of two muscle fibers, depending on the lengths of their respective axon terminals. If the two muscle fibers under study are widely separated, this in turn might cause fluctuation of the interpotential interval. It might be expected, therefore, that the longer interpotential interval would result in the greater jitter. In normal muscles, however, jitter values are independent of the interpotential interval if the latter does not exceed 4 ms. In most recordings interpotential intervals are less than 1 ms, and changes in conduction time caused by prior discharge largely cancel out between the two potentials. Thus, jitter is primarily attributable to variability in neuromuscular transmission time. This view is further supported by the observation that nonparalytic doses of d-tubocurarine, known to block end-plate depolarization, cause jitter to increase without changing the shape and amplitude of the single muscle fiber potentials.[8] In pathologic conductions in which the interpotential interval may be on the order of many milliseconds, however, variability in the propagation velocity may contribute to the jitter.

## Determination of jitter

To determine jitter, the oscilloscope settings and the techniques for needle manipulation are the same as for fiber density determination. Once paired single fiber potentials fulfilling the criteria are identified, the first of the paired responses is set to trigger the oscilloscope so that the variability in the interpotential interval is seen as a changing delay of the second potential of the pair. Electromyographic jitter may be calculated in several ways. Ekstedt, Nilsson, and Stålberg[13] recommend that the jitter be expressed as the Mean Value of Consecutive Difference (MCD) rather than the standard deviation (SD) about the mean interpotential interval (MIPI). The SD is less suitable, because it measures not only the short-term random variability but also the slow variation of MIPI reflecting fluctuation in propagation velocity. In contrast, the MCD measures only the short-term variation, without the superimposed slow changes, and has the additional advantage of being more easily calculated. Jitter values expressed by the MCD remain the same during continuous activity lasting up to one hour.[13]

The most commonly used method for determination of electromyographic jitter is photographic superimposition of 10 consecutive discharges with a sweep speed of 200 μs per cm or faster (Fig. 15-5). If the first potential triggers the oscilloscope, then the jitter is measured by the variability of a series of second potential, which follows within approximately one millisecond. After 10 paired discharges are recorded, the latency difference between the baseline intersection points of the earliest and latest second potentials is measured. This time range of 10 discharges (R10) is collected for 5 different sampling sites from the same muscle and averaged. The mean range ($MR_{10}$) is then converted to the estimated MCD by multiplying by a conversion factor of 0.37, as described by Ekstedt, Nilsson and Stålberg;[13] i.e., estimated MCD = $MR_{10} \times 0.37$. It has been shown that the value obtained by this formula gives a good approximation to the actual MCD, which can be calculated using a computer program.[21]

## Normal and abnormal jitter values

Table 15-2 summarizes the jitter values for various muscles as reported by Stålberg and Trontelj,[34] who use a very fast sweep speed with the time resolution of 0.3 μs. Jitter measurements may show a different range and higher mean value than those listed if recorded with less time resolution. Thus, it is necessary for each laboratory to establish its own normal ranges. Values are correlated with the age of the subject and the individual muscles tested. The jitter value is relatively constant below the age of 70 in the extensor digitorum communis, whereas it increases around the age of 50 in the tibialis anterior, probably secondary to neurogenic change.[33] In normal muscles, jitter values are the same regardless of the innervation rates or of the recording site relative to the end-plate zone.

Jitter is dependent on the temperature of the muscle, increasing 2 to 3 μs per °C as the temperature falls from 36 to 32°C, followed by a more rapid increase of about 7.5 μs per °C thereafter.[35] Despite an increase in the jitter value, cooling is associated with a reduced decrement of the compound muscle action potentials to a train of stimuli. A number of factors may contribute to the apparent discrepancy. Defective release of transmitter at low temperatures would explain increased jitter and reduced decrement, since with fewer quanta released by the first impulse, more quanta are available for subsequent release. Increases in temperature between 35 and 38°C do not normally change the jitter value.

In normal muscles, jitter may be increased during ischemia or following administration of curare. Jitter is increased not only in diseases of neuromuscular transmission[11] but also in many other conditions associated with conduction abnormalities of nerve and muscle.[30] Increased jitter may result from abnormally low end-plate potentials (EPP) or from a decreased excitability of the muscle fiber membrane. In general, transmission block is preceded by increases in jitter which typically exceed 80 to 100 μs.

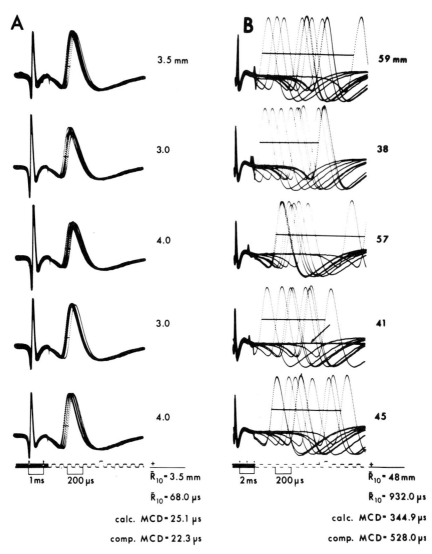

A

3.5 mm

3.0

4.0

3.0

4.0

1ms    200 μs    $\bar{R}_{10}$ = 3.5 mm

$\bar{R}_{10}$ = 68.0 μs

calc. MCD = 25.1 μs

comp. MCD = 22.3 μs

B

59 mm

38

57

41

45

2ms    200 μs    $\bar{R}_{10}$ = 48mm

$\bar{R}_{10}$ = 932.0 μs

calc. MCD = 344.9 μs

comp. MCD = 528.0 μs

Manual calculation of the jitter

Figure 15-5

Manual calculation of jitter in a normal (A) and abnormal (B) action potential pair. Five groups of 10 superimpositions are made and ranges of interpotential interval variation are measured for each group. The mean value is then calculated and multiplied by 0.37 to obtain an approximation to Mean Value of Consecutive Difference (calc MCD), which is comparable to the result determined by a computer (comp MCD). (From Stålberg and Trontelj,[34] with permission.)

## CLINICAL APPLICATION

Single fiber electromyography (SFEMG) can now be recorded using a commercially available system or with minor modification of the conventional units of electromyography. Stålberg and his colleagues have simplified the method so that, with a little extra training, it can be conducted as part of routine electromyography.[34] Although the technique appears to have clinical and research applications for lower motor neuron disorders and diseases of muscle, it is perhaps most useful, from an electrodiagnostic point of view, as a test for disorders of neuromuscular transmission.[11, 29, 36]

TABLE 15-2 Jitter in normal subjects ($\mu$s)

| Muscles | Number of potential pairs | MCD—pooled data | | SD of MCD values from individual subjects | | Upper normal limit close to mean $+3SD$ |
|---|---|---|---|---|---|---|
| | | mean | SD | mean | SD | |
| frontalis (range of means for individual subjects) | 258 | 20.4 (15.7–29.2) | 8.8 | 6.2 (5.5–8.7) | 2.3 | 45 |
| biceps | 125 | 15.6 | 5.9 | | | 35 |
| extensor digitorum communis (range of means for individual subjects) | 759 | 24.6 (16.5–32.0) | 10.6 | 8.3 (2.3–12.4) | 3.2 | 55 |
| rectus femoris | 73 | 31.0 | 12.6 | | | (65)* |
| tibialis anterior | 153 | 32.1 | 15.0 | | | (75)* |
| extensor digitorum brevis | 29 | 85.3 | 68.6 | | | none |

Jitter (MCD) in different muscles of normal subjects, age 10–70 years.
*Since the data are not gaussian distributed, a more appropriate upper normal limit is 60 $\mu$s.
(From Stålberg and Trontelj,[34] with permission.)

## Motor neuron disease and peripheral neuropathy

Various processes affecting the anterior horn cell have been studied.[37] Among motor neuron diseases, fiber density is most increased in the chronic disorders with marked collateral sprouting, for example, chronic spinal muscular atrophy. The duration of the action potential is increased, suggesting a mixture of hypertrophic and atrophic fibers and slowly conducting, newly formed, nerve sprouts. In contrast, rapidly progressive diseases such as amyotrophic lateral sclerosis are characterized by increased jitter and blocking. Stålberg and his colleagues note that SFEMG may be used to characterize the functional status of the motor unit and may help in establishing the diagnosis and prognosis. The study is sometimes abnormal in clinically asymptomatic muscles, even if conventional electromyography is not revealing. Thus, it may be useful in early detection of motor neuron disease.

Disorders of the peripheral nerves are, in general, also associated with increased jitter, occasional blocking, and increased fiber density.[30] These findings seem to be particularly prominent during the process of reinnervation, having been observed, for example, up to one year after autogenous facial muscle transplants.[18] Stålberg and his colleagues have suggested that abnormalities of SFEMG result in part from reinnervation, when seen in patients with polyneuropathies and motor neuron disease, and perhaps also in those with polymyositis and muscular dystrophy. Not all the polyneuropathies are affected similarly, however. Studying the extensor digitorum communis, Thiele and Stålberg[39] noted that fiber density, duration, jitter, and blocking were all increased in patients with alcoholic neuropathy but not in those with diabetic or uremic neuropathy. This may reflect on-going reinnervation of the former, but the exact reason for the discrepancy is not known. Increased jitter values have also been demonstrated in patients with multiple sclerosis, suggesting peripheral nervous system involvement in this disease.[40]

## Myasthenia gravis and myasthenic syndrome

In normal muscles, increased jitter may be found in 1 of 20 recorded potentials.[35] Thus, neuromuscular transmission is considered abnormal only if 2 or more potential pairs of 20 recordings show increased jitter or blocking. Jitter values within any one muscle in a patient with myasthenia gravis may be normal or increased. If the jitter is greater than 100 μs, intermittent blocking may occur.[38] Abnormalities are usually found in more than 30 percent of recorded potential pairs in the extensor digitorum communis. In ocular myasthenia, however, abnormalities may occur only in the facial muscles and not necessarily in the extensor digitorum communis.[23, 38] In about 25 percent of patients with myasthenia gravis the fiber density is slightly increased above the normal range.

Stålberg, Trontelj, and Schwartz[38] emphasize that disturbances of neuromuscular transmission can be detected by means of SFEMG before symptoms are present, and that the diagnosis of myasthenia gravis can be excluded if the jitter is normal in a clinically weak muscle. In their series, increased jitter or blocking was found in the hypothenar muscles in all 40 patients with mild to moderate generalized myasthenia gravis, even though the conventional nerve stimulation technique revealed equivocal results in 40 percent of these cases. Similarly, 127 to 131 patients demonstrated defective neuromuscular transmission by SFEMG, whereas less than 50 percent of these patients showed an abnormality by the conventional nerve stimulation technique in a series reported by Sanders, Howard, and Johns.[23] The SFEMG of the extensor digitorum communis was abnormal in 8 of 24 asymptomatic, first-degree relatives of 12 patients with juvenile myasthenia gravis. In this group, jitter was increased on the average of 5 out of 20 potential pairs, and abnormalities were seen in 25 percent of all recordings, in contrast to 75 percent in clinically symptomatic patients.[38]

The SFEMG abnormalities are well correlated with symptomatic changes in serial studies of the same individuals. Administration of edrophonium (Tensilon) improves abnormal jitter and decreases blocking, although it does not affect initially normal jitter. A therapeutic dosage of anticholinesterase medication may correct jitter in myasthenia. In some cases, however, recovery from total block in a number of fibers after treatment may give an apparent increase in jitter values. In a healthy subject, anticholinesterase does not affect the jitter value. Indeed, a normal jitter value was found in a patient who had received the medication for years for a mistaken diagnosis of myasthenia gravis.[34] The SFEMG may occasionally return to normal during spontaneous remission or after thymectomy, but most of these patients still show increased jitter without blocking.[34]

The myasthenic syndrome is also associated with increased jitter as high as 500 μs, with the interpotential interval ranging up to 2 ms for 50 discharges.[24, 25] In this syndrome the degree of blocking and jitter values decrease as the stimulation rate increases, and the transmission worsens following rest. These findings contrast with those typically seen in patients with myasthenia gravis. Blocking tends to occur with higher jitter values in the myasthenic syndrome than in myasthenia gravis. In accordance with changes seen in Type II fiber grouping,[20] fiber density has been reported to be slightly increased in this syndrome.[34]

## Dystrophy and myositis

In Duchenne dystrophy, fiber density is markedly increased. In one series,[29] it was 3.5 in contrast to 1.45 in normal muscle. In the late stage, fiber density was less, although still above normal. Jitter was increased in about 30 percent of the recordings in each muscle, and occasional blocking was noted in 10 percent of the recordings with increased jitter.[31] Interestingly, some potential pairs showed jitter values below the normal range. Stålberg has suggested that the potential pairs with reduced jitter are generated by split muscle fibers that share a common innervation zone. This view is supported by the observation that, when subjected to d-tubocurarine or other agents that inhibit neuromuscular transmission, blocking always occurs simultaneously in the paired potentials. This is not the case with ordinary potential pairs.

Patients with limb-girdle dystrophy have also been shown to have increased fiber density, but to a lesser degree than in Duchenne dystrophy.[28] In this series, jitter was increased in 54 percent of the recordings in clinically weak muscles, and blocking occurred in less than 10 percent. The findings in facioscapulohumeral dystrophy were similar to those in patients with limb-girdle dystrophy.[28] The pathophysiology of these SFEMG abnormalities is not clear. Increased jitter may be related to altered propagation time in the muscle fibers as demonstrated by Stålberg.[26] Increased fiber density may be attributable to reinnervation of a portion of the muscle fiber separated from the end-plate by transverse lesions, as shown in Duchenne dystrophy by Desmedt and Borenstein.[5] Alternatively, it may result from new innervation of regenerating muscle fibers or splitting of muscle fibers.[27]

In polymyositis, a portion of the affected muscle fiber is separated from its motor end-plate by a segmental degeneration. This probably accounts for the presence of denervation potentials in this disorder. The denervated portion of the muscle fiber may then be reinnervated by collateral sprouts. The SFEMG shows increased fiber density, jitter, and blocking, perhaps as the result of reinnervation of previously degenerated muscle segments.[19]

# REFERENCE SOURCES

1.  ADRIAN, ED AND BRONK, DW: *The discharge of impulses in motor nerve fibres. Part II. The frequency of discharge in reflex and voluntary contractions.* J Physiol (Lond) 67:119, 1929.

2.  BORENSTEIN, S AND DESMEDT, JE: *Local cooling in myasthenia. Improvement of neuromuscular failure.* Arch Neurol 32:152, 1975.

3.  BUCHTHAL, F, GULD, C, AND ROSENFALCK, P: *Multielectrode study of the territory of a motor unit.* Acta Physiol Scand 39:83, 1957.

4.  DAHLBÄCK, LO, EKSTEDT, J, AND STÅLBERG, E: *Ischemic effects on impulse transmission to muscle fibers in man.* Electroenceph Clin Neurophysiol 29:579, 1970.

5.  DESMEDT, JE AND BORENSTEIN, S: *Regeneration in Duchenne muscular dystrophy. Electromyographic evidence.* Arch Neurol 33:642, 1976.

6.  EKSTEDT, J: *Human single muscle fiber action potentials.* Acta Physiol Scand (suppl 226)61:1, 1964.

7.  EKSTEDT, J AND STÅLBERG, E: *A method of recording extracellular action potentials of single muscle fibres and measuring their propagation velocity in voluntarily activated human muscle.* Bulletin of the American Association of Electromyography and Electrodiagnosis 10:16, 1963.

8.  EKSTEDT, J AND STÅLBERG, E: *The effect of non-paralytic doses of D-tubocurarine on individual motor end-plates in man, studied with a new electrophysiological method.* Electroenceph Clin Neurophysiol 27:557, 1969.

9.  EKSTEDT, J AND STÅLBERG, E: *How the size of the needle electrode leading-off surface influences the shape of the single muscle fibre action potential in electromyography.* Computer Prog Biomed 3:204, 1973.

10. EKSTEDT, J AND STÅLBERG, E: *Single fibre electromyography for the study of the microphysiology of the human muscle.* In DESMEDT, JE (ED): *New Developments in Electromyography and Clinical Neurophysiology,* Vol 1. Karger, Basel, 1973, pp 89–112.

11. EKSTEDT, J AND STÅLBERG, E: *Single muscle fibre electromyography in myasthenia gravis.* In KUNZE, K AND DESMEDT, JE (EDS): *Studies in Neuromuscular Diseases.* Proceedings of the International Symposium (Giessen) Karger, Basel, 1975, pp 157–161.

12.  EKSTEDT, J, HÄGGQVIST, P, AND STÅLBERG, E: *The construction of needle multi-electrodes for single fiber electromyography.* Electroenceph Clin Neurophysiol 27:540, 1969.

13.  EKSTEDT, J, NILSSON, G, AND STÅLBERG, E: *Calculation of the electromyographic jitter.* J Neurol Neurosurg Psychiatry 37:526, 1974.

14.  ELMQVIST, D, ET AL: *An electrophysiological investigation of neuromuscular transmission in myasthenia gravis.* J Physiol (Lond) 174:417, 1964.

15.  GATH, I AND STÅLBERG, E: *Frequency and time domain characteristics of single muscle fibre action potentials.* Electroenceph Clin Neurophysiol 39:371, 1975.

16.  GATH, I AND STÅLBERG, E: *On the volume conduction in human skeletal muscle: In situ measurements.* Electroenceph Clin Neurophysiol 43:106, 1977.

17.  GATH, I AND STÅLBERG, E: *The calculated radial decline of the extracellular action potential compared with in situ measurements in the human brachial biceps.* Electroenceph Clin Neurophysiol 44:547, 1978.

18.  HAKELIUS, L AND STÅLBERG, E: *Electromyographical studies of free autogenous muscle transplants in man.* Scand J Plast Reconstr Surg 8:211, 1974.

19.  HENRIKSSON, KG AND STÅLBERG, E: *The terminal innervation pattern in polymyositis: A histochemical and SFEMG study.* Muscle and Nerve 1:3, 1978.

20.  HENRIKSSON, KG, ET AL: *Clinical, neurophysiological and morphological findings in Eaton Lambert syndrome.* Acta Neurol Scand 56:117, 1977.

21.  MIHELIN, M, TRONTELJ, JV AND TRONTELJ, JK: *Automatic measurement of random interpotential intervals in single fibre electromyography.* Int J Bio-Med Comp 6:181, 1975.

22.  PAYAN, J: *The blanket principle: A technical note.* Muscle and Nerve 1:423, 1978.

23.  SANDERS, DB, HOWARD, JF, JR, AND JOHNS, TR: *Single-fiber electromyography in myasthenia gravis.* Neurology (New York) 29:68, 1979.

24.  SCHWARTZ, MS AND STÅLBERG, E: *Myasthenia gravis with features of the myasthenic syndrome. An investigation with electrophysiologic methods including single-fiber electromyography.* Neurology (Minneap) 25:80, 1975.

25.  SCHWARTZ, MS AND STÅLBERG, E: *Myasthenic syndrome studied with single fiber electromyography.* Arch Neurol 32:815, 1975.

26.  STÅLBERG, E: *Propagation velocity in human muscle fibers in situ.* Acta Physiol Scand (suppl 287)70:1, 1966.

27.  STÅLBERG, E: *Single fibre electromyography for motor unit study in man.* In SHAHANI, M (ED): *The Motor System: Neurophysiology and Muscle Mechanisms.* Elsevier, Amsterdam, 1976, pp 79–92.

28.  STÅLBERG, E: *Electrogenesis in human dystrophic muscle.* In ROWLAND, LP (ED): *Pathogenesis of Human Muscular Dystrophies.* Excerpta Medica, Amsterdam, 1977.

29.  STÅLBERG, E: *Neuromuscular transmission studied with single fibre electromyography.* Acta Anaesth Scand (suppl 70):112, 1978.

30.  STÅLBERG, E AND EKSTEDT, J: *Single fibre EMG and microphysiology of the motor unit in normal and diseased human muscle.* In DESMEDT, JE (ED): *New Developments in Electromyography and Clinical Neurophysiology,* Vol 1. Karger, Basel, 1973, pp 113–129.

31.  STÅLBERG, E AND THIELE, B: *Transmission block in terminal nerve twigs: A single fibre electromyographic finding in man.* J Neurol Neurosurg Psychiatry 35:52, 1972.

32.  STÅLBERG, E AND THIELE, B: *Motor unit fibre density in the extensor digitorum communis muscle. Single fibre electromyographic study in normal subjects at different ages.* J Neurol Neurosurg Psychiatry 38:874, 1975.

33.  STÅLBERG, E AND TRONTELJ, JV: *Demonstration of axon reflexes in human motor nerve fibres.* J Neurol Neurosurg Psychiatry 33:571, 1970.

34.  STÅLBERG, E AND TRONTELJ, J: *Single Fibre Electromyography.* The Miraville Press Limited, Old Woking, Surrey, U.K., 1979.

35.  STÅLBERG, E, EKSTEDT, J, AND BROMAN, A: *The electromyographic jitter in normal human muscles.* Electroenceph Clin Neurophysiol 31:429, 1971.

36.  STÅLBERG, E, EKSTEDT, J, AND BROMAN, A: *Neuromuscular transmission in myasthenia gravis studied with single fibre electromyography.* J Neurol Neurosurg Psychiatry 37:540, 1974.

37. STÅLBERG, E, SCHWARTZ, MS, AND TRONTELJ, JV: *Single fibre electromyography in various processes affecting the anterior horn cell.* J Neurol Sci 24:403, 1975.

38. STÅLBERG, E, TRONTELJ, JV, AND SCHWARTZ, MS: *Single-muscle-fiber recording of the jitter phenomenon in patients with myasthenia gravis and in members of their families.* Ann NY Acad Sci 274:189, 1976.

39. THIELE, B AND STÅLBERG, E: *Single fibre EMG findings in polyneuropathies of different aetiology.* J Neurol Neurosurg Psychiatry 38:881, 1975.

40. WEIR, A, HANSEN, S, AND BALLANTYNE, JP: *Single fibre electromyographic jitter in multiple sclerosis.* J Neurol Neurosurg Psychiatry 42:1146, 1979.

# PART
# 5

# TESTS FOR
# LESS ACCESSIBLE REGIONS
# OF THE NERVOUS SYSTEM

# 16

# THE BLINK REFLEX

The mechanically or electrically elicited blink reflex has been studied extensively.[13, 15, 18, 44, 47, 60, 65, 69, 70, 76, 77] The response is analogous to the corneal reflex tested in ordinary clinical practice, but the use of an oscilloscope display allows a more meaningful assessment with accurate quantitative analysis.[1, 52, 62, 79] Stimulation of the supraorbital nerve elicits two temporally separate responses of the orbicularis oculi, an early R1 and a late R2 component (Fig. 16-1). Of the two, R1 is evoked only on the side of stimulation as a pontine reflex,[29, 76] whereas R2 is recorded bilaterally with unilateral stimulation. The R2 response is presumably relayed through a more complex route including the pons and lateral medulla.[11, 24, 40, 61, 80]

The more reproducible R1 provides a better means for assessing nerve conduction of the reflex pathways. Analysis of R2, however, helps determine whether the lesion affects the afferent (trigeminal nerve) or efferent arc (facial nerve) of the reflex.[23, 40] A lesion of the trigeminal nerve delays or diminishes R2 bilaterally when the affected side is stimulated (afferent involvement). A lesion of the facial nerve alters R2 only on the affected side regardless of the side of stimulation (efferent involvement). Parenthetically, this distinction between an afferent and efferent delay of R2 resembles the clinical analysis of the pupillary light reflex.

## DIRECT VERSUS REFLEX RESPONSES

### Stimulation of the facial nerve

Determination of nerve excitability consists of applying shocks of increasing intensity and inspecting the visible contraction of the facial muscles. The normal threshold has been reported to be 3.0 to 8.0 mA. However, individual variation in skin resistance, skin temperature, and the anatomic course of the facial nerve makes it impossible to set a reliable standard. Comparisons with the unaffected nerve on the opposite side reduce the number of variables to a minimum. In healthy subjects, differences between left and right are usually less than 2.0 mA. After complete section of the nerve at a proximal site, distal excitability remains normal up to four days. However, complete loss of excitability occurs by the end of the first week, when the nerve undergoes wallerian degeneration. Hence, normal excitability during the first week after onset suggests a good prognosis for recovery.[22]

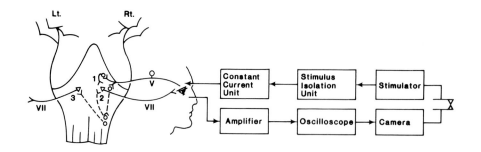

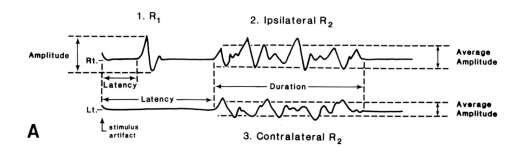

1. R₁ 2. Ipsilateral R₂

Amplitude

Average Amplitude

Average Amplitude

3. Contralateral R₂

**A**

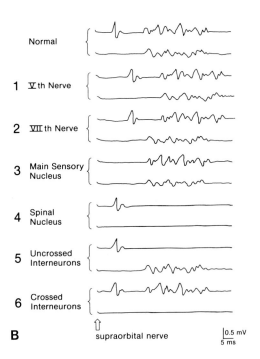

Normal

1 Ⅴth Nerve

2 Ⅶth Nerve

3 Main Sensory Nucleus

4 Spinal Nucleus

5 Uncrossed Interneurons

6 Crossed Interneurons

supraorbital nerve

0.5 mV
5 ms

**B**

As opposed to nerve excitability testing by visual inspection of contracting muscle, electrical recording of muscle action potentials allows a quantitative assessment. Stimulating the facial nerve with the cathode placed just anterior to the mastoid process elicits compound muscle action potentials in the facial muscles (Fig. 16-2). Designated as the direct response, it contrasts with the reflex responses of the orbicularis oculi elicited by stimulation of the trigeminal nerve. Its latency is measured from the stimulus artifact to the beginning of the evoked potential. Determination of nerve excitability, although no longer widely practiced, may supplement studies of the direct response.[14]

The amplitude of the direct response varies substantially from one subject to the next. Thus, the comparison between the sides in the same individual is more meaningful than the absolute value. An amplitude reduction to one half that of the response on the normal side suggests distal degeneration. More important, serial determinations reveal progressive amplitude changes as an increasing number of axons degenerate (Fig. 16-3). As illustrated in Chapter 7 (see Fig. 7-1), a strong shock applied in this region may inadvertently activate the masseter muscle, since its motor point lies near the stimulus point. In this instance, visual inspection allows discrimination of the contracting muscle and the presence of unintended volume-conducted potentials.

## Stimulation of the trigeminal nerve

Stimulation of the trigeminal nerve elicits reflex contraction of the orbicularis oculi. In contrast to the direct response, which provides a measure of distal nerve excitability, the blink reflex reflects the integrity of the afferent and efferent pathways including the proximal segment of the facial nerve. As mentioned earlier, a single shock to the supraorbital nerve evokes two separate contractile responses of the orbicularis oculi. The latency of R1 represents the conduction time along the trigeminal and facial nerve and pontine relay. R2 is less reliable for this purpose, because of inherent latency variability from one trial to the next. Furthermore, the latency of R2 reflects excitability of interneurons and synaptic transmission in addition to axonal conduction.

Subjects lie supine on a bed in a warm room with the eyes open or gently closed. Surface electrodes are used for stimulation of the nerve and recording of the evoked muscle action potentials.[44] We place the recording electrode ($G_1$) on the upper or lower lateral aspect of the orbicularis oculi with a reference electrode ($G_2$) on the temple or the lateral surface of the nose and a ground electrode under the chin or around the arm (Fig. 16-4). The supraorbital, infraorbital, or mental nerve is stimulated with the cath-

←─────────────────────────────────────────────

Figure 16-1

(A) Top: Stimulation and recording arrangement for the blink reflex. The presumed pathway of R1 through the pons (1) and direct and consensual R2 through the pons and lateral medulla (2 and 3) are schematically indicated. Dotted lines indicate the presence of multiple interneurons. The primary afferents of R1 and R2 are shown as one fiber in the illustration. This and other details of central connections of these reflexes are not known. Bottom: A typical oscilloscope recording of the blink reflex after right-sided stimulation. Note an ipsilateral R1 response and bilateral simultaneous R2 responses. (From Kimura,[37] with permission.) (B) Five basic types of blink reflex abnormalities. From top to bottom, the finding suggests a conduction abnormality of the (1) afferent pathway along the trigeminal nerve; (2) efferent pathway along the facial nerve; (3) main sensory nucleus or pontine interneurons to the facial nucleus (1 in part A); (4) spinal tract and nucleus or medullary interneurons to the facial nuclei on both sides; (5) uncrossed medullary interneurons to the ipsilateral facial nucleus (2 of part A); and (6) crossed medullary interneurons to the contralateral facial nucleus (3 of part A). Increased latencies of R1 are usually seen with involvement of the reflex arc itself, whereas the loss or diminution of R1 or R2 may occur not only with lesions directly affecting the reflex pathway but also with distant lesions indirectly influencing the excitability of the interneurons and motor neurons.

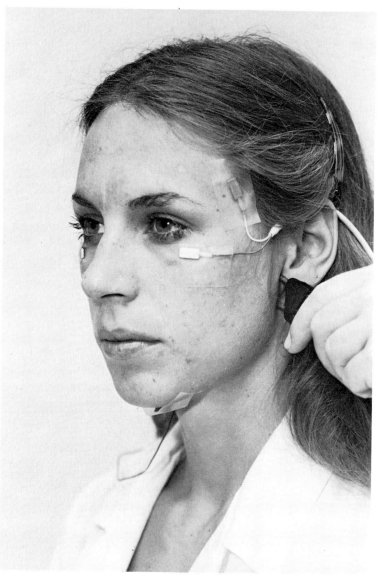

Figure 16-2

Technique for recording the direct response. The facial nerve is stimulated percutaneously with the cathode placed just anterior to the mastoid process. The muscle action potentials may be recorded from any muscles of the face. When tested in conjunction with the blink reflex, the active electrode ($G_1$) is placed on the orbicularis oculi and the reference electrode ($G_2$) on the temple or the side of the nose. In contrast to the blink reflex, the direct response, of course, is recorded only unilaterally on the side of stimulus.

ode placed over the respective foramen on one side. A two channel machine allows simultaneous recording from the orbicularis oculi on both sides. Assessment of facial synkinesis described later in this chapter requires two pairs of recording electrodes on the same side of the face, one pair over the orbicularis oculi and the other over the orbicularis oris or platysma.[3, 45]

Shocks of optimal intensity elicit maximum and nearly stable responses with repeated trials. We use the same intensity on each side in order to compare relative

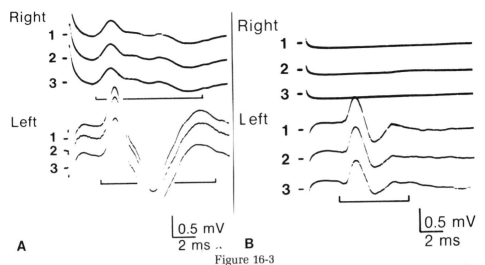

Figure 16-3

Direct response on the right (top three tracings) and left (bottom three tracings) in a patient with traumatic facial diplegia. (A) The compound muscle action potential recorded from the right orbicularis oculi was normal in latency but significantly reduced in amplitude when compared with the opposite side. This finding indicated that a substantial number of axons had already degenerated distally on the right. Distal excitability of the left facial nerve was considered normal despite clinical weakness. (Compare part B.) (B) A repeat study in one week. No evoked potential could be recorded from the right orbicularis oculi, indicating total distal degeneration of the right facial nerve. The compound muscle action potential recorded from the left orbicularis oculi was considerably smaller than the one obtained a week earlier, suggesting the beginning of delayed degeneration. A follow up examination a week later showed no direct response on either side (see Fig. 7-1).

excitability of the reflexes elicited by right-sided and left-sided stimulation. The reflex latency of R1 is measured from the stimulus artifact to the initial deflection of the evoked potential. For each subject at least eight responses are measured and the shortest latency is determined. The latency ratios of R1 to the direct response (R/D ratio) provide a means to compare the conduction through the distal segment of the facial nerve with that of the entire reflex arc, which includes the trigeminal nerve and the proximal segment of the facial nerve.

If R1 is absent or not reproducible with single shocks of appropriate intensities, we use paired stimuli with an interstimulus interval of 3 to 5 ms to facilitate the response and determine the shortest latency. A pair of stimuli usually consists of a subthreshold conditioning shock to subliminally excite the motor neurons and a supramaximal test stimulus (Figs. 16-5 and 16-6 A and B). Since the recorded response is elicited by the second and not the first stimulus, the latency is determined from the second shock artifact.

Determining the latency of R1 requires control of stimulus artifact, since $G_1$ and $G_2$ lie only a few centimeters away from the cathode. Using a conventional amplifier, R1 tends to be coincident with the stimulus artifact even though its latency is in the order of 10 ms. Usual care in reducing surface spread of stimulus current, however, helps accomplish optimal recording of short latency responses. We use a specially designed amplifier with a short blocking time (0.1 ms) and low internal noise (0.5 $\mu$V RMS at bandwidth of 2 KHz) developed to minimize the problem of stimulus artifact. Details of this amplifier have been described elsewhere[81] and are discussed in Appendix 2B. Frequency response ranges from 20 Hz to 32 KHz for recording either the R1 or R2 components.

In addition to electrical stimulation of the supraorbital nerve, a mechanical tap over the glabella elicits the blink reflex.[20, 47, 76] We use a specially constructed reflex

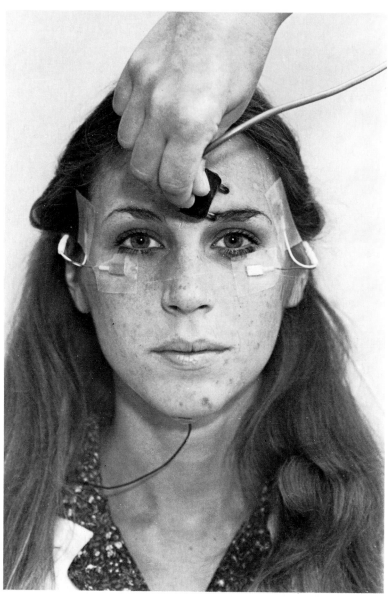

Figure 16-4

Technique for recording the blink reflex. The supraorbital nerve is stimulated percutaneously with the cathode placed over the supraorbital foramen on one side. The muscle action potentials are recorded simultaneously from the right and left orbicularis oculi. The active recording electrode ($G_1$) is placed over either the inferior or superior portion of the orbicularis oculi near the outer canthus and the reference electrode ($G_2$) on the temple or the side of the nose. The shock artifact may be reduced considerably if an optimal position of the stimulating electrodes is selected by rotating the anode around the cathode.

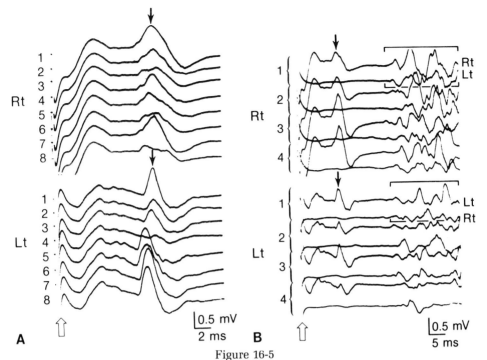

Figure 16-5

(A) R1 components recorded from the orbicularis oculi after stimulation of the supraorbital nerve by single supramaximal stimuli (top four trials on each side) or by paired stimuli with interstimulus interval of 5 ms (bottom four trials on each side). The first of the paired stimuli was a subthreshold shock that subliminally primed the motor neuron pool. The second stimulus was a supramaximal shock that activated the reflex and triggered the oscilloscope sweep. (From Kimura,[37] with permission.) (B) Simultaneous recording from ipsilateral (upper tracing in each frame) and contralateral (lower tracing) orbicularis oculi after unilateral stimulation of the supraorbital nerve either with single shocks (top two trials on each side) or with paired shocks (bottom two trials on each side). The first of the paired stimuli was a subthreshold shock, whereas the second stimulus was a supramaximal shock that triggered the oscilloscope sweep. Note unilateral R1 (arrows) recorded only in the upper tracing in each frame and bilateral R2 (brackets) in both upper and lower tracings. Slight variability of R2 in latency and amplitude is not uncommon in normal subjects. (From Kimura,[37] with permission.)

hammer with a built in microswitch that closes on impact and triggers a sweep. Other pressure-sensitive devices are also available commercially. Although the stimulus is a gentle tap, this is a cutaneous rather than a stretch reflex, probably relayed via the same polysynaptic reflex pathways as the electrically elicited blink reflex. However, in contrast to unilateral electrical stimulation, the glabellar tap elicits the R1 component bilaterally, allowing instantaneous comparison between the two sides (Fig. 16-6C). The latency of R1 is a few milliseconds greater when elicited by a glabellar tap as compared with an electrical stimulation. The discrepancy seems only partly accounted for by additional length of the afferent arc from the glabella to the supraorbital foramen.

The R2 component elicited by a glabellar tap provides confirmation of an afferent or efferent abnormality of the electrically elicited R2. A glabellar tap stimulates the right and left trigeminal nerves simultaneously, each of which activates the facial nuclei on both sides to elicit bilateral R2 responses. A consistent latency or amplitude difference between simultaneously recorded right- and left-sided R2 indicates a delay or block in the facial nerve, or in the final common path. A lesion affecting the afferent arc does not alter R2 on either side owing to crossed afferent input from the unaffected

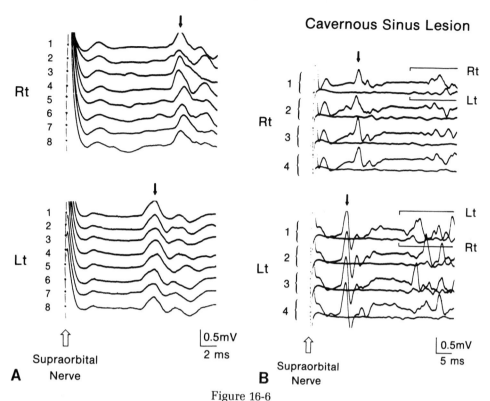

Cavernous Sinus Lesion

Figure 16-6

Blink reflex in a 68-year-old man with a mass lesion involving the right anterior cavernous sinus. (A) R1 (arrow) obtained with the same stimulation and recording arrangements as in Figure 16-5A. Note substantially increased latency of R1 on the right. (B) R2 (bracket) recorded as in Figure 16-5B. With right-sided stimulation, R2 is delayed and small in amplitude, bilaterally. With left-sided stimulation, R2 is normal on both sides. These findings suggest a lesion involving the afferent arc of the reflex pathway on the right. (Compare Figure 16-1B.)

side (Fig. 16-6C). A glabellar tap is better tolerated by some patients and causes no shock artifacts. In our experience, however, electrical stimulation of the supraorbital nerve generally provides more precise information.

# NORMAL VALUES IN ADULTS AND INFANTS

Table 16-1 shows the normal latency range of the direct response, R1, R/D ratio, and R2 elicited by stimulation of the supraorbital nerve in 83 healthy subjects, 7 to 86 years of age (average age, 37) and in 30 full-term neonates.[35, 42] In the 113 subjects, R1 was recorded in all but three infants. Its latency in neonates was significantly greater than that in adults, despite the considerably shorter reflex arc in the former. Unlike the consistent response in adults, R2 is difficult to elicit in infants[9, 25] and was recorded in only 20 of 30 neonates, mostly on the side ipsilateral to the stimulus.[42] Both direct and reflex responses vary considerably in amplitude from one individual to the next. In 60 nerves from 30 healthy subjects, 7 to 67 years of age, the average values were 1.21 ± 0.77 mV (mean ± SD), 0.38 ± 0.23 mV, 0.53 ± 0.24 mV, and 0.49 ± 0.24 mV for direct response, R1, ipsilateral R2, and contralateral R2, respectively.[44]

In 50 other healthy subjects, 12 to 77 years of age (average age 40), the infraorbital and mental nerves were tested in addition to the supraorbital nerve on each side of the

# Cavernous Sinus Lesion

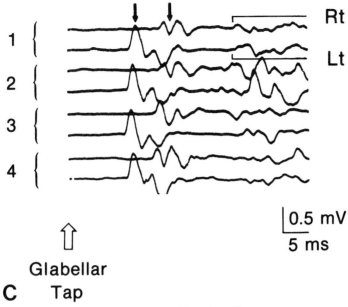

Figure 16-6 (*Continued*)

(C) R1 (arrow) and R2 (bracket) after a glabellar tap. Note a delayed R1 on the right in conjunction with a normal R2, bilaterally. Because of crossed and uncrossed input from the trigeminal nerve, a unilateral lesion involving the afferent arc results in no alteration of R2 when elicited by a glabellar tap.

face. The reflex response was recorded from the orbicularis oculi on both sides. Stimulation of the supraorbital nerve elicited both R1 and R2 regularly. When the infraorbital nerve was stimulated R2 was present in all, but R1 was inconsistent. Stimulation of the mental nerve elicited R2 inconsistently and R1 only rarely. The latencies of R1 and R2 were similar for the supraorbital and infraorbital nerves. However, R2 elicited by stimulation of the mental nerve was considerably greater in latency.

## Upper and lower limits of normal values

We use the mean latency plus three standard deviations as the upper limit of normal. The direct response is considered delayed if it exceeds 4.1 ms, and R1 is delayed if it exceeds 13.0 ms. Additionally, the latency of the direct response should not vary more than 0.6 ms between the two sides in one subject and that of R1 should not vary more than 1.2 ms. The R/D ratio is considered abnormal if its falls outside the range of 2.6 to 4.6, two standard deviations above and below the mean in normals.

With stimulation of the supraorbital nerve, R2 latency should not exceed 40 ms on the side of stimulus and 41 ms on the contralateral side. Two types of comparison are possible. First, the ipsilateral and the contralateral R2 simultaneously evoked by stimulation on one side should not vary more than 5 ms in latency. Secondly, a latency difference between R2 evoked by right-sided stimulation and corresponding R2 evoked by left-sided stimulation should not exceed 7 ms. With stimulation of the infraorbital and mental nerves, the upper limit is 41 ms and 50 ms, respectively, on the side of stimulus and 42 ms and 51 ms, respectively, on the contralateral side.

**TABLE 16-1 Normal subjects and patients with polyneuropathies and multiple sclerosis (mean ± SD)**

| Category | Number of patients | Direct response right and left Combined | | | R1 right and left combined | | | Direct response ms | R1 ms | R/D ratio | Ipsilateral R2 ms | Contralateral R2 ms |
|---|---|---|---|---|---|---|---|---|---|---|---|---|
| | | Abs | Delay | Nl | Abs | Delay | Nl | | | | | |
| Normal adults | 83 | 0 | 0 | 166 | 0 | 0 | 166 | 2.9 ± 0.4 | 10.5 ± 0.8 | 3.6 ± 0.5 | 30.5 ± 3.4 | 30.5 ± 4.4 |
| Normal neonates | 60 | 0 | 0 | 120 | 6 | 0 | 114 | 3.3 ± 0.4 | 12.1 ± 1.0 | 3.7 ± 0.4 | 35.9 ± 2.5 | often absent |
| Guillain-Barré syndrome | 90 | 12 | 63 | 105 | 20 | 78 | 82 | 4.2 ± 2.1 | 15.1 ± 5.9 | 3.9 ± 1.3 | 37.4 ± 8.9 | 37.7 ± 8.4 |
| Chronic inflammatory polyneuropathy | 14 | 4 | 13 | 11 | 7 | 13 | 8 | 5.8 ± 2.6 | 16.4 ± 6.4 | 3.1 ± 0.5 | 39.5 ± 9.4 | 42.0 ± 10.3 |
| Fisher syndrome | 4 | 0 | 0 | 8 | 0 | 1 | 7 | 2.7 ± 0.2 | 10.7 ± 0.8 | 3.9 ± 0.4 | 31.8 ± 1.3 | 31.4 ± 1.9 |
| Hereditary motor sensory neuropathy Type I | 62 | 9 | 88 | 27 | 0 | 105 | 19 | 6.7 ± 2.7 | 17.0 ± 3.7 | 2.8 ± 0.9 | 39.5 ± 5.7 | 39.3 ± 6.4 |
| Hereditary motor sensory neuropathy Type II | 17 | 0 | 0 | 34 | 1 | 0 | 33 | 2.9 ± 0.4 | 10.1 ± 0.6 | 3.6 ± 0.6 | 30.1 ± 3.8 | 30.1 ± 3.7 |
| Diabetic polyneuropathy | 86 | 2 | 20 | 150 | 1 | 17 | 154 | 3.4 ± 0.6 | 11.4 ± 1.2 | 3.4 ± 0.5 | 33.7 ± 4.6 | 34.8 ± 5.3 |
| Multiple sclerosis with clinical pontine signs | 62 | 0 | 0 | 124 | 1 | 44 | 79 | 2.9 ± 0.5 | 12.3 ± 2.7 | 4.3 ± 0.9 | 35.8 ± 8.4 | 37.7 ± 8.0 |

(Modified from Kimura.[37])

# NEUROLOGIC DISORDERS
# WITH ABNORMAL BLINK REFLEX

Tables 16-1 through 16-3 summarize a ten-year experience with the blink reflex in our laboratory.[30, 32, 33, 35, 40, 42, 43, 46, 49] The findings in each category will be briefly summarized below.

## Trigeminal neuralgia and paratrigeminal syndrome

The trigeminal nerve constitutes the afferent arc of the reflex pathway.[46, 60] In patients with trigeminal neuralgia, R1 was abnormal in 7 and normal in 89. Since 3 of the 7 had undergone nerve avulsion prior to the test, only 4 of 93 patients with idiopathic trigeminal neuralgia showed a block or slowing of R1. These findings suggest that nerve conduction tends to be normal along the first division of the trigeminal nerve in this disorder. In contrast, 10 of 17 patients with tumor, infection, or other demonstrable causes for facial pain showed significant delay of R1 on the affected side (Fig. 16-6a). In these patients, R2 was often, although not always, delayed bilaterally when the affected side was stimulated, indicating involvement of the afferent arc of the blink reflex (Fig. 16-6b). Normal conduction along the distal segment of the facial nerve tended to increase the R/D ratio.

## Bell's palsy

Blink reflex latencies reflect the conduction along the entire length of the facial nerve, including the interosseous portion involved in Bell's palsy.[43, 44, 64, 66, 69, 71] Thus, abnormalities were detected in all 144 patients during the first week of Bell's palsy, although they were not necessarily apparent at the onset. (In two patients not included in this study, however, the blink reflex remained normal throughout the entire course of minimal unilateral facial weakness lasting one to two days, perhaps representing an unusually mild form of Bell's palsy.) All patients showed delayed or absent R1 on the paretic

**TABLE 16-2 Affected and normal sides in patients with unilateral neurologic diseases (mean ± SD)**

| | Number of patients | Direct response ms | R1 ms | R/D ratio | Ipsilateral R2 ms | Contralateral R2 ms |
|---|---|---|---|---|---|---|
| Trigeminal neuralgia | | | | | | |
| Affected side | 89 | 2.9 ± 0.4 | 10.6 ± 1.0 | 3.7 ± 0.6 | 30.4 ± 4.4 | 31.6 ± 4.5 |
| Normal side | 89 | 2.9 ± 0.5 | 10.5 ± 0.9 | 3.7 ± 0.6 | 30.5 ± 4.2 | 31.1 ± 4.7 |
| Paratrigeminal syndrome | | | | | | |
| Affected side | 17 | 3.1 ± 0.5 | 11.9 ± 1.8 | 3.9 ± 1.0 | 36.0 ± 5.5 | 37.2 ± 5.7 |
| Normal side | 17 | 3.2 ± 0.6 | 10.3 ± 1.1 | 3.4 ± 0.6 | 33.7 ± 3.5 | 34.8 ± 4.1 |
| Bell's palsy | | | | | | |
| Affected side | 100 | 2.9 ± 0.6 | 12.8 ± 1.6 | 4.4 ± 0.9 | 33.9 ± 4.9 | 30.5 ± 4.9 |
| Normal side | 100 | 2.8 ± 0.4 | 10.2 ± 1.0 | 3.7 ± 0.6 | 30.5 ± 4.3 | 34.0 ± 5.4 |
| Acoustic neuroma | | | | | | |
| Affected side | 26 | 3.2 ± 0.7 | 14.0 ± 2.7 | 4.6 ± 1.7 | 38.2 ± 8.2 | 36.6 ± 8.2 |
| Normal side | 26 | 2.9 ± 0.4 | 10.9 ± 0.9 | 3.8 ± 0.5 | 33.1 ± 3.5 | 35.3 ± 4.5 |
| Wallenberg syndrome | | | | | | |
| Affected side | 23 | 3.2 ± 0.6 | 10.9 ± 0.7 | 3.6 ± 0.6 | 40.7 ± 4.6 | 38.4 ± 7.1 |
| Normal side | 23 | 3.2 ± 0.4 | 10.7 ± 0.5 | 3.4 ± 0.4 | 34.0 ± 5.7 | 35.1 ± 5.8 |

## TABLE 16-3 Direct response and R1 and R2 of the blink reflex

| Disorders | Direct response | R1 | R2 |
|---|---|---|---|
| Trigeminal neuralgia | Normal | Normal (95%) | Normal |
| Paratrigeminal syndrome | Normal | Abnormal on the affected side (59%) | Abnormal on both sides when affected side stimulated (afferent type) |
| Bell's palsy | Normal unless distal segment degenerated | Abnormal on the affected side (99%) | Abnormal on the affected side regardless of the side of the stimulus (efferent type) |
| Acoustic neuroma | Normal unless distal segment degenerated | Abnormal on the affected side (85%) | Afferent and/or efferent type |
| Guillain-Barré syndrome | Abnormal (42%) | Abnormal (54%) | Afferent and/or efferent type |
| Hereditary motor sensory neuropathy Type I | Abnormal (78%) | Abnormal (85%) | Afferent and/or efferent type |
| Diabetic polyneuropathy | Abnormal (13%) | Abnormal (10%) | Afferent and/or efferent type |
| Multiple sclerosis | Normal | Abnormal with pontine or lateral medullary lesion | Afferent and/or efferent type |
| Wallenberg syndrome | Normal | Normal or borderline | Afferent type |
| Facial hypesthesia | Normal | Abnormal with lesions of the trigeminal nerve or pons | Afferent type |
| Comatose state, Akinetic mutism & Locked-in syndrome | Normal | Abnormal with pontine lesion; reduced excitability in acute supratentorial lesion | Absent on both sides regardless of side of stimulus |

side of the face. In addition, R2 was affected on the paretic side, regardless of the side of stimulation, consonant with efferent involvement.

In 100 of 127 patients tested serially, the previously absent R1 or R2 returned, while the direct response remained relatively normal. This indicates recovery of conduction across the involved segment without substantial distal degeneration (Fig. 16-7). These patients generally showed good clinical recovery within a few months after onset. The latency of R1, however, was increased, on the average, by more than 2 ms initially, suggesting demyelination of the involved segment. The R/D ratios were much greater than in normals, indicating conduction abnormalities in the proximal segment of the facial nerve. The latency of R1 decreased during the second month and returned to normal during the third or fourth months (Fig. 16-8). In the remaining 27 patients, the direct response was markedly diminished without return of the reflex response during the first two weeks, indicating distal degeneration.[45]

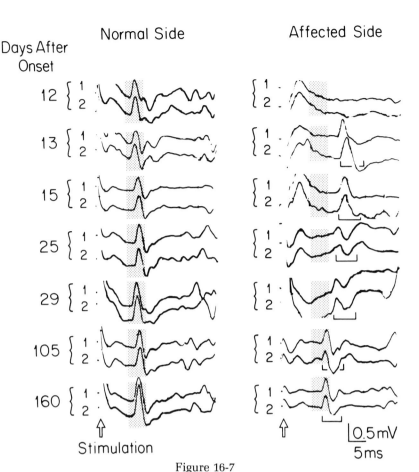

Days After
Onset

Normal Side | Affected Side

Stimulation

$\lfloor$0.5mV

5ms

Figure 16-7

Serial changes of R1 in a 16-year-old girl with Bell's palsy on the right. Two consecutive tracings were recorded on each side to show consistency of R1 on a given day. On the affected side, R1 was delayed when it first appeared on the 13th day of onset but recovered progressively thereafter. Shaded areas indicate normal range (mean ± 3 SD in 83 subjects). (From Kimura,[36] with permission.)

## Synkinesis of facial muscles

Both R1 and R2 components of the blink reflex are normally recorded in the orbicularis oculi alone and only rarely, if at all, in other facial muscles.[21, 76] During aberrant axon regeneration, however, fibers that originally innervated the orbicularis oculi are misdirected to other facial muscles.[45] Under such circumstances, the blink reflex will be present in muscles other than the orbicularis oculi and thus serve as a sign of aberrant reinnervation (Fig. 16-9).

Synkinetic movements detected by this means can be clearly distinguished from volitional movements. Also the size of the evoked potentials reflects the extent of aberrant reinnervation. In 26 of 29 patients tested at least four months after total facial nerve degeneration, an aberrant blink reflex was recorded in the orbicularis oris on the affected side. One of the remaining 3 had injury only to a peripheral branch of the facial nerve and experienced return of function with no evidence of synkinesis. In the other 2, the affected side of the face remained totally paralyzed with no evidence of any regeneration. Thus, synkinetic movements ultimately occur in nearly all cases following

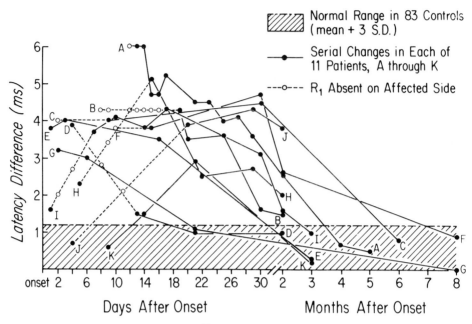

Figure 16-8

Serial changes in difference of R1 latency between normal and paretic sides in 11 patients recovering without nerve degeneration (A through K) seen early in course of disease and followed periodically. In general, nerve conduction is relatively normal at onset but deteriorates during the first week. Shaded area indicates normal range of difference of R1 latency between two sides in the same individuals (mean ± SD in 83 subjects). (From Kimura, Giron, and Young,[43] with permission.)

degeneration of the facial nerve provided that the lesion is not too distal and that the facial nerve does regenerate.

## Hemifacial spasm

Patients with hemifacial spasm also exhibit clinical and electrical evidence of synkinetic movements.[3, 8, 17, 35, 53, 82] In these cases the appearance of the blink reflex in muscles other than the orbicularis oculi may simply indicate hyperexcitability at the facial nucleus or ephaptic activation of motor axons not normally involved in blinking. Unlike the constant aberrant responses seen after peripheral facial paresis,[45] successive aberrant responses in hemifacial spasm vary in latency and waveform.[3] The blink reflex reveals no evidence of synkinesis in essential bleopharospasm, focal seizures, or facial myokymia.

## Acoustic neuroma

A cerebellopontine angle tumor frequently compresses the trigeminal and facial nerves, as well as brain stem structures. Since these are the afferent, efferent, and central pathways of the blink reflex, respectively, the reflex test is of unique diagnostic value.[6, 15, 41, 49, 68, 75] In 33 patients included in this review, the direct response was absent in 7, including 5 tested only after surgical sacrifice of the facial nerve. Of the remaining 26

## Blink Reflex After Aberrant Regeneration
## of the Facial Nerve

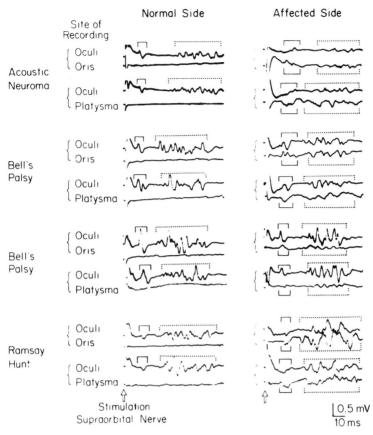

Figure 16-9

The blink reflex in the orbicularis oris and platysma in four patients following various diseases of the facial nerve. When the affected side of the face was stimulated, both R1 (small bracket) and R2 (dotted bracket) were elicited in the orbicularis oris as well as in the platysma, indicating widespread synkinetic movements. The blink reflex was elicited only in the orbicularis oculi on the normal side of the face, which thus served as a control in each patient. (From Kimura, Rodnitzky, and Okawara,[45] with permission.)

patients, R1 was absent on the affected side in 5, delayed in 17, and normal in 4. Abnormalities of R2 indicated efferent, afferent, and mixed patterns in 6, 6, and 7 patients, respectively. R2 was normal in the remaining 7 cases.

## Polyneuropathy

Facial or trigeminal nerve involvement in various polyneuropathies affects the blink reflex (Fig. 16-10A). Although R2 begins clearly after R1 in normal subjects, this distinction becomes unclear in a demyelinative neuropathy in which R1 is temporally dispersed (Fig. 16-10B). In neuropathy the ipsilateral and contralateral R2 are of nearly identical latency. Thus, a simultaneously recorded contralateral R2 helps to identify the apparent initial portion of the ipsilateral response as containing a delayed R1 continuous with R2 (Fig. 16-10C).

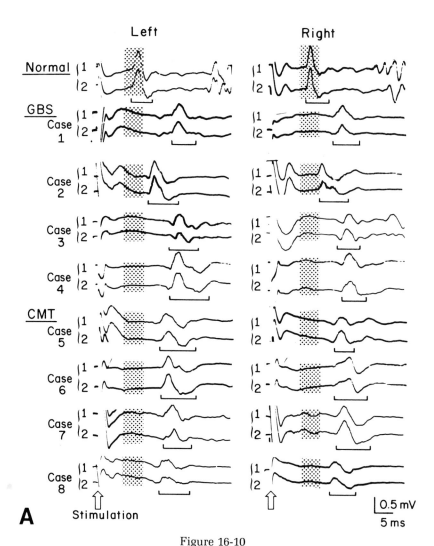

Left     Right

Normal

GBS
Case 1

Case 2

Case 3

Case 4

CMT
Case 5

Case 6

Case 7

Case 8

**A** Stimulation

0.5 mV

5 ms

Figure 16-10

(A) Bilateral delay of R1 in four patients with the Guillain-Barré syndrome (GBS) and four patients with hereditary motor and sensory neuropathy Type I or hypertrophic type of Charcot-Marie-Tooth disease (CMT). Two tracings were recorded on each side in each subject. The top tracings are from a normal control with shaded areas indicating the normal range. (From Kimura,[36] with permission.)

The findings in each category will be briefly described below.[37] In the Guillain-Barré syndrome, chronic inflammatory polyneuropathy, and hereditary motor and sensory neuropathy Type I, or the hypertrophic type of Charcot-Marie-Tooth disease, the direct and R1 responses were either absent or delayed in a majority of patients. The incidence of abnormality was considerably less in diabetic polyneuropathy. In the Fisher syndrome, the direct and R1 responses were normal in all except one patient, who had peripheral facial palsy associated with delayed R1 on the affected side. In hereditary motor and sensory neuropathy Type II or neuronal type of Charcot-Marie-Tooth disease, the studies were normal in all except one patient, who had an absent R1 on one side. The average latencies of the direct and R1 responses were markedly increased in the Guillain-Barré syndrome, chronic inflammatory polyneuropathy, and hereditary motor and sensory neuropathy Type I, increased to a much lesser degree in

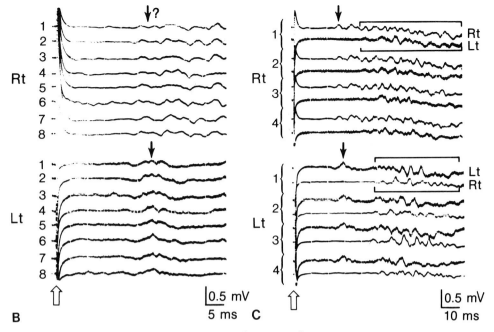

Figure 16-10 (*Continued*)

(B) R1 in a 55-year-old woman with chronic peripheral neuropathy and monoclonal gammopathy. Stimulation and recording arrangements are the same as in Figure 16-5A. However, a slower sweep was required to record a substantially delayed and temporally dispersed R1 in this patient. (C) R1 and R2 in the same patient shown in part b. Stimulation and recording arrangements are the same as in Figure 16-5B. However, a slower sweep was required to record delayed R2. Of interest was the continuity between R1 and R2 components on the right with no clear separation between them. Distinction between R1 and R2 could be made solely on the basis of the contralateral R2 recorded simultaneously.

diabetic polyneuropathy, and normal in the Fisher syndrome and hereditary motor and sensory neuropathy Type II (see Table 16-1). The latency ratio of R1 to the direct response showed a mild increase in the Guillain-Barré syndrome, a moderate decrease in hereditary motor and sensory neuropathy Type I and chronic inflammatory polyneuropathy, and a mild decrease in diabetic polyneuropathy. Although latencies of R2 were commonly within the normal range when analyzed individually, the average value was significantly greater in the neuropathies than in controls.

## Multiple sclerosis

Alterations of the electrically elicited blink reflex may result from disorders of the central reflex pathways. Of various lesions affecting the brain stem, the delay of R1 is most conspicuous in multiple sclerosis,[28, 29, 35, 48, 50, 59, 63] reflecting the slowing of impulse propagation associated with demyelination.[54, 72, 83] The incidence of blink reflex abnormality varies a great deal, depending on the selection of patients. In general, the longer the history of clinical symptoms is, the higher is the rate of abnormality.

In our earlier study of 260 patients, mostly suffering from long-standing disease,[35] R1 was delayed in 96 of 145 patients (66 percent) who clinically had disseminated lesions as well as episodes of remission and exacerbation (Fig. 16-11). The abnormality was found in 32 of 57 patients (56 percent) known to have either multiple sites of involvement without relapse or a history of recurrence of a localized lesion. The R1 component was affected in 17 of the remaining 58 patients (29 percent) in whom the

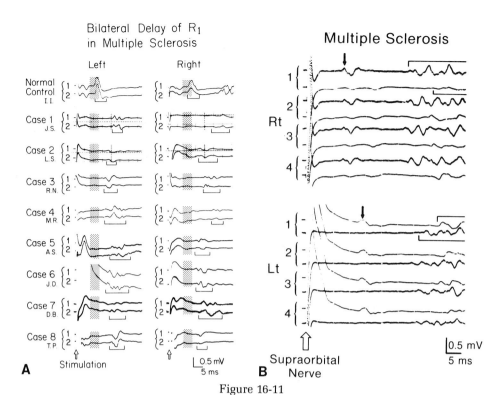

Figure 16-11

(A) Delayed R1 on both sides in multiple sclerosis. Two tracings were recorded on each side in each subject to show consistency of R1 response. The top tracings are from a normal control, with shaded areas indicating the normal range (mean $\pm$ 3 SD in 83 subjects). In addition to obvious increases in latency, R1 obtained in these patients is temporally dispersed and very irregular in waveform when compared with that in the normal control. None of these patients had unequivocal pontine signs clinically, although mild horizontal nystagmus was present in cases 1, 2, 5, 6, and 7. (From Kimura,[35] with permission.) (B) R1 and R2 in a 35-year-old woman with multiple sclerosis and mild facial and abducens paresis on the left. Stimulation and recording arrangements are the same as in Figure 16-5B. With right-sided stimulation R1 is normal and R2 is delayed contralaterally, whereas with left-sided stimulation R1 is slowed and R2 is delayed ipsilaterally. This finding suggests a lesion involving the efferent arc of the reflex on the left, i.e., intrapontine portion of the facial nerve. (Compare Figure 16-1B.) (From Kimura,[36] with permission.)

diagnosis was suspected but not clinically established. In the same 260 patients, R1 was abnormal in 49 of 63 patients with clinical evidence of pontine lesions (78 percent), 50 of 104 with other brain stem lesions (57 percent), and 37 of 93 with neither brain stem signs nor symptoms (40 percent).

In the 63 patients with clinical signs of pontine lesions, the average latency of R1 was substantially greater than that in normals, but less than in patients with the Guillain-Barré syndrome and Charcot-Marie-Tooth disease (Fig. 16-12). Since the direct response was normal in multiple sclerosis, the R/D ratio was significantly increased. Hyperthermia did not induce significant changes in mean reflex latency, amplitude, or duration in patients with multiple sclerosis, including those with unequivocal blink reflex abnormalities before warming.[67]

Comparable results were reported in similar studies of multiple sclerosis by Namerow and Etemadi,[59] Lyon and Van Allen,[50] Lowitzsch and associates,[48] and Paty and associates.[63] In a more recent study, Khoshbin and Hallett[28] found delayed R1 in 41 percent and 18 percent of patients with definite and possible diagnoses, respectively. The lower rates of abnormality are consistent with our current findings in a series of

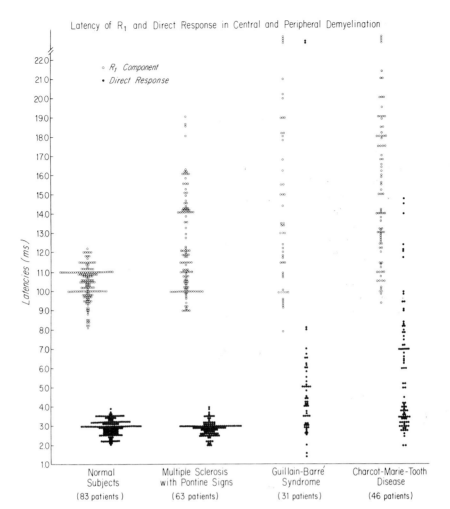

Figure 16-12

Latency distribution of the direct response and R1 of the blink reflex in normals and in patients with central or peripheral demyelination of the reflex pathways. The direct response is slowed in Charcot-Marie-Tooth disease and to a slightly lesser extent in the Guillain-Barré syndrome, but remains normal in multiple sclerosis. Delay of R1 is comparable between two polyneuropathies but slightly less in multiple sclerosis. (From Kimura,[36] with permission.)

patients referred for electrophysiologic testing soon after the onset of their symptoms.[27] The blink reflex with its shorter central pathway detects fewer abnormalities than visual, somatosensory, or brain stem auditory evoked potentials in multiple sclerosis. However, a delayed R1 is valuable in localizing a lesion to the pons and establishing subclinical dissemination of pathology.

## Wallenberg syndrome

Alteration of R2 is commonly associated with lesions affecting the lateral medulla, as demonstrated in patients with the Wallenberg syndrome.[40, 61] As shown in Table 16-2, the average latency of R1 was normal in this syndrome; although when analyzed individually, the values were sometimes slightly greater on the affected side than on the normal side. When the affected side of the face was stimulated, both ipsilateral and contralateral R2 were absent in 7, reduced in amplitude in 6, and significantly delayed in 10 (Fig. 16-13). With stimulation on the normal side, R2 was normal bilaterally in 20 of 23 patients. The remaining 3 patients showed normal R2 only on the side of stimulation.[61] The findings were essentially the same whether the supraorbital, infraorbital, or mental nerve was tested.

## Facial hypesthesia

Afferent delay of R2 is by no means specific to the Wallenberg syndrome, since a similar alteration may occur in patients with contralateral hemispheric lesions.[12, 20, 34, 57] An afferent impairment of R2 is seen commonly, although not exclusively, with sensory disturbances of the face. Thus, the electrically elicited blink reflex may be used to quantitatively substantiate corneal reflex changes in the assessment of facial sensation.[2] In equivocal cases, the right and left sides of the face are alternately stimulated every 5 to 10 seconds. With this maneuver, apparent asymmetry based on random variations tends to shift from one side to the other.

Of 6 patients with bilateral trigeminal neuropathy, R1 was slowed or absent bilaterally in 3 and normal in the others, whereas R2 was delayed or difficult to elicit regardless of the side of stimulation in 4 and normal in the remainder. In 19 patients with unilateral disease of either the trigeminal nerve (10) or brain stem (9), R1 was

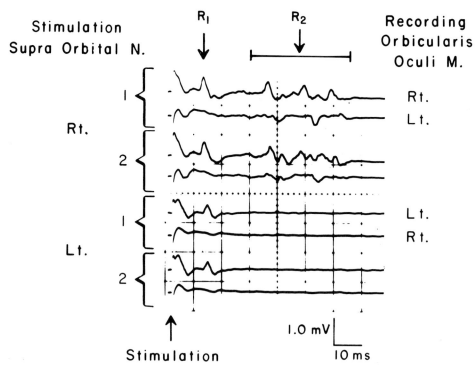

Figure 16-13

Left lateral medullary syndrome. Two successive stimuli were given on the right (top two pairs) followed by two successive stimuli on the left (bottom two pairs). R2 was absent bilaterally when the side of the lesion (left) was stimulated, although R1 was normal. (Compare Figure 16-17.) (From Kimura and Lyon,[40] with permission.)

absent on the affected side in 6, delayed in 7, and normal in the others. When the affected side was stimulated, R2 was bilaterally absent or small in 4, delayed in 7, and normal in the rest (Fig. 16-14). The response was generally smaller when the sensory loss was more complete, and stimulation of an anesthetic part of the face elicited no R2.

# ANALYSIS OF THE R1 COMPONENT

## Direct involvement of the reflex arc

R1 of the blink reflex shows increased latency in diseases associated with demyelination either centrally[29, 32, 35, 48, 58, 59] or peripherally affecting the trigeminal nerve,[46, 60] facial nerve,[43, 44, 64, 66, 69, 71] or both.[6, 15, 30, 41, 49] Posterior fossa tumors may affect R1 either by compressing the cranial nerves extra-axially or by involvement of the brain stem itself.[10, 31, 41]

## Effect of lesions outside the reflex pathway

Alteration of R1 does not necessarily indicate a pathologic process of the reflex arc itself, since edema or other indirect effects of lesions outside the primary reflex pathway may also contribute.[35] A reversible block of R1 may occur in comatose patients when the brain stem is severely depressed with acute supratentorial lesions or massive drug intoxication.[51] Using a glabellar tap, a significant increase in latency of R1 was described in patients with acute hemispheric strokes.[20] The changes were transient, recovering almost completely within a few days. In contrast, the latency of electrically elicited R1 usually remains normal even during acute stages of hemispheric disease, provided an adequate stimulus is given to compensate for reduced excitability of the reflex pathway.[12, 26, 34]

In some patients with acute supranuclear lesions, single electric shocks on the contralateral side may elicit R1 only partially or not at all. An apparent increase in

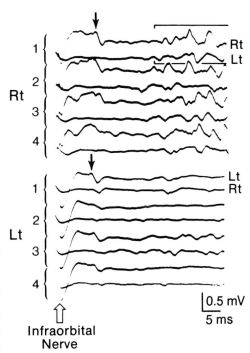

Figure 16-14
R1 and R2 elicited by stimulation of the infra-orbital nerve in a 39-year-old woman with syringobulbia. Stimulation and recording arrangements are the same as in Figure 16-5B, although the stimulus was delivered to the infraorbital instead of supraorbital nerve. Note a normal R1 and absent R2 when the hypesthetic (left) side of the face was stimulated.

latency of R1 results if a submaximal stimulus fails to activate the fastest conducting fibers. In this instance, paired stimuli with an interstimulus interval of 3 to 5 ms usually elicit a maximal R1 with normal latency.[31, 34, 35] Thus, once R1 is fully activated, its latency generally indicates the conduction characteristics of the reflex arc itself rather than excitability effects of a remote lesion. In particular, a delay of R1 by several milliseconds is difficult to explain on the basis of altered excitability alone. In these cases, the reflex response may be mediated by smaller, slower conducting fibers, because larger myelinated fibers are substantially blocked or because conduction is generally slowed across a demyelinated area.

## Degree of slowing

In the central demyelination of multiple sclerosis, the average latency of R1 is 12.3 ± 2.7 ms (mean ± SD) as compared with 15.1 ± 5.9 ms in the Guillain-Barré syndrome and 17.0 ± 3.7 ms in hereditary motor and sensory neuropathy Type 1 or hypertrophic type of Charcot-Marie-Tooth disease. These findings presumably reflect that demyelination in multiple sclerosis is restricted to a short segment in the pons. The average latency of R1 in Bell's palsy due to focal involvement of the facial nerve (12.8 ± 1.6 ms) is very close to that found in multiple sclerosis. In most patients with trigeminal neuralgia, the reflex latency is normal. In contrast, the paratrigeminal syndrome is frequently associated with significant conduction abnormalities of the trigeminal nerve and slowing of R1.

The degree of slowing in the direct response and R1 is much the same in Charcot-Marie-Tooth disease and the Guillain-Barré syndrome (see Figs. 16-10A and 16-12), but the decreased R/D ratio found in the former suggests that slowing of facial nerve conduction is more distal than proximal. In the latter, the average R/D ratio is slightly increased indicating more proximal involvement of the facial nerve, provided, of course, that the trigeminal nerve is relatively intact. The R/D ratio is also significantly increased in multiple sclerosis and the paratrigeminal syndrome in which conduction of the facial nerve is normal. The ratio is also increased in Bell's palsy, unless the facial nerve has degenerated distally.

# ANALYSIS OF THE R2 COMPONENT
## Direct and remote effect on polysynaptic pathways

As mentioned earlier, abnormalities of R2 can usually be categorized as either afferent or efferent in type. However, some brain stem lesions may give rise to a more complex pattern (see Fig. 16-1B). Stimulation on one side may reveal unilateral abnormality of R2 either ipsilateral or contralateral to the stimulus, whereas stimulation on the opposite side may show R2 to be normal, absent, or delayed bilaterally, or affected unilaterally but not on the same side as implicated by the contralateral stimulation. Unlike R1, R2 is regularly altered not only by lesions directly affecting the reflex pathways as in the Wallenberg syndrome[40, 61] but also by lesions indirectly influencing the excitability of the polysynaptic connections (Fig. 16-15). Thus, R2 is absent, or if present, markedly diminished or delayed in any comatose state (Fig. 16-16), regardless of the site of lesion.[51, 56] It is also substantially affected by a hemispheric lesion (Fig. 16-17) showing either an afferent or efferent pattern of delay, perhaps depending on the site of involvement.[12, 20, 26, 34, 57]

## Level of consciousness and perception of pain

The state of arousal alters the excitability of R2 and, to a lesser extent, R1.[5, 7, 13, 19, 38, 39, 73, 74, 78] The R2 component is markedly reduced during synchronized sleep,

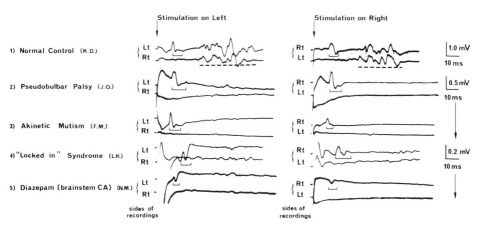

Figure 16-15

Absence of R2 in various neurologic disorders. The stimulus was delivered to the supraorbital nerve. When R2 was absent with an ordinary shock of 10 to 20 mA and 0.1 ms duration, the intensity was slowly advanced up to 40 mA and 0.5 ms duration. Note virtual absence of R2 regardless of the side of stimulation in cases 2 through 5. R1 was normal in cases 2, 3, and 5, and markedly delayed in case 4. (From Kimura,[32] with permission.)

but significantly higher in rapid eye movement (REM) sleep than in stages II, III, or IV. The level of excitability in REM sleep is about the same as in stage I, but slightly less than in full wakefulness. The R2 component may be absent, whereas R1 remains normal or nearly normal in some alert but immobile patients with features of the locked-in syndrome, in alert and ambulatory patients with pseudobulbar palsy, and in alert patients given therapeutic dosages of diazepam (Valium), which presumably blocks the multisynaptic reflex arc.[32]

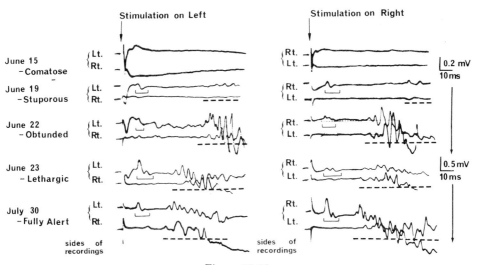

Figure 16-16

R1 and R2 in a patient recovering from herpes simplex encephalitis. The stimulus was delivered to the supraorbital nerve. The intensity of the shock was advanced to a level above which the evoked potential remained constant. Both R1 and R2 were absent on June 9 (not shown) and on June 15 when the patient was comatose. R1 was normal but R2 was markedly delayed and diminished on June 19 when the patient was responsive but stuporous. Note the progressive recovery in amplitude and latency of R2 contemporaneous with her improvement to full alertness in July. (From Kimura,[32] with permission.)

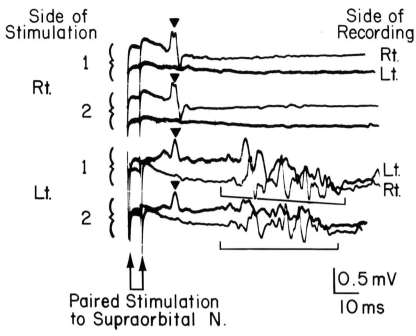

## Lt. Cerebral Stroke
### Absent R₂ to Paired Stimuli on Rt. Side of Face

Side of Stimulation

Side of Recording

Rt.

1

Rt.
Lt.

2

Lt.

1

Lt.
Rt.

2

Paired Stimulation to Supraorbital N.

0.5 mV
10 ms

Figure 16-17

Left cerebral stroke. Stimulation and recording arrangements are the same as in Figure 16-13. Paired stimuli (shocks of 0.1 ms and 15 mA separated by 7 ms) were delivered to the supraorbital nerve. To show consistency of the responses, two successive trials are shown on each side. When the affected (right) side of the face was stimulated, R1 was normal but R2 was absent, as shown in the top two trials. (Compare Figure 16-13.) (From Kimura,[34] with permission.)

Both ipsilateral and contralateral R2 components are significantly smaller with stimulation on a hypesthetic area of the face than with stimulation on the corresponding area of the normal side. But, whereas sensory deficits of the face are often associated with alteration of R2, the reverse is not always true. Indeed, similar reduction of R2 occurs in pure motor hemiplegia.[4, 12, 20, 34] In these cases, it is possible that minor sensory deficits are not detected clinically. It is more likely, however, that certain supratentorial lesions outside the somatosensory pathways can cause inhibition or reduced facilitation of the reflex pathways.

## Altered excitability of interneurons

Finally, R2 habituates readily in normals but not in patients with Parkinson's disease, whether tested clinically (the glabellar sign) or electromyographically.[55, 66, 70] The paired shock technique reveals the effect of a single cutaneous conditioning stimulus on this reflex (Fig. 16-18). Dissociation between the recovery curves of the oligosynaptic R1 and polysynaptic R2 components may be considered an index of excitability changes at the interneuron level.[33] As R2 but not R1 is profoundly suppressed by a conditioning stimulus in normals, diffuse reduction of excitability must occur predominantly at the interneuron rather than at the motor neuron, which is the final common path of both reflex-

# ORBICULARIS OCULI REFLEX TO PAIRED STIMULI

## Normal Control

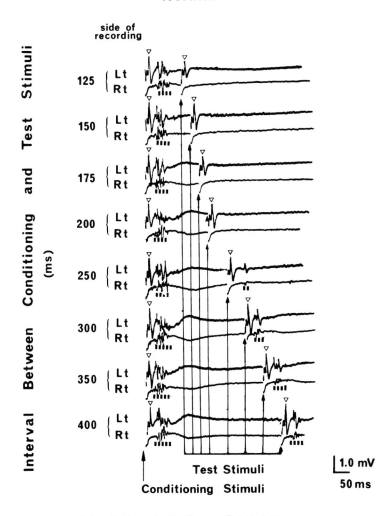

Stimulation - Left Supra Orbital Nerve

Figure 16-18

Normal control. Paired shocks (arrows) were delivered to the left supraorbital nerve with time intervals ranging from 125 to 400 ms between test and conditioning stimuli. R1 of the test response was slightly suppressed at time intervals of 125 to 175 ms but was, thereafter, relatively constant and equal in amplitude to the conditioning response. R2 of the test response was absent up to the time interval of 200 ms and then recovered slowly. (From Kimura,[33] with permission.)

es. The suppression of R2 in normals occurs whether the conditioning and test stimuli are delivered in the same or in different, ipsilateral or contralateral trigeminal cutaneous fields.[33]

In Parkinson's disease, the recovery curve of R1 is normal. However, the suppression of R2 following a conditioning stimulus is significantly less when compared with controls. The recovery curve of R2 indicates that physiologic suppression of interneurons, which normally takes place following a cutaneous conditioning stimulus, fails to occur in Parkinson's disease. Additionally, the latency of R2 in response to a single maximal stimulus is significantly shorter in advanced cases of Parkinson's disease when compared with controls. These findings suggest that in this disease interneurons but not motor neurons are primarily hyperactive. In contrast, diminution of R2 component in Huntington's chorea represents the opposite extreme and probably reflects a decreased interneuronal activity secondary to overinhibition of dopaminergic receptors.[16]

# REFERENCE SOURCES

1. ACCORNERO, N, ET AL: *Corneal reflex elicited by electrical stimulation of the human cornea.* Neurology (New York) 30:782, 1980.

2. ASHWORTH, B AND TAIT, GBW: *Trigeminal neuropathy in connective tissue disease.* Neurology (Minneap) 21:609, 1971.

3. AUGER, RG: *Hemifacial spasm: Clinical and electrophysiologic observations.* Neurology (New York) 29:1261, 1979.

4. BARRON, SA, HEFFNER, RR, JR, AND ZWIRECKI, R: *A familial mitochondrial myopathy with central defect in neural transmission.* Arch Neurol 36:553, 1979.

5. BECK, U, SCHENCK, E, AND ISCHINGER, TH: *Spinale und bulbäre Reflexe im Schlaf beim Menschen.* Arch Psychiatr Nervenkr 217:157, 1973.

6. BENDER, LF, MAYNARD, FM, AND HASTINGS, SV: *The blink reflex as a diagnostic procedure.* Arch Phys Med Rehabil 50:27, 1969.

7. BOELHOUWER, AJW AND BRUNIA, CHM: *Blink reflexes and the state of arousal.* J Neurol Neurosurg Psychiatry 40:58, 1977.

8. BOHNERT, B AND STÖHR, M: *Beitrag zum Spasmus facialis.* Arch Psychiatr Nervenkr 224:11, 1977.

9. CLAY, SA AND RAMSEYER, JC: *The orbicularis oculi reflex in infancy and childhood. Establishment of normal values.* Neurology (Minneap) 26:521, 1976.

10. CLAY, SA AND RAMSEYER, JC: *The orbicularis oculi reflex: Pathologic studies in childhood.* Neurology (Minneap) 27:892, 1977.

11. CSÉCSEI, G: *Facial afferent fibers in the blink reflex of man.* Brain Res 161:347, 1979.

12. DEHEN, H, ET AL: *Blink reflex in hemiplegia.* Electroenceph Clin Neurophysiol 40:393, 1976.

13. DESMEDT, JE AND GODAUX, E: *Habituation of exteroceptive suppression and of exteroceptive reflexes in man as influenced by voluntary contraction.* Brain Res 106:21, 1976.

14. DEVI, S, ET AL: *Prognostic value of minimal excitability of facial nerve in Bell's palsy.* J Neurol Neurosurg Psychiatry 41:649, 1978.

15. EISEN, A AND DANON, J: *The orbicularis oculi reflex in acoustic neuromas: A clinical and electrodiagnostic evaluation.* Neurology (Minneap) 24:306, 1974.

16. ESTEBAN, A AND GIMÉNEZ-ROLDÁN, S: *Blink reflex in Huntington's Chorea and Parkinson's disease.* Acta Neurol Scand 52:145, 1975.

17. FERGUSON, IT: *Electrical study of jaw and orbicularis oculi reflexes after trigeminal nerve surgery.* J Neurol Neurosurg Psychiatry 41:819, 1978.

18. FERRARI, E AND MESSINA, C: *Osservazioni elettrofisiologiche sui riflessi trigemino-facciali nell'uomo: L' "abitudine" della componente polisinaptica.* Estratto da Rivista Di Neurologia 38:84, 1968.

19. FERRARI, E AND MESSINA, C: *Blink reflexes during sleep and wakefulness in man.* Electroenceph Clin Neurophysiol 32:55, 1972.

20. FISHER, MA, SHAHANI, BT, AND YOUNG, RR: *Assessing segmental excitability after acute rostral lesions: II. The blink reflex.* Neurology (New York) 29:45, 1979.

21. GANDIGLIO, G AND FRA, L: *Further observations on facial reflexes.* J Neurol Sci 5:273, 1967.

22. GILLIATT, RW AND TAYLOR, JC: *Electrical changes following section of the facial nerve.* Proc R Soc Med 52:1080, 1959.

23. GOOR, C AND ONGERBOER DE VISSER, BW: *Jaw and blink reflexes in trigeminal nerve lesions. An electrodiagnostic study.* Neurology (Minneap) 26:95, 1976.

24. HIRAOKA, M AND SHIMAMURA, M: *Neural mechanisms of the corneal blinking reflex in cats.* Brain Res 125:265, 1977.

25. HOPF, HC, HUFSCHMIDT, HJ, AND STRÖDER, J: *Development of the "trigeminofacial" reflex in infants and children.* Ann Paediat 204:52, 1965.

26. KAPLAN, PE AND KAPLAN, C: *Blink reflex: Review of methodology and its application to patients with stroke syndromes.* Arch Phys Med Rehabil 61:30, 1980.

27. KAYAMORI, R, YAMADA, T, AND KIMURA, H: *Brainstem auditory evoked potential and blink reflex in multiple sclerosis* (in preparation).

28. KHOSHBIN, S AND HALLETT, M: *Multimodality evoked potentials and blink reflex in multiple sclerosis.* Neurology 31:138, 1981.

29. KIMURA, J: *Alteration of the orbicularis oculi reflex by pontine lesions. Study in multiple sclerosis.* Arch Neurol 22:156, 1970.

30. KIMURA, J: *An evaluation of the facial and trigeminal nerves in polyneuropathy: Electrodiagnostic study in Charcot-Marie-Tooth disease, Guillain-Barré syndrome, and diabetic neuropathy.* Neurology (Minneap) 21:745–752, 1971.

31. KIMURA, J: *Electrodiagnostic study of brainstem strokes.* Stroke 2:576, 1971.

32. KIMURA, J: *The blink reflex as a test for brain-stem and higher central nervous system functions.* In DESMEDT, JE (ED): New Developments in Electromyography and Clinical Neurophysiology, Vol 3. Karger, Basel, 1973, pp 682–691.

33. KIMURA, J: *Disorder of interneurons in parkinsonism—The orbicularis oculi reflex to paired stimuli.* Brain 96:87, 1973.

34. KIMURA, J: *Effect of hemispheral lesions on the contralateral blink reflex.* Neurology (Minneap) 24:168, 1974.

35. KIMURA, J: *Electrically elicited blink reflex in diagnosis of multiple sclerosis—Review of 260 patients over a seven-year period.* Brain 98:413, 1975.

36. KIMURA, J: *Clinical uses of the electrically elicited blink reflex.* In DESMEDT, JE (ED): Brain and spinal mechanisms of movement control in man: New developments and clinical applications. Raven Press, New York, 1982 (in press).

37. KIMURA, J: *Conduction abnormalities of the facial and trigeminal nerves in polyneuropathy.* Muscle and Nerve, 1982 (in press).

38. KIMURA, J AND HARADA, O: *Excitability of the orbicularis oculi reflex in all night sleep: Its suppression in non-rapid eye movement and recovery in rapid eye movement sleep.* Electroenceph Clin Neurophysiol 33:369, 1972.

39. KIMURA, J AND HARADA, O: *Recovery curves of the blink reflex during wakefulness and sleep.* J Neurol 213:189, 1976.

40. KIMURA, J AND LYON, LW: *Orbicularis oculi reflex in the Wallenberg syndrome: Alteration of the late reflex by lesions of the spinal tract and nucleus of the trigeminal nerve.* J Neurol Neurosurg Psychiatry 35:228, 1972.

41. KIMURA, J AND LYON, LW: *Alteration of orbicularis oculi reflex by posterior fossa tumors.* J Neurosurg 38:10, 1973.

42. KIMURA, J, BODENSTEINER, J, AND YAMADA, T: *Electrically elicited blink reflex in normal neonates.* Arch Neurol 34:246, 1977.

43. KIMURA, J, GIRON, LT, JR, AND YOUNG, SM: *Electrophysiological study of Bell Palsy. Electrically elicited blink reflex in assessment of prognosis.* Arch Otolaryngol 102:140, 1976.

44. KIMURA, J, POWERS, JM, AND VAN ALLEN, MW: *Reflex response of orbicularis oculi muscle to supraorbital nerve stimulation. Study in normal subjects and in peripheral facial paresis.* Arch Neurol 21:193, 1969.

45. KIMURA, J, RODNITZKY, RL, AND OKAWARA, S: *Electrophysiologic analysis of aberrant regeneration after facial nerve paralysis.* Neurology (Minneap) 25:989, 1975.

46. KIMURA, J, RODNITZKY, RL, AND VAN ALLEN, MW: *Electrodiagnostic study of trigeminal nerve. Orbicularis oculi reflex and masseter reflex in trigeminal neuralgia, paratrigeminal syndrome, and other lesions of the trigeminal nerve.* Neurology (Minneap) 20:574, 1970.

47. KUGELBERG, E: *Facial reflexes.* Brain 75:385, 1952.

48. LOWITZSCH, K, ET AL: *Visual pattern evoked responses and blink reflexes in assessment of multiple sclerosis diagnosis. A clinical study of 135 multiple sclerosis patients.* J Neurol 213:17, 1976.

49. LYON, LW AND VAN ALLEN, MW: *Alteration of the orbicularis oculi reflex by acoustic neuroma.* Arch Otolaryngol 95:100, 1972.

50. LYON, LW AND VAN ALLEN, MW: *Orbicularis oculi reflex. Studies in internuclear ophthalmoplegia and pseudointernuclear ophthalmoplegia.* Arch Ophthalmol 87:148, 1972.

51. LYON, LW, KIMURA, J, AND MCCORMICK, WF: *Orbicularis oculi reflex in coma: Clinical, electrophysiological, and pathological correlations.* J Neurol Neurosurg Psychiatry 35:582, 1972.

52. MAGLADERY, JW AND TEASDALL, RD: *Corneal reflexes: An electromyographic study in man.* Arch Neurol 5:269, 1961.

53. MARTIN, RC: *Late results of facial nerve repair.* Ann Otolaryngol 64:859, 1955.

54. MCDONALD, WI AND SEARS, TA: *The effects of experimental demyelination on conduction in the central nervous system.* Brain 93:583, 1970.

55. MESSINA, C: *L'abitudine dei riflessi trigemino-facciali in parkinsoniani sottoposti a trattamento con L-DOPA.* Riv Neurol 40:327, 1970.

56. MESSINA, C AND MICALIZZI, V: *I riflessi trigemino-facciali nel corso del coma insulinico.* Acta Neurologica 25:357, 1970.

57. MESSINA, C AND QUATTRONE, A: *Comportamento dei riflessi trigemino-facciali in soggetti con lesioni emisferiche.* Riv Neurol 43:379, 1973.

58. NAMEROW, NS: *Observations of the blink reflex in multiple sclerosis.* In DESMEDT, JE (ED): *New Developments in Electromyography and Clinical Neurophysiology,* Vol 3. Karger, Basel, 1973, pp 692–696.

59. NAMEROW, NS AND ETEMADI, A: *The orbicularis oculi reflex in multiple sclerosis.* Neurology (Minneap) 20:1200, 1970.

60. ONGERBOER DE VISSER, BW AND GOOR, C: *Electromyographic and reflex study in idiopathic and symptomatic trigeminal neuralgias: Latency of the jaw and blink reflexes.* J Neurol Neurosurg Psychiatry 37:1225, 1974.

61. ONGERBOER DE VISSER, BW AND KUYPERS, HGJM: *Late blink reflex changes in lateral medullary lesions. An electrophysiological and neuro-anatomical study of Wallenberg's syndrome.* Brain 101:285, 1978.

62. ONGERBOER DE VISSER, BW, MELCHELSE, K, AND MEGENS, PHA: *Corneal reflex latency in trigeminal nerve lesions.* Neurology (New York) 27:1164, 1977.

63. PATY, DW, ET AL: *Chronic progressive myelopathy: Investigation with CSF electrophoresis, evoked potentials, and CT scan.* Ann Neurol 6:419, 1979.

64. PENDERS, C AND BONIVER, R: *Exploration électrophysiologique du réflexe de clignement dans la paralysie faciale a frigore.* J Otolaryngol 34:17, 1972.

65. PENDERS, CA AND DELWAIDE, PJ: *Le réflexe de clignement chez l'homme. Particularités électrophysiologiques de la réponse précoce.* Arch Int Physiol Biochem 77:351, 1969.

66. PENDERS, CA AND DELWAIDE, PJ: *Interet de l'exploration du reflexe de clignement en cas de paralysie faciale.* Electromyography 11:149, 1971.

67. RODNITZKY, RL AND KIMURA, J: *The effect of induced hyperthermia on the blink reflex in multiple sclerosis.* Neurology (New York) 28:431, 1978.

68. ROSSI, D, ET AL: *Blink reflexes in posterior fossa lesions.* J Neurol Neurosurg Psychiatry 42:465, 1979.

69. RUSHWORTH, G: *The effects of cranial nerve pathology on the blink reflexes.* Trans Ophthalmol Soc 82:549, 1962.

70. RUSHWORTH, G: *Observations on blink reflexes.* J Neurol Neurosurg Psychiatry 25:93, 1962.

71. SCHENCK, E AND MANZ, F: *The blink reflex in Bell's Palsy.* In DESMEDT, JE (ED): *New Developments in Electromyography and Clinical Neurophysiology,* Vol 3. Karger, Basel, 1973.

72. SEARS, TA, BOSTOCK, H, AND SHERATT, M: *The pathophysiology of demyelination and its implications for the symptomatic treatment of multiple sclerosis.* Neurology (New York) 28:21, 1978.

73. SHAHANI, B: *Effects of sleep on human reflexes with a double component.* J Neurol Neurosurg Psychiatry 31:574, 1968.

74. SHAHANI, B: *The human blink reflex.* J Neurol Neurosurg Psychiatry 33:792, 1970.

75. SHAHANI, BT AND PARKER, SW: *Electrophysiological studies in patients with cerebellarpontine angle lesions.* Neurology (New York) 29:582, 1979.

76. SHAHANI, BT AND YOUNG, RR: *Human orbicularis oculi reflexes.* Neurology (Minneap) 22:149, 1972.

77. SHAHANI, BT AND YOUNG, RR: *The blink, H, and tendon vibration reflexes.* In GOODGOLD, J AND EBERSTEIN, A (EDS): *Electrodiagnosis of Neuromuscular Diseases,* ed 2. Williams & Wilkins, Baltimore, 1977, pp 245–263.

78. SILVERSTEIN, LD, GRAHAM, FK, AND CALLOWAY, JM: *Preconditioning and excitability of the human orbicularis oculi reflex as a function of state.* Electroenceph Clin Neurophysiol 48:406, 1980.

79. THATCHER, DB AND VAN ALLEN, MW: *Corneal reflex latency.* Neurology (Minneap) 21:735, 1971.

80. TRONTELJ, MA AND TRONTELJ, JV: *Reflex arc of the first component of the human blink reflex: A single motoneurone study.* J Neurol Neurosurg Psychiatr 41:538, 1978.

81. WALKER, DD AND KIMURA, J: *A fast-recovery electrode amplifier for electrophysiology.* Electroenceph Clin Neurophysiol 45:789, 1978.

82. WARTENBERG, R: *Associated movements in the oculomotor and facial muscles.* Arch Neurol Psychiatry 55:439, 1946.

83. WAXMAN, SG AND BRILL, MH: *Conduction through demyelinated plaques in multiple sclerosis: Computer simulations of facilitation by short internodes.* J Neurol Neurosurg Psychiatry 41:408, 1978.

# CHAPTER
# 17

# THE F-WAVE

Conventional nerve conduction studies seldom contribute to the investigation of more proximal lesions. To study the entire length of the sensory nerve, one may record somatosensory cerebral evoked potentials (SEP).[9] Motor conduction along the most proximal segment can be assessed by measurement of the F-wave, a late muscle potential that results from the backfiring of antidromically activated anterior horn cells. This possibility was first explored in patients with Charcot-Marie-Tooth disease,[38] and the technique has been applied to a variety of neurologic disorders since then.[6, 18, 19, 42, 43, 45, 46, 49, 51, 58, 59, 62, 63, 64, 88]

Inherent variability of the latency and configuration makes F-wave determination less precise than the measurement of the direct compound muscles action potential or the M-response. Nonetheless, the technique is a useful supplement to conventional nerve conduction studies. Delay of the F-wave often clearly exceeds the normal range of variability, especially in demyelinating polyneuropathies. In addition to determination of F-wave latencies, calculation of conduction velocities and the F-ratio permits comparison of conduction in the proximal versus the distal nerve segments.[42, 43] The F-wave also provides a measure of motor neuron excitability that presumably determines the probability of a recurrent response in individual axons. This section will review the rapidly accumulating data on F-wave determination and discuss its clinical value and limitations.[44]

# PHYSIOLOGY OF THE F-WAVE

## Recurrent versus reflexive activation of the motor neuron

A supramaximal electric shock delivered to a nerve often elicits a late response, called the F-wave, in the innervated muscle.[54] The F-wave occurs after the direct motor potential, or the M-response. With more proximal stimulation, the latency of the M-response increases, whereas that of the F-wave decreases (Fig. 17-1). This indicates that the impulse to elicit the F-wave first travels away from the recording electrodes toward the spinal cord before it returns to activate distal muscles.

# F Waves — Left Median Nerve

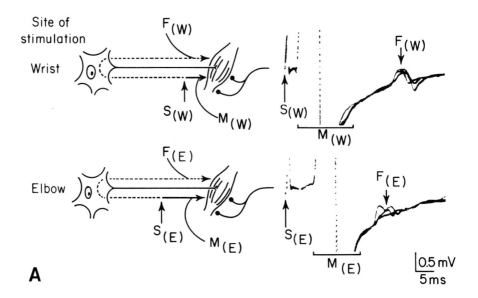

**A**

0.5 mV
5 ms

# F Waves — Left Tibial Nerve

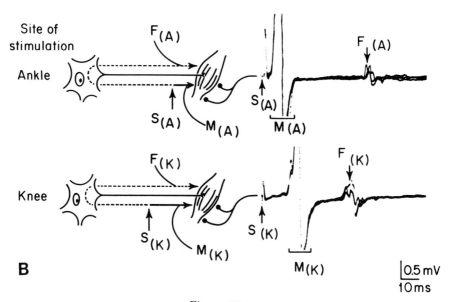

**B**

0.5 mV
10 ms

### Figure 17-1

(A) Normal M-response (horizontal brackets) and F-wave (small arrows) recorded from the thenar muscles through surface electrodes. Sites of supramaximal stimulus to the median nerve are shown. Three consecutive traces are superimposed for each. As the stimulus was moved from the wrist to the elbow, the latency of the M-response increased; whereas that of the F-wave decreased. The figures on the left are schematic illustrations showing the centrifugal (solid arrows) and centripetal (dotted arrows) impulses carrying the M-response and F-wave, respectively. (Modified from Kimura.[38]) (B) Normal M-response (horizontal brackets) and F-wave (small arrows) recorded from the abductor hallucis through surface electrodes. Supramaximal stimulus was delivered to the tibial nerve at the ankle (top tracing) and knee (bottom tracing). Three consecutive traces are superimposed for each. As the stimulus was moved from ankle to knee, the latency of the M-response increased, whereas that of the F-wave decreased. (From Kimura, Bosch, and Lindsay,[46] with permission.)

Since the original description by Magladery and McDougal,[54] who designated the late response as the F-wave (presumably because it was initially recorded from intrinsic foot muscles), different authors have debated whether it is a reflex response[33, 52, 54] or a recurrent discharge of antidromically activated motor neurons,[8, 55, 56, 78] or both.[28, 29] The presence of the F-wave in deafferented limbs[55, 56] and after transverse myelotomy[57] strongly suggests that it depends in part on backfiring of motor neurons. Single-fiber electromyography (SFEMG) studies[78, 80] have also shown that the occurrence of the F-wave requires prior activation of the motor axon. Although evidence of its recurrent nature is accumulating, reflex components may still contribute.

## Block of antidromic or orthodromic impulse

Motor neurons subject to recurrent activation fire only infrequently after a series of direct motor responses.[72] Thus, although antidromic and orthodromic activation of motor neurons are physiologically the same,[4, 13] additional mechanisms must prevent the motor neurons from generating the recurrent response with every stimulus.[13, 65] Recurrent discharges occur in only a limited number of motor units, in part because the antidromic impulse fails to enter the somata of some of the motor neurons.[53] This type of block often takes place at the axon hillock where membrane characteristics change, but it may also occur more distally in the myelinated segment of the axons.

The impulse may also be blocked during orthodromic propagation of the spike potential generated in the soma-dendrite membrane (SD spike). The antidromically activated SD spike travels orthodromically only if the axon hillock can be depolarized again. Subliminally excited soma-dendrite membrane facilitates antidromic activation of the SD spike, resulting in increased probability of a recurrent response. Conversely, excessive depolarization of the soma-dendrite membrane may lead to early generation of the SD spike, which cannot be propagated across the still depolarized axon hillock. The two opposing effects of subliminal depolarization of motor neurons have clinical implications: slight voluntary excitation of the motor neuron pool may enhance F-wave activation, but excessive effort may have the reverse effect.

## Latency and amplitude of the F-wave

Blockage at the initial segment probably occurs more commonly in the smaller, lower threshold motor neurons which are more rapidly depolarized.[35, 37] Preferential activation of the larger motor neurons may result if Renshaw cells inhibit the smaller motor neurons more effectively.[14, 15, 32] Hence recurrent discharges occur, at least in part, in the larger motor neurons with faster conducting axons. This in turn provides a rationale for using the minimal latency of the F-wave as a measure of the fastest conducting fibers.

Since a particular set of physiologic conditions is required for generation of a recurrent discharge, the latency of successive F-waves from single muscle fibers varies narrowly between 10 to 30 $\mu$s.[72] Parenthetically, the latency of consecutive H-reflexes from single muscle fibers may fluctuate by as much as 2.5 ms, primarily because of variation in synaptic transmission as will be discussed in Chapter 18. When recording from a muscle as a whole, however, the latency variability of consecutive F-waves far exceeds that of the H-reflex. This is primarily because recurrent discharges occur in different groups of motor neurons with successive supramaximal stimuli, whereas reflexive activation involves the same motor neurons, if a series of submaximal shocks remain constant in intensity.

The amplitude and frequency of the F-wave provide a measure of motor neuron excitability, but the relationship is physiologically complex.[17, 20, 21, 22, 23] No recurrent discharge occurs when an antidromic impulse produces subliminal depolarization in hypoexcitable cells. On the other hand, F-wave may also fail to occur in hyperexcitable cells which may discharge too rapidly during the refractory period of the initial axon segments. Recording with surface electrodes, greater F-wave potentials are recruited with higher stimulus intensities.[87] However, no consistent correlation exists between the latency and amplitude of the F-wave.

# AXON REFLEX

## Physiologic characteristics

The axon reflex is another late potential which was originally described as the intermediate latency response because it usually appears between the M-response and F-wave.[26] It presumably occurs only in the presence of collateral sprouting in the proximal portion of the nerve. If a submaximal stimulus excites one branch of the axon but not the other, the antidromic impulse propagates up to the point of branching and turns around to proceed distally along a second branch. Shocks of higher intensity which also activate the collateral distally abolish the response, since the descending turn around impulse collides with the antidromic impulse in the second branch (Fig. 17-2A and B).

The axon reflex most commonly appears with stimulation of the median or ulnar nerve at the wrist, or the peroneal or tibial nerve at the ankle. Proximal stimulation above the origin of the collateral sprout produces only an M-response (Fig. 17-2C). Thus, series of stimuli applied along the course of the nerve may localize the site of bifurcation. Collateral sprouting, however, does not always occur at the level of the lesion, but frequently well below the actual site of involvement.[26] If distal and proximal stimuli elicit the same axon reflex, the conduction velocity can be determined for the short intersegment of that particular axon (Fig. 17-2D).

The axon reflex has a constant latency and waveform, presumably because it originates from the same portion of a single motor unit innervated by a collateral sprout. The lack of synaptic connection along the pathway allows the axon reflex to follow repetitive submaximal stimulation up to 40 per second. The point of axonal branching and the conduction velocity of the two branches of the axon involved determine the latency of the axon reflex. It is usually, but not always, intermediate between those of the M-response and F-wave. The unmyelinated regenerating collateral sprout may conduct the ascending or descending impulses of an axon reflex much slower than the intact axons that relay the F-wave. We have encountered occasional axon reflexes that follow rather than precede the F-wave (Fig. 17-2A and C).

## Clinical significance

The axon reflex may resemble other late potentials such as those elicited ephaptically or those caused by repetitive discharges in the nerve trunk. These components, however, fail to follow high repetition rates and tend to vary in latency and waveform. A late potential may also result from a scattered motor response because of slow conduction in pathologic nerves. However, the latency of the axon reflex decreases while that of a temporally dispersed M-response increases with proximal stimulation (Figs. 17-2D and 17-3). Finally, the F-wave varies in latency and waveform and appears with supramaximal stimuli, which normally abolish the axon reflex altogether.

The axon reflex occurs in patients with neurogenic atrophy and rarely, if at all, in healthy individuals. The axon reflex has been observed in patients with tardy ulnar palsy, brachial plexus lesions, diabetic neuropathy, Charcot-Marie-Tooth disease, facial neuropathy, amyotrophic lateral sclerosis, and cervical root lesions.[25, 26, 69, 70] In a recent large scale survey, Roth[67, 68] concludes that this sign of nerve regeneration abounds in chronic neuropathies and entrapment syndromes. The diagnostic value of the axon reflex remains to be seen.

# DETERMINATION OF F-WAVE LATENCY

## Recording procedures

A supramaximal stimulus applied at practically any point along the course of a nerve elicits the F-wave. Placing the anode distal to the cathode or off the nerve trunk avoids anodal block of the antidromic impulse. The recording electrode ($G_1$) is placed over the motor point of the tested muscle and the reference electrode ($G_2$) over the tendon. An optimal display of F-waves requires an amplifier gain of 200 or 500 $\mu$V per cm and an oscilloscope sweep of 5 or 10 ms per cm, depending on the nerve length and stimulus point. These recording parameters truncate and compress the simultaneously recorded M-response into the initial portion of the tracing. Thus, one must study the M-response and F-wave separately, using different gains and time bases.

F-wave latencies measured from the stimulus artifact to the beginning of the evoked potential vary by a few milliseconds from one stimulus to the next. Hence, we display at least sixteen trials on a storage oscilloscope, automatically shifting successive sweeps vertically (Fig. 17-4). An adequate study requires more than ten F-waves clearly identified among these trials. In addition to the minimal latency, we determine the longest latency to assess the degree of scatter among consecutive F-waves, which provides a measure of temporal dispersion.[60]

Slight voluntary contraction often enhances the F-wave and is a maneuver employed in our laboratory. If voluntary impulses collide with antidromic activity in all axons, then the F-wave obviously cannot occur. Instead, reflexively activated impulses may elicit a late muscle response, since the motor axons are cleared of the antidromic impulse, which would ordinarily collide with the descending potentials. Thus, the late response produced by this type of activation may be contaminated by the H-reflex.[34, 82] However, with slight voluntary contractions, the relative number of axons carrying voluntary impulses at any given moment is very small.[41] The antidromic impulse will then reach the cell body in a majority of axons and generate recurrent discharges. Hence, the minimal latency of the late response recorded during mild voluntary contraction may be taken as representative of the fastest motor conduction to and from the spinal cord.

## Distal versus proximal stimulation

With distal stimulation at the wrist or ankle the motor conduction time along the entire length of the nerve may be determined. The accumulated delays allow detection of mild slowing in a diffusely affected nerve in proportion to the length of the activated pathway. Thus, relatively mild slowing may escape detection by conventional motor nerve conduction studies but appear as delayed F-waves. However, increased latency of the F-wave by itself is not specific to proximal conduction abnormalities. Such localization requires comparison of F-wave and M-response latencies with more proximal stimulation.

The F-wave first travels in the centripetal direction toward the spinal cord before it is transmitted distally to activate the muscle. With more proximal stimulation, the F-wave moves closer to the M-response, because the latency of the M-response increases, whereas that of the F-wave decreases. The F-wave occurs clearly after the M-response with stimulation at the wrist, elbow, ankle, and knee. With axillary stimulation, however, the M-response is superimposed on the F-wave.[38, 39] In this instance, simultaneous stimulation at the axilla and wrist helps to isolate the F-wave. With this technique, the orthodromic impulse from the axilla and the antidromic impulse from the wrist collide, leaving the M-response from the wrist and the F-wave from the axilla intact. These two remaining evoked muscle potentials do not overlap, allowing detection of the F-wave elicited by axillary stimulation.[38]

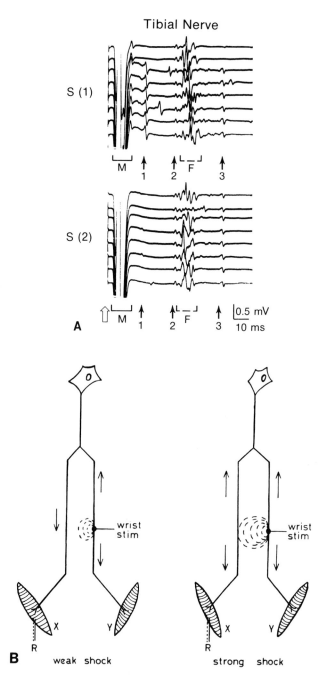

Figure 17-2

(A) 51-year-old man with low back pain. The right tibial nerve was stimulated at the ankle with weak shocks, S(1), and strong shocks, S(2). A series of eight trials were displayed simultaneously with stepwise vertical shift of the baseline. This type of display facilitates the selection of the minimal latency F-wave, while at the same time allowing careful assessments of all the individual late responses. Of the three axon reflexes indicated by small arrows, 1, 2, and 3, only the earliest response was eliminated with shocks of higher intensity. (B) Collateral sprouting in the proximal part of the nerve. The axon reflex is generated by weak stimulation but is eliminated by collision with the antidromic impulse when shock intensity is increased. (From Fullerton and Gilliatt,[26] with permission.)

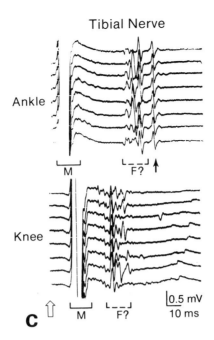

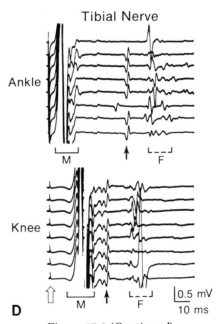

Figure 17-2 (Continued)

(C) The left tibial nerve was stimulated at the ankle and knee in the same patient as in part A. The axon reflex (arrow) that followed the F-wave with distal stimulation was eliminated with proximal stimulation. (D) 50-year-old man with recurrent backaches following laminectomy. The tibial nerve was stimulated at the ankle and knee. The latency of the axon reflex (arrow) was shortened by moving the stimulating electrode up the nerve trunk from the ankle to the knee. This indicates that propagation of the impulse is first in the proximal direction.

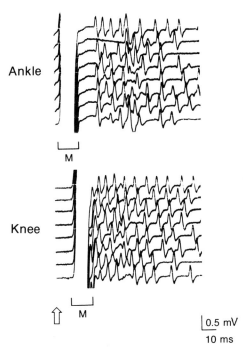

**Tibial Nerve**

Ankle

Knee

M

M

0.5 mV

10 ms

**Figure 17-3**
Incidental finding of unusual repetitive discharges resembling axon reflexes in a 38-year-old man with history of right pelvic fracture. The right tibial nerve was stimulated at the ankle and knee. The onset latency of the repetitive discharge was shortened with proximal as opposed to distal stimulation as expected for an axon reflex.

Using the collision technique, we have shown that the decrease in latency of the F-wave nearly equals the increase in latency of the M-response, when the stimulating point moves from the wrist to the elbow and then to the axilla. This observation allows the prediction of F-wave latency from the axilla without actual measurement, as it must equal the sum of the latencies of the F-wave and M-response elicited by distal stimulation minus the latency of the M-response evoked by axillary stimulation.[45] Or, $F(A) = F(W) + M(W) - M(A)$, where $F(A)$ and $F(W)$ are latencies of the F-waves from the axilla and wrist, respectively, and $M(A)$ and $M(W)$ are latencies of the corresponding M-responses from the same stimulus points.[3, 85]

To make clinical studies simple and brief, our routine procedures include study of the F-wave only with stimulation at the wrist and elbow for the median and ulnar nerves, and at the ankle and knee for the tibial and peroneal nerves. When necessary, we calculate the latency of the F-wave from any proximal sites by the equation described above. The F-wave may also occur after stimulation of the facial nerve,[71] but inadvertent stimulation of neighboring trigeminal afferent fibers may simultaneously activate reflex responses.[81]

# MOTOR CONDUCTION
# TO AND FROM THE SPINAL CORD

## Central latency

Central latency or conduction time from the stimulus point to and from the spinal cord equals F − M, where F and M are latencies of the F-wave and M-response, respectively (Fig. 17-5). Subtracting an estimated delay of 1.0 ms for the turn around time at the cell and dividing by two, $(F-M-1)/2$ represents the conduction time along the proximal segment from the stimulus site to the spinal cord. It is also postulated that the F-wave

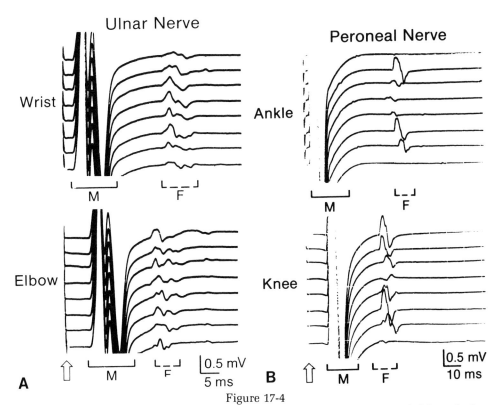

**Figure 17-4**

(A) Eight consecutive tracings showing normal M-responses and F-waves recorded from the hypothenar muscles after stimulation of the ulnar nerve at the wrist and elbow. (B) Eight consecutive tracings showing normal M-responses and F-waves recorded from the extensor digitorum brevis after stimulation of the peroneal nerve at the ankle and knee.

with the shortest latency travels in the fastest conducting motor fibers, and, therefore, is directly comparable to the M-response.

No information is available for the exact central delay at the anterior horn cells in man.[80] However, animal data indicate a delay of nearly 1.0 ms.[30, 53, 65] Furthermore, the absolute refractory period of the fastest human motor fibers lasts about 1.0 ms or slightly less.[40, 47] If recurrent discharge occurs earlier, the impulse cannot propagate distally because of refractoriness at the initial segment of the axon. For the F-wave of minimal latency, therefore, the turn around time is at least 1.0 ms and possibly greater.

A given F-wave represents only a portion of the motor axons available for activation of the M-response. The interval of a few milliseconds between the earliest and latest F-wave probably results from the difference between the fast and slow conducting motor fibers. The fastest fibers are studied by recording many F-waves and selecting the shortest F-wave latency.[6, 18, 38, 46, 49, 63] In some diseased nerves, however, surviving fibers that contribute to the M-response may not generate antidromic impulses. Thus, F-waves may not occur at all in the presence of an M-response. In less extreme instances, fast conducting fibers may be blocked proximally. F-waves then appear only in slow conducting fibers, while faster conducting fibers still contribute to the M-response, thus resulting in the false impression of proximal slowing.

The error, however, must be small if the increase in latency of the M-response equals the decrease in latency of the F-wave when the stimulus is moved proximally.[38, 46, 55, 63] One can test this relationship simply by comparing the sum of the F-latency and M-latency at distal and proximal stimulus sites. This observation indicates that the

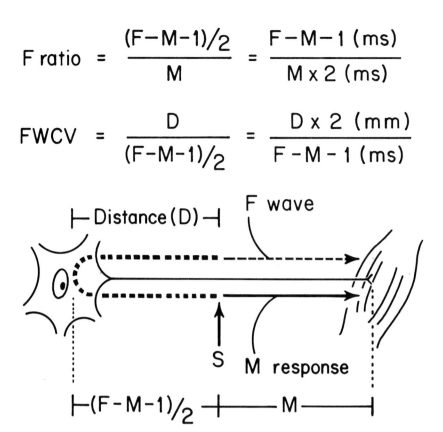

$$\text{F ratio} = \frac{(F-M-1)/2}{M} = \frac{F-M-1 \ (ms)}{M \times 2 \ (ms)}$$

$$\text{FWCV} = \frac{D}{(F-M-1)/2} = \frac{D \times 2 \ (mm)}{F-M-1 \ (ms)}$$

Figure 17-5

The latency difference between F-wave and M-response represents the passage of a motor impulse to and from the cord through the proximal segment. Considering an estimated minimal delay of 1.0 ms at the motor neuron pool, the proximal latency from the stimulus site to the cord is expressed as $(F-M-1)/2$, where F and M are latencies of F-wave and M-response, respectively. The FWCV in the segment to and from the spinal cord is calculated as $(D \times 2)/(F-M-1)$, where D is the distance from the stimulus site to the cord and $(F-M-1)/2$, the time required to cover the length D. The ratio between conduction time in the proximal segment to the cord and that of the remaining distal segment to the muscle is calculated as follows: F ratio $= (F-M-1)/2M$, where $(F-M-1)/2$ and M represent proximal and distal latencies, respectively. (From Kimura,[43] with permission.)

F-wave of minimal latency travels in the centripetal direction with the same speed as the centrifugal impulse of the earliest portion of the M-response. Thus, the same group of motor fibers, or at least those with the same conduction characteristics, contribute to the F-wave and the fastest components of M-response. This in turn provides a rationale for the direct latency comparison of these two muscle potentials.[42]

## F-wave conduction velocity

The F-wave conduction velocity (FWCV) can be calculated in the upper extremities based on the surface distance from the stimulus point to the C-7 spinous process via the axilla and midclavicular point.[38, 43] Likewise, a surface measurement is necessary to determine the distance from the stimulus site to the T-12 spinous process by way of the knee and greater trochanter of the femur in the lower extremities.[46] Estimation of the nerve length allows calculation of conduction velocity in the segment to and from the spinal cord as follows: FWCV $= (D \times 2)/(F-M-1)$, where D is the distance from the stimulus site to the cord, and $(F-M-1)/2$ is the time required to cover the length (Fig. 17-5).

Assessment of F-wave latencies requires determination of surface distances to adjust for differing nerve lengths. The height of the patient may be used for this purpose if a normogram is available.[79] The estimated length of a nerve segment by surface measurement correlates well with its F-wave latency. In a study of the lower extremities, observations in five cadavers showed good agreement between surface determinations and actual lengths of nerves.[46] No such data are available for the upper extremities. Absolute F-wave latencies may suffice in studying those extremities of average length.[7] The value of latency determination is enhanced if one compares the right and left sides in the same subject or one nerve with another in the same extremity (Tables 17-1 and 17-2).[42, 86]

## F-ratio

Proximal nerve compression syndromes may be assessed by the F/M ratio, where F and M are latencies of the F-wave and M-response, respectively.[18, 19] A similar ratio, $(F-M-1)/2M$, compares the conduction time from the cord to the stimulus site, represented by $(F-M-1)/2$, with that of the remaining distal nerve segment to the muscle, indicated by M. For this purpose, the median and ulnar nerves are stimulated at the elbow with the cathode at the volar crease and 3 cm above the medial epicondyle, respectively. The tibial and peroneal nerves are stimulated at the popliteal fossa and immediately above the head of the fibula, respectively. Designated the F-ratio, it provides a simple means to evaluate conduction characteristics of the proximal versus distal segment (Fig. 17-5). The F-ratio circumvents the need for nerve length determination but assumes the same proportion for the proximal and distal lengths of the extremity among different individuals.[43]

F-ratios are close to unity with stimulation at the elbow and knee, indicating equal conduction times to the cord and to the muscle from the site of stimulation (Table 17-1). This finding suggests faster conduction proximally, since the proximal segment is longer, whether estimated by surface determination or measured directly in cadavers.[46] Human studies of FWCV have also suggested faster conduction proximally than distally.[6, 38, 45, 46, 49, 58, 63] However, an experimental study of baboons has shown slower conduction of single motor axons in the brachial plexus than in the peripheral nerves.[5]

# THE F-WAVE IN HEALTH AND DISEASE

## Clinical value and limitations

Clinical uses of the F-wave suffer from inherent latency variability from one trial to the next. Determination of the shortest latency after a large number of trials partially circumvents this uncertainty. Recording as many as 100 F-waves at each stimulus site proved useful in special studies[64] but not practical in routine clinical applications. Calculation of central latency, F-wave conduction velocity (FWCV), and the F-ratio requires certain assumptions. But, a study is valid if one uses the same equations to establish the normal values for evaluating patients. We use the latency differences between two sides or between two nerves in the same limb in a unilateral disorder affecting a single nerve. Absolute latencies are used for assessing the entire course of the nerve in a diffuse process, and FWCV and the F-ratio for comparison between proximal and distal segments (Tables 17-1 and 17-2).

Abnormalities of the F-wave occur in Charcot-Marie-Tooth disease,[38, 46, 59] Guillain-Barré syndrome,[43, 45, 49] diabetic polyneuropathy,[6, 48] uremic polyneuropathy,[61, 62] alcoholic neuropathy,[51] entrapment neuropathies,[18, 86] amyotrophic lateral sclerosis,[1] and radiculopathies.[19, 24] Of these, the F-wave is perhaps most useful in patients with poly-

TABLE 17-1 F-waves in normal subjects[1]

| Number of nerves tested | Site of stimulation | F-wave latency to recording site ms | Difference between right and left ms | Central latency[2] to and from the spinal cord ms | Difference between right and left ms | Conduction velocity[3] to and from the spinal cord m/s | F-ratio[4] between proximal and distal segment |
|---|---|---|---|---|---|---|---|
| 122 median nerves from 61 subjects | wrist | 26.6 ± 2.2 (31)[6] | 0.95 ± 0.67 (2.3)[6] | 23.0 ± 2.1 (27)[6] | 0.93 ± 0.62 (2.2)[6] | 65.3 ± 4.7 (56)[7] | |
| | elbow | 22.8 ± 1.9 (27) | 0.76 ± 0.56 (1.9) | 15.4 ± 1.4 (18) | 0.71 ± 0.52 (1.8) | 67.8 ± 5.8 (56) | 0.98 ± 0.08 (0.82–1.14)[6,7] |
| | axilla[5] | 20.4 ± 1.9 (24) | 0.85 ± 0.61 (2.1) | 10.6 ± 1.5 (14) | 0.85 ± 0.58 (2.0) | | |
| 130 ulnar nerves from 65 subjects | wrist | 27.6 ± 2.2 (32) | 1.00 ± 0.83 (2.7) | 25.0 ± 2.1 (29) | 0.84 ± 0.59 (2.0) | 65.3 ± 4.8 (55) | |
| | above elbow | 23.1 ± 1.7 (27) | 0.68 ± 0.48 (1.6) | 16.0 ± 1.2 (18) | 0.73 ± 0.52 (1.8) | 65.7 ± 5.3 (55) | 1.05 ± 0.09 (0.87–1.23) |
| | axilla[5] | 20.3 ± 1.6 (24) | 0.73 ± 0.54 (1.8) | 10.4 ± 1.1 (13) | 0.76 ± 0.52 (1.8) | | |
| 120 peroneal nerves from 60 subjects | ankle | 48.4 ± 4.0 (56) | 1.42 ± 1.03 (3.5) | 44.7 ± 3.8 (52) | 1.28 ± 0.90 (3.1) | 49.8 ± 3.6 (43) | |
| | above knee | 39.9 ± 3.2 (46) | 1.28 ± 0.91 (3.1) | 27.3 ± 2.4 (32) | 1.18 ± 0.89 (3.0) | 55.1 ± 4.6 (46) | 1.05 ± 0.09 (0.87–1.23) |
| 118 tibial nerves from 59 subjects | ankle | 47.7 ± 5.0 (58) | 1.40 ± 1.04 (3.5) | 43.8 ± 4.5 (53) | 1.52 ± 1.02 (3.6) | 52.6 ± 4.3 (44) | |
| | knee | 39.6 ± 4.4 (48) | 1.25 ± 0.92 (3.1) | 27.6 ± 3.2 (34) | 1.23 ± 0.88 (3.0) | 53.7 ± 4.8 (44) | 1.11 ± 0.11 (0.89–1.33) |

1. Mean ± standard deviation (SD) in the same patients shown in Tables 6-1, 6-3, 6-9, and 6-11.
2. Central latency = F−M, where F and M are latencies of F-wave and M-response, respectively.
3. Conduction velocity = 2D/(F−M−1), where D is the distance from the stimulus point to the C-7 or T-12 spinous process.
4. F-ratio = (F−M−1)/2M with stimulation with the cathode on the volar crease at the elbow (median), 3 cm above the medial epicondyle (ulnar), just above the head of the fibula (peroneal), and in the popliteal fossa (tibial).
5. F(A) = F(E) + M(E) − M(A), where F(A) and F(E) are latencies of F-wave with stimulation at the axilla and elbow, respectively, and M(A) and M(E) are latencies of the corresponding M-response.
6. Upper limits of normal calculated as mean + 2SD.
7. Lower limits of normal calculated as mean − 2SD.

## TABLE 17-2 Comparison between two nerves in the same limb[1]

| Site of stimulation | F-wave latency to recording site | | | Central latency[2] to and from the spinal cord | | |
|---|---|---|---|---|---|---|
| | Median nerve ms | Ulnar nerve ms | Difference ms | Median nerve ms | Ulnar nerve ms | Difference ms |
| wrist | 26.6 ± 2.3 (31)[3] | 27.2 ± 2.5 (32)[3] | 1.00 ± 0.68 (2.4)[3] | 23.3 ± 2.2 (28)[3] | 24.5 ± 2.4 (29)[3] | 1.24 ± 0.75 (2.7)[3] |
| elbow | 22.9 ± 1.8 (26) | 23.0 ± 1.7 (26) | 0.84 ± 0.55 (1.9) | 15.5 ± 1.4 (18) | 16.0 ± 1.2 (18) | 0.79 ± 0.65 (2.1) |
| | Peroneal nerve ms | Tibial nerve ms | Difference ms | Peroneal nerve ms | Tibial nerve ms | Difference ms |
| ankle | 47.7 ± 4.0 (55) | 48.1 ± 4.2 (57) | 1.68 ± 1.21 (4.1) | 43.6 ± 4.0 (52) | 44.1 ± 3.9 (52) | 1.79 ± 1.20 (4.2) |
| knee | 39.6 ± 3.7 (47) | 40.1 ± 3.7 (48) | 1.71 ± 1.19 (4.1) | 27.1 ± 2.9 (33) | 28.0 ± 2.7 (33) | 1.75 ± 1.07 (3.9) |

1. Mean ± standard deviation (SD) in the same patients shown in Tables 6–2 and 6–10.
2. Central latency = F−M, where F and M are latencies of F-wave and M-response, respectively.
3. Upper limits of normal calculated as mean +2SD.

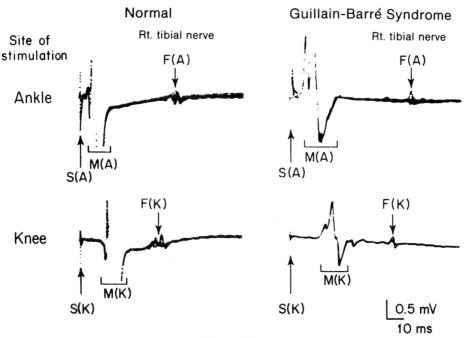

Figure 17-6

M-response (open brackets) and F-wave (small arrows) recorded from the abductor hallucis in two subjects. Three consecutive traces are superimposed for each. Compared with the control, the F-wave in the patient with the Guillain-Barré syndrome was increased in latency. The M-response was normal in latency, although reduced in amplitude.

neuropathies, particularly those associated with prominent proximal pathology (Figs. 17-6, 17-7, and 17-8). In the early diagnosis of more localized nerve lesions such as radiculopathies, the remaining normal segment tends to dilute a conduction delay across the much shorter segment. Thus, relatively mild abnormalities encountered in these conditions may not alter F-wave latency above and beyond its inherent variability.

The F-wave may provide a means to assess motor neuron excitability. According to Eisen and Odusote,[17] the average amplitude of 32 F-waves was 1 percent of the M-response in normals. This value significantly increased in patients with spasticity, primarily because the F-wave became more persistent. The largest F-wave, 4.5 percent of the M-response in normals, did not increase in the patient group with chronic paraparesis. It is conceivable that average as well as maximal amplitude of the F-wave is determined by the degree, duration, and type of spasticity.[27] We have recorded unusually large F-waves in association with clinical spasticity in occasional patients with upper motor neuron signs (Fig. 17-9). In these instances, reflex components may contribute to the late response, especially if the patient has prominent hyperreflexia. The amplitude of the F-wave also increases in disorders of the lower motor neuron, presumably because regenerated axons supply an increased number of muscle fibers.[73]

## Charcot-Marie-Tooth Disease

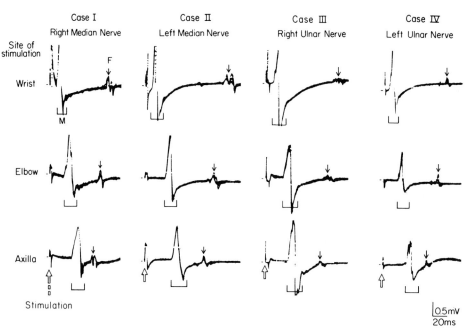

Figure 17-7

M-response (horizontal brackets) and F-wave (small arrows) recorded from the thenar (cases 1 and 2) and hypothenar muscles (cases 3 and 4) in patients with hereditary motor and sensory neuropathy Type I or hypertrophic type of Charcot-Marie-Tooth disease. Sites of supramaximal stimulus to the median and ulnar nerves are shown. Three consecutive traces are superimposed for each. A slower sweep speed (20 ms/cm instead of 5 ms/cm used for controls) was necessary to record these potentials, because latencies of both the M-response and the F-wave were markedly increased in these cases. Because of slowing in nerve conduction, the M-response and the F-wave were distinctly separate, even when stimulation was delivered at the axilla, rendering the collision technique unnecessary. (From Kimura,[38] with permission.)

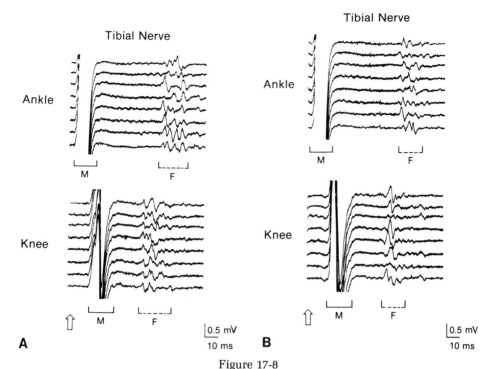

Figure 17-8

A 44-year-old man with adrenoleukodystrophy and diffuse weakness. The tibial nerve was stimulated at the ankle and knee on the right (A) and left (B). The F-waves recorded from the abductor hallucis were increased in latency and duration, showing marked temporal dispersion. Conventional motor nerve conduction studies were normal. (Compare Figure 17-4B.)

## Normal values

Tables 17-1 and 17-2 summarize the normal latencies and derived values of the F-wave described in the preceding section for the major nerves of the extremities. Compared with earlier results,[38, 46] F-wave latencies are slightly shorter in this series, because the stimulus site of the median and ulnar nerves at the wrist is three centimeters more proximal than the distal crease of the wrist used in earlier studies. In addition, we now elicit three times as many F-waves at each stimulus site. Slight voluntary facilitation routinely employed also increases the chance of recording the fastest conducting fibers. Two standard deviations above and below the mean are taken as the normal limits.

## Charcot-Marie-Tooth disease

Both the M-response and F-wave are difficult to elicit in the lower extremities[46, 59] and, if present, are markedly slowed in the upper extremities. These findings support the clinical impression that the lower extremities are more severely diseased (Table 17-3). Mildly affected nerves may show slow motor conduction in the distal segment and normal conduction in the proximal segment.[38] In advanced cases, conduction abnormalities affect both segments equally. A bimodal distribution of motor nerve conduction velocities (MNCV)[76, 77] supports the dichotomous separation of hereditary motor and sensory neuropathy Types I and II[11, 12] or hypertrophic and neuronal types of Charcot-Marie-Tooth disease, respectively. A number of intermediate values exist in latency of the F-wave as shown in the present series (Fig. 17-10), probably reflecting the extremes of the diseases.

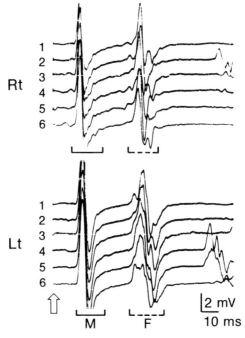

Figure 17-9

Unusually large F-waves recorded from the extensor digitorum brevis after supramaximal stimulation of the peroneal nerve at the knee in a 39-year-old man with chronic tetanus. Six consecutive trials are shown on each side to show consistency of the response. The average amplitude of six consecutive F-waves was 57 percent and 43 percent of the corresponding M-response on the right and left, respectively. Despite supramaximal stimulation, reflex components may have contributed to the late response in view of clinical hyperreflexia. (From Risk, et al,[66] with permission.)

## Guillain-Barré syndrome

Conduction abnormalities may involve any segment of the peripheral nerve in this syndrome (Table 17-4). However, the disease commonly affects the most proximal, possibly radicular, portion of the nerve, and the most distal or terminal segment and relatively spares the main nerve trunk in early stages.[2, 43, 45, 49] The MNCV may be normal in 15 to 20 percent of cases tested within the first few days of onset.[16, 36, 50] Some of these patients may have axonal neuropathies but others probably have the lesion too proximal to detect using ordinary techniques. In these cases, the F-wave is typically absent initially during acute stages of illness when the MNCVs are normal. The return of the previously absent F-wave indicates recovery of conduction across the proximal segment. The F-wave latency, however, is initially considerably increased, suggesting demyelination of the involved segment (Fig. 17-10).

In many patients the average F-ratio remains normal, indicating that the nerves are affected to the same degree above and below the stimulus site at the elbow and knee. This does not necessarily mean that conduction is uniformly slowed along the entire length of the peripheral nerve. In our series, slowing of FWCV in the cord-to-axilla occurred more frequently than slowing in the elbow-to-wrist segment for both the median and ulnar nerves. But, in calculating the F-ratio, a marked increase in terminal latency may compensate for the prominent proximal slowing.

## Diabetic neuropathy

Clinical observations in diabetics have repeatedly shown that neuropathic symptoms usually appear in the distal extremities. Distally predominant symptoms, however, do

### TABLE 17-3 Charcot-Marie-Tooth disease (mean ± SD)

| Number of nerves tested | Sites of stimulation | M-latency ms | F-latency ms | MNCV between two stimulus sites m/s | FWCV from cord to stimulus site m/s |
|---|---|---|---|---|---|
| 36 median nerves | wrist | 6.4 ± 3.0 | 55.6 ± 26.1 | 30.4 ± 14.6 | 33.7 ± 14.6 |
| | elbow | 15.6 ± 7.8 | 46.1 ± 21.4 | 38.9 ± 20.2 | 36.4 ± 14.9 |
| | axilla | 22.2 ± 10.6 | 39.3 ± 17.8 | | 38.4 ± 16.8 |
| 31 ulnar nerves | wrist | 5.2 ± 2.9 | 55.5 ± 35.1 | 38.0 ± 18.3 | 39.2 ± 18.7 |
| | below elbow | 13.1 ± 7.9 | 48.2 ± 29.8 | 36.6 ± 19.3 | 40.2 ± 19.0 |
| | above elbow | 18.0 ± 10.6 | 40.7 ± 27.2 | 42.5 ± 22.1 | 42.3 ± 20.8 |
| | axilla | 21.3 ± 14.0 | 37.3 ± 23.6 | | 43.7 ± 18.9 |
| 10 peroneal nerves | ankle | 5.6 ± 1.3 | 52.8 ± 10.6 | 40.7 ± 15.2 | 47.2 ± 6.9 |
| | knee | 15.0 ± 4.8 | 50.8 ± 19.1 | | 41.6 ± 6.8 |
| 12 tibial nerves | ankle | 5.4 ± 1.4 | 62.8 ± 21.3 | 40.3 ± 14.9 | 42.9 ± 14.2 |
| | knee | 16.2 ± 6.3 | 52.5 ± 15.3 | | 43.9 ± 12.3 |

not necessarily indicate a distal pathologic process, since probability models can reproduce a distal sensory deficit on the basis of randomly distributed axonal dysfunction.[83] In diabetics, F-wave latencies are increased and FWCVs are decreased over both proximal and distal segments.[6, 48] The average value and distribution of the F-ratio, however, indicate distally prominent conduction abnormalities despite slowing along the entire length of the nerve (Fig. 17-11).

## Entrapment syndromes

Patients with the carpal tunnel syndrome show a reduced F-ratio for the median nerve.[48] In our series, the value was nearly the same as in diabetics and significantly smaller than in control patients (Fig. 17-11). The slope of a regression line plotting the distal and proximal latencies was similar to that in diabetic neuropathy, but significantly different when compared with the control group. F-waves show significant abnormalities in ulnar compression neuropathies. Differences between minimum and

### TABLE 17-4 Guillain-Barré syndrome (mean ± SD)

| Number of nerves tested | Sites of stimulation | M-latency ms | F-latency ms | MNCV between two stimulus sites m/s | FWCV from cord to stimulus site m/s |
|---|---|---|---|---|---|
| 58 median nerves | wrist | 5.8 ± 3.1 | 38.1 ± 12.7 | 48.2 ± 12.1 | 48.6 ± 11.1 |
| | elbow | 11.2 ± 4.8 | 32.6 ± 9.9 | 55.5 ± 14.1 | 49.1 ± 11.4 |
| | axilla | 14.5 ± 5.7 | 29.4 ± 9.5 | | 47.5 ± 14.5 |
| 40 ulnar nerves | wrist | 4.0 ± 2.0 | 36.8 ± 8.6 | 52.2 ± 10.7 | 48.1 ± 9.7 |
| | below elbow | 8.3 ± 2.5 | 32.1 ± 7.1 | 47.7 ± 12.0 | 47.4 ± 9.6 |
| | above elbow | 11.2 ± 3.5 | 29.7 ± 8.7 | 56.8 ± 14.9 | 47.4 ± 10.7 |
| | axilla | 13.7 ± 4.8 | 27.2 ± 6.2 | | 48.0 ± 12.3 |
| 39 peroneal nerves | ankle | 7.6 ± 4.8 | 59.9 ± 11.5 | 43.0 ± 8.2 | 42.5 ± 8.7 |
| | knee | 16.9 ± 5.8 | 50.6 ± 10.3 | | 43.9 ± 11.8 |
| 29 tibial nerves | ankle | 5.6 ± 2.3 | 56.4 ± 10.6 | 43.3 ± 9.0 | 42.7 ± 8.8 |
| | knee | 14.6 ± 3.8 | 47.9 ± 9.4 | | 43.8 ± 9.9 |

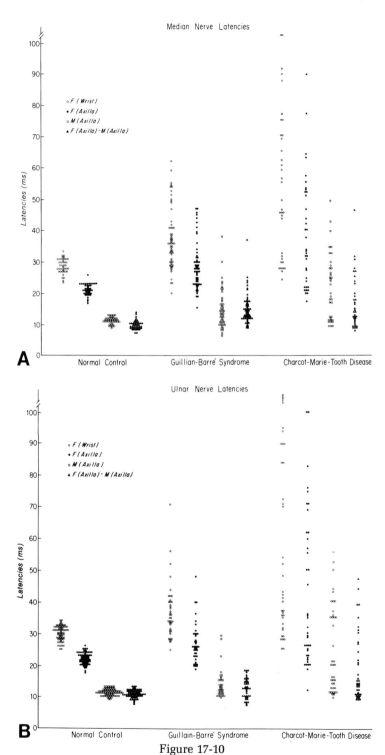

Figure 17-10

Latencies of F-wave and M-response for median (A), ulnar (B), peroneal (C), and tibial nerves (D) in normal subjects, patients with the Guillain-Barré syndrome (GBS), and patients with Charcot-Marie-Tooth disease (CMT). Only those nerves for which both F-wave and M-response were elicited are included. Sites of nerve stimulation are indicated in the key.

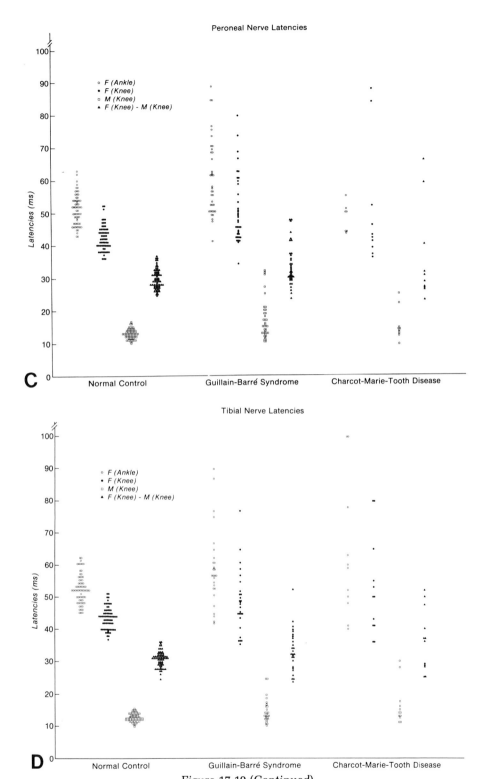

Figure 17-10 (Continued)

The difference in latency between F-wave and M-response (triangles) is the central latency required for passage of the impulses to and from the spinal cord. (From Kimura,[36] with permission.)

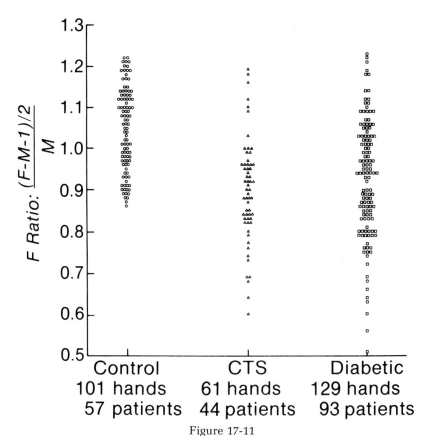

Figure 17-11

F-ratio of the median nerve in the control group, carpal tunnel syndrome (CTS), and diabetic polyneuropathy (DPN). Significantly reduced ratios in both disease groups indicate disproportionate slowing of motor conduction distally. (From Kimura,[36] with permission.)

maximum F-wave latencies may provide a sensitive indicator for early detection of this syndrome.[74, 75]

## Plexopathy and radiculopathy

F-wave assessments have been useful in patients with root injuries,[18, 19, 24, 79] but the F-wave is usually normal in mild cases of radiculopathy, especially if the lesion primarily affects the sensory fibers. The F-wave is also normal in the thoracic outlet syndrome with predominantly vascular symptoms,[42, 74, 75] although the neuronal type, or classical thoracic outlet syndrome does affect the F-wave latency.[10, 31, 84, 86] We have often encountered normal F-waves in clinically unequivocal cases of brachial or lumbosacral plexopathy. Thus, normal F-wave latencies do not preclude the presence of radicular or plexus lesions, and the F-wave determination seems less helpful than might have been expected on theoretical grounds in early diagnosis of these conditions.[42] However, unequivocal delay of the F-wave in conjunction with normal motor conduction distally is a sign of a proximal lesion (Fig. 17-12). Comparison of F-wave latencies between the right and left sides in the same subject may provide a reliable means of assessing unilateral radicular or plexus lesions.[42] Further work is necessary to prove or disprove such a contention, however.

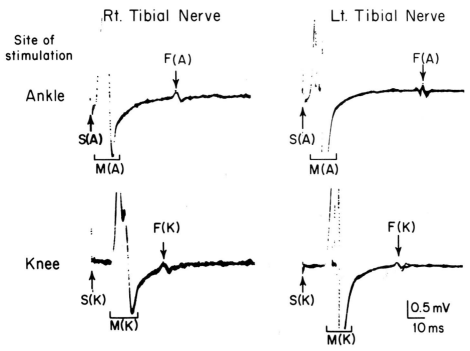

# Left Sacral Plexus Lesion

Figure 17-12

M-response (open brackets) and F-wave (small arrows) recorded from the abductor hallucis after stimulation of the tibial nerve at the ankle and knee in a patient with sacral plexus lesion on the left. The F-wave was increased in latency on the affected side as compared with the normal side.

# REFERENCE SOURCES

1.  ARGYROPOULOS, CJ, PANAYIOTOPOULOS, CP, AND SCARPALEZOS, S: *F- and M-wave conduction velocity in amyotrophic lateral sclerosis*. Muscle and Nerve 1:479, 1978.

2.  ASBURY, AK, ARNASON, BG, AND ADAMS, RD: *The inflammatory lesion in idiopathic polyneuritis: Its role in pathogenesis*. Medicine 48:173, 1969.

3.  BABA, M, NARITA, S, AND MATSUNAGA, M: *F-wave conduction velocity from the spinal cord to the axilla without using collision technique. A simplified method*. Electromyogr Clin Neurophysiol 20:19, 1980.

4.  BROCK, LG, COOMBS, JS, AND ECCLES, JC: *Intracellular recording from antidromically activated motoneurones*. J Physiol (Lond) 122:429, 1953.

5.  CLOUGH, JFM, KERNELL, D, AND PHILLIPS, CG: *Conduction velocity in proximal and distal portions of forelimb axons in the baboon*. J Physiol (Lond) 198:167, 1968.

6.  CONRAD, B, ASCHOFF, JC, AND FISCHLER, M: *Der diagnostische Wert der F-Wellen-Latenz*. J Neurol 210:151, 1975.

7.  DAUBE, JR: *F-wave and H-reflex measurements*. American Academy of Neurology, Special Course #16, Clinical Electromyography, Chicago, 1979.

8.  DAWSON, GD AND MERTON, PA: *"Recurrent" discharges from motoneurones*. XXth International Physiological Congress, Brussels, 1956.

9.  DESMEDT, JE AND NOËL, P: *Average cerebral evoked potentials in the evaluation of lesions of the sensory nerves and of the central somatosensory pathway*. In DESMEDT, JE (ED): *New*

Developments in Electromyography and Clinical Neurophysiology, Vol 2. Karger, Basel, 1973, pp 352–371.

10. DORFMAN, LJ: F-wave latency in the cervical-rib-and-band syndrome. Muscle and Nerve 2:158, 1979.

11. DYCK, PJ: Inherited neuronal degeneration and atrophy affecting peripheral motor, sensory, and autonomic neurons. In DYCK, PJ, THOMAS, PK, AND LAMBERT, EH (EDS): Peripheral Neuropathy, Vol 2. WB Saunders, Philadelphia, 1975.

12. DYCK, PJ AND LAMBERT, EH: Lower motor and primary sensory neuron diseases with peroneal muscular atrophy. II. Neurologic, genetic, and electrophysiologic findings in various neuronal degenerations. Arch Neurol 18:619, 1968.

13. ECCLES, JC: The central action of antidromic impulses in motor nerve fibres. Pflügers Archiv 260:385, 1955.

14. ECCLES, JC: The inhibitory control of spinal reflex action. Electroenceph Clin Neurophysiol (suppl 25):20, 1967.

15. ECCLES, JC, ET AL: Distribution of recurrent inhibition among motoneurones. J Physiol (Lond) 159:479, 1961.

16. EISEN, A AND HUMPHREYS, P: The Guillain-Barré syndrome. A clinical and electrodiagnostic study of 25 cases. Arch Neurol 30:438, 1974.

17. EISEN, A AND ODUSOTE, K: Amplitude of the F wave: A potential means of documenting spasticity. Neurology (New York) 29:1306, 1979.

18. EISEN, A, SCHOMER, D, AND MELMED, C: The application of F-wave measurements in the differentiation of proximal and distal upper limb entrapments. Neurology (Minneap) 27:662, 1977.

19. EISEN, A, SCHOMER, D, AND MELMED, C: An electrophysiological method for examining lumbosacral root compression. J Canad des Sciences Neurologiques 4:117, 1977.

20. FISHER, MA: Electrophysiological appraisal of relative segmental motoneurone pool excitability in flexor and extensor muscles. J Neurol Neurosurg Psychiatry 41:624, 1978.

21. FISHER, MA: F waves: Comments on the central control of recurrent discharges. Muscle and Nerve 2:406, 1979.

22. FISHER, MA: F-response latency-duration correlations: An argument for the orderly antidromic activation of motoneurons. Muscle and Nerve 3:437, 1980.

23. FISHER, MA, SHAHANI, BT, AND YOUNG, RR: Assessing segmental excitability after acute rostral lesions. I. The F response. Neurology (New York) 28:1265, 1978.

24. FISHER, MA, ET AL: Clinical and electrophysiological appraisal of the significance of radicular injury in back pain. J Neurol Neurosurg Psychiatry 41:303, 1978.

25. FULLERTON, PM AND GILLIATT, RW: Intermediate latency responses to nerve stimulation. Electroenceph Clin Neurophysiol 17:94, 1964.

26. FULLERTON, PM AND GILLIATT, RW: Axon reflexes in human motor nerve fibres. J Neurol Neurosurg Psychiatry 28:1, 1965.

27. GARCIA-MULLIN, R AND MAYER, RF: H reflexes in acute and chronic hemiplegia. Brain 95:559, 1972.

28. GASSEL, MM: Monosynaptic reflexes (H-reflex) and motoneurone excitability in man. Dev Med Child Neurol 11:193, 1969.

29. GASSEL, MM AND WIESENDANGER, M: Recurrent and reflex discharges in plantar muscles of the cat. Acta Physiol Scand 65:138, 1965.

30. GASSEL, MM, MARCHIAFAVA, PL, AND POMPEIANO, O: Modulation of the recurrent discharge of alpha motoneurons in decerebrate and spinal cats. Arch Ital Biol 103:1, 1965.

31. GILLIATT, RW, ET AL: Peripheral nerve conduction in patients with a cervical rib and band. Ann Neurol 4:124, 1978.

32. GRANIT, R, PASCOE, JE, AND STEG, G: The behavior of tonic α and γ motoneurones during stimulation of recurrent collaterals. J Physiol (Lond) 138:381, 1957.

33. HAGBARTH, KE: Spinal withdrawal reflexes in the human lower limbs. J Neurol Neurosurg Psychiatry 23:222, 1960.

34. HAGBARTH, KE: *Post-tetanic potentiation of myotatic reflexes in man.* J Neurol Neurosurg Psychiatry 25:1, 1962.

35. HENNEMAN, E, SOMJEN, G, AND CARPENTER, DO: *Excitability and inhibitibility of motoneurons of different sizes.* J Neurophysiol 28:599, 1965.

36. HUMPHREY, JG: *Motor nerve conduction studies in the Landry-Guillain-Barré syndrome (acute ascending polyneuropathy).* Electroenceph Clin Neurophysiol 17:96, 1964.

37. KERNELL, D: *Input resistance, electrical excitability, and size of ventral horn cells in cat spinal cord.* Science 152:1637, 1966.

38. KIMURA, J: *F-wave velocity in the central segment of the median and ulnar nerves. A study in normal subjects and in patients with Charcot-Marie-Tooth disease.* Neurology (Minneap) 24:539, 1974.

39. KIMURA, J: *Collision technique. Physiologic block of nerve impulses in studies of motor nerve conduction velocity.* Neurology (Minneap) 26:680, 1976.

40. KIMURA, J: *A method for estimating the refractory period of motor fibers in the human peripheral nerve.* J Neurol Sci 28:485, 1976.

41. KIMURA, J: *Electrical activity in voluntarily contracting muscle.* Arch Neurol 34:85, 1977.

42. KIMURA, J: *Clinical value and limitations of F-wave determination. A comment. Letter to the Editor.* Muscle and Nerve 1:250, 1978.

43. KIMURA, J: *Proximal versus distal slowing of motor nerve conduction velocity in the Guillain-Barré syndrome.* Ann Neurol 3:344, 1978.

44. KIMURA, J: *F-wave determination in nerve conduction studies.* In DESMEDT, JE (ED): *Brain and spinal mechanisms of movement control in man: New developments in clinical applications.* Raven Press, New York, 1982 (in press).

45. KIMURA, J AND BUTZER, JF: *F-wave conduction velocity in Guillain-Barré syndrome. Assessment of nerve segment between axilla and spinal cord.* Arch Neurol 32:524, 1975.

46. KIMURA, J, BOSCH, P, AND LINDSAY, GM: *F-wave conduction velocity in the central segment of the peroneal and tibial nerves.* Arch Phys Med Rehabil 56:492, 1975.

47. KIMURA, J, YAMADA, T, AND RODNITZKY, RL: *Refractory period of human motor nerve fibres.* J Neurol Neurosurg Psychiatry 41:784, 1978.

48. KIMURA, J, YAMADA, T, AND STEVLAND, NP: *Distal slowing of motor nerve conduction velocity in diabetic polyneuropathy.* J Neurol Sci 42:291, 1979.

49. KING, D AND ASHBY, P: *Conduction velocity in the proximal segments of a motor nerve in the Guillain-Barré syndrome.* J Neurol Neurosurg Psychiatry 39:538, 1976.

50. LAMBERT, EH AND MULDER, DW: *Nerve conduction in the Guillain-Barré syndrome.* Electroenceph Clin Neurophysiol 17:86, 1964.

51. LEFEBVRE D'AMOUR, M, ET AL: *The importance of studying sural nerve conduction and late responses in the evaluation of alcoholic subjects.* Neurology (New York) 29:1600, 1979.

52. LIBERSON, WT, ET AL: *Comparison of conduction velocities of motor and sensory fibers determined by different methods.* Arch Phys Med Rehabil 47:17, 1966.

53. LLOYD, DPC: *The interaction of antidromic and orthodromic volleys in a segmental spinal motor nucleus.* J Neurophysiol 6:143, 1943.

54. MAGLADERY, JW AND McDOUGAL, DB, JR: *Electrophysiological studies of nerve and reflex activity in normal man. 1. Identification of certain reflexes in the electromyogram and the conduction velocity of peripheral nerve fibres.* Bull Johns Hopkins Hosp 86:265, 1950.

55. MAYER, RF AND FELDMAN, RG: *Observations on the nature of the F wave in man.* Neurology (Minneap) 17:147, 1967.

56. McLEOD, JG AND WRAY, SH: *An experimental study of the F wave in the baboon.* J Neurol Neurosurg Psychiatry 29:196, 1966.

57. MIGLIETTA, OE: *The F response after transverse myelotomy.* In DESMEDT, JE (ED): *New Developments in Electromyography and Clinical Neurophysiology,* Vol 3. Karger, Basel, 1973, pp 323–327.

58. MÜLLER, D: *Die Bestimmung der F-Wellengeschwindigkeit am N. Ulnaris Gesunder.* Psychiatr Neurol Med Psychol 27:619, 1975.

59. PANAYIOTOPOULOS, CP: *F-wave conduction velocity in the deep peroneal nerve: Charcot-Marie-Tooth disease and dystrophia myotonica.* Muscle and Nerve 1:37, 1978.

60. PANAYIOTOPOULOS, CP: *F chronodispersion: A new electrophysiologic method.* Muscle and Nerve 2:68–72, 1979.

61. PANAYIOTOPOULOS, CP AND LAGOS, G: *Tibial nerve H-reflex and F-wave studies in patients with uremic neuropathy.* Muscle and Nerve 3:423, 1980.

62. PANAYIOTOPOULOS, CP AND SCARPALEZOS, S: *F-wave studies on the deep peroneal nerve. Part 2. 1. Chronic renal failure 2. Limb-girdle muscular dystrophy.* J Neurol Sci 31:331, 1977.

63. PANAYIOTOPOULOS, CP, SCARPALEZOS, S, AND NASTAS, PE: *F-wave studies on the deep peroneal nerve. Part 1. Control subjects.* J Neurol Sci 31:319, 1977.

64. PANAYIOTOPOULOS, CP, SCARPALEZOS, S, AND NASTAS, PE: *Sensory (1a) and F-wave conduction velocity in the proximal segment of the tibial nerve.* Muscle and Nerve 1:181, 1978.

65. RENSHAW, B: *Influence of discharge of motoneurons upon excitation of neighboring motoneurons.* J Neurophysiol 4:167, 1941.

66. RISK, WS, ET AL: *Chronic tetanus: Clinical report and histochemistry of muscle.* Muscle and Nerve 4:363, 1981.

67. ROTH, G: *Intravenous regeneration of lower motor neuron- 1. Study of 1153 motor axon reflexes.* Electromyograph Clin Neurophysiol 18:225, 1978.

68. ROTH, G: *Intravenous regeneration. The study of motor axon reflexes.* J Neurol Sci 41:139, 1979.

69. SATOYOSHI, E, DOI, Y, AND KINOSHITA, M: *Pseudomyotonia in cervical root lesions with myelopathy. A sign of the misdirection of regenerating nerve.* Arch Neurol 27:307, 1972.

70. SAWHNEY, BB AND KAYAN, A: *A study of axon reflexes in some neurogenic disorders.* Electromyography 10:297, 1970.

71. SAWHNEY, BB AND KAYAN, A: *A study of the F wave from the facial muscles.* Electroenceph Clin Neurophysiol 30:261, 1971.

72. SCHILLER, HH AND STÅLBERG, E: *F responses studied with single fibre EMG in normal subjects and spastic patients.* J Neurol Neurosurg Psychiatry 41:45, 1978.

73. SHAHANI, BT, POTTS, F, AND DOMINGUE, J: *F response studies in peripheral neuropathies.* Neurology (New York) 30:409, 1980.

74. SHAHANI, BT, ET AL: *Maximal-minimal motor nerve conduction and F response studies in normal subjects and patients with ulnar compression neuropathies.* Muscle and Nerve 3:182, 1980.

75. SHAHANI, BT, ET AL: *Electrophysiological studies in "thoracic outlet syndrome."* Muscle and Nerve 3:182, 1980.

76. THOMAS, PK AND CALNE, DB: *Motor nerve conduction velocity in peroneal muscular atrophy: Evidence for genetic heterogeneity.* J Neurol Neurosurg Psychiatry 37:68, 1974.

77. THOMAS, PK, CALNE, DB, AND STEWART, G: *Hereditary motor and sensory polyneuropathy (peroneal muscular atrophy).* Ann Hum Genet 38:111, 1974.

78. THORNE, J: *Central responses to electrical activation of the peripheral nerves supplying the intrinsic hand muscles.* J Neurol Neurosurg Psychiatry 28:482, 1965.

79. TONZOLA, RF, ET AL: *Usefulness of electrophysiological studies in the diagnosis of lumbosacral root disease.* Ann Neurol 9:305, 1981.

80. TRONTELJ, JV: *A study of the F response by single fibre electromyography.* In DESMEDT, JE (ED): *New Developments in Electromyography and Clinical Neurophysiology, Vol 3.* Karger, Basel, 1973, pp 318–322.

81. TRONTELJ, JV AND TRONTELJ, M: *F-responses of human facial muscles. A single motoneurone study.* J Neurol Sci 20:211, 1973.

82. UPTON, ARM, McCOMAS, AJ, AND SICA, REP: *Potentiation of 'late' responses evoked in muscles during effort.* J Neurol Neurosurg Psychiatry 34:699, 1971.

83. WAXMAN, SG, ET AL: *Probability of conduction deficit as related to fiber length in random-distribution models of peripheral neuropathies.* J Neurol Sci 29:39, 1976.

84.  WEBER, RJ AND PIERO, DL: *F wave evaluation of thoracic outlet syndrome: A multiple regression derived F wave latency predicting technique.* Arch Phys Med Rehabil 59:464, 1978.

85.  WU, Y, ET AL: *Axillary F central latency: A simple electrodiagnostic technique for proximal neuropathy.* Arch Phys Med Rehabil, 1982 (in press).

86.  WULFF, CH AND GILLIATT, RW: *F waves in patients with hand wasting caused by a cervical rib and band.* Muscle and Nerve 2:452, 1979.

87.  YATES, SK AND BROWN, WF: *Characteristics of the F response: A single motor unit study.* J Neurol Neurosurg Psychiatr 42:161, 1979.

88.  YOUNG, RR AND SHAHANI, BT: *Clinical value and limitations of F-wave determination.* Letter to the editor. Muscle and Nerve 1:248, 1978.

# CHAPTER 18

# THE H-REFLEX AND OTHER LATE RESPONSES

Nerve stimulation techniques commonly used in an electromyography laboratory are traditionally applicable to the distal segments of the peripheral nerves. More recently, several neurophysiologic methods have been introduced as tests of the proximal nerve segments as well as the central nervous system. Of potential interest are the blink reflex and F-wave described in previous chapters. One can also explore different levels of the nervous system using the H-reflex, T-reflex, tonic vibration reflex, and silent period. These techniques assess conduction characteristics along the entire course of the axon as well as motor neuron excitability.

The H-reflex has long been used as a clinical test, and its practical value in certain neurologic disorders is now well established. The other techniques have also been extensively studied physiologically, but their clinical applications have been limited. Nonetheless, these methods are promising as a means of quantitating clinical observation. This chapter will review the basic physiology and some clinical applications of these newer techniques for regions of the nervous system not accessible to conventional diagnostic methods.

## H-REFLEX AND T-REFLEX

The muscle stretch reflex of the triceps surae provides a measure of motor neuron excitability in spasticity and other neurologic phenomena. However, clinical observation does not objectively quantitate the briskness, the velocity, and the bilateral symmetry of these responses. Electrophysiologic recordings of the stretch reflex after a mechanical tap to the Achilles tendon or after direct electrical stimulation of the 1A afferent fibers of the tibial nerve do offer these advantages. The electrically elicited spinal monosynaptic reflex (H-reflex) was originally described by Hoffmann,[59] and further investigated by Magladery and associates,[82, 83] Paillard,[102] and many others. The H-reflex is equivalent in many respects to the monosynaptic reflex elicited by a mechanical tap to the tendon (T-reflex), since the same motor neuron pool is activated in both responses. But, since the stimulus for the H-reflex bypasses the muscle spindles, comparison between the H- and T-reflexes provides an indirect means to assess spindle sensitivity controlled by the gamma motor system.[8]

# H-reflex versus F-wave

In clinical tests, the H-reflex must be distinguished from the F-wave. An H-reflex may be elicited by stimulation of the ulnar nerve in newborn infants and during the first year of life.[57, 126] In adults, the reflex is normally limited to the calf muscles and flexor carpi radialis at rest.[20] However, mild voluntary contraction may prime the motor neuron pool sufficiently for reflex activation in other antigravity muscles and, to a lesser extent, in physiologic flexors of both upper and lower extremities.[29, 44, 120] The limited distribution of the H-reflex contrasts with a much wider representation of the F-wave, which occurs in practically any distal limb muscle.

The effect of increasing stimulus intensity from subthreshold to supramaximal levels also distinguishes the H-reflex from the F-wave (Fig. 18-1). H-reflex amplitude increases initially as the stimulus is raised from the subthreshold to submaximal range. As the M-response begins to appear with further increases in shock intensity, the H-reflex diminishes progressively and is eventually replaced by the F-wave when the stimulus strength becomes supramaximal. Thus, the H-reflex is best elicited by a stimulus submaximal for the M-response, whereas the F-wave occurs with shocks of supramaximal intensity. However, not all late responses recorded with submaximal intensity are of reflex origin, since, if any motor axons are activated by the stimulus, the antidromic impulse in those axons can generate recurrent discharges.

Possible mechanisms for the extinction of the H-reflex with increasing stimulus intensity include: (1) collision of the reflex impulse with antidromic activity in the alpha motor axon;[59, 81] (2) refractoriness of the axon hillock secondary to preceding passage of the antidromic impulse;[40] and (3) Renshaw inhibition mediated by motor neuron axon collaterals via internuncial cells to the same and neighboring alpha motor neurons.[24, 107, 127, 130]

Consecutive F-waves characteristically vary in latency and waveform, as they represent recurrent discharges of different groups of motor neurons with different con-

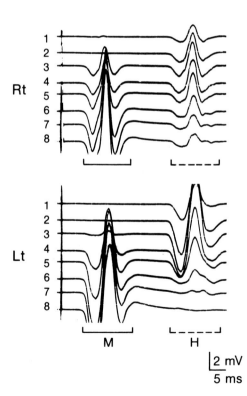

Figure 18-1

H-reflex recorded from the soleus after stimulation of the tibial nerve at the knee. Shock intensity was gradually increased from subthreshold level (1) to supramaximal stimulation (8). Note initial increase and subsequent decrease in amplitude of the reflex potential with successive stimuli of progressively higher intensity. The H-reflex normally disappears with shocks of supramaximal intensity that elicit a maximal M-response.

duction characteristics. In contrast, H-reflexes remain constant in response to repetitive stimuli as each trial activates the same motor neuron pool (Fig. 18-2). When recording from single motor fibers, however, the latency variability of consecutive H-reflexes far exceeds that of the F-waves. As mentioned earlier, this reflects greater variability in single axon synaptic transmission compared with the variability in turn around time for a recurrent discharge.[115, 127] The latency of successive H-reflexes recorded from single muscle fibers of the human triceps surae varied up to 2.5 ms.[127]

## Recording procedures

For routine determination of reflex latencies, the H-reflex is recorded from the soleus with the patient supine or prone on an examining table (Fig. 18-3). For an accurate analysis of the amplitude or force of the reflex response, the subjects sit upright in a modified dental chair that is preferably equipped with a potentiometer for monitoring the movement of the feet and a force transducer to measure the torque.[66] To relax the calf muscles, the knee is supported by a soft cushion and semiflexed at about 120 degrees. The angle of the ankle joint is kept constant at about 110 degrees. One pair of recording electrodes is placed along the longitudinal axis of the calf, the active electrode ($G_1$) being 2 cm distal to the insertion of the gastrocnemius on the Achilles tendon and the reference electrode ($G_2$), 3 cm further distally. Alternatively, $G_1$ may be placed over the soleus just medial to the tibia, one half the distance from the tibial tubercle to the medial malleolus, with $G_2$ over the Achilles tendon medial and proximal to the medial malleolus.[12] The H-reflex is recorded as a triphasic potential with initial positivity in the former arrangement, and as a diphasic potential with initial negativity in the latter. A second pair of electrodes placed over the belly of the anterior tibialis muscle 3 cm apart, along the longitudinal axis and near midline, monitors the antagonistic muscle. A ground electrode is located between the stimulation and recording electrodes.

We use two different types of stimuli: (1) an electrical shock applied to the tibial nerve at the popliteal fossa (H-reflex); and (2) a mechanical tap of the Achilles tendon with a conventional reflex hammer fitted to trigger the oscilloscope (T-reflex). Stimulus conditions must be standardized to obtain reproducible reflexes. Intensities of me-

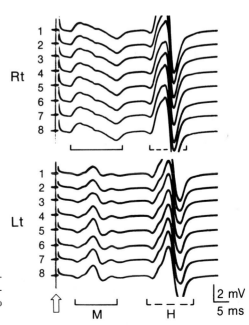

**Figure 18-2**
H-reflex from the soleus after stimulation (arrow) of the tibial nerve at the knee. Eight consecutive trials are shown on each side to show consistency of the response.

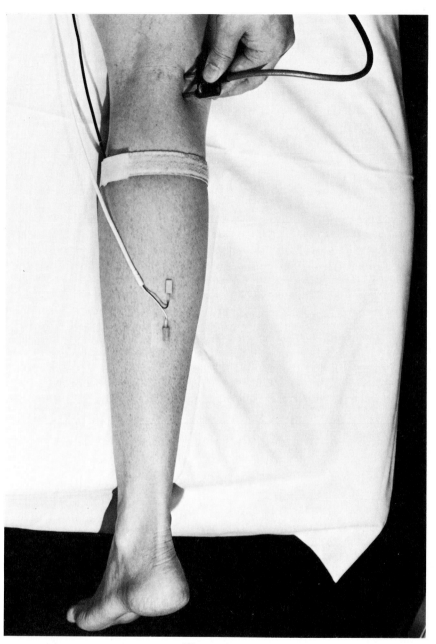

Figure 18-3

Recording of the H-reflex from the soleus. A pair of surface electrodes is placed along the midline of the calf muscle with the active ($G_1$) electrode 2 cm distal to the insertion of the gastrocnemius and the inactive electrode ($G_2$) 3 cm further distally. The tibial nerve is stimulated at the popliteal fossa with the cathode placed 2 cm proximal to the anode.

chanical and electrical stimuli are adjusted individually to obtain the maximal responses. To maintain the temperature along the nerve at 35 to 37°C, the skin temperature above the popliteal nerve is kept at 34°C.

Studies under isometric conditions measure the force of induced muscle contraction (myogram) with a force transducer placed against the foot plate. Isotonic conditions allow determination of the degree and rate of foot displacement (motogram), using a potentiometer mounted on the axis of the foot plate. In each series, muscle action potentials of the soleus and anterior tibialis are simultaneously recorded (electromyogram). The latencies of the H- and T-reflexes are measured from the stimulus artifact to the onset of the initial negative or positive deflection. Additional parameters commonly determined include H max/M max, where H max and M max are the maximal amplitude of the H-reflex and M-response, respectively; and T max/M max, where T max is the maximal amplitude of the T-reflex elicited by a brief stretch of the Achilles tendon.

## Excitability and recovery curve

The amplitudes of the H- and T-reflexes depend upon the strength of the mechanical or electrical stimuli as well as the excitability of the alpha motor neurons. If the stimulus is kept constant, variations in the amplitude of the evoked response provide a measure of excitability changes in the soleus motor neuron.[91, 95, 118] Supraspinal influences on the H-reflex have been extensively investigated.[95] The response in the lower limb is significantly influenced by postural changes of the upper limb.[18] Caloric stimulation of the labyrinth facilitates the H-reflex bilaterally and approximately symmetrically.[15, 16] Sleep, in general, depresses the H-reflex, but a much greater reduction occurs during the rapid eye movement period.[57]

In the paired shock technique, alterations in motor neuron excitability are induced by a conditioning stimulus.[17, 30, 41, 70, 102, 103, 136] With shocks of suprathreshold intensity, some motor neurons discharge in response to the conditioning stimulus and others do not. Those motor neurons activated by the conditioning stimulus become less responsive to the test stimulus because of Renshaw and other inhibitory mechanisms. However, the motor neurons that are subliminally primed by the conditioning stimulus are more easily excited by the test stimulus. The presence of these two opposing factors complicates the evaluation of excitability changes of the motor neuron pool when using a suprathreshold conditioning stimulus.[53]

A subthreshold conditioning stimulus applied to the tibial nerve causes an early facilitation lasting up to 25 ms, a period of depression lasting 25 to 75 ms, and late facilitation lasting about 300 ms (Fig. 18-4). Initial facilitation is attributed to excitatory postsynaptic potentiation in subliminally excited alpha motor neurons.[124, 125] Subsequent depression is presumably caused by presynaptic inhibition or transmitter depletion. Late facilitation, seen bilaterally with unilateral conditioning,[111] results from interaction of cutaneous segmental or long loop reflexes.[31, 32]

Selective cutaneous stimulation of the peroneal or tibial nerve can also be used to assess supranuclear control of the H-reflex.[105] In normal subjects, it results in marked reduction of the H-reflex at an interstimulus interval of about 100 ms.[31, 32, 64, 65] This physiologic inhibition is significantly reduced in Parkinsonian rigidity.[87] In patients with corticospinal lesions, conditioning cutaneous stimulation facilitates the H-reflex, whereas it would inhibit the reflex in normal subjects. The paired shock technique of the H-reflex has also been used to study reciprocal inhibition[3, 96, 98, 135] and reflex interactions.[51, 80]

## Clinical value of latency measurement

H-reflex latency is a measure of conduction velocity in the proximal segment of the tibial nerves.[43] It increases in patients with various polyneuropathies. In diabetics this measurement rivals the conventional nerve conduction studies in detecting early neuropathic abnormalities.[132, 133] The test also appears to be a sensitive indicator of the mild neuropathies associated with alcoholism[134] or uremia,[50] and of maturational changes in the proximal versus distal segment of the tibial nerve.[131]

Reflex changes occur with lumbar and sacral root compression. Although the usefulness of the T-reflex in the study of nerve root compression was described some

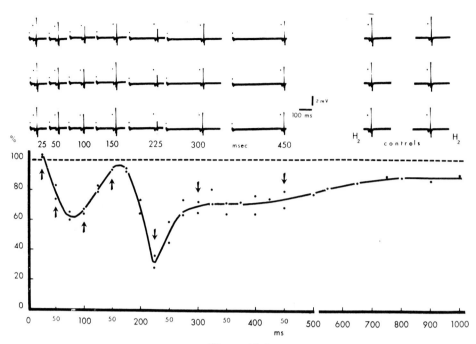

Figure 18-4

Conditioning of an H-reflex by a subliminal H-reflex stimulus. In the upper half are specimen records which are arranged in groups of three for each experimental situation. To the right are three $H_2$ control reflexes before and after the conditioning series. To the left are groups of three conditioned $H_2$ reflexes at testing intervals of 25, 50, 100, 150, 225, 300, and 450 ms as indicated below. The $S_1$ stimulus was just below the threshold for evoking an H-reflex, while the $S_2$ stimulus was just below the threshold for an M-response. Below is plotting of the mean of the three $H_2$ reflexes at each testing interval (abscissa), the mean sizes being expressed as percentages of the mean $H_2$ reflex controls. (From Táboříková and Sax,[125] with permission.)

time ago,[84] application of the H-reflex for this purpose has been popularized only during recent years.[9, 19, 116] The H-reflex recorded from the triceps surae is primarily mediated by the S-1 nerve root. Therefore, like the clinical ankle stretch reflex, the H-reflex of the triceps surae helps differentiate S-1 versus L-5 radiculopathy. The H-reflex recorded from the extensor digitorum longus by common peroneal nerve stimulation may be abnormal in patients with L-5 radiculopathy.[19]

Table 18-1 summarizes the normal values in our laboratory. In assessing a unilateral lesion, the latency difference between the two sides is the most sensitive measure of the T- or H-reflex (Fig. 18-5). Braddom and Johnson[9] conclude that unilateral absence or a right-left latency difference greater than 1.5 ms supports the diagnosis of S-1 radic-

### TABLE 18-1 H-reflex[1]

| Amplitude[2] mV | Difference between right and left mV | Latency[3] ms | Difference between right and left ms |
|---|---|---|---|
| 2.4 ± 1.4 | 1.2 ± 1.2 | 29.5 ± 2.4 (35)[4] | 0.6 ± 0.4 (1.4)[4] |

1. Mean ± standard deviation (SD) in the same 59 patients shown in Table 6-9.
2. Amplitude of the evoked response measured from the baseline to negative peak.
3. Latency measured to the onset of the evoked response.
4. Upper limits of normal calculated as mean + 2SD.

ulopathy. This finding should be interpreted in clinical context and should not be taken of itself as sufficient evidence of a herniated disc or of a need for laminectomy.[37]

# THE JAW REFLEX

The jaw reflex, or masseteric T-reflex, is activated by sudden stretching of the muscle spindles from a sharp tap to the mandible.[38, 76] Electric stimulation of the masseter nerve also elicits a masseteric H-reflex.[34] This reflex, relayed via the mesencephalic nucleus of the trigeminal nerve, reflects conduction through the midbrain. The so-called motor root of the trigeminal nerve contains the sensory fibers of the muscle spindle and motor axons to the extrafusal muscle fibers that constitute the afferent and efferent arcs of the masseter reflex, respectively. The cell bodies of the proprioceptive spindle afferents lie in the mesencephalic trigeminal nucleus. The collateral branches from these cells make monosynaptic connection with the motor neurons of the trigeminal nerve located in the pons. The physiology of the jaw reflex differs considerably from that of the spinal monosynaptic reflex. For example, muscle vibration that inhibits the soleus T- and H-reflexes potentiates the masseteric T- and H-reflexes.[35]

## Methods and normal values

The jaw reflex is ordinarily elicited by a mechanical tap over the mandible. The closure of a microswitch attached to the percussion hammer triggers the oscilloscope sweep. The reflex responses are recorded simultaneously from the right and left masseter muscles. Since reflex latencies vary with successive trials, comparison of simultaneously recorded right-sided and left-sided responses is more meaningful than absolute values. Reflex amplitude is also quite variable both in the same subjects and among individuals.

Amplitude increases proportionally with the weight supported by the mandible and with Jendrassik facilitation.[52] The amplitude ratio between simultaneously record-

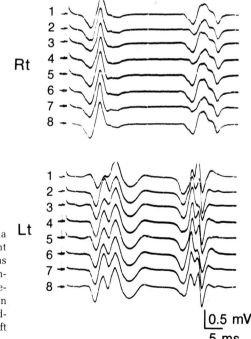

Figure 18-5
H-reflex in a 77-year-old man with cauda equina syndrome. The recording arrangement is the same as for Figure 18-2. The reflex was delayed by more than 2 ms on the right compared with the left. The central latency as determined by the latency difference between the M-response and H-reflex was also considerably greater on the right than on the left side.

ed right-sided and left-sided responses is, however, relatively constant.[74] Ongerboer de Visser and Goor,[100] who use a needle recording electrode, consider the test abnormal in patients with consistent unilateral absence of the reflex, a difference of more than 0.5 ms between the latencies of the two sides, or bilateral absence of the reflex up to the age of 70 years. Table 18-2 summarizes normal values in our laboratory.[74]

## Clinical applications

The jaw reflex is perhaps less frequently used as a diagnostic test than the electrically elicited blink reflex. Its applications are limited by the difficulty in standardizing the mechanical stimulus and in regulating the tonus of the masseter for optimal reflex activation (Fig. 18-6). However, a unilateral delay or absence of this reflex suggests a lesion of the trigeminal nerve if the brain stem is intact.[74, 114] Electromyography of the masseter is also of great value in documenting the presence of denervation. Its clinical value is amplified by simultaneous use of the reflex studies, which enables one to measure conduction along the trigeminal nerve.[99] Goodwill and O'Tuama,[39] using the jaw reflex as a test of midbrain function, found absence or increased latency in 12 out of an unselected series of 32 patients with multiple sclerosis.

## Masseteric silent period

A jaw reflex elicited during voluntary clenching is immediately followed by a brief pause in the electromyographic activity of the masseter (Fig. 18-7). This inactivity, referred to as the masseteric silent period (SP), lasts about 30 ms in normal subjects.[123] The masseteric SP also occurs after acoustic or electric stimulation of the tongue, gums, oral mucosa, or the belly of the masseter.[36, 93, 117] Central pathways for this inhibition are probably crossed and uncrossed, since a unilateral stimulus causes SP on both sides.[101] Analogous SP occurs in limb muscles following electrical stimulation of the nerve, as will be discussed later in this chapter.

The force and direction of the tap and the magnitude of jaw clenching significantly influence the masseteric SP. In particular, a decrease in voluntary muscle contraction results in a significant increase in SP duration. Thus, stimulus and subject variables must be standardized if the SP is to be a meaningful test of the masticatory system.[92] Some patients with tetanus lack the masseteric SP.[109, 110, 123] Conversely, the duration of the masseteric SP is prolonged in patients with the temporomandibular joint syndrome.[4]

# THE TONIC VIBRATION REFLEX

In contrast to the phasic activity of T- and H-reflexes mentioned earlier, the tonic stretch reflex in postural and volitional movements has been difficult to study electro-

TABLE 18-2 Jaw reflex[1]

| Amplitude[2] mV | Amplitude ratio (large/small) | Latency[3] ms | Difference between right and left ms |
|---|---|---|---|
| 0.22 ± 0.24 | 1.44 ± 0.42 | 7.1 ± 0.6 (9.0)[4] | 0.27 ± 0.15 (0.8)[4] |

1. Mean ± standard deviation (SD) in 20 healthy subjects.
2. Amplitude of the evoked response measured from the baseline to negative peak.
3. Latency measured to the onset of the evoked response.
4. Upper limits of normal calculated as mean + 3SD.
(Modified from Kimura, Rodnitzky, and Van Allen.[74])

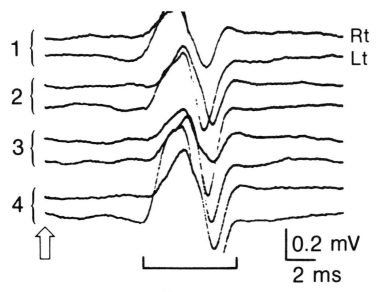

Figure 18-6

Jaw reflex recorded simultaneously from right (top tracing of each frame) and left (bottom) masseter after a mechanical tap on the chin (open arrow). Four trials are taken to show consistency of the response.

physiologically.[42] A vibratory stimulus applied to a tendon or a muscle excites the muscle spindles selectively and produces a sustained contraction of the muscle.[23, 47, 67] This tonic vibration reflex (TVR) in many respects simulates a tonic stretch reflex,[35, 49, 97] although skin mechanoreceptors may also contribute.[1, 27] Hence, the TVR provides a means to test motor neuron reaction to tonic rather than phasic stimuli.[21, 25, 56, 60, 77, 129] A small vibrator[26] attached over the tendon that oscillates at 150 Hz with an approximate amplitude of 0.5 to 1.5 mm elicits the TVR. Intervals of at least 10 seconds should separate the stimuli to avoid cumulative depression of the reflex activities evoked segmentally. The response is recorded using surface electrodes placed over the belly ($G_1$) and tendon ($G_2$) of the muscle.

## Normal and abnormal response

The motor effects of tonic vibration include:[5] (1) active and sustained muscle contraction;[26, 46, 77, 78, 85, 88] (2) reciprocal inhibition of motor neurons innervating antagonistic muscles;[13, 45, 78] and (3) suppression of the T- and H-reflexes (Fig. 18-8).[13, 14, 85, 112] The TVR involves more than a simple, spinal neural arc.[54] Studies in cat gastrocnemius muscle before and after lesions at preselected neural sites indicate that for generation of TVR an intact neural axis caudal to the midcolliculus is required; facilitatory pathways ascend ipsilaterally in the ventral quadrant of the spinal cord; the lateral vestibular nucleus and pontine reticular formation provide essential facilitation; and the medullary reticular formation is a source of inhibition.[2, 10, 33, 106]

Abnormalities of the TVR occur in patients with a variety of motor disorders.[6, 10, 13, 22, 69, 77, 119] These abnormalities include: (1) absence or diminution of the TVR in paretic muscles when the ventral quadrant of the spinal cord is involved; (2) loss of voluntary control over the TVR; (3) more abrupt development and termination of the TVR than in normals; (4) loss or diminution in TVR-induced suppression of the T- and H-reflexes; (5) asymmetries of the TVR between corresponding muscles in the two limbs; and (6) imbalances of the TVR between two antagonistic muscles within the

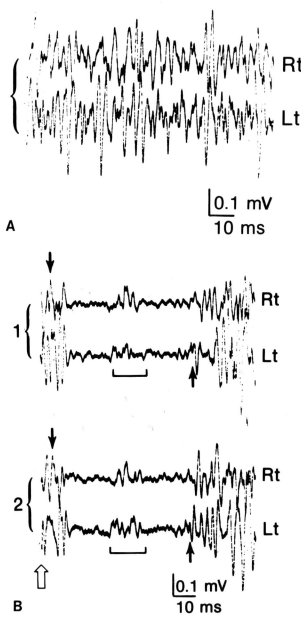

Figure 18-7

(A) Voluntary contraction of the masseter. Electromyography was recorded simultaneously from right (top tracing) and left (bottom) sides using two pairs of surface electrodes placed on the belly of the muscle (G₁) and under the chin (G₂) on each side. (B) Silent period (SP) of the masseter. The recording arrangement is the same as for part A but the mechanical tap was applied to the chin at the beginning of the sweep (open arrow). Electrical activity ceases immediately following the jaw reflex (arrows from top) elicited by the stimulus. Small volitional potentials (brackets) appear in the midst of the SP before the return of full volitional activity (arrows from bottom) in approximately 80 ms after the tap.

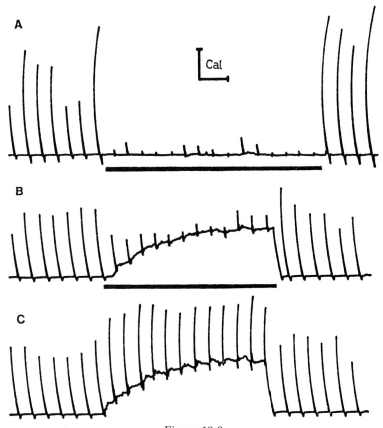

Figure 18-8

Effects of continuous muscle vibration: suppression of stretch reflexes and the tonic vibration reflex (TVR) in a normal subject. A: Vibration of the quadriceps while knee reflexes are elicited every 5 seconds. Knee reflexes are depressed during the period of vibration (black bar) even without the development of tonic contraction, probably because of the spread of the vibration wave to flexor muscles. B: Suppression of knee reflexes accompanying a tonic contraction induced by vibration. C: voluntary contraction of quadriceps in the same subject as B, without suppression of knee reflexes Calibration: vertical 0.4 kg for A, 0.6 kg for B and C. Horizontal, 10 seconds. (From De Gail, Lance, and Neilson,[13] with permission.)

same limb. Responses to vibratory stimuli have also been used to assess reciprocal inhibition, presynaptic inhibition, and central control of voluntary movements.

## Clinical applications

Clinical applications include early detection of incipient weakness, subclinical rigidity, spasticity, and involuntary movements such as tremors, clonus, and choreoathetosis.[46, 77] Responses to tonic vibration vary from patient to patient, depending upon the site of spinal cord lesions. If it were possible to predict which patients typically display all or any of the above effects, TVR would be useful for localization of a lesion.[7]

A large number of papers have appeared describing the effect of tonic vibration on spasticity or rigidity.[46, 47, 48, 61, 77] In most reported series, vibration produced beneficial effects. These include: (1) increased voluntary power of a weak muscle; (2) reduced resistance of the spastic antagonist; and (3) increased range of motion.[7] Unfortunately, these positive effects last only for the duration of vibration, which is limited to a few minutes by frictional generation of heat. Nonetheless, the technique holds therapeutic promise for patients with a spinal cord injury.

# THE SILENT PERIOD

Despite continued effort, action potentials of a voluntarily contracting muscle are transiently suppressed following electric stimulation of the nerve innervating that muscle.[58] This period of electrical inactivity, designated the silent period (SP), results from several physiologic mechanisms.[117] The SP induced by electric stimulation[94, 117] or by unloading the muscle spindles[121] has been studied in normal subjects[55, 90] and in patients with neurologic disorders.[79]

## Potentials that break through the silent period

Electrical suppression during the SP is not absolute and can be interrupted by increasing voluntary muscle contraction. Two separate potentials appear. At high levels of

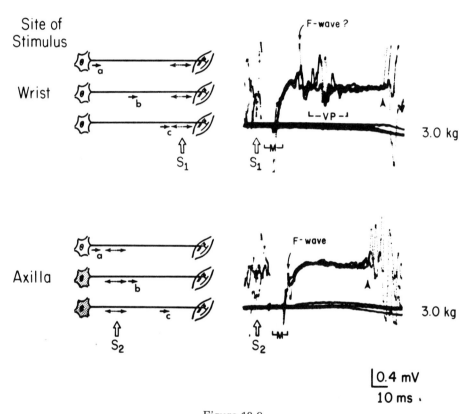

Figure 18-9
Simultaneous recording of muscle force of 3.0 kg (straight line) and the silent period (SP) from the voluntarily contracting first dorsal interosseous muscle (three trials superimposed). The SP was broken by the voluntary potential (VP) with a stimulus at the wrist but not with stimulus at the axilla, indicating greater inhibition of motor neurons with proximal than distal nerve stimulation. With distal stimulation, most antidromic activity is extinguished by collision with voluntary impulses, a, b, and c, before reaching the motor neuron pool. With proximal stimulation antidromic activity, escaping collision, presumably invades recurrent axon collaterals and inhibits the motor neurons (shaded). (From Kimura,[73] with permission.)

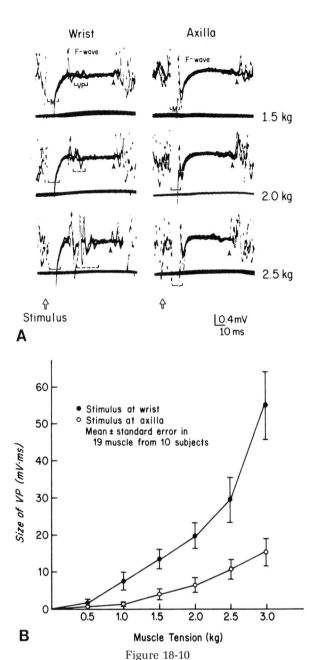

Figure 18-10

(A) Stimulation and recording as in Figure 18-9 at muscle tension ranging from 1.5 to 2.5 kg. Stimulating at the wrist, the voluntary potential (VP) became progressively greater in size at increasingly higher muscle forces. With stimulation at the axilla, no VP was recorded at any level of muscle force, but the duration of the silent period (SP) was shortened as the muscle force was increased. (From Kimura,[73] with permission.) (B) Muscle tension and the size of the VP breaking through the SP. For muscle forces of 1.0 kg and above, the VP was significantly larger with stimulus at the wrist than at the axilla, indicating that motor neurons were more inhibited by proximal as opposed to distal nerve stimulation during voluntary muscle contraction. The difference in inhibitory effects of proximal versus distal stimulation became progressively larger as the muscle force was increased. (From Kimura,[73] with permission.)

muscle contraction, where the antidromic activity collides with voluntary impulses in most axons, the first potential consists mainly of the H-reflex.[89, 120] However, at low levels of muscle contraction, where few voluntary impulses are present, the first potential represents the F-wave, because substantial antidromic activity reaches the central motor neuron pool.[72] The second potential, which appears in the middle of the SP, is designated the voluntary potential (VP). It is attributed to either descending volitional or polysynaptic reflexive inputs to motor neurons.[128] Alternatively, the VP may in part represent transcortical reflex activity following brief stretching of arm muscles.[28, 86] It is totally or partially abolished in hemiparetic patients, and repetitive trains of stimuli have a strong facilitatory effect.[11]

## Physiologic mechanisms

Pierrot-Deseilligny and Bussel[104] have demonstrated in man that Renshaw inhibition[108] occurs following the passage of an orthodromic impulse via the H-reflex pathway. In the cat, antidromic impulses produce Renshaw inhibition more effectively than orthodromic impulses.[113] It is thus likely that in man the middle portion of the SP is at least in part caused by antidromic invasion of the Renshaw loop. The VP tends to appear when Renshaw inhibition is decreased because of reduced antidromic invasion of the central motor neuron pool.[73] Thus, the appearance of VP is favored by weaker stimuli that activate fewer motor axons and consequently produce less of an inhibitory Renshaw effect.[117]

Even with supramaximal stimulation, not all antidromic impulses generated by nerve stimulation reach the central motor neuron pool; during voluntary muscle contraction some of them are extinguished by collision with orthodromic voluntary impulses. Increased voluntary effort increases the probability of collision, because more axons carry orthodromic impulses at the time of stimulation.[71, 72] Stimulation of the nerve distally also enhances this probability, because the chance of collision increases in proportion to the length of the nerve segment between the stimulus site and the cell body of the motor neuron (Fig. 18-9). Thus, with greater voluntary effort and with weaker and more distal nerve stimulation, both antidromic invasion and the recurrent inhibition of motor neurons responsible for the SP are decreased (Fig. 18-10).

Besides Renshaw inhibition, other mechanisms such as unloading of the muscle spindle[68, 94, 122] and activation of the Golgi tendon organ[41] during muscle contraction contribute to the SP.[117] Ascending cutaneous volleys may also influence the SP, although to produce a well-defined SP, a high intensity stimulus is required.[75] Sensory nerve stimulation could generate a reproducible SP, presumably through either group 1B afferent fibers from tendon organs or through ascending reflex pathways.[62, 63] In this case, proximal stimulation, which activates more afferent fibers, would be more likely than distal stimulation to inhibit motor neurons, and thus enhance the SP.

# REFERENCE SOURCES

1. ABBRUZZESE, G, ET AL: *Excitation from skin receptors contributing to the tonic vibration reflex in man.* Brain Res 150:194, 1978.

2. ANDREWS, C, KNOWLES, L, AND HANCOCK, J: *Control of the tonic vibration reflex by the brain stem reticular formation in the cat.* J Neurol Sci 18:217, 1973.

3. BATHIEN, N AND RONDOT, P: *Reciprocal continuous inhibition in rigidity of parkinsonism.* J Neurol Neurosurg Psychiatry 40:20, 1977.

4. BESSETTE, R, BISHOP, B, AND MOHL, N: *Duration of masseteric silent period in patients with TMJ syndrome.* J Appl Physiol 30:864, 1971.

5. BISHOP, B: *Vibratory stimulation. Part I. Neurophysiology of motor responses evoked by vibratory stimulation.* Phys Ther 54:1273, 1974.

6. BISHOP, B: *Vibratory stimulation. Part II. Vibratory stimulation as an evaluation tool.* Phys Ther 55:28, 1975.

7. BISHOP, B: *Vibratory stimulation. Part III. Possible applications of vibrations in treatment of motor dysfunctions.* Phys Ther 55:139, 1975.

8. BISHOP, B, ET AL: *A quantitative assessment of gamma-motoneuron contribution to the Achilles tendon reflex in normal subjects.* Arch Phys Med Rehabil 49:145, 1968.

9. BRADDOM, RI AND JOHNSON, EW: *Standardization of H reflex and diagnostic use in S1 radiculopathy.* Arch Phys Med Rehabil 55:161, 1974.

10. BURKE, D, ET AL: *Spasticity, decerebrate rigidity and the clasp-knife phenomenon: An experimental study in the cat.* Brain 95:31, 1972.

11. CONRAD, B AND ASCHOFF, JC: *Effects of voluntary isometric and isotonic activity on late transcortical reflex components in normal subjects and hemiparetic patients.* Electroenceph Clin Neurophysiol 42:107, 1977.

12. DAUBE, JR: *F-wave and H-reflex measurements.* American Academy of Neurology, Course #16, Clinical Electromyography, 1979, pp 93–101.

13. DE GAIL, P, LANCE, JW, AND NEILSON, PD: *Differential effects on tonic and phasic reflex mechanisms produced by vibration of muscles in man.* J Neurol Neurosurg Psychiatry 29:1, 1966.

14. DELWAIDE, PJ: *Différences d'organisation fonctionnelle des arcs myotatiques du quadriceps et du court biceps chez l'homme.* Revue Neurologique (Paris) 128:39, 1973.

15. DELWAIDE, PJ: *Excitability of lower limb myotatic reflex arcs under the influence of caloric labyrinthine stimulation. Analysis of the postural effects in man.* J Neurol Neurosurg Psychiatry 40:970, 1977.

16. DELWAIDE, PJ AND JUPRELLE, M: *The effects of caloric stimulation of the labyrinth on the soleus motor pool in man.* Acta Neurol Scand 55:310, 1977.

17. DELWAIDE, PJ, CORDONNIER, M, AND CHARLIER, M: *Functional relationships between myotatic reflex arcs of the lower limb in man: Investigation by excitability curves.* J Neurol Neurosurg Psychiatry 39:545, 1976.

18. DELWAIDE, PJ, FIGIEL, C, AND RICHELLE, C: *Effects of postural changes of the upper limb on reflex transmission in the lower limb. Cervicolumbar reflex interactions in man.* J Neurol Neurosurg Psychiatry 40:616, 1977.

19. DESCHUYTERE, J AND ROSSELLE, N: *Diagnostic use of monosynaptic reflexes in L5 and S1 root compression.* In DESMEDT, JE (ED): *New Developments in Electromyography and Clinical Neurophysiology,* Vol 3. Karger, Basel, 1973, pp 360–366.

20. DESCHUYTERE, J, ROSSELLE, N, AND DE KEYSER, C: *Monosynaptic reflexes in the superficial forearm flexors in man and their clinical significance.* J Neurol Neurosurg Psychiatry 39:555, 1976.

21. DESMEDT, JE AND GODAUX, E: *Vibration-induced discharge patterns of single motor units in the masseter muscle in man.* J Physiol (Lond) 253:429, 1975.

22. DIMITRIJEVIC, MR, ET AL: *Reflex effects of vibration in patients with spinal cord lesions.* Neurology (New York) 27:1078, 1977.

23. DINDAR, F AND VERRIER, M: *Studies on the receptor responsible for vibration induced inhibition of monosynaptic reflexes in man.* J Neurol Neurosurg Psychiatry 38:155, 1975.

24. ECCLES, JC: *The inhibitory control of spinal reflex action.* Electroenceph Clin Neurophysiol (suppl 25):20, 1967.

25. EKLUND, G: *Some physical properties of muscle vibrators used to elicit tonic proprioceptive reflexes in man.* Acta Soc Med Upsal 76:271, 1971.

26. EKLUND, G AND HAGBARTH, KE: *Motor effects of vibratory muscle stimuli in man.* Electroenceph Clin Neurophysiol 19:619, 1965.

27. EKLUND, G, HAGBARTH, KE, AND TOREBJÖRK, E: *Exteroceptive vibration-induced finger flexion reflex in man.* J Neurol Neurosurg Psychiatry 41:438, 1978.

28. EVARTS, EV: *Sensorimotor cortex activity associated with movements triggered by visual as compared to somesthetic inputs.* In SCHMITT, FO AND WORDEN, FG (EDS): *The Neurosciences, Third Study Program.* MIT Press, Cambridge, Mass, 1974, pp 327–337.

THE H-REFLEX AND OTHER LATE RESPONSES

29. GARCIA, HA, FISHER, MA, AND GILAI, A: *H reflex analysis of segmental reflex excitability in flexor and extensor muscles.* Neurology (New York) 29:984, 1979.

30. GARCIA-MULLIN, R AND MAYER, RF: *H reflexes in acute and chronic hemiplegia.* Brain 95:559, 1972.

31. GASSEL, MM AND OTT, KH: *Local sign and late effects on motoneuron excitability of cutaneous stimulation in man.* Brain 93:95, 1970.

32. GASSEL, MM AND OTT, KH: *Patterns of reflex excitability change after widespread cutaneous stimulation in man.* J Neurol Neurosurg Psychiatry 36:282, 1973.

33. GILLIES, JD, BURKE, DJ, AND LANCE, JW: *Tonic vibration reflex in the cat.* J Neurophysiol 34:252, 1971.

34. GODAUX, E AND DESMEDT, JE: *Human masseter muscle: H- and tendon reflexes. Their paradoxical potentiation by muscle vibration.* Arch Neurol 32:229, 1975.

35. GODAUX, E AND DESMEDT, JE: *Evidence for a monosynaptic mechanism in the tonic vibration reflex of the human masseter muscle.* J Neurol Neurosurg Psychiatry 38:161, 1975.

36. GODAUX, E AND DESMEDT, JE: *Exteroceptive suppression and motor control of the masseter and temporalis muscles in normal man.* Brain Res 85:447, 1975.

37. GOODGOLD, J: *H reflex.* (Letter to the editor). Arch Phys Med Rehabil 57:407, 1976.

38. GOODWILL, CJ: *The normal jaw reflex: Measurement of the action potential in the masseter muscles.* Ann Phys Med 9:183, 1968.

39. GOODWILL, CJ AND O'TUAMA, L: *Electromyographic recording of the jaw reflex in multiple sclerosis.* J Neurol Neurosurg Psychiatry 32:6, 1969.

40. GOTTLIEB, GL AND AGARWAL, GC: *Extinction of the Hoffmann reflex by antidromic conduction.* Electroenceph Clin Neurophysiol 41:19, 1976.

41. GRANIT, R: *Reflex self-regulation of muscle contraction and autogenetic inhibition.* J Neurophysiol 13:351, 1950.

42. GRANIT, R: *The functional role of the muscle spindle's primary end organs.* Proc R Soc Med (Lond) 61:69, 1968.

43. GUIHENEUC, P AND BATHIEN, N: *Two patterns of results in polyneuropathies investigated with the H reflex. Correlation between proximal and distal conduction velocities.* J Neurol Sci 30:83, 1976.

44. GUIHENEUC, P AND GINET, J: *Etude du reflexe de Hoffmann obtenu au niveau du muscle quadriceps de sujets humains normaux.* Electroenceph Clin Neurophysiol 36:225, 1974.

45. HAGBARTH, KE: *EMG studies of stretch reflexes in man.* Electroenceph Clin Neurophysiol (suppl 25):74, 1967.

46. HAGBARTH, KE: *The effect of muscle vibration in normal man and in patients with motor disorders.* In DESMEDT, JE (ED): *New Developments in Electromyography and Clinical Neurophysiology,* Vol 3. Karger, Basel, 1973, pp 428–443.

47. HAGBARTH, KE AND EKLUND, G: *Motor effects of vibratory muscle stimuli in man.* In GRANIT, R (ED): *Proceedings of the First Nobel Symposium: Muscle Afferents and Motor Control.* Almqvist and Wiksell, Stockholm, 1966, pp 177–186.

48. HAGBARTH, KE AND EKLUND, G: *The muscle vibrator—A useful tool in neurological therapeutic work.* Scand J Rehabil Med 1:26, 1969.

49. HAGBARTH, KE, HELLSING, G, AND LÖFSTEDT, L: *TVR and vibration-induced timing of motor impulses in the human jaw elevator muscles.* J Neurol Neurosurg Psychiatry 39:719, 1976.

50. HALAR, EM, ET AL: *H-reflex latency in uremic neuropathy: Correlation with NCV and clinical findings.* Arch Phys Med Rehabil 60:174, 1979.

51. HAMANN, WC AND MORRIS, JGL: *Effect of stretching the patella tendon on voluntary and reflex contractions of the calf muscles in man.* Exper Neurol 55:405, 1977.

52. HANNAM, AG: *Effect of voluntary contraction of the masseter and other muscles upon the masseteric reflex in man.* J Neurol Neurosurg Psychiatry 35:66, 1972.

53. HAYES, KC, ET AL: *Assessment of the H-reflex excitability curve using a cubic spline function.* Electroenceph Clin Neurophysiol 46:114, 1979.

54. HENDRIE, A AND LEE, RG: *Selective effects of vibration on human spinal and long-loop reflexes.* Brain Res 157:369, 1978.

55. HIGGINS, DC AND LIEBERMAN, JS: *The muscle silent period: Variability in normal man.* Electroenceph Clin Neurophysiol 24:176, 1968.

56. HIRAYAMA, K, ET AL: *Separation of the contributions of voluntary and vibratory activation of motor units in man by cross-correlograms.* Jpn J Physiol 24:293, 1974.

57. HODES, R: *Effects of age, consciousness, and other factors on human electrically induced reflexes (EIRs).* Electroenceph Clin Neurophysiol (suppl 25):80, 1967.

58. HOFFMANN, P: *Demonstration eines Hemmungsreflexes im menschlichen Rückenmark.* Zeitschrift für Biologie 70:515, 1919.

59. HOFFMANN, P: *Untersuchungen über die Eigenreflexe (Sehnenreflexe) menschlicher Muskeln.* Springer, Berlin, 1922.

60. HOMMA, S: *A survey of Japanese research on muscle vibration.* In DESMEDT, JE (ED): *New Developments in Electromyography and Clinical Neurophysiology,* Vol 3. Karger, Basel, 1973, pp 463–468.

61. HOMMA, S, ISHIKAWA, K, AND STUART, DG: *Motoneuron responses to linearly rising muscle stretch.* Am J Phys Med 49:290, 1970.

62. HUFSCHMIDT, HJ: *Wird die Silent period nach direkter Muskelreizung durch die Golgi-Sehnenorgane ausgelöst?* Pflügers Arch 271:35, 1960.

63. HUFSCHMIDT, HJ AND LINKE, D: *A damping factor in human voluntary contraction.* J Neurol Neurosurg Psychiatry 39:536, 1976.

64. HUGON, M: *Methodology of the Hoffmann reflex in man.* In DESMEDT, JE (ED): *New Developments in Electromyography and Clinical Neurophysiology,* Vol 3. Karger, Basel, 1973.

65. HUGON, M AND BATHIEN, N: *Influence de la stimulation du nerf sural sur divers réflexes monosynaptiques de l'homme.* J Physiol (Paris) 59:244, 1967.

66. HUGON, M, ET AL: *A discussion of the methodology of the triceps surae T- and H-reflexes.* In DESMEDT, JE (ED): *New Developments in Electromyography and Clinical Neurophysiology,* Vol 3. Karger, Basel, 1973, pp 773–780.

67. JACK, JJB AND ROBERTS, RC: *The role of muscle spindle afferents in stretch and vibration reflexes of the soleus muscle of the decerebrate cat.* Brain Res 146:366, 1978.

68. JACOBS, MB, ET AL: *Antagonist EMG temporal patterns during rapid voluntary movement.* Neurology (Minneap) 30:36, 1980.

69. KANDA, K, HOMMA, S, AND WATANABE, S: *Vibration reflex in spastic patients.* In DESMEDT, JE (ED): *New Developments in Electromyography and Clinical Neurophysiology,* Vol 3. Karger, Basel, 1973, pp 469–474.

70. KATZ, R, ET AL: *Conditioning of H reflex by a preceding subthreshold tendon reflex stimulus.* J Neurol Neurosurg Psychiatry 40:575, 1977.

71. KIMURA, J: *A method for estimating the refractory period of motor fibers in the human peripheral nerve.* J Neurol Sci 28:485, 1976.

72. KIMURA, J: *Electrical activity in voluntarily contracting muscle.* Arch Neurol 34:85, 1977.

73. KIMURA, J: *Recurrent inhibition of motoneurons during the silent period in man.* In DESMEDT, JE (ED): *Brain and Spinal Mechanisms of Movement Control in Man: New Developments and Clinical Applications.* Raven Press, New York, 1982 (in press).

74. KIMURA, J, RODNITZKY, RL, AND VAN ALLEN, MW: *Electrodiagnostic study of trigeminal nerve. Orbicularis oculi reflex and masseter reflex in trigeminal neuralgia, paratrigeminal syndrome, and other lesions of the trigeminal nerve.* Neurology (Minneap) 20:574, 1970.

75. KRANZ, H, ADORJANI, C, AND BAUMGARTNER, G: *The effect of nociceptive cutaneous stimuli on human motoneurons.* Brain 96:571, 1973.

76. KUGELBERG, E: *Facial reflexes.* Brain 75:385, 1952.

77. LANCE, JW, BURKE, D, AND ANDREWS, CJ: *The reflex effects of muscle vibration. Studies of tendon jerk irradiation, phasic reflex inhibition and the tonic vibration reflex.* In DESMEDT, JE (ED): *New Developments in Electromyography and Clinical Neurophysiology,* Vol 3. Karger, Basel, 1973, pp 444–462.

78. LANCE, JW, DE GAIL, P, AND NEILSON, PD: *Tonic and phasic spinal cord mechanisms in man.* J Neurol Neurosurg Psychiatry 29:535, 1966.

79. LAXER, K AND EISEN, A: *Silent period measurement in the differentiation of central demyelination and axonal degeneration.* Neurology (Minneap) 25:740, 1975.

**THE H-REFLEX AND OTHER LATE RESPONSES**

80. LUNDBERG, A, MALMGREN, K, AND SCHOMBURG, ED: *Group II excitation in motoneurones and double sensory innervation of extensor digitorum brevis.* Acta Physiol Scand 94:398, 1975.

81. MAGLADERY, JW AND McDOUGAL, DB, JR: *Electrophysiological studies of nerve and reflex activity in normal man. I. Identification of certain reflexes in the electromyogram and the conduction velocity of peripheral nerve fibres.* Bull Johns Hopkins Hosp 86:265, 1950.

82. MAGLADERY, JW, ET AL: *Electrophysiological studies of nerve and reflex activity in normal man. IV. The two-neurone reflex and identification of certain action potentials from spinal roots and cord.* Bull Johns Hopkins Hosp 88:499, 1951.

83. MAGLADERY, JW, ET AL: *Electrophysiological studies of reflex activity in patients with lesions of the nervous system. 1. A comparison of spinal motoneurone excitability following afferent nerve volleys in normal persons and patients with upper motor neurone lesions.* Bull Johns Hopkins Hosp 91:219, 1952.

84. MALCOLM, DS: *A method of measuring reflex times applied in sciatica and other conditions due to nerve-root compression.* J Neurol Neurosurg Psychiatry 14:15, 1951.

85. MARSDEN, CD, MEADOWS, JC, AND HODGSON, HJF: *Observations on the reflex response to muscle vibration in man and its voluntary control.* Brain 92:829, 1969.

86. MARSDEN, CD, MERTON, PA, AND MORTON, HB: *Is the human stretch reflex cortical rather than spinal?* Lancet 1:759, 1973.

87. MARTINELLI, P AND MONTAGNA, P: *Conditioning of the H reflex by stimulation of the posterior tibial nerve in Parkinson's disease.* J Neurol Neurosurg Psychiatry 42:701, 1979.

88. MATTHEWS, PBC: *Reflex activation of the soleus muscle of the decerebrate cat by vibration.* Nature 209:204, 1966.

89. McCOMAS, AJ, SICA, REP, AND UPTON, ARM: *Excitability of human motoneurones during effort.* J Physiol (Lond) 210:145, 1970.

90. McLELLAN, DL: *The electromyographic silent period produced by supramaximal electrical stimulation in normal man.* J Neurol Neurosurg Psychiatry 36:334, 1973.

91. McLEOD, JG AND WALSH, JC: *H reflex studies in patients with Parkinson's disease.* J Neurol Neurosurg Psychiatry 35:77, 1972.

92. McNAMARA, DC, ET AL: *Duration of the electromyographic silent period following the jaw-jerk reflex in human subjects.* J Dent Res 56:660, 1977.

93. MEIER-EWERT, K, GLEITSMANN, K, AND REITER, F: *Acoustic jaw reflex in man: Its relationship to other brain-stem and microreflexes.* Electroenceph Clin Neurophysiol 36:629, 1974.

94. MERTON, PA: *The silent period in a muscle of the human hand.* J Physiol (Lond) 114:183, 1951.

95. MILNER-BROWN, SH, GIRVIN, JP, AND BROWN, WF: *The effects of motor cortical stimulation on the excitability of spinal motoneurons in man.* J Canad des Sciences Neurologiques 2:245, 1975.

96. MIZUNO, Y, TANAKA, R, AND YANAGISAWA, N: *Reciprocal group I inhibition on triceps surae motoneurons in man.* J Neurophysiol 34:1010, 1971.

97. MODDEL, G, BEST, B, AND ASHBY, P: *Effect of differential nerve block on inhibition of the monosynaptic reflex by vibration in man.* J Neurol Neurosurg Psychiatry 40:1066, 1977.

98. MORIN, C AND PIERROT-DESEILLIGNY, E: *Role of Ia afferents in the soleus motoneurones inhibition during a tibialis anterior voluntary contraction in man.* Exp Brain Res 27:509, 1977.

99. ONGERBOER DE VISSER, BW AND GOOR, C: *Electromyographic and reflex study in idiopathic and symptomatic trigeminal neuralgias: Latency of the jaw and blink reflexes.* J Neurol Neurosurg Psychiatry 37:1255, 1974.

100. ONGERBOER DE VISSER, BW AND GOOR, C: *Jaw reflexes and masseter electromyograms in mesencephalic and pontine lesions: An electrodiagnostic study.* J Neurol Neurosurg Psychiatry 39:90, 1976.

101. ONGERBOER DE VISSER, BW AND GOOR, C: *Cutaneous silent period in masseter muscles: A clinical and electrodiagnostic evaluation.* J Neurol Neurosurg Psychiatry 39:674, 1976.

102. PAILLARD, J: *Réflexes et Régulations d'Origine Proprioceptive chez l'Homme. Etude Neurophysiologique et Psychophysiologique.* Arnette, Paris, 1955.

103. PAILLARD, J: *Functional organization of afferent innervation of muscle studied in man by monosynaptic testing.* Am J Phys Med 38:239, 1959.

104. PIERROT-DESEILLIGNY, E AND BUSSEL, B: *Evidence for recurrent inhibition by motoneurons in human subjects.* Brain Res 88:105, 1975.

105. PIERROT-DESEILLIGNY, E, BUSSEL, B, AND MORIN, C: *Supraspinal control of the changes induced in H-reflex by cutaneous stimulation, as studied in normal and spastic man.* In DESMEDT, JE (ED): *New Developments in Electromyography and Clinical Neurophysiology,* Vol 3. Karger, Basel, 1973, pp 550–555.

106. POMPEIANO, O AND BARNES, CD: *Response of brain stem reticular neurons to muscle vibration in the decerebrate cat.* J Neurophysiol 34:709, 1971.

107. RENSHAW, B: *Influence of the discharge of motoneurons upon excitation of neighboring motoneurons.* J Neurophysiol 4:167, 1941.

108. RENSHAW, B: *Central effects of centripetal impulses in axons of spinal ventral roots.* J Neurophysiol 9:191, 1946.

109. RICKER, K, EYRICH, K, AND ZWIRNER, R: *Seltenere Formen von Tetanuserkrankung. Klinische und elektromyographische Untersuchung.* Arch Psychiatr Nervenkr 215:75, 1971.

110. RISK W, ET AL: *Chronic tetanus: Clinical report and histochemistry of muscle.* Muscle and Nerve 4:363, 1981.

111. ROBINSON, KL, MCILWAIN, JS, AND HAYES, KC: *Effects of H-reflex conditioning upon the contralateral alpha motoneuron pool.* Electroenceph Clin Neurophysiol 46:65, 1979.

112. RUSHWORTH, G AND YOUNG, RR: *The effect of vibration on tonic and phasic reflexes in man.* J Physiol (Lond) 185:63, 1966.

113. RYALL, RW, ET AL: *Excitation of Renshaw cells in relation to orthodromic and antidromic excitation of motoneurons.* J Neurophysiol 35:137, 1972.

114. SCHENK, E AND BECK, U: *Somatic brain stem reflexes in clinical neurophysiology.* Electromyogr Clin Neurophysiol 15:107, 1975.

115. SCHILLER, HH AND STÅLBERG, E: *F responses studied with single fibre EMG in normal subjects and spastic patients.* J Neurol Neurosurg Psychiatry 41:45, 1978.

116. SCHUCHMANN, JA: *H reflex latency in radiculopathy.* Arch Phys Med Rehabil 59:185, 1978.

117. SHAHANI, BT AND YOUNG, RR: *Studies of the normal human silent period.* In DESMEDT, JE (ED): *New Developments in Electromyography and Clinical Neurophysiology,* Vol 3. Karger, Basel, 1973, pp 589–602.

118. SICA, REP, MCCOMAS, AJ, AND UPTON, ARM: *Impaired potentiation of H-reflexes in patients with upper motoneurone lesions.* J Neurol Neurosurg Psychiatry 34:712, 1971.

119. SOMERVILLE, J AND ASHBY, P: *Hemiplegic spasticity: Neurophysiologic studies.* Arch Phys Med Rehabil 59:592, 1978.

120. STANLEY, EF: *Reflexes evoked in human thenar muscles during voluntary activity and their conduction pathways.* J Neurol Neurosurg Psychiatry 41:1016, 1978.

121. STRUPPLER, A: *Silent period.* Electromyogr Clin Neurophysiol 15:163, 1975.

122. STRUPPLER, A, LANDAU, WM, AND MEHLS, O: *Analyse des Entlastungsreflexes am Menschen.* Pflügers Arch 313:155, 1969.

123. STRUPPLER, A, STRUPPLER, E, AND ADAMS, RD: *Local tetanus in man. Its clinical and neurophysiological characteristics.* Arch Neurol 8:162, 1963.

124. TÁBOŘÍKOVÁ, H: *Fraction of the motoneurone pool activated in the monosynaptic H-reflexes in man.* Nature 209:206, 1966.

125. TÁBOŘÍKOVÁ, H AND SAX, DS: *Conditioning of H-reflexes by a preceding subthreshold H-reflex stimulus.* Brain 92:203, 1969.

126. THOMAS, JE AND LAMBERT, EH: *Ulnar nerve conduction velocity and H-reflex in infants and children.* J Applied Physiol 15:1, 1960.

127. TRONTELJ, JV: *A study of the H-reflex by single fibre EMG.* J Neurol Neurosurg Psychiatry 36:951, 1973.

128. UPTON, ARM, MCCOMAS, AJ, AND SICA, REP: *Potentiation of 'late' responses evoked in muscles during effort.* J Neurol Neurosurg Psychiatry 34:699, 1971.

129. VAN BOXTEL, A: *Selective effects of vibration on monosynaptic and late EMG responses in human soleus muscle after stimulation of the posterior tibial nerve or a tendon tap.* J Neurol Neurosurg Psychiatry 42:995, 1979.

130. VEALE, JL AND REES, S: *Renshaw cell activity in man.* J Neurol Neurosurg Psychiatry 36:674, 1973.

131. VECCHIERINI-BLINEAU, MF AND GUIHENEUC, P: *Electrophysiological study of the peripheral nervous system in children. Changes in proximal and distal conduction velocities from birth to age 5 years.* J Neurol Neurosurg Psychiatry 42:753, 1979.

132. WAGER, EW, JR AND BUERGER, AA: *A linear relationship between H-reflex latency and sensory conduction velocity in diabetic neuropathy.* Neurology (Minneap) 24:711, 1974.

133. WAGER, EW, JR AND BUERGER, AA: *H-reflex latency and sensory conduction velocity in normal and diabetic subjects.* Arch Phys Med Rehabil 55:126, 1974.

134. WILLER, JC AND DEHEN, H: *Le reflexe h du muscle pedieux: Etude au cours des neuropathies alcooliques latentes.* Electroenceph Clin Neurophysiol 42:205, 1977.

135. YANAGISAWA, N, TANAKA, R, AND ITO, Z: *Reciprocal Ia inhibition in spastic hemiplegia of man.* Brain 99:555, 1976.

136. YAP, CB: *Spinal segmental and long-loop reflexes on spinal motoneurone excitability in spasticity and rigidity.* Brain 90:887, 1967.

# CHAPTER
# 19

# SOMATOSENSORY EVOKED POTENTIALS

Conventional sensory nerve conduction studies deal with the more distal portions of the peripheral nerve, since the proximal segments are not easily accessible to stimulating electrodes. In contrast, studies of somatosensory evoked potential (SEP) allow assessment of the entire length of the somatosensory pathways. Early SEP work dealt primarily with changes in amplitude and waveform in diseases affecting the cerebrum or spinal cord.[56, 81, 96, 99] More recent studies have emphasized evaluation of central neural conduction by determining latencies of the SEP recorded over the spine[10, 19, 21, 23, 28, 39, 64, 74, 85] or the scalp.[24, 27, 82]

This chapter will review recording techniques and normal values and discuss neural sources of spinal and scalp-recorded SEPs. The most extensively studied have been those following stimulation of the median nerve. In contrast, only limited information is available for responses obtained with stimulation of the lower extremities. Possible clinical applications will also be outlined at the end, although further studies are still needed to elucidate its practical value and limitations as a diagnostic test in an electromyographic laboratory.

## TECHNIQUES AND GENERAL PRINCIPLES

### Nomenclature

Considerable confusion exists in the analysis of somatosensory evoked potentials (SEP), because various authors have used different systems to describe the same waveforms. There are two major nomenclature principles: (1) components are either described or numbered by their sequence, such as CP for spinal potential recorded in the cervical region, and IP, NI, PI, and NII for initial positive, and subsequent negative and positive scalp-recorded potentials; or (2) components are specified by polarity and average peak latency to the nearest millisecond, for example, cervical $N_{13}$ or scalp-recorded $P_{14}$, $N_{17}$, $P_{20}$, and $N_{29}$ as recommended by a committee at the International Symposium on Cerebral Evoked Potentials in Man held in Brussels in 1974.[29] Unfortunately, the latency of the same component varies individually, reflecting the different lengths of the somatosensory pathways. Despite this problem, there is no better system available at this time. The various peaks could ideally be identified according to the respective neural sources, but the exact generator sites of most peaks still remain to be determined.

For the purpose of this discussion, the spinal potential recorded from cervical region (CP) after stimulation of the median nerve at the wrist (Fig. 19-1) is divided into four components, $Pc_9$ ($N_9$), $N_{11}$, $N_{13}$, and $N_{14}$ (Fig. 19-2A).[101] The earliest component is negative in polarity, relative to the ear reference electrode, but positive when recorded with a noncephalic reference; thus, the name positive cervical potential, $Pc_9$ (Fig. 19-2B). The initial positive peak (IP) of scalp-recorded SEPs (see Fig. 19-1) is divided into four positive peaks $P_9$, $P_{11}$, $P_{13}$, and $P_{14}$, using the knee reference (Fig. 19-2A). When referenced to the ear, the IP consists only of $P_{13}$ and/or $P_{14}$, since the first two peaks are nearly isopotential between the scalp and ear (Fig. 19-2C). These four peaks of the cervical and scalp-recorded SEPs normally occur within the first 15 ms. Intermediate and late components of scalp-recorded SEPs during the next 100 ms consist of $N_{17}$, $P_{20}$, $N_{29}$, $P_{40}$, and $N_{60}$ in the frontal area, and $N_{20}$, $P_{26}$, $N_{34}$, $P_{40}$, and $N_{60}$ in the parietal area or, according to the other nomenclature, NI, PI, NII, PII, and NIII (Fig. 19-2D).

Of all the peaks of peroneal or tibial evoked scalp-recorded potentials, the most consistently elicited are $P_{35}$, after stimulation of the peroneal nerve at the knee and $P_{40}$ after stimulation of the tibial nerve at the ankle (Fig. 19-3A).[30, 71] Earlier components corresponding to the short latency peaks of the median SEP are harder to register. However, three positive peaks, $P_{17}$, $P_{24}$, and $P_{31}$ regularly occur preceding $P_{40}$ of the tibial SEP, if 4000 to 6000 trials are averaged (Fig. 19-3B). These short latency components are analogous to the $P_9$, $P_{11}$, and $P_{14}$ of median SEPs (Fig. 19-3C and D). Evoked potentials recorded from the lumbosacral region in response to peroneal or tibial nerve stimulation show two well-defined negative peaks (Fig. 19-4). The first peak originates from a traveling wave of depolarization in afferent fibers in the cauda equina, and the second peak is derived as a standing potential in the spinal cord.[85] These two peaks may be referred to as cauda potential and cord potential, respectively.

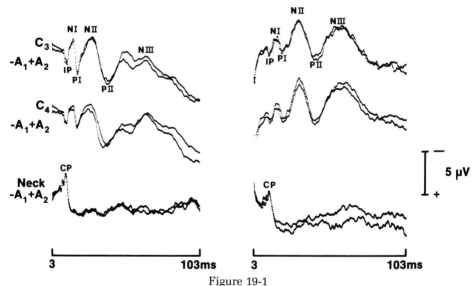

Figure 19-1

Somatosensory evoked potentials in two normal subjects after simultaneous stimulation of both median nerves at the wrist. From top to bottom the responses were recorded from the left ($C_3$) and right ($C_4$) central regions of the scalp and the midneck, all referenced to the connected ears. The initial positive potential (IP) and cervical potential (CP) recorded at this sweep speed may be equated with $P_{13}$ and/or $P_{14}$ and $N_{13}$ and/or $N_{14}$, respectively. The subsequent negative and positive peaks, NI, PI, NII, PII, and NIII, correspond to centrally recorded $N_{19}$, $P_{23}$, $N_{32}$, $N_{18}$, $P_{22}$, $N_{30}$, $P_{40}$, and $N_{60}$. (From Yamada, et al,[106] with permission.)

# Stimulation

Any sensory nerve may be stimulated electrically or mechanically at any level to elicit cerebral or spinal SEPs.[34, 79, 86, 88] In the upper extremities it is common to apply electrical stimulation to the median nerve at the wrist. In the lower extremities, the peroneal nerve may be best stimulated at the knee and the tibial nerve at the ankle, where they are relatively superficial. It is customary to adjust the shock intensity to obtain a small twitch of the innervated muscle. Dealing with the somatosensory pathway, we are of course interested in sensory and not motor impulses. It is assumed that all the large myelinated sensory fibers are activated if a muscle twitch occurs, because these sensory fibers are in general more easily excitable than the motor fibers. If possible, somatic stimuli should be specified in milliamperes above muscle twitch threshold.[29] Pulses from a stimulus isolation unit are usually square waves of 0.1 to 0.2 ms duration and 150 to 300 V or, depending on the resistance, approximately 5 to 30 mA, using surface electrodes. With needle electrodes inserted subcutaneously over and perpendicular to the nerve for stimulation, the required current, of course, is significantly less.[72]

The frequency of stimulation and number of stimuli vary a great deal, depending on whether early or late components are being studied. Spinal potentials and short latency components of scalp-recorded SEP require a higher number of trials for adequate recording. For short latency potentials one set of trials consists of up to 4000 stimuli given at frequencies of up to 4 per second.[72] Most subjects tolerate a higher frequency poorly. Slower rates are necessary to yield more distinct late components. To record the entire evoked potential during the 200 to 250 ms after the stimulus, one set of tests usually consists of a total of 200 to 400 stimuli delivered randomly every 1 to 2 seconds.

Early SEP studies focused on the presence or absence of asymmetry between the evoked potentials recorded from the right and left hemispheres after contralateral stimulation of the median nerve.[56, 81, 82, 94, 96, 99] More recent studies emphasize the clinical application of simultaneous bilateral stimulation.[105] We recommend using right, left, and bilateral stimulation. Each side should be stimulated independently in order to delineate unilateral abnormalities of short latency components, which are represented bilaterally. Long latency responses show obvious asymmetry to unilateral stimulation, since the ipsilateral components are minimal compared with the contralateral components. Bilateral stimulation elicits symmetric responses of all the SEP components between the two hemispheres in normal subjects (see Fig. 19-1). Thus, it allows comparison of simultaneously rather than consecutively recorded responses, which may vary from one trial to the next.

# Recording

Experimental investigators agree that one should use as many recording channels as available, because the SEP components have different scalp distributions. For clinical testing, however, one to four recording channels suffice, with either needle or surface electrodes placed over the optimal recording sites according to the international 10–20 system (Fig. 19-5A). In this system, electrodes are spaced either 10 or 20 percent of the total distance between nasion and inion in the sagittal plane, and between right and left preauricular points in the coronal plane.[58] The use of percentages rather than absolute distances provides flexibility for normal variations in head size and shape. The anatomic relationship between electrodes placed according to the 10–20 system and cortical landmarks has been delineated.[61] The $C_3$ electrode, for instance, lies within ± 1 cm of the central sulcus (Fig. 19-5B).

The active scalp electrodes ($G_1$) commonly selected are $P_3$, $P_4$, $C_3$, or $C_4$ contralateral to the side of stimulus for median-evoked SEPs, and $C_1$ (midpoint between $C_3$ and

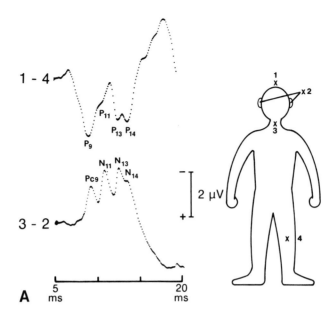

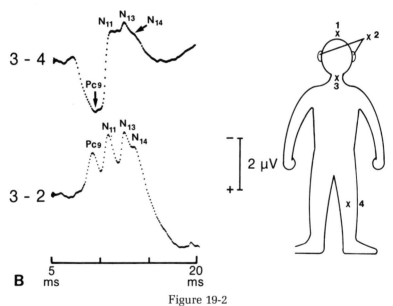

Figure 19-2

(A) Simultaneous recording from $C_z$ (1) referenced to knee (4) and low cervical (3) electrode referenced to ear (2) after stimulation of the median nerve at the wrist in a normal subject. Four positive peaks, $P_9$, $P_{11}$, $P_{13}$, and $P_{14}$ recorded at $C_z$ were nearly identical in latency to four negative peaks, $N_9$ ($Pc_9$), $N_{11}$, $N_{13}$, and $N_{14}$ recorded at the low cervical electrode. (Compare with parts B and C.) (From Yamada, Kimura, and Nitz,[101] with permission.) (B) Simultaneous recording from a low cervical (3) electrode with knee (4) and ear (2) references after stimulation of the median nerve at the wrist in a normal subject. The initial positive peak, $Pc_9$, was followed by three negative peaks, $N_{11}$, $N_{13}$, and $N_{14}$, using a knee reference, but $Pc_9$ appeared as a negative peak and $N_{11}$ and $N_{14}$ were better delineated when an ear reference was used. (From Yamada, Kimura, and Nitz,[101] with permission.)

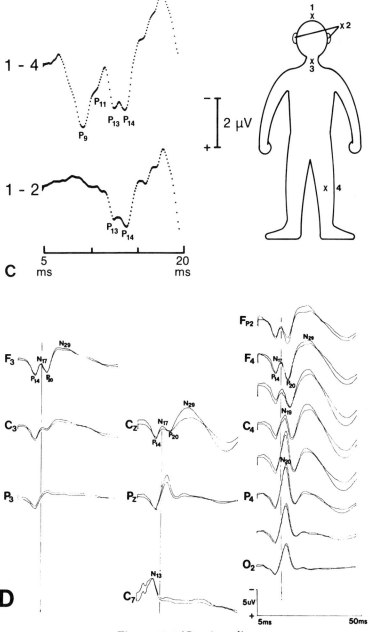

Figure 19-2 (*Continued*)

(C) Simultaneous recording from $C_z$ (1) with knee (4) and ear (2) references after stimulation of the median nerve at the wrist in a normal subject. Four positive peaks, $P_9$, $P_{11}$, $P_{13}$, and $P_{14}$ were recorded at $C_z$ when using a knee reference, but $P_9$ and $P_{11}$ were absent with an ear reference recording. (From Yamada, Kimura, and Nitz,[101] with permission.) (D) Topographic display of scalp-recorded potentials to stimulation of the left median nerve. Electrode placement was in accordance with the 10-20 International System with a neck electrode, $C_7$, placed just above the C-7 spinous process. Frontal $N_{17}$ ($F_{Pz}$, $F_4$) preceded central $N_{19}$ ($C_4$) and parietal $N_{20}$ ($P_4$) contralateral to the stimulus. $N_{17}$ also appeared at the vertex ($C_z$) and frontal and central areas ipsilaterally ($F_3$, $C_3$). (From Kimura and Yamada,[68] with permission.)

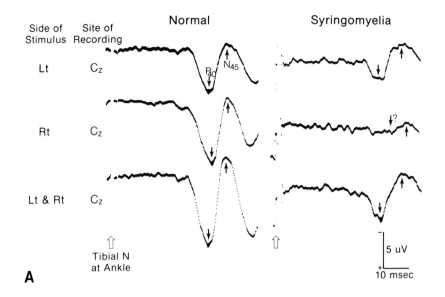

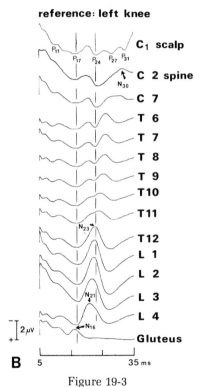

Figure 19-3

(A) Scalp-recorded somatosensory evoked potentials (SEP) referenced to the combined ears after stimulation of the tibial nerve at the ankle in a normal subject (left) and a patient with syringomyelia (right) with loss of vibration sense in the right leg. The tibial nerve was stimulated at the ankle either unilaterally or bilaterally. For both subjects, 1000 trials were summated using a sampling time of 200 $\mu$s. The use of ear reference precluded recording of either the short latency positive peaks, $P_{17}$, $P_{24}$, and $P_{31}$, or the subsequent negative peak, $N_{37}$, preceding $P_{40}$. Note the minimal response to right-sided stimulation in the patient (middle tracing on the right). (B) Tibial SEPs recorded from a scalp lead and longitudinally placed electrodes over a spine. The first two positive peaks, $P_{11}$ and $P_{17}$, were recorded along the entire spine. The gluteal lead registered $P_{11}$ and a negative peak, $N_{16}$, which slightly preceded $P_{17}$. The third component, $P_{24}$, extended caudally to the T-9 vertebral level, and replaced by negativity, $N_{23}$, best recorded at the T-12 level. A negative peak, $N_{30}$, recorded at the C-2 vertebral level slightly preceded $P_{31}$. (From Yamada, Machida, and Kimura,[102] with permission.)

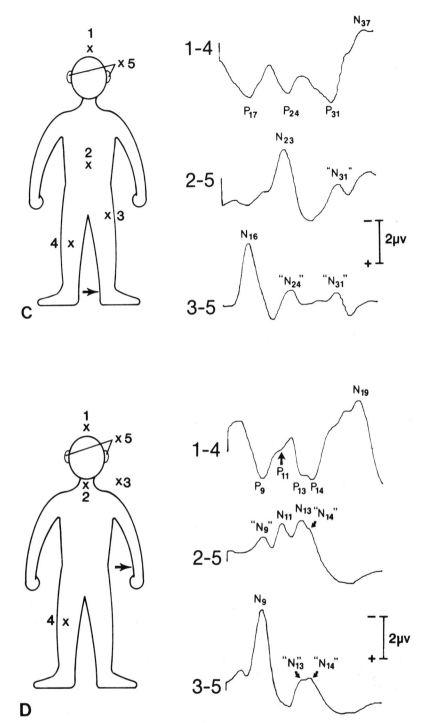

Figure 19-3 (*Continued*)

(*C* and *D*) Comparison between the tibial and median SEPs. Scalp-recorded $P_{17}$, $P_{24}$, and $P_{31}$ of the tibial SEP are analogous to $P_9$, $P_{11}$, and $P_{14}$ of the median SEP. A similar relationship exists between the gluteal potential, $N_{16}$, and shoulder potential, $N_9$, and between $N_{23}$ recorded at the T-12 vetebral level and $N_{11}$ recorded at the C-7 level. Positivity at the reference electrode is in part responsible for "$N_9$", "$N_{13}$", and "$N_{14}$" of the median SEP, and "$N_{24}$" and "$N_{31}$", of the tibial SEP.

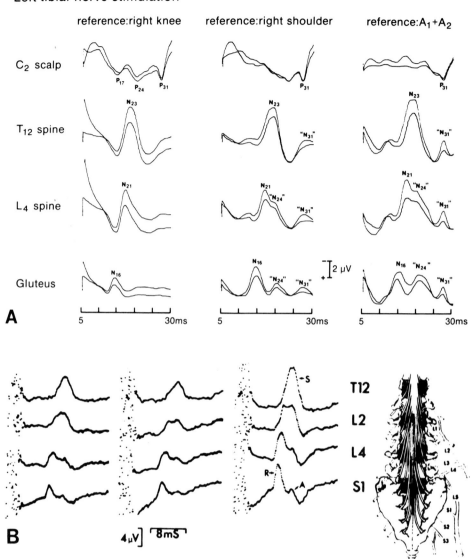

## Left tibial nerve stimulation

Figure 19-4

(A) Potentials recorded over the scalp, at the thoracic and lumbar spines, and near the gluteal fold after stimulation of the left tibial nerve at the ankle. The scalp peaks, $P_{17}$, $P_{24}$, and $P_{31}$ (left, top) are far field potentials from the sciatic nerve, conus medullaris, and probably brain stem, respectively. The corresponding peaks recorded from the gluteal fold (right, bottom) represent negative discharge near the source of the generator ($N_{16}$) and far field potentials recorded by an active reference electrode ("$N_{24}$", "$N_{31}$"). The first lumbar potential ($N_{21}$) probably originates from the cauda equina. The second ("$N_{23}$") and the third ("$N_{31}$") peaks in the right and middle columns represent conus and brain stem potentials registered by an active reference electrode. In the left column, neither the second nor the third peak is seen, since the knee reference electrode is not active. (B) Surface recording of lumbosacral evoked potentials after stimulation of the right (left column), left (middle column), and bilateral (right column) tibial nerves at the popliteal fossae using a common reference electrode at the T-6 vetebral level. The spinal (S) and double-peaked (R and A) cauda equina potentials are indicated. On the right is a diagram of the lower spine and pelvis. The shaded areas indicate the location of recording electrodes at T-12, L-2, L-4, and S-1 vertebral levels. All traces are averages of 64 responses. (From Dimitrijevic, et al,[28] with permission.)

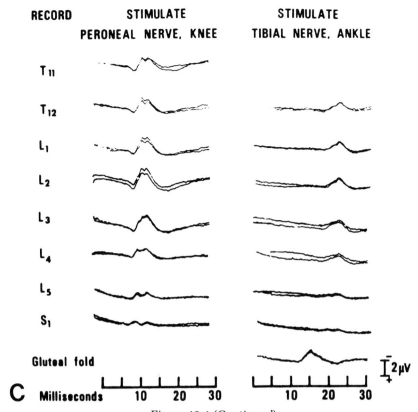

**RECORD**     **STIMULATE**            **STIMULATE**

**PERONEAL NERVE, KNEE**      **TIBIAL NERVE, ANKLE**

$T_{11}$

$T_{12}$

$L_1$

$L_2$

$L_3$

$L_4$

$L_5$

$S_1$

Gluteal fold

**C**   Milliseconds    10    20    30      10    20    30    $2\mu V$

Figure 19-4 (*Continued*)

(C) Cauda (first) and cord (second) peaks in spinal evoked potentials recorded from multiple spinal levels in one subject. The responses in the left column are a result of peroneal nerve stimulation, and those in the right column are a result of tibial nerve stimulation. Each of the superimposed traces is the average of 128 responses. The reference electrode is over the iliac crest contralateral to the side of stimulation. For comparison, a potential is recorded from an electrode over the sciatic nerve at the gluteal fold in response to tibial nerve stimulation (last trace of right column). (From Phillips and Daube,[85] with permission.)

$C_z$), $C_2$ (midpoint between $C_4$ and $C_z$), or $C_z$ for peroneal- or tibial-evoked SEPs. A common reference electrode ($G_2$) usually lies at $F_z$, the chin, or connecting the ears, $A_1$ and $A_2$. However, the knee reference best delineates the earliest scalp components, that is, $P_9$ and $P_{11}$ of median SEPs[72] or $P_{17}$ and $P_{24}$ of tibial SEPs.[102] To record cervical SEPs, $G_1$ is placed on the neck at the high or low cervical spines with $G_2$ connecting the ears. Simultaneous bilateral stimulation is usually more effective in eliciting unequivocal responses. Cervical potentials and early peaks of the scalp-recorded SEPs are registered in a majority of subjects when the median nerve is stimulated but are more difficult to detect after stimulation of the peroneal or tibial nerve.

In most subjects, spinal potentials can clearly be detected from the lumbosacral spinous process after unilateral or bilateral stimulation of the peroneal or tibial nerve.[21, 22, 23, 28, 64, 74, 85] Lumbosacral SEPs are recorded with $G_1$ placed anywhere over the spinous processes of L-1 through S-1, and $G_2$ over the T-6 spinous process or iliac crest. With this electrode arrangement, $G_2$ is not entirely neutral and registers an approaching positive field as mentioned later. The recorded potentials are of maximum amplitude over the upper lumbar vertebrae, but the two negative peaks representing cauda and cord potentials are separated maximally over the low lumbar and upper sacral vertebrae.[85] Recordings can also be made from electrodes at thoracic and cervical levels, but SEPs obtained are inconsistent and of much reduced amplitude.

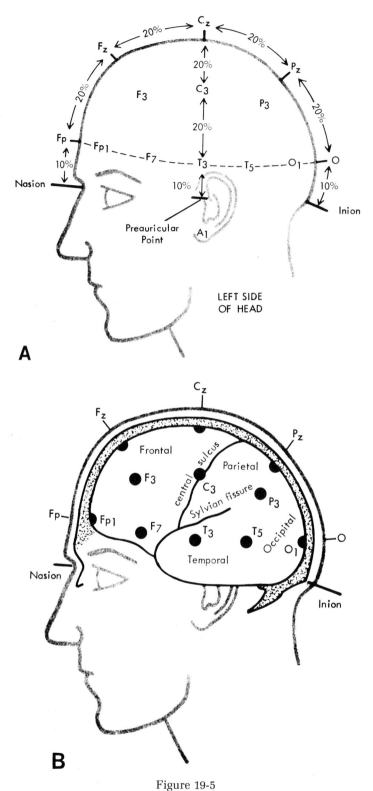

Figure 19-5

(A) The 10–20 system. Electrodes are placed either 10 percent or 20 percent of the total distance between skull landmarks. (From Harner and Sannit, with permission.) (B) Relationship between central sulcus, sylvian fissure, lobes of the brain, and electrode positions. (From Harner and Sannit,[58] with permission.)

The evoked potential generally becomes larger with greater distance between the active and reference electrodes. However, background noise also increases with greater interelectrode distance. In our experience,[102] the positive farfield potentials extend over the entire trunk, head, and arm as the negative impulses ascend along the peripheral nerve, spinal cord, and brain stem. Thus, any reference electrode placed rostral to the knee is to a greater or lesser extent active with approaching field of positivity when the tibial or peroneal nerve is stimulated. The size and shape of spinal potentials of course depend on the relative activity of the reference electrode. Unless a knee reference is used, spurious peaks generated by an active reference may confuse SEP analysis, especially if this possibility is overlooked.

Evoked spinal potentials have also been recorded in man using subdural[41-44] or epidural recording techniques,[12, 90, 91] but surface recordings are more practical for clinical use in an electromyography laboratory.

## Averaging procedure

Electrode potentials are enhanced $10^4$ to $10^5$ times by a differential amplifier with 3 dB frequency cutoff of about 1 Hz to 3KHz. The data are either fed directly into a computer or averager for on-line analysis or stored on FM magnetic tape for later off-line analysis. The memory core available, number of channels employed, and the duration of total sweep for each channel determine the sampling rate. In general, an adequate analysis requires analog to digital (A/D) conversion of 8 to 10 bits accuracy and sweeps of 100 to 500 $\mu$s per address, which provide 10 to 2 points per ms, respectively. For the study of late components, a sampling rate as slow as 1 to 2 ms per address may suffice.

To obtain a clean SEP recording, one must exclude from averaging those trials contaminated by the electrocardiogram (ECG), muscle potentials, movement, and other interference. This requires studying each tracing separately and selecting only good trials or using a computer program for automatic editing. In our laboratory, the edit program at a sampling rate of 100 to 500 $\mu$s per address automatically rejects any samples with five successive equal points, which usually indicate an overloaded response or mistrigger. A more commonly used amplitude criterion eliminates trials with unrealistically large potentials exceeding a predetermined level. The number of rejected trials is greater with the knee than with the ear reference, because ECG and other artifacts are more prominent in the former. We use a computer program to provide random triggering of the stimulus, while automatically avoiding the ECG artifact. The computer detects QRS complexes (or other overloaded artifacts exceeding the duration of 100 ms) and triggers the stimulus with a random time delay of 0 to 200 ms following the overloaded period. A low-frequency filter setting of from 30 to 100 Hz largely eliminates ECG T-waves.

Analyzing small neural responses requires high amplitude resolution in computer averaging. If we divided the sum by the actual count, small peaks would be eliminated. To circumvent this difficulty, we use a computer program to determine the smallest divisor that will retain the largest point within the display range.[97] The sum is divided by this artificial trial count, and a correction factor is applied to the computer measurement of the data, so that the amplitude displayed is the actual averaged amplitude. Typically, the divisors are one-fifteenth of the actual trial count.

# NEURAL SOURCES OF VARIOUS PEAKS

## Stimulation of the median nerve

Since Cracco's earlier report,[18] several studies have confirmed the presence of short latency somatosensory evoked potentials (SEPs) in man[15, 20, 25, 62, 72] as well as in animals.[8, 60, 98] To delineate the field distribution of the short latency components, SEPs may be recorded simultaneously from the scalp and cervical electrodes (see Fig. 19-2). Different investigators have described nearly identical waveform and distribution of scalp-recorded and cervical SEPs, without necessarily postulating the same neural sources for various components. Desmedt and Cheron [25, 26] have recently provided a comprehensive review of this subject. As mentioned earlier, short latency median SEPs are divided into four scalp recorded peaks, $P_9$, $P_{11}$, $P_{13}$, and $P_{14}$, and four corresponding cervical components, $Pc_9$, $(N_9)$, $N_{11}$, $N_{13}$, and $N_{14}$ in our laboratory.

The earliest scalp potential, $P_9$, probably originates from a distal portion of the brachial plexus.[7, 20, 72] Recording from the neck using a scalp reference, Jones[62] noted a negative peak with a latency of 9 ms and concluded that it also represented activity occurring in the brachial plexus. Although negative relative to the ear, this cervical potential is clearly positive in reference to the knee (see Fig. 19-2B). The field distribution of the first component is diagonally oriented with negativity at the shoulder and axilla and positivity over the entire scalp and neck (Fig. 19-6). It is not known why the propagating impulse is recorded as if it were a standing potential at this level. The electrical field may alter abruptly, however, as the impulse enters the brachial plexus, because of the change in anatomic orientation of the impulse, branching of the nerve, or alteration of the surrounding volume conductor.[68, 101]

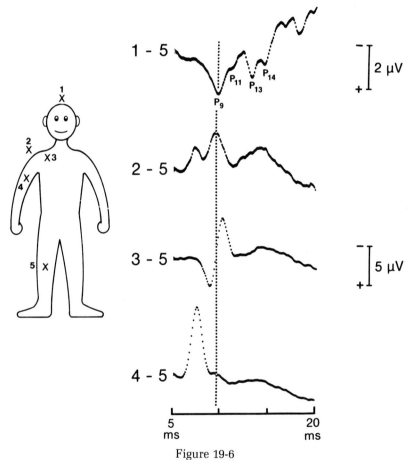

Figure 19-6

Relationship between scalp (1) recorded $P_9$ and potentials recorded at shoulder (2), Erb's point (3), and 5 cm distal to the axilla (4). The positive peak, $P_9$, at the scalp corresponded in latency to the negative peak recorded from the shoulder. (From Yamada, Kimura, and Nitz,[101] with permission.)

Our scalp-recorded $P_{11}$ is probably the same as $P_{12}$ of Kritchevsky and Wiederholt,[72] who postulated that the dorsal column or medial lemniscus might be the source of this potential. Others [39, 76] observed a negative cervical potential of the same latency and suggested that this was a postsynaptic cord potential. Jones,[62] however, proposed a generator site of $N_{11}$ at a region immediately adjacent to or just within the spinal cord. Various investigators [59, 76] noted that the potential analogous to $N_{11}$ was of greatest amplitude over the C-7 spinal process. We have also observed progressive decrease in amplitude of $P_{11}$ from the scalp to the high cervical region, eventually being replaced by a negative peak, $N_{11}$, at the low cervical area (Fig. 19-7).

An estimated mean conduction time from wrist to seventh cervical spine is 10 to 11 ms.[35, 71] Thus, the latency of $P_{11}$ or $N_{11}$ is barely enough to allow the sensory impulse to reach the spinal cord. The neural source of this component, therefore, must be near the entry into the cervical spinal cord.[101] This view is further supported by a close relationship of $N_{11}$ with the activity recorded from the lateral neck on the side of stimulation. It is thus likely that $N_{11}$ is generated at the entry into the spinal cord, and $P_{11}$ is the positive end of the field recorded at a distance. Desmedt and Cheron[26] also found that $N_{11}$ started upon arrival of the peripheral nerve volley at the spinal cord and interpreted $P_{11}$ as volume-conducted action potentials ascending the dorsal column. On the other hand, in two patients with cervical cord and medullary lesions studied by Anziska and Cracco,[6] this potential had an abnormally prolonged latency. Therefore, these authors suggest that it probably arises either in the spinal cord or lower brain stem. Its exact neural origin remains to be elucidated.

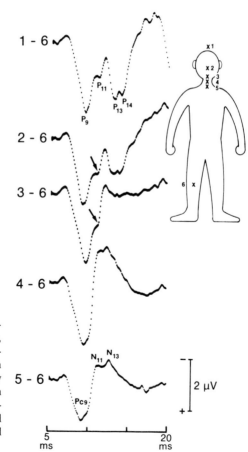

**Figure 19-7**

Responses from longitudinally placed electrodes at $C_z$ (1), $O_z$ (2), and high (3), mid (4), and low (5) cervical regions with knee reference. The amplitude of $P_{11}$ from $C_z$ to high cervical electrode (arrows) and replaced by negatively, $N_{11}$, at low cervical electrode. In contrast, the positive field of the first component extended from $C_z$ ($P_9$) to low cervical electrode ($Pc_9$). (From Yamada, Kimura, and Nitz,[101] with permission.)

The third positive potential [20, 72] is often bilobed, suggesting that it may have two different generator sources. In our laboratory, we regard this bilobed potential as two distinct components, $P_{13}$ and $P_{14}$. In contrast to the small and often equivocal $P_{13}$, $N_{13}$ is the largest negative component of the cervical potential. Jones[62] described the same negative potential as of spinal cord or brain stem origin. Desmedt and Cheron,[25, 26] using a noncephalic reference, noted that $P_{13}$ was generated above the foramen magnum and not at the level of the neck. The SEPs recorded from the nucleus ventralis caudalis in man consisted of monophasic or diphasic potentials with mean onset latency of 13.8 ms.[13] In the monkey, the potential analogous to $P_{13}$ seems to originate in the medial lemniscus.[8] We found the maximum negativity of this component at cervical level decreasing in amplitude rostrally and caudally.[101] We believe, therefore, that $N_{13}$ probably originates in the cervical spinal cord or cuneate nucleus and $P_{13}$ is a far field potential recorded at a distance, although the exact relationship between $N_{13}$ and $P_{13}$ remains unknown.[6] Cracco,[19] observing a slight delay of $N_{13}$ at higher cervical electrode placement, suggested the presence of a traveling wave. Similar latency changes occurred in some, but not all, of our subjects.[71]

Earlier studies using an ear reference described the initial positive potential with a latency of 13 to 17 ms.[1, 2, 18, 53] This potential, which probably corresponds to $P_{14}$ of the current nomenclature, was thought to originate in the thalamus.[20, 72] Similarly, $N_{14}$ of the cervical potential was attributed to neural discharges in the thalamus or brain stem.[62] More recent studies, however, have demonstrated that $P_{14}$ was intact in patients with lesions in the thalamus[59, 80] or midbrain[15] and in some patients with cerebral death,[5] suggesting a more caudal location of the neural source. This potential appears as a positive peak not only over the scalp but also at the nasopharyngeal electrode (Fig. 19-8), suggesting a more caudal generator site.[101] Detailed topographic data led Desmedt and Cheron[25] to conclude that $P_{14}$ originates in the medial lemniscus rather than above the thalamus. Unlike $N_{11}$ and $N_{13}$, $N_{14}$ is barely detectable from the cervical spine, indicating a neural source rostral to the cervical spine. These observations suggest that $N_{14}$ originates in the brain stem, and $P_{14}$ is a far field potential from the same origin.

We believe that a negative field near the generator site is responsible for the cervical potentials and that the scalp-recorded far field potential is primarily, although perhaps not exclusively, attributable to an approaching field of positivity from the same source.[100] Presumed neural generators corresponding to the beginning of each short latency peak are (1) the entry to the brachial plexus ($Pc_9$ and $P_9$); (2) the entry to the spinal cord ($N_{11}$ and $P_{11}$); (3) ascending volley of the cervical cord or synaptic discharge of cuneate nucleus ($N_{13}$ and $P_{13}$); and (4) the entry to the medial lemniscus ($N_{14}$ and $P_{14}$). Our findings also indicate that short latency SEPs are best delineated for clinical application by combined recording from the scalp with a noncephalic reference and from the neck with a cephalic reference.[101]

Following the $P_{14}$ which is distributed diffusely over the entire scalp, there is a small but distinct negative peak, $N_{17}$, recorded bilaterally in the frontal region.[26, 68] In contrast, the first major negative peaks, $N_{19}$ and $N_{20}$, recorded from the central and parietal region, respectively, are contralateral to the side of stimulation. The frontal negative peak, $N_{17}$, is also recorded consistently from the vertex and ipsilateral central electrode, and occasionally from the contralateral central area preceding the major negative peak, $N_{19}$. The topography of $N_{17}$ and $N_{19}$ suggests that these are two distinct peaks of separate neural origin (see Fig. 19-2D). If $P_{14}$ arises in the medial lemniscus, then it is likely that $N_{17}$ is generated subcortically, possibly reflecting a thalamic positive potential. However, the origins of $N_{17}$, subsequent peaks, and their field distributions remain to be elucidated.

Allison and associates[3] have suggested that $N_{20}$ is the first cortical potential and that $N_{20}$ and $N_{30}$ may have separate cortical generators because of their different potential distributions. Recent topographic studies of the short latency peaks do not support the hypothesis of dipole relationship between parietal $N_{20}$ and frontal $P_{20}$. The latencies

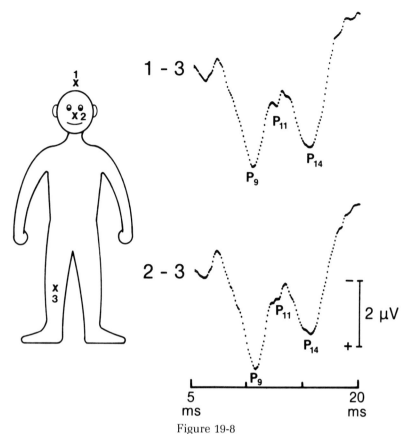

Figure 19-8

Responses from $C_z$ (1) and nasopharyngeal electrode (2). Note the positivity of $P_{14}$ in both tracings. This is in contrast to the negative peak, $N_{14}$, of the cervical potentials. (From Yamada, Kimura, and Nitz,[101] with permission.)

of the two are close but not the same, the $P_{20}$ having slightly later onset than the $N_{20}$.[26, 68] Further, negative-positive peaks subsequent to $P_{14}$ are shortest in latency at the frontal electrodes ($N_{17}$, $P_{20}$, $N_{29}$), showing a progressive delay toward the central ($N_{19}$, $P_{23}$, $N_{32}$) and parietal areas ($N_{20}$, $P_{26}$, $N_{34}$). The topographic specificity for various SEP components suggests the presence of a separate neural generator in each cortical location.

The last negative peak, $N_{60}$, appears entirely distinct from the preceding peaks. This component is more widely distributed over the cortex and shows greater temporal variability than the earlier peaks. It is likely that $N_{60}$ is mediated through a nonspecific polysynaptic pathway in contrast to the preceding peaks relayed by specific oligosynaptic routes.

## Stimulation of the peroneal and tibial nerves

Neural generators of the scalp-recorded peroneal or tibial SEP (see Fig. 19-3A, B, and C) remain to be elucidated. With the use of a knee reference contralateral to the side of stimulation, short latency tibial SEPs after stimulation of the nerve at the ankle consist of six positive peaks, $P_{11}$, $P_{17}$, $P_{21}$, $P_{24}$, $P_{27}$, and $P_{31}$.[102] Of these, $P_{17}$, $P_{24}$, and $P_{31}$ are the most consistent components. Only $P_{31}$ occurs regularly when the ear or shoulder serves as the reference, and $P_{24}$ and $P_{31}$ if referenced to the iliac crest. These findings indicate that the entire trunk and head are active and not suitable as a reference. Although $P_{17}$,

$P_{24}$, and $P_{31}$ are the same regardless of the position of the recording electrodes, the subsequent negative peak appears earlier over the ipsilateral ($N_{35}$) than contralateral hemisphere ($N_{37}$), possibly representing two independent generator sources.

Simultaneous recording from the peripheral nerve, spine, and scalp suggests that early components of the scalp-recorded SEPs are far field potentials, which originate from the sensory impulse ascending in the peripheral nerve, spinal cord, and brain stem (see Fig. 19-3B and C). Presumable generator sources are the popliteal fossa for $P_{11}$, entry to the sacral plexus for $P_{17}$, cauda equina for $P_{21}$, entry to the conus medullaris for $P_{24}$, rostral spinal cord for $P_{27}$, and brain stem for $P_{31}$. Subsequent negative and positive peaks, $N_{35}$ (or $N_{37}$) and $P_{40}$, probably represent thalamic or cortical discharges, but their neural sources have not been elucidated. We do not know as yet why the traveling impulse gives rise to SEP peaks with apparent temporal relationships to its entry to the sacral plexus and spinal cord. Our findings indicate, however, that the presence of a standing potential does not necessarily imply nonpropagating neural discharges such as those that occur at synapses in relay nuclei.[68]

Lumbosacral potentials recorded from the surface after stimulation of peroneal or tibial nerve consist of two negative components (see Fig. 19-4A).[10, 23, 28, 39, 64, 85] Dimitrijevic and associates[28] stimulated the tibial nerve at the knee and recorded two types of evoked potentials from T-12, L-2, L-4, and S-1 vertebral levels using a common reference electrode at the T-6 vertebral level (see Fig. 19-4B). Of the two, the spinal wave (S-wave) was a predominantly negative potential maximal at the T-12 vertebral level (lower end of the spinal cord). The other component, recorded at L-4, L-5, or S-1 vertebral level, was bilobed. They postulated that the first of the double peaks represented neural activity ascending in dorsal roots of the cauda equina (R-wave), whereas the second peak might be composed of dromic and antidromic discharges in the ventral roots (A-wave) with a possible contribution from slow fibers in the dorsal roots. The second potential may also reflect, at least in part, activity at the reference electrode that becomes positive ($P_{24}$) coincidental with the negative peak ($N_{23}$) at T-12, representing a lumbosacral potential (see Fig. 19-3B).

Phillips and Daube[85] also identified two well-defined negative peaks in the evoked potentials recorded from the lumbosacral region in response to electrical stimuli applied to the peroneal or tibial nerves (see Fig. 19-4C). The latency of the early peak increased progressively, but that of the second peak remained constant, as the active recording electrode $G_1$ was moved rostrally from sacral to upper lumbar levels. Thus, latency separation between peaks was maximal in recordings from the lower lumbar and upper sacral sites. The first peak probably represents a traveling wave ascending in the nerve roots of the cauda equina (cauda peak) and the second peak may be a standing potential generated in the lumbosacral region of the spinal cord (cord peak). The cord peak appears to be presynaptic in origin because it is stable to paired stimulation with very short interstimulus intervals.

The spinal evoked potential from stimulation of the sciatic nerve in the monkey consists of predominantly negative triphasic propagated potentials recorded at all spinal levels and greatest in amplitude over the cauda equina and caudal spinal cord.[45]

# PATHWAYS FOR SOMATOSENSORY POTENTIALS

## Dorsal column-medial lemniscal system and other central pathways

In most early clinical studies abnormal somatosensory evoked potentials (SEP) were noted only if vibration or position sense was impaired in patients with lesions of the spinal cord,[51, 56, 57] cerebral hemisphere,[99] or brain stem.[82] These findings suggested that all SEP components might be dependent upon the integrity of the dorsal column-medial lemniscal system in man.[56, 82] However, activity carried in the anterolateral column may also reach the cortex in monkeys as well as in man.[4, 11, 84] Indeed, Katz, Martin, and Blackburn[65] showed that stimulation with an intensity great enough to activate both large and small diameter fibers in the peroneal nerve produced SEPs even after transection of the dorsal column and spinocervical tract in cats. More recent clinical observation described below is consistent with the experimental evidence that multiple somatosensory pathways are operant.

If NI and NII are mediated by two separate central pathways, they may be affected independently. We have seen abnormalities of NII or subsequent peaks when early components were normal (Figs. 19-9 and 19-10), in patients with lesions of the brain stem, cervical cord, or brachial plexus.[104] We have also encountered selective involvement of the early peaks with intact NII and subsequent components in multiple sclerosis (Figs. 19-11, 19-12, and 19-13). Although rare, this dissociation is difficult to explain by the traditional view that successive peaks of the SEP represent progressively rostral levels along the course of a unitary somatosensory pathway.

## Peripheral pathways and the effect of tourniquet-induced ischemia

Studying the effect of ischemia and mechanical stimulations, Shimada and Nakanishi[89] found that an SEP was elicitable by pinprick but not by touch or tactile tap when vibration and touch sensations were lost. Pratt and associates[86] showed that mechanically evoked potentials were of lower amplitude and contained fewer components than the electrically evoked events, suggesting that the electrical stimulus activates more fibers synchronously than a mechanical stimulus. These findings support the contention of Tsumoto and associates[96] that NI may be related to the position-vibration sense,

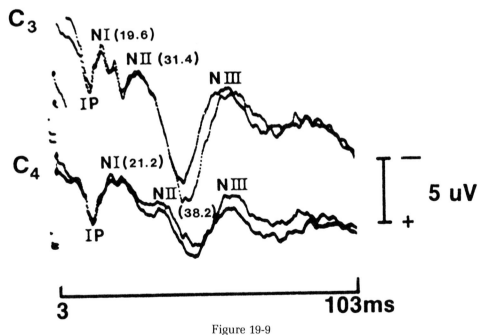

Figure 19-9
Scalp-recorded potential to bilateral stimulation of the median nerve in a 33-year-old man with traumatic avulsion of C-8, T-1, and probably T-2 roots on the left. A large meningocele was demonstrated at the C-7 vertebral level by myelography. The IP and NI were within normal range but NII was significantly delayed on the right (C$_4$). Despite the delay of NII, NIII was well preserved on the affected side.

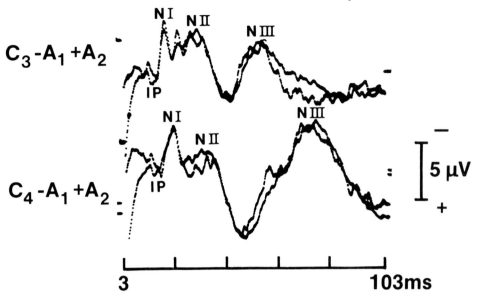

Figure 19-10

Scalp-recorded potential to bilateral stimulation of the median nerve in a 46-year-old woman with multiple sclerosis. Note a slight delay of the IP and NI and far greater delay of NII and NIII on the right (C₄). (From Yamada, et al,[106] with permission.)

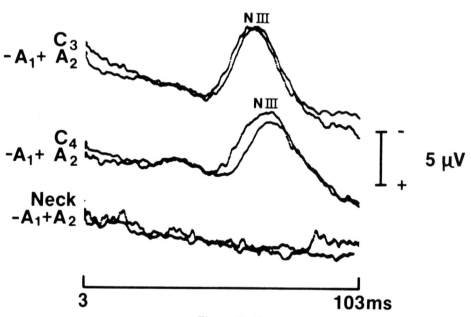

Figure 19-11

Scalp-recorded and cervical potentials to bilateral stimulation of the median nerve in a 47-year-old man with multiple sclerosis. The initial positive and first two negative peaks of the scalp-recorded potential were absent and the cervical potential was equivocal. Despite the absence of these early components, a late peak, NIII, was well preserved. (From Yamada, et al,[106] with permission.)

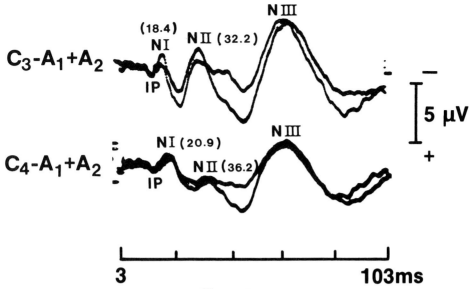

Figure 19-12

Scalp-recorded potential to bilateral stimulation of the median nerve in a 59-year-old woman with multiple sclerosis. The IP and NIII were normal. In contrast, NI and NII were both significantly delayed on the right (C₄). (From Yamada, et al,[106] with permission.)

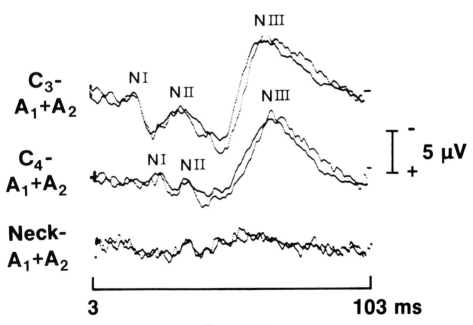

Figure 19-13

Scalp-recorded potential to bilateral stimulation of the median nerve in a 55-year-old woman with multiple sclerosis. Initial positive peak of both the scalp-recorded potential and the cervical potential was absent, and NI was substantially delayed on the right (C₄). Nonetheless, the subsequent peaks, NII and NIII were normal.

whereas NII is attributable to the pain-temperature sense. We have also seen occasional patients with impairment of pain-temperature sense alone who show depressed or absent NII even if NI was relatively preserved.[105]

It has been generally held that all SEP components are mediated exclusively by the fast conducting, large myelinated sensory fibers in the peripheral nerve. To test this hypothesis, we studied the effect of tourniquet-induced ischemia on SEP.[103] During the course of this reversible peripheral nerve dysfunction, one of the most consistent findings was the early diminution of Erb's potential. The change in Erb's potential coincided with a nearly parallel diminution in amplitude of the early SEP peaks ($P_9$, $P_{14}$, and NI) with relative sparing of the amplitude of the later components (PI, NII, PII, and NIII). In contrast, latencies of the late peaks were significantly more delayed than those of the early peaks (Fig. 19-14).

The brief effect of an inflated cuff on nerve is probably caused by ischemia rather than mechanical compression, since the largest myelinated fibers are the first to

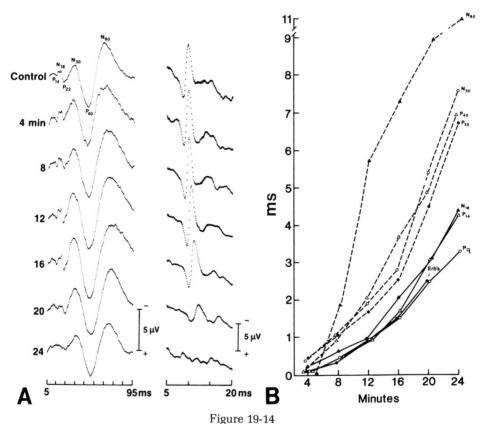

Figure 19-14

(A) Sequential changes of scalp-recorded somatosensory evoked potentials (left) and Erb's potential (right) during ischemia in a normal subject. The initial positive and negative components, $P_{14}$ and NI ($N_{18}$), were affected along with Erb's potentials earlier than the later components, PI ($P_{22}$), NII ($N_{30}$), PII ($P_{40}$), and NIII ($N_{60}$). The ischemia-sensitive peaks were no longer present after 24 minutes, when the ischemia-resistant peaks were still relatively intact. (From Yamada, Muroga, and Kimura,[103] with permission.) (B) Effect of ischemia on the somatosensory evoked potentials and Erb's potential. The change in latency in milliseconds (ordinate) was plotted against duration of ischemia in minutes (abscissa). There was a clear dissociation in the time course of latency change between the ischemia-sensitive components (Erb's potential, $P_9$, $P_{14}$, and $N_{18}$) and the ischemia-resistant components ($P_{22}$, $N_{30}$, $P_{40}$, and $N_{60}$). (From Yamada, Muroga, and Kimura,[103] with permission.)

fail.[16, 48, 49, 50, 83] Most sensitive to ischemia is the potential recorded from Erb's point which is subserved primarily by large myelinated fibers. Since $P_9$, $P_{14}$, and NI are as sensitive to ischemia as Erb's potential, these early components are probably mediated by large afferent fibers as well. In contrast, PI and later components have different characteristics and may be mediated through independent routes, possibly involving different first-order afferent fibers, for example, smaller myelinated fibers.

An alternative explanation may be that central amplification compensates for peripheral conduction block. Sensory nerve potentials represent highly synchronous activity and may be sensitive to even slight desynchronization in peripheral neuropathy.[52] In contrast, the cortex, operating as an integrator, may be able to generate a sizable evoked response after several synaptic relays, even if the corticopetal input is severely desynchronized.[24] Therefore, a few large afferent fibers that survive the effects of ischemia may be sufficient to evoke late SEPs even when Erb's potential and early SEPs are no longer elicitable. In severe sensory neuropathy, the peripheral nerve potential may be unrecordable, while SEP peaks are delayed but preserved.

Although the mechanism remains to be determined, our data document that selective amplitude abnormalities of the short latency SEP can occur in disorders of the peripheral nerve. Similarly the late components may show disproportionately greater latency increases than the early components, even though the conduction abnormalities are limited to the peripheral nerve. In clinical use of SEPs, these possibilities must always be considered before concluding that abnormalities are manifestations of a central nervous system disease.

## Measurement of conduction time

At least two separate trials with the same stimulus setting should be analyzed for consistency. Onset and peak latencies and peak-to-peak amplitudes are ordinarily measured. Tables 19-1, 19-2, and 19-3 summarize the average peak latencies of median and tibial SEPs.

**TABLE 19-1 Short latency somatosensory evoked potentials after stimulation of the median nerve in 34 normal subjects**

| Components | Latency (left and right combined) | | | Latency difference between left and right | | |
|---|---|---|---|---|---|---|
| | number identified | mean ± SD (ms) | mean + 3SD | number identified | mean ± SD (ms) | mean + 3SD |
| Erb's Potential | 68 | 9.8 ± 0.8 | 12.2 | 34 | 0.4 ± 0.2 | 1.0 |
| P9* | 68 | 9.1 ± 0.6 | 10.9 | 34 | 0.4 ± 0.2 | 1.0 |
| N11 | 43 | 11.2 ± 0.6 | 13.0 | 19 | 0.4 ± 0.3 | 1.3 |
| N13* | 68 | 13.2 ± 0.9 | 15.9 | 34 | 0.5 ± 0.4 | 1.7 |
| P14 | 55 | 14.1 ± 0.9 | 16.8 | 25 | 0.5 ± 0.4 | 1.7 |
| NI | 68 | 18.3 ± 1.5 | 22.8 | 34 | 0.5 ± 0.5 | 2.0 |
| P9–P11 | 43 | 2.2 ± 0.3 | 3.1 | 19 | 0.2 ± 0.2 | 0.8 |
| N11–13 | 43 | 1.9 ± 0.4 | 3.1 | 19 | 0.2 ± 0.2 | 0.8 |
| N13–14 | 55 | 1.0 ± 0.4 | 2.2 | 25 | 0.3 ± 0.2 | 0.9 |
| P14–N18 | 55 | 4.2 ± 0.9 | 6.9 | 25 | 0.7 ± 0.5 | 2.2 |
| P9–N13* | 68 | 4.0 ± 0.4 | 5.2 | 34 | 0.3 ± 0.3 | 1.2 |
| N13–NI | 68 | 5.1 ± 0.9 | 7.8 | 34 | 0.6 ± 0.5 | 2.1 |

*These components are consistently elicited in normal subjects and therefore most useful in evaluating patients. (From Yamada, et al,[106] with permission.)

## TABLE 19-2 Intermediate and long latency somatosensory evoked potentials after stimulation of the median nerve in 34 normal subjects

| Components | Latency (left and right combined) | | | Latency difference between left and right | | |
|---|---|---|---|---|---|---|
| | number identified | mean ± SD (ms) | mean + 3SD | number identified | mean ± SD (ms) | mean + 3SD |
| NI | 68 | 18.1 ± 1.6 | 22.9 | 34 | 0.4 ± 0.4 | 1.6 |
| PI | 68 | 22.8 ± 2.3 | 29.7 | 34 | 0.6 ± 0.4 | 1.8 |
| NII | 68 | 31.6 ± 2.6 | 39.4 | 34 | 0.5 ± 0.4 | 1.7 |
| PII | 68 | 43.6 ± 3.6 | 54.4 | 34 | 0.6 ± 0.5 | 2.1 |
| NIII | 64 | 62.8 ± 9.3 | 90.7 | 32 | 1.5 ± 1.1 | 4.8 |

(From Yamada, et al,[106] with permission.)

The conduction time over the somatosensory pathways consists of two parts, peripheral and central latencies. The peripheral latency covers the distal part of the first neuron from the stimulus site to the spinal cord entry. The central latency corresponds to the central part of the first neuron up to the dorsal column nuclei, lemniscal system, and thalamocortical fibers, including at least three synapses. The central latencies for median and peroneal nerves represent the sensory pathways to the cortex from the cervical enlargement (C-7 spine) and conus medullaris (T-12 spine), respectively. The difference between the two provides the spinal cord conduction from the conus medullaris to the cervical enlargement.[30, 31] To determine central latencies from overall SEP latencies, one must first estimate the conduction time along the peripheral pathway.

The peripheral sensory latency to the spinal cord may be estimated by spinal potentials recorded over the C-7 and T-12 spines in the upper and lower extremities, respectively. One can also estimate the peripheral latency by measuring the motor conduction through use of the F-wave and M-response. As described in Chapter 17, the motor latency from the stimulus site to the spinal cord is calculated by the equation $(F-M-1)/2$, where F and M are latencies of F-wave and M-response, respectively.[30, 31, 35, 66, 67, 70] The motor latency is then converted to a sensory latency by the ratio SNCV/MNCV for the median nerve, where SNCV and MNCV are sensory and motor nerve conduction velocities in the elbow-to-wrist segment.

## TABLE 19-3 Scalp-recorded positive components (A) and negative peaks (B) registered in the gluteus and along the spine after stimulation of the tibial nerve

| (A) Components | Scalp | | | | | |
|---|---|---|---|---|---|---|
| Recording Site | $P_{11}$ | $P_{17}$ | $P_{21}$ | $P_{24}$ | $P_{27}$ | $P_{31}$ |
| Mean ± SD (ms) | 11.4 ± 2.7 | 17.3 ± 1.9 | 20.8 ± 1.9 | 23.8 ± 2.0 | 27.4 ± 2.1 | 31.2 ± 2.1 |
| Number recorded | 22 | 40 | 21 | 39 | 30 | 40 |
| Number tested | 40 | 40 | 40 | 40 | 40 | 40 |

| (B) Components | Gluteus | L-4 | T-12 | C-7 | C-2 |
|---|---|---|---|---|---|
| Recording Site | $N_{16}$ | $N_{21}$ | $N_{23}$ | $N_{28}$ | $N_{30}$ |
| Mean ± SD (ms) | 16.4 ± 3.2 | 20.9 ± 2.2 | 23.2 ± 2.1 | 27.6 ± 1.8 | 30.2 ± 1.9 |
| Number recorded | 20 | 40 | 40 | 18 | 25 |
| Number tested | 22 | 40 | 40 | 22 | 26 |

(From Yamada, Machida, and Kimura,[102] in preparation).

In the above discussion, we assumed that SEP components are mediated by large myelinated, fast conducting fibers. However, changes in conduction characteristics of slower conducting fibers, not assessed by conventional nerve conduction studies, could conceivably alter the latency and waveform of SEPs. The spinal conduction time calculated by this method varies considerably from one subject to the next, in part because of cumulative error from various latency determinations.[30, 36, 71] Thus the currently available technique is of limited value as a routine diagnostic test for spinal cord conduction.[71]

# CLINICAL APPLICATION

## Lesions of the peripheral nerve

Desmedt[24] has summarized clinical uses of somatosensory evoked potentials (SEP) for a wide variety of neurologic disorders. Conventional study of sensory nerve conduction velocity consists of recording sensory nerve potentials at the wrist, elbow, and axilla after electrical stimulation to the fingers. This method fails to provide direct assessment of sensory fibers proximal to the axilla. It is also limited technically by the small amplitude of sensory potentials recorded in diseased nerves, especially in pediatric patients.[87] Electrical stimulation of a mixed nerve trunk may elicit larger proximal nerve potentials. However, not only skin and joint afferents are activated, but also muscle afferents and antidromic motor impulses. Scalp-recorded or spinal SEPs are, however, free of motor components even though a mixed nerve is stimulated.

SEPs serve clinically to evaluate the proximal nerve segment from the axilla to the spinal cord.[27] The F-wave is also useful in assessing this segment but relates solely to motor fibers. SEPs are of diagnostic value in brachial plexopathy or radiculopathy, especially if only sensory nerve fibers are involved.[40, 55, 63, 92] Eisen and Elleker[34] have shown that SEP measurement is feasible for sensory studies of the median, ulnar, radial, musculocutaneous, sural, superficial peroneal, and saphenous nerves. Simultaneous recording of sensory nerve action potential allows comparison of peripheral and central sensory conduction times.

## Lesions of the spinal cord and brain stem

SEPs are uniquely suited for the evaluation of diseases involving the posterior column or the larger fibers in dorsal roots and sensory nerves. In Friedreich's ataxia, the sural nerve conducts at normal velocity.[33] However, its potentials are much reduced in size and often unrecordable.[32, 78] The SEP has shown slowed peripheral as well as central sensory conductions in this condition.[27] Abnormalities of SEPs have been described in subacute combined degeneration.[47] In syringomyelia (Fig. 19-3A) SEPs may be abnormal with clinical sensory loss, even though sensory nerve conduction studies remain unaffected.[46] SEPs also provide useful data in patients with vascular lesions of the brain stem.[27]

## Multiple sclerosis

Symptoms and signs of multiple sclerosis are generally related to blocked and impaired conduction in central nerve fibers across areas of demyelination. Namerow[81] showed that the SEPs evoked by median nerve stimulation were abnormal and delayed in multiple sclerosis patients in whom there was impairment of position and/or vibration sense. Because the peripheral nerves are essentially normal in multiple sclerosis,[17] the delay in SEP latencies indicates conduction abnormalities along the central somatosensory pathways. The SEP can uncover clinically silent lesions and document dissemination of disease site when clinical signs are confined to a single lesion.[27] More recently, Dorfman, Bosley, and Cummins[31] were able to localize the level of the sensory disturbance to either the spinal or the supraspinal segment of the somatosensory pathway. Reduced spinal conduction velocity correlated with clinical evidence of spinal cord malfunction, but abnormalities were encountered also in some cases with no signs of myelopathy.

The overall incidence of abnormal scalp-recorded SEPs in multiple sclerosis ranges from 50 to 86 percent.[9, 14, 27, 54, 73, 95] In one study,[7] abnormal SEPs were found in 25 out of 26 patients with definite diagnoses using scalp-recorded short latency positive peaks and the initial negative peak. Recording short latency SEP ($N_{13}$) from the neck, abnormalities occurred in 58 percent of the total patient group with suspected or established diagnoses, and in 94 percent of those with a definite diagnosis.[75] Others[93] reported 59 percent and 69 percent, respectively. In another series, the cervical response was abnormal in 41 percent of patients with a suspected diagnosis and 87 percent of these with a definite diagnosis.[38] The cervical potential was greatly disorganized after heating in many patients with multiple sclerosis.[77] Using the latency difference between cervical and scalp-recorded negative peaks (equivalent to our cervical $N_{13}$-scalp NI interwave peak), the incidences of abnormality were 68 percent overall and 83 percent in the definite group.[37]

We also studied SEP in 52 patients, 29 with definite and 23 with probable diagnoses of multiple sclerosis.[106] In 39 patients who had unequivocal alterations of the SEP, changes of short (up to $N_{18}$) and long latency (after $N_{18}$) components were compared. Both were affected in 28 patients, whereas the abnormality was limited to the long latency SEPs in the remaining 11 patients. These findings indicate that a substantial number of SEP abnormalities may be overlooked if the test is determined solely on the basis of short latency components. Further, questionable changes of short latency SEPs could be corroborated by significant asymmetries in the long latency components. Thus long latency SEPs are a useful adjunct in evaluating multiple sclerosis patients, especially if bilateral stimulation is used.

## Clinical value and limitations

Electrodiagnostic studies of the somatosensory system have previously been limited largely to measurement of sensory nerve conduction velocities in the more distal portions of the peripheral nerve. SEPs elicited after stimulation of a peripheral nerve can be used for assessment of the entire length of the somatosensory pathway. Clinical application was impeded until recently, because few medical centers were equipped to detect these small potentials against larger background cortical activity. The availability of mini-computers and averagers, however, has now made it feasible to record SEPs as a diagnostic test for anatomic regions not accessible by ordinary methods.

With unilateral stimulation, slight SEP changes may be attributed to intertrial variability, but bilateral stimulation allows simultaneous evaluation of sensory input to both hemispheres.[105] Since the neuroanatomic substrates of the SEP peaks are still unknown, clinical localization of lesions based on this test requires extreme care. For example, with involvement of the peripheral nerve, selective reduction in amplitude of the early SEPs may occur in association with relative preservation of the late SEPs. Or, the late peaks may show disproportionately greater latency increases than the early peaks.[69, 103]

Various SEP components may not be transmitted via a single pathway but may be mediated through independent routes, possibly involving different first order afferent fibers. Alternatively, central amplification may compensate for peripheral axonal loss so that partial block of the peripheral nerve may not significantly change the SEP. These and other uncertainties must be resolved before the SEP can be considered a reliable diagnostic tool for the precise localization of sensory lesions. Nonetheless, the combined application of both short and long latency SEPs promises to provide maximum information in evaluating the peripheral, as well as central, somatosensory system.

# REFERENCE SOURCES

1. ABRAHAMIAN, HA, ET AL: *Effects of thiopental on human cerebral evoked responses.* Anesthesiology 24:650, 1963.

2. ALLISON, T, ET AL: *The effects of barbiturate anesthesia upon human somatosensory evoked responses.* Electroenceph Clin Neurophysiol (suppl 24):68, 1963.

3. ALLISON, T, ET AL: *On the neural origin of early components of the human somatosensory evoked potential.* In DESMEDT, JE (ED): *Progress in Clinical Neurophysiology,* Vol 7. Karger, Basel, 1980, pp 51–68.

4. ANDERSSON, SA, NORRSELL, K, AND NORRSELL, U: *Spinal pathways projecting to the cerebral first somatosensory area in the monkey.* J Physiol (Lond) 225:589, 1972.

5. ANZISKA, BJ AND CRACCO, RQ: *Short latency somatosensory evoked potentials in brain dead patients.* Arch Neurol 37:222, 1980.

6. ANZISKA, BJ AND CRACCO, RQ: *Short latency somatosensory evoked potentials: Studies in patients with focal neurological disease.* Electroenceph Clin Neurophysiol 49:227, 1980.

7. ANZISKA, B, ET AL: *Somatosensory far field potentials: Studies in normal subjects and patients with multiple sclerosis.* Electroenceph Clin Neurophysiol 45:602, 1978.

8. AREZZO, J, LEGATT, AD, AND VAUGHAN, HG, JR: *Topography and intracranial sources of somatosensory evoked potentials in the monkey. I. Early components.* Electroenceph Clin Neurophysiol 46:155, 1979.

9. BAKER, JB, ET AL: *Evoked potentials as an aid to the diagnosis of multiple sclerosis.* Neurology (Minneap) 18:286, 1968.

10. BARAN, EM: *Evoked spinal responses in man (abstr).* Electroenceph Clin Neurophysiol 45:16P, 1978.

11. BLACKBURN, JG, PEROT, PL, AND KATZ, S: *Effects of low spinal transection on somatosensory evoked potentials from forelimb stimulation (abstr).* Fed Proc 33:400, 1974.

12. CACCIA, MR, UBIALI, E, AND ANDREUSSI, L: *Spinal evoked responses recorded from the epidural space in normal and diseased humans.* J Neurol Neurosurg Psychiatry 39:962, 1976.

13. CELESIA, GG: *Somatosensory evoked potentials recorded directly from human thalamus and Sm I cortical area.* Arch Neurol 36:399, 1979.

14. CHIAPPA, KH: *Pattern shift visual, brainstem auditory, and short-latency somatosensory evoked potentials in multiple sclerosis.* Neurology (New York) 30:110, 1980.

15. CHIAPPA, KH, CHOI, SK, AND YOUNG, RR: *Short-latency somatosensory evoked potentials following median nerve stimulation in patients with neurological lesions.* In DESMEDT, JE (ED): *Progress in Clinical Neurophysiology,* Vol 7. Karger, Basel, 1980, pp 264–281.

16. CLARK, D, HUGHES, J, AND GASSER, HS: *Afferent function in the group of nerve fibers of slowest conduction velocity.* Am J Physiol 114:69, 1935.

17. CONRAD, B AND BECHINGER, D: *Sensorische und motorische Nervenleitgeschwindigkeit und distale Latenz bei Multipler Sklerose.* Arch Psychiatr Nervenkr 212:140, 1969.

18. CRACCO, RQ: *The initial positive potential of the human scalp-recorded somatosensory evoked response.* Electroenceph Clin Neurophysiol 32:623, 1972.

19. CRACCO, RQ: *Spinal evoked response: Peripheral nerve stimulation in man.* Electroenceph Clin Neurophysiol 35:379, 1973.

20. CRACCO, RQ AND CRACCO, JB: *Somatosensory evoked potential in man: Far field potentials.* Electroenceph Clin Neurophysiol 41:460, 1976.

21. CRACCO, JB, CRACCO, RQ, AND GRAZIANI, LJ: *The spinal evoked response in infants and children.* Neurology (Minneap) 25:31, 1975.

22. CRACCO, JB, CRACCO, RQ, AND STOLOVE, R: *Spinal evoked potential in man: A maturational study.* Electroenceph Clin Neurophysiol 46:58, 1979.

23.   DESMEDT, JE: *Somatosensory cerebral evoked potentials in man.* In RÉMOND, A (ED): *Handbook of Electroencephalography and Clinical Neurophysiology,* Vol 9. Elsevier, Amsterdam, 1971, pp 55–82.

24.   DESMEDT, JE: *Clinical Uses of Cerebral, Brainstem and Spinal Somatosensory Evoked Potentials.* In DESMEDT, JE (ED): *Progress in Clinical Neurophysiology,* Vol 7. Karger, Basel, 1980.

25.   DESMEDT, JE AND CHERON, G: *Central somatosensory conduction in man: Neural generators and interpeak latencies of the far-field components recorded from neck and right or left scalp and earlobes.* Electroenceph Clin Neurophysiol 50:382, 1980.

26.   DESMEDT, JE AND CHERON, G: *Somatosensory evoked potentials to finger stimulation in healthy octogenarians and in young adults: Wave forms, scalp topography and transit times of parietal and frontal components.* Electroenceph Clin Neurophysiol 50:404, 1980.

27.   DESMEDT, JE AND NOËL, P: *Average cerebral evoked potentials in the evaluation of lesions of the sensory nerves and of the central somatosensory pathway.* In DESMEDT, JE (ED): *New Developments in Electromyography and Clinical Neurophysiology,* Vol 2. Karger, Basel, 1973, pp 352–371.

28.   DIMITRIJEVIC, MR, ET AL: *Evoked spinal cord and nerve root potentials in humans using a non-invasive recording technique.* Electroenceph Clin Neurophysiol 45:331, 1978.

29.   DONCHIN, E, ET AL: *Publication criteria for studies of evoked potentials (EP) in man.* In DESMEDT, JE (ED): *Attention, voluntary contraction and event-related cerebral potentials in man. Progress in Clinical Neurophysiology,* Vol 1. Karger, Basel, 1977, pp 1–11.

30.   DORFMAN, LJ: *Indirect estimation of spinal cord conduction velocity in man.* Electroenceph Clin Neurophysiol 42:26, 1977.

31.   DORFMAN, LJ, BOSLEY, TM, AND CUMMINS, KL: *Electrophysiological localization of central somatosensory lesions in patients with multiple sclerosis.* Electroenceph Clin Neurophysiol 44:742, 1978.

32.   DYCK, P, LAMBERT, EH, AND NICHOLS, PC: *Quantitative measurements of sensation related to compound action potential and number and sizes of myelinated and unmyelinated fibers of sural nerve in health, Friedreich's ataxia, hereditary sensory neuropathy, and tabes dorsalis.* In RÉMOND, A (ED): *Handbook of Electroencephalography and Clinical Neurophysiology,* Vol 9. Elsevier, Amsterdam, 1971, pp 83–118.

33.   DYCK, PJ, ET AL: *Histologic and teased-fiber measurements of sural nerve in disorders of lower motor and primary sensory neurons.* Mayo Clin Proc 43:81, 1968.

34.   EISEN, A AND ELLEKER, G: *Sensory nerve stimulation and evoked cerebral potentials.* Neurology (New York) 30:1097, 1980.

35.   EISEN, A AND NUDLEMAN, K: *F-wave and cervical somatosensory response conduction from the seventh cervical spinous process to cortex in multiple sclerosis.* J Canad Sciences Neurologiques 5:289, 1978.

36.   EISEN, A AND NUDLEMAN, K: *Cord to cortex conduction in multiple sclerosis.* Neurology (New York) 29:189, 1979.

37.   EISEN, A AND ODUSOTE, K: *Central and peripheral conduction times in multiple sclerosis.* Electroenceph Clin Neurophysiol 48:253, 1980.

38.   EISEN, A, ET AL: *Short-latency somatosensory responses in multiple sclerosis.* Neurology (New York) 29:827, 1979.

39.   EL-NEGAMY, E AND SEDGWICK, EM: *Properties of a spinal somatosensory evoked potential recorded in man.* J Neurol Neurosurg Psychiatry 41:762, 1978.

40.   EL-NEGAMY, E AND SEDGWICK, EM: *Delayed cervical somatosensory potentials in cervical spondylosis.* J Neurol Neurosurg Psychiatry 42:238, 1979.

41.   ERTEKIN, C: *Human evoked electrospinogram.* In DESMEDT, JE (ED): *New Developments in Electromyography and Clinical Neurophysiology,* Vol 2. Karger, Basel, 1973.

42.   ERTEKIN, C: *Studies on the human evoked electrospinogram. I. The origin of the segmental evoked potentials.* Acta Neurol Scand 53:3, 1976.

43.   ERTEKIN, C: *Studies on the human evoked electrospinogram. II. The conduction velocity along the dorsal funiculus.* Acta Neurol Scand 53:21, 1976.

44. ERTEKIN, C: *Evoked electrospinogram in spinal cord and peripheral nerve disorders.* Acta Neurol Scand 57:329, 1978.

45. FELDMAN, MH, ET AL: *Spinal evoked potential in the monkey.* Ann Neurol 7:238, 1980.

46. FINCHAM, RW AND CAPE, CA: *Sensory nerve conduction in syringomyelia.* Neurology (Minneap) 18:200, 1968.

47. FINE, EJ AND HALLETT, M: *Neurophysiological study of subacute combined degeneration.* J Neurol Sci 45:331, 1980.

48. FOWLER, TJ AND OCHOA, J: *Unmyelinated fibres in normal and compressed peripheral nerves of the baboon: A quantitative electron microscopic study.* Neuropathol Appl Neurobiol 1:247, 1975.

49. FOWLER, TJ, DANTA, G, AND GILLIATT, RW: *Recovery of nerve conduction after a pneumatic tourniquet: Observations on the hind-limb of the baboon.* J Neurol Neurosurg Psychiatry 35:638, 1972.

50. FOX, JL AND KENMORE, PI: *The effect of ischemia on nerve conduction.* Exp Neurol 17:403, 1967.

51. GIBLIN, DR: *Somatosensory evoked potentials in healthy subjects and in patients with lesions of the nervous system.* Ann NY Acad Sci 112:93, 1964.

52. GILLIATT, RW AND SEARS, TA: *Sensory nerve action potentials in patients with peripheral nerve lesions.* J Neurol Neurosurg Psychiatry 21:109, 1958.

53. GOFF, WR, ROSNER, BS, AND ALLISON, T: *Distribution of cerebral somatosensory evoked responses in normal man.* Electroenceph Clin Neurophysiol 14:697, 1962.

54. GREEN, JB, PRICE, R, AND WOODBURY, SG: *Short-latency somatosensory evoked potentials in multiple sclerosis. Comparison with auditory and visual evoked potentials.* Arch Neurol 37:630, 1980.

55. GRISOLIA, JS AND WIEDERHOLT, WC: *Short latency somatosensory evoked potentials from radial, median and ulnar nerve stimulation in man.* Electroenceph Clin Neurophysiol 50:375, 1980.

56. HALLIDAY, AM: *Changes in the form of cerebral evoked responses in man associated with various lesions of the nervous system.* Electroenceph Clin Neurophysiol (suppl 25):178, 1967.

57. HALLIDAY, AM AND WAKEFIELD, GS: *Cerebral evoked potentials in patients with dissociated sensory loss.* J Neurol Neurosurg Psychiatry 26:211, 1963.

58. HARNER, PF AND SANNIT, T: *A review of the international ten-twenty system of electrode placement.* Grass Instrument Co., Quincy, Mass, 1974.

59. HUME, AL AND CANT, BR: *Conduction time in central somatosensory pathways in man.* Electroenceph Clin Neurophysiol 45:361, 1978.

60. IRAGUI-MADOZ, VJ AND WIEDERHOLT, WC: *Far field somatosensory evoked potentials in the cat.* Electroenceph Clin Neurophysiol 43:646, 1977.

61. JASPER, HH: *The ten twenty electrode system of the International Federation.* Electroenceph Clin Neurophysiol 10:371, 1958.

62. JONES, SJ: *Short latency potentials recorded from the neck and scalp following median nerve stimulation in man.* Electroenceph Clin Neurophysiol 43:853, 1977.

63. JONES, SJ: *Investigation of brachial plexus traction lesions by peripheral and spinal somatosensory evoked potentials.* J Neurol Neurosurg Psychiatry 42:107, 1979.

64. JONES, SJ AND SMALL, DG: *Spinal and sub-cortical evoked potentials following stimulation of the posterior tibial nerve in man.* Electroenceph Clin Neurophysiol 44:299, 1978.

65. KATZ, S, MARTIN, HF, AND BLACKBURN, JG: *The effects of interaction between large and small diameter fiber systems on the somatosensory evoked potential.* Electroenceph Clin Neurophysiol 45:45, 1978.

66. KIMURA, J: *F-wave velocity in the central segment of the median and ulnar nerves. A study in normal subjects and in patients with Charcot-Marie-Tooth disease.* Neurology (Minneap) 24:539, 1974.

67. KIMURA, J: *A method for estimating the refractory period of motor fibers in the human peripheral nerve.* J Neurol Sci 28:485, 1976.

68. KIMURA, J AND YAMADA, T: *Short latency somatosensory evoked potentials following median nerve stimulation.* Ann NY Acad Sci 388:689, 1982.

69. KIMURA, J, ET AL: *Neural pathways of somatosensory evoked potentials, clinical implications.* In BUSER, P (ED) *Contemporary Clinical Neurophysiology* (EEG suppl 36). Elsevier, Amsterdam, 1982 (in press).

70. KIMURA, J, BOSCH, P, AND LINDSAY, GM: *F-wave conduction velocity in the central segment of the peroneal and tibial nerves.* Arch Phys Med Rehabil 56:492, 1975.

71. KIMURA, J, YAMADA, T, AND KAWAMURA, H: *Central latencies of somatosensory cerebral evoked potentials.* Arch Neurol 35:683, 1978.

72. KRITCHEVSKY, M AND WIEDERHOLT, WC: *Short-latency somatosensory evoked potentials.* Arch Neurol 35:706, 1978.

73. LEHMANN, D, GABATHULER, U, AND BAUMGARTNER, G: *Right/left differences of median nerve evoked scalp potentials in multiple sclerosis.* J Neurol 221:15, 1979.

74. LIBERSON, WT AND KIM, KC: *The mapping out of evoked potentials elicited by stimulation of the median and peroneal nerves.* Electroenceph Clin Neurophysiol 15:721, 1963.

75. MASTAGLIA, FL, BLACK, JL, AND COLLINS, DWK: *Visual and spinal evoked potentials in diagnosis of multiple sclerosis.* Br Med J 2:732, 1976.

76. MATTHEWS, WB, BEAUCHAMP, M, AND SMALL, DG: *Cervical somato-sensory evoked responses in man.* Nature 252:230, 1974.

77. MATTHEWS, WB, READ, DJ, AND POUNTNEY, E: *Effect of raising body temperature on visual and somatosensory evoked potentials in patients with multiple sclerosis.* J Neurol Neurosurg Psychiatry 42:250, 1979.

78. McLEOD, JG: *An electrophysiological and pathological study of peripheral nerves in Friedreich's ataxia.* J Neurol Sci 12:333, 1971.

79. NAKANISHI, T, TAKITA, K, AND TOYOKURA, Y: *Somatosensory evoked responses to tactile tap in man.* Electroenceph Clin Neurophysiol 34:1, 1973.

80. NAKANISHI, T, ET AL: *The initial positive component of the scalp-recorded somatosensory evoked potential in normal subjects and in patients with neurological disorders.* Electroenceph Clin Neurophysiol 45:26, 1978.

81. NAMEROW, NS: *Somatosensory evoked responses in multiple sclerosis patients with varying sensory loss.* Neurology (Minneap) 18:1197, 1968.

82. NOËL, P AND DESMEDT, JE: *Somatosensory cerebral evoked potentials after vascular lesions of the brain-stem and diencephalon.* Brain 98:113, 1975.

83. OCHOA, J, FOWLER, TJ, AND GILLIATT, RW: *Anatomical changes in peripheral nerves compressed by a pneumatic tourniquet.* J Anat 113:433, 1972.

84. PEROT, PL, JR: *The clinical use of somatosensory evoked potentials in spinal cord injury.* In *Clinical Neurosurgery.* Proceedings of the Congress of Neurological Surgeons, Williams & Wilkins, Baltimore, 1973, pp 367–381.

85. PHILLIPS, LH, II AND DAUBE, JR: *Lumbosacral spinal evoked potentials in humans.* Neurology (New York) 30:1175, 1980.

86. PRATT, H, ET AL: *Mechanically and electrically evoked somatosensory potentials in normal humans.* Neurology (New York) 29:1236, 1979.

87. ROBERTSON, WC, JR AND LAMBERT, EH: *Sensory nerve conduction velocity in children using cerebral evoked potentials.* Arch Phys Med Rehabil 59:1, 1978.

88. SCHRAMM, J: *Clinical experience with the objective localization of the lesion in cervical myelopathy.* In GROTE, W, ET AL (EDS): *Advances in Neurosurgery, Surgery of Cervical Myelopathy Infantile Hydrocephalus: Long-Term Results,* Vol 8. Springer-Verlag, Berlin, 1980, pp 26–32.

89. SHIMADA, Y AND NAKANISHI, T: *Somatosensory evoked responses elicited by mechanical stimulations in man.* Adv Neurol Sci (Tokyo) 23:282, 1979.

90. SHIMIZU, H, ET AL: *Slow cord dorsum potentials elicited by descending volleys in man.* J Neurol Neurosurg Psychiatry 42:242, 1979.

91. SHIMOJI, K, ET AL: *Evoked spinal electrogram in a quadriplegic patient.* Electroenceph Clin Neurophysiol 35:659, 1973.

92. SIIVOLA, J, ET AL: *Brachial plexus and radicular neurography in relation to cortical evoked*

responses. J Neurol Neurosurg Psychiatry 42:1151, 1979.

93. SMALL, DG, MATTHEWS, WB, AND SMALL, M: *The cervical somatosensory evoked potential (SEP) in the diagnosis of multiple sclerosis.* J Neurol Sci 35:211, 1978.

94. TAMURA, K: *Ipsilateral somatosensory evoked responses in man.* Folia Psychiatr Neurol Jpn 26:83, 1972.

95. TROJABORG, W AND PETERSEN, E: *Visual and somatosensory evoked cortical potentials in multiple sclerosis.* J Neurol Neurosurg Psychiatry 42:323, 1979.

96. TSUMOTO, T, ET AL: *Cerebrovascular disease: Changes in somatosensory evoked potentials associated with unilateral lesions.* Electroenceph Clin Neurophysiol 35:463, 1973.

97. WALKER, D, KIMURA, J, AND YAMADA, T: *Maximization of amplitude resolution in computer averaging.* (In preparation).

98. WIEDERHOLT, WC AND IRAGUI-MADOZ, VJ: *Far field somatosensory potentials in the rat.* Electroenceph Clin Neurophysiol 42:456, 1977.

99. WILLIAMSON, PD, GOFF, WR, AND ALLISON, T: *Somato-sensory evoked responses in patients with unilateral cerebral lesions.* Electroenceph Clin Neurophysiol 28:566, 1970.

100. WOODBURY, JW: *Potentials in a volume conductor.* In RUCH, TC, ET AL (EDS): Neurophysiology, ed 2. W.B. Saunders, Philadelphia, 1965, pp 85–91.

101. YAMADA, T, KIMURA, J, AND NITZ, DM: *Short latency somatosensory evoked potentials following median nerve stimulation in man.* Electroenceph Clin Neurophysiol 48:367, 1980.

102. YAMADA, T, MACHIDA, M, AND KIMURA, J: *Far field somatosensory evoked potentials after stimulation of the tibial nerve in man.* Neurology (New York) (in press).

103. YAMADA, T, MUROGA, T, AND KIMURA, J: *The effect of tourniquet induced ischemia on somatosensory evoked potentials.* Neurology (New York) 31:1524, 1981.

104. YAMADA, T, WILKINSON, JT, AND KIMURA, J: *Are there multiple pathways for the short and long latency SEPs?* Electroenceph Clin Neurophysiol 51:43P, 1981.

105. YAMADA, T, ET AL: *Somatosensory-evoked potentials elicited by bilateral stimulation of the median nerve and its clinical application.* Neurology (New York) 28:218, 1978.

106. YAMADA, T, ET AL: *Short and long latency somatosensory evoked potentials in multiple sclerosis.* Arch Neurol 29:88, 1982.

# PART 6

# DISORDERS OF THE SPINAL CORD AND PERIPHERAL NERVOUS SYSTEM

# 20

# DISEASES
# OF THE MOTOR NEURON

Of the wide range of disorders that affect the spinal cord, the most commonly encountered in an electromyographic laboratory are degenerative diseases of the anterior horn cells. Various classifications have been proposed for this group of disorders, but those based on clinical as well as genetic factors seem to be the most satisfactory until the basic biochemical defects are uncovered.[68] Classic motor neuron disease is characterized by combined involvement of the upper and lower motor neurons. This definition includes progressive bulbar palsy and progressive muscular atrophy, in addition to the more common amyotrophic lateral sclerosis and its variant, primary lateral sclerosis. In contrast, the spinal muscular atrophies may be defined as a group of genetically determined disorders causing degeneration of the anterior horn cells with no corticospinal tract involvement.

The motor neurons in the spinal cord may be affected selectively or in conjunction with the corticospinal tracts in a number of other conditions, including infectious and toxic disorders. Although rare since the development of a vaccine in the 1950s, poliomyelitis still occurs in the tropics and, less frequently, in the United States. With diminishing public awareness of the need for vaccination new epidemics may occur. The residual of old poliomyelitis remains relatively common but often difficult to diagnose. Experimental anterior horn cell disease has been caused by aluminum, vincristine, and acetyl ethyl tetramethyl tetralin. Syringomyelia is another classic neurologic disorder that affects the spinal cord. The disease is often misdiagnosed as motor neuron disease, because cutaneous touch sensation may be completely normal. Careful sensory examination will, however, reveal a selective loss of pain perception in the involved cervical or lumbosacral dermatomes.

This section will discuss the clinical features of certain diseases of the spinal cord with emphasis on disorders of the anterior horn cells commonly evaluated by electromyography and nerve conduction studies. Readers interested in more comprehensive clinical reviews are referred to existing texts.[14, 79, 118]

## MOTOR NEURON DISEASE

This group of disorders is characterized by degeneration of upper and lower motor neurons.[105] The etiology is unknown, although the possibilities of infectious or toxic agents have been extensively explored. The various syndromes described as separate nosologic entities under this heading are probably all part of a disease spectrum dependent on the sites of maximal neuronal involvement. Most are considered sporadic disorders, although 5 to 10 percent are familial with an autosomal dominant pattern of inheritance. In patients with amyotrophic lateral sclerosis, the features of upper and lower motor neuron involvement are evident, whereas patients with progressive muscular atrophy present with only lower motor neuron impairment. In contrast, prominent corticospinal tract signs without lower motor neuron involvement suggest primary lateral sclerosis. Progressive bulbar palsy is characterized by prominent brain stem dysfunction and spasticity of the extremities.

Electromyography and nerve stimulation techniques are of value in the differential diagnosis of these disease entities. Reduced recruitment suggests loss of motor neurons. Fibrillation potentials appear after the disease process has been present for at least two to three weeks. Large amplitude, long duration motor unit potentials develop later as the consequence of reinnervation. The clinical severity of the disease correlates approximately with the magnitude and distribution of fibrillation potentials and the degree of reduction in amplitude of the compound muscle action potentials. Slowing of motor nerve conduction velocity may occur, but sensory action potentials remain normal in the vast majority of cases.

# Amyotrophic lateral sclerosis

The adjective amyotrophic is used here to imply muscle wasting as a result of an anterior horn cell disorder, although the term is also used to describe any neurogenic atrophy, including those resulting from radicular lesions or localized injuries of the peripheral nerve. The disease has a prevalence rate of 2 to 7 and an incidence rate of 1.4 per 100,000 population.[9, 74] It usually begins in the fifth to seventh decades, affecting men two to four times as frequently as women. The disease is of unknown etiology. Genetic, toxic, and viral causes have been postulated, but none has been proven.[70, 75, 83, 100]

Pathologically, amyotrophic lateral sclerosis is characterized by relatively selective degeneration of the motor cells in the spinal cord and brain stem and to a much lesser extent in the cortex. The most extensive cellular damage occurs in the cervical and lumbar levels, primarily affecting the large, rather than small motor cells. The most commonly affected brain stem motor nuclei are those of the 10th, 11th, and 12th cranial nerves and, less frequently, those of the 5th and 7th nerves. Although rare, the nuclei of the 3rd, 4th, and 6th cranial nerves may also be involved.[52] Secondary degeneration of the corticospinal tracts occurs consistently in the lateral and ventral funiculi of the spinal cord. Indeed, some degeneration of the lateral portion of the spinal cord is often seen even in the absence of clinical upper motor neuron signs. Although the anterior horn cells and the corticospinal tracts appear to be the most severely affected, a wide spectrum of involvement of the entire spinal cord is common.

The disease may appear at any age, but onset is usually between 50 and 60 years of age.[85] The most common early symptom is distal weakness of the extremities. Although initial manifestations typically are asymmetric or limited to only one extremity, the disease often progresses rapidly to involve muscles of the trunk and those innervated by the cranial nerves. Bulbar signs tend to appear late in the course of the disease, but in up to one third of the patients, the initial symptoms are dysarthria and dysphagia.[12] Aching and other vague sensory complaints are not uncommon, but they are associated with no clear loss of sensation. Pathologic examination of the peripheral nerves has revealed some abnormalities of sensory axons, but they are not an essential part of the disease.[30] Spasms and cramps of the leg muscles are common early symptoms, often appearing after exercise and also at night. Urinary symptoms are rare at the onset of the disease, but a neurogenic bladder may develop terminally. Pathologic laughter and crying may occur as a manifestation of pseudobulbar palsy at some stage of the illness.

Clinical signs include widespread atrophy affecting the muscles of the extremities and face, usually in proportion to the degree of weakness. The extraocular muscles are not clinically involved, but the tongue is commonly affected. A majority of patients have hyperreflexia with ankle clonus in severe cases. Extensor plantar responses may or may not be present. The disease progresses without remission and death usually occurs in two to three years, most often as a result of respiratory difficulties. However, a less severe prognosis may be more common than was previously thought; perhaps as many as 20 percent of all patients with motor neuron disease have a more benign course with survival in excess of five years.[14] In the slow form, bulbar signs are often absent in the early stages, but other clinical features are the same as in the more classic variety. Slow motor neuron disease resembles the Kugelberg-Welander form of spinal muscular atrophy in its time course but does not show the proximal atrophy characteristic of the latter condition. The signs and symptoms may appear to wax and wane, presumably because of reinnervation and collateral sprouting. In one study,[116] 32 of 74 patients showed a fluctuating course.

Fasciculations may be observed. Often the patients are unaware of spontaneous muscle twitchings (insensible fasciculations). A paucity of fasciculations may suggest slow progression of the illness,[91] but abundant fasciculations do not necessarily imply a worse prognosis. The fasciculations considered characteristic of anterior horn cell degeneration not uncommonly occur in healthy subjects as well. They are usually seen in the calf or intrinsic hand muscles, especially after strong contraction. They are not associated with muscle weakness or atrophy, nor are they accompanied by electromyographic evidence of denervation.

The diagnosis of motor neuron disease should be made with considerable care because of its universal fatality. Clinical diagnosis depends on the combined features of widespread muscular atrophy, weakness, and fasciculations, and evidence of damage to corticospinal and bulbar tracts. Differential diagnoses include any condition associated with diffuse muscle atrophy. A syndrome clinically resembling amyotrophic lateral sclerosis has been reported in association with lead intoxication[11] and chronic mercurialism,[65] although the latter may represent a sensorimotor polyneuropathy secondary to organic mercury toxicity. Cervical spondylosis and developmental anomalies in the region of the foramen magnum may simulate the disease closely, with presenting symptoms of muscular weakness in the upper extremities and evidence of spasticity in the lower extremities. Diagnostic problems arise when motor neuron disease and cervical or lumbar spondylosis coexist, since sensory symptoms of radiculopathy alter the picture of pure motor dysfunction. A myelogram is useful to exclude these diagnostic possibilities. Serum levels of muscle enzymes may be elevated to two or three times normal in about half of the patients;[119] hence, their elevation does not exclude the diagnosis.

Degeneration of the anterior horn cells results in denervation of muscle fibers, which are then reinnervated by collateral sprouts from surviving motor neurons.[123] Muscle biopsies show characteristic changes of denervation atrophy with fiber grouping, which is best demonstrated histochemically in fresh frozen specimens. The intermyofibrillar network and cellular architecture of the fibers are relatively intact,[17] although myopathic changes may appear, presumably as part of the denervation process.[1] The grouping of fiber types is taken to represent a compensatory mechanism of denervated muscle.[28] Type I grouping correlates with the best prognosis, whereas a high density of atrophic fibers implies the worst prognosis.[93] A quantitative study of the terminal innervation ratio and fiber type grouping has shown that collateral reinnervation is less efficient in amyotrophic lateral sclerosis than in the more slowly progressing Charcot-Marie-Tooth disease.[114]

Electromyographic abnormalities found during various stages of the illness reflect the sequence of pathologic changes in the muscle. Diffuse denervation gives rise to fibrillation potentials and positive sharp waves (see Fig. 13-7 top left). Fasciculation potentials are presumably caused by motor neuron irritability.[23, 77, 103] The distribution of findings is typically asymmetric, particularly early. The presence of both large and small fibrillation potentials is suggestive of both recent and chronic denervation. Many motor unit potentials are polyphasic and some show late components. Their average amplitude is greater than normal and abnormally large potentials are commonly seen.[18] In general, motor unit potentials are reduced in number, recruit poorly, and produce a less-than-full interference pattern (see Figs. 12-8 bottom left and 12-9).

A large number of patients with amyotrophic lateral sclerosis complain of easy fatigability. This is generally attributed to impairment of neuromuscular transmission.[78, 86, 109] Indeed, many patients with a rapidly progressive form of the disease show defects in neuromuscular transmission with slow repetitive nerve stimulation and small unstable motor unit potentials with temporal amplitude variability during needle examination (see Fig. 13-12). Motor unit potentials are usually of stable configuration in the relatively chronic forms. In a recent series, 67 percent of 55 patients with the established diagnosis showed a decremental response.[22] A larger decrement occurred in muscles showing atrophy and in those with frequent fasciculations. As in myasthenia gravis, the abnormality was reduced with local cooling or after administration of edrophonium (Tensilon). Post-tetanic exhaustion was also observed. Neuromuscular transmission defects may be secondary to decreased trophic function of the neuron.

Additional physiologic findings include enlarged motor unit territories[36] and increased fiber density and jitter values determined by single fiber electromyography (SFEMG).[112] These subtle signs of reinnervation and immature motor nerve terminals may occur in muscle showing no abnormalities either clinically or by conventional needle examination. Despite active reinnervation, progressive denervation produces a deteriorating clinical course. In one study,[51] a computer-assisted quantitative measure of motor unit function revealed that reinnervation was only sufficient to compensate for up to 50 percent loss of the motor neuron pool. The study also showed no difference in the electrophysiologic parameters between amyotrophic lateral sclerosis and progressive muscular atrophy.

In the vast majority of cases, sensory action potentials remain normal in amplitude and latency. If they are low, it is usually from another disorder. Motor nerve conduction velocities may be normal, or slightly slowed, if the muscle action potential is reduced in amplitude. However, the values are rarely less than 70 to 80 percent of the normal lower limits. Hausmanowa-Petrusewicz and associates,[55] in an electrophysiologic and histologic study, found little or no change in maximal conduction velocity at any clinical stage and concluded that at least part of the fastest conducting fibers were preserved for a long time. However, some fibers conducted at a velocity much below that of normal slow fibers; hence, the scatter of velocities was increased. Hansen and Ballantyne[51] found neither pathologically slowed conduction nor evidence to indicate preferential loss of fast motor neurons. Increased excitability of the spinal motor neuron pool results in a higher incidence of the H-reflex in the soleus after stimulation of the tibial nerve. Unlike in normals, the H-reflex also appears in the intrinsic hand muscles after stimulation of the ulnar or median nerve, and in the extensor digitorum or tibialis anterior after stimulation of the peroneal nerve.[91]

A variety of focal or diffuse neuropathic disorders may mimic amyotrophic lateral sclerosis electrophysiologically. A set of criteria proposed by Lambert[77] to support the diagnosis includes (1) fibrillation and fasciculation in muscles of the lower and the upper extremities, or in the extremities and the head; (2) reduction in number and increase in amplitude and duration of motor unit action potentials; (3) normal electrical excitability of the surviving motor nerve fibers; (4) motor fiber conduction velocity within the normal range in nerves of relatively unaffected muscles and not less than 70 percent of the average normal value according to age in nerves of more severely affected muscles; and (5) normal excitability and conduction velocity of afferent nerve fibers even in severely affected extremities.

In typical cases, the electrophysiologic findings are often asymmetric and multifocal. The abnormalities must be present in at least three muscles innervated by different nerves and spinal roots in at least three extremities; the head may be counted as one extremity. This is particularly important in differentiating amyotrophic sclerosis from a syrinx or spondylosis in which the involvement is confined to the upper limbs. The muscles selected for examination should be free of compressive neuropathies, most notably, median nerve at the wrist or ulnar nerve at the elbow. Thus, for example, the flexor pollicis longus is a better choice than the thenar or hypothenar muscles. Similarly, denervation of the extensor digitorum brevis may be secondary to nerve compression by a tight shoe. Studies should include, in addition to electromyography, sensory as well as motor conduction measurements and, when appropriate, tests of neuromuscular transmission. Sparing of sensory nerves should be demonstrated in one of the weaker extremities. Evidence of defective neuromuscular transmission with either repetitive stimulation or SFEMG suggests active disease with immature end-plates secondary to recent reinnervation, and hence, a poor prognosis.

## Progressive muscular atrophy

In this rare syndrome of Aran-Duchenne, clinical signs and symptoms implicate only the anterior horn cells, although the corticospinal tract may also be involved pathologically. The majority of cases occur sporadically, but familial incidence is reported in a small percentage, and these patients have a more benign course. Atrophy and weakness of the extremities develop without accompanying features of spasticity or other evidence of upper motor neuron involvement. Asymmetric wasting and weakness of the intrinsic hand muscles are common presenting signs. This is followed by atrophy of shoulder girdle, bulbar, and lower extremity muscles. Less commonly, the clinical signs may initially resemble Charcot-Marie-Tooth disease or peroneal nerve palsy, if the anterior compartment of the leg is preferentially involved in the early stages. Diaphragmatic paralysis, although rare, may occur, causing respiratory insufficiency as a prominent presenting symptom.[92] Wasting and weakness become generalized, but the stretch reflexes usually remain normal or slightly decreased. The disease runs a slower course than classic amyotrophic lateral sclerosis but is nonetheless steadily progressive without remission, leading to eventual demise, often from aspiration pneumonia.

## Progressive bulbar palsy

If signs and symptoms predominate in muscles innervated by the medulla, then the name progressive bulbar palsy may be appropriate.[2, 49] The presence of disease in siblings suggests an autosomal recessive form of inheritance.[5] The disease usually begins in the fifth or sixth decade with initial symptoms of progressive dysarthria and dysphagia. The tongue becomes atrophic with visible fasciculations. Troublesome signs include pooling of saliva, nasal regurgitation of fluids, and inability to chew or swallow. A majority of these patients will eventually develop signs of pseudobulbar palsy, indicating involvement of higher levels of the brain stem or cerebral cortex. Regardless of the initial symptoms, which may be localized, widespread involvement of motor neurons occurs in the terminal stage.

## Primary lateral sclerosis

This is another variation of amyotrophic lateral sclerosis with clinical features reflecting on the distribution of pathology. The syndrome of primary lateral sclerosis results from selective changes of the corticospinal and corticobulbar tracts with little involvement of the anterior horn cells. The clinical signs include spasticity, diffuse hyperreflexia, Babinski signs, and pseudobulbar palsy. Atrophy and weakness of distal musculature are conspicuously absent. The disease may present with a spastic paraparesis simulating cord compression.

## Disorders with geographic predilection

A few geographic foci of motor neuron disease have been described in the literature. These include the island of Guam,[13] Kii Peninsula of Japan,[108] and Ryuku Island south of Japan.[69] The Guamanian motor neuron disease in the Chamorro population[46] is characterized by a high familial incidence. It is estimated that nearly 10 percent of the adult population of the island die of the disease. The parkinsonian-dementia complex is another disease that affects the same population, but no etiologic relationship between the two entities has been established.

# SPINAL MUSCULAR ATROPHY

In the 1968 classification proposed by the World Commission on Neuromuscular Disease,[44] spinal muscular atrophy included infantile spinal muscular atrophy (Werdnig-Hoffmann disease), arthrogryposis multiplex secondary to anterior horn cell disease, juvenile spinal muscular atrophy (Kugelberg-Welander disease), and scapuloperoneal spinal muscular atrophy. A more recent subdivision[31] includes distal spinal muscular atrophy, juvenile progressive bulbar palsy (Fazio-Londe disease), and facioscapulohumeral spinal muscular atrophy. Although the term spinal muscular atrophy is now widely used to describe these entities, the unfortunate choice of the word spinal may be a source of clinical confusion. It is used here to distinguish diseases of anterior horn cells from those of nerve root or peripheral nerves and not to exclude cases with bulbar involvement, which are commonly seen in many of these entities. Indeed, in few of these conditions is the disease limited to the spinal cord.[79] Spinal muscular atrophy is one of the most devastating genetically determined neurologic disorders in childhood. In a series of 108 patients seen in the Mayo Clinic between 1955 and 1975, the mortality rate was 31 percent with a mean age of 65 months at the time of death.[73] Furthermore, unassisted ambulation was possible in only 35 percent of these patients.

It is still not entirely settled whether various subdivisions represent independent disease entities or different parts of the spectrum in the same disorder.[88, 106] At least two distinct categories exist clinically as well as genetically: the rapidly progressive infantile form, or Werdnig-Hoffmann disease, which leads to death before three years of age,[97] and the late childhood or juvenile form generally called the Kugelberg-Welander syndrome.[16, 34, 45, 94] An intermediate type with onset between 3 and 18 months of age has also been described.[26, 89] Despite overlap in the age of onset, the course of the disease and age of death appear distinctly different among the infantile, juvenile, and intermediate forms. Table 20-1 summarizes these and other features useful in separating the three types of spinal muscular atrophy.[68]

In addition, disease with adult onset has been reported as a variant of the more common and relatively benign late juvenile type.[16, 34, 89, 115] A recent survey of the occurrence of this variety over a ten-year period in northeast England, however, suggests that it too may be a distinct clinical and genetic entity.[99] The distribution of affected muscles distinguishes amyotrophic lateral sclerosis with distal weakness from the adult form of spinal muscular atrophy with more proximal involvement. Another form called juvenile amyotrophic lateral sclerosis occurs in older children and is characterized by late onset, rapid progression and the presence of both upper and lower motor neuron signs.[90, 111]

| Type | Age (Usual) onset | survival | Ability to sit without support* | Fasciculations of skeletal muscles | Serum creatine kinase |
|------|------|------|------|------|------|
| Infantile | <9 months | < 4 years | never | +/− | normal |
| Intermediate | 3–18 months | >4 years | usually | +/− | usually normal |
| Juvenile | >2 years | adulthood | always | + + | often raised |
| Adult | >30 years | 50 years + | always | + + | often raised |

*At some time during the course of the illness.

(From Kloepfer and Emery,[68] with permission.)

The electromyographic findings in various types of spinal muscular atrophy are similar and consist of fibrillation potentials, positive sharp waves, fasciculations, large motor unit potentials, and a reduced interference pattern.[3, 15, 45, 57, 76, 81, 82] In rapidly progressing infantile spinal muscular atrophy, electromyography suggests a mixture of denervation and regeneration with small motor unit potentials that vary temporally in configuration.

## Infantile spinal muscular atrophy

This disease, first described by Werdnig[120] and Hoffmann,[59] is inherited as an autosomal recessive trait with a significantly higher rate of consanguinity among the parents of affected children compared with controls. The estimated incidence is 1 in 15,000 to 1 in 25,000 live births in Britain.[97] In one third, the disease is already manifest at birth as decreased fetal movements or congenital arthrogryposis.[96] In the remainder, onset usually occurs by 3 months, and certainly before 6 months, after birth with delayed developmental milestones. Death from pneumonia occurs often before the first birthday and usually by the age of 3 years, although not all cases of neurogenic muscular atrophy starting in infancy have this malignant course.[26] In chronic childhood spinal muscular atrophy, clinical signs first appear at about 6 months, but occasionally as late as 8 years of age, and the median age at death is later than 10 years.[16, 33, 45, 98]

The clinical features consist of progressive muscle weakness and atrophy of the trunk and extremities. Hypotonia and feeding difficulties are common. Previously developed motor skills are lost. Characteristically, the infants lie motionless with limbs abducted in the frog-leg position. They are unable to hold their head up or sit, and they have difficulty with any type of locomotion. Fasciculations may be observed in the tongue in about half of the patients and, much less frequently, in the atrophic muscles of the limbs. Skeletal deformities and contractures are uncommon at birth,[96] but children with the chronic form of spinal muscular atrophy may develop kyphoscoliosis, contractures of the joints, and dislocation of the hip as the disease progresses. Bulbar signs appear later in the course of the rapidly progressive illness. The facial muscles are affected only mildly, if at all. Thus, the infant usually shows an alert expression, despite severe generalized hypotonia. The stretch reflexes are reduced or absent. Sphincter functions remain normal, and the sensory system is unaffected, even in the terminal stages of illness.

The level of serum creatine (CK) may be elevated in the chronic form. Muscle biopsy reveals characteristic changes with sheets of round atrophic fibers intermixed with clumps of large hypertrophic fibers, which are all histochemically Type I when evaluated with the adenosine triphosphatase reaction. The chronic form shows fiber type grouping and large Type II fibers.

Electromyography reveals widespread fibrillation potentials and sharp positive waves in many muscles, with the incidence reaching 100 percent in one study.[54] Fibrillation potentials may be considerably less prominent, depending on the progression and severity of the disease.[73] Fasciculation potentials may be recorded but are generally infrequent. Studying 30 patients with infantile spinal muscular atrophy, Buchthal and Olsen[15] found regularly discharging potentials occurring at a rate of 5 to 15 impulses per second in 75 percent of the patients, irrespective of their age, duration and severity of the disease, or biopsy findings. It was noted that these spontaneously discharging motor units could be activated and graded voluntarily. This activity has not always been observed in subsequent series.

A reduced number of motor unit potentials are recruited, reflecting the loss of anterior horn cells. The interference pattern is incomplete with a limited number of potentials discharging at a rapid rate. In extreme instances, only one or two motor units fire at 40 to 50 impulses per second. Consistent with collateral sprouting and high fiber density, many motor unit potentials are increased in amplitude and duration. The territories of the motor units are also enlarged. Some potentials are, however, normal in size and some others are even smaller than normal. The low amplitude, short duration potentials are variable in amplitude and waveform, presumably reflecting unstable neuromuscular transmission of the regenerating axons. In advanced stages, the motor unit potentials are either abnormally large or small, with no normal units between the two extremes.[54]

Motor nerve conduction velocities are normal or nearly normal, but compound muscle action potentials are significantly reduced. Amplitude was less than 50 percent of normal in 94 percent of the patients in one study.[73] Mildly slowed conduction velocity[84] can be attributed to the loss of fast conducting axons. Repetitive stimulation at either slow or fast rates shows a decrementing motor response, suggesting defective neuromuscular transmission during ongoing reinnervation. In contrast to the motor responses, sensory nerve studies usually reveal normal amplitudes and velocities. However, minor abnormalities of the sensory nerves have been reported electrophysiologically[102] as well as histologically.[19] Rare cases of infantile neuronal degeneration clinically resemble infantile spinal muscular atrophy but are characterized by markedly decreased conduction velocity. Thus, nerve conduction studies are of value in documenting a demyelination neuropathy as part of the widespread extensive neuronal degeneration in this disorder.[113]

## Juvenile spinal muscular atrophy

Wohlfart, Fex, and Eliasson[124] and Kugelberg and Welander[72] first described a juvenile form of spinal muscular atrophy. The disease, inherited in an autosomal dominant or recessive fashion, is characterized by proximal muscle weakness and atrophy commencing in the lower extremities.[31, 32, 45, 56, 57, 89] Two thirds of the patients have a family history of the disease. The disease progresses more slowly with less predilection for proximal muscles in the dominantly than the recessively inherited cases.[16, 95, 125] Compared with the infantile form it has a later onset, with the initial symptoms appearing throughout childhood or adolescence, but most commonly between the ages of 5 and 15 years. The extensor muscles of the hip and knees are the first affected; the shoulder girdle muscles are involved later.

The patient characteristically shows a lordotic posture with protuberant abdomen, hyperextended knees, and hypertrophic calves. Fasciculations are seen in the proximal muscles in one half of the cases. They are also seen in the tongue, but very rarely. The legs are generally more involved than the arm. Distal muscles tend to be spared, except in the advanced stages. Involvement of the cranial musculature is rare, although ptosis has been described. Muscle stretch reflexes are usually reduced or absent, but some patients have normal or even increased reflexes despite atrophy. Babinski signs may be noted in some cases. The disease follows a relatively benign course with frequent survival into adulthood, although most patients are confined to a wheelchair by their mid-30s. Patients with chronic neurogenic quadriceps amyotrophy have been described as a forme fruste of Kugelberg-Welander disease.[10, 41] These cases must be differentiated from polymyositis and muscular dystrophy.[117, 118]

Serum enzymes such as CK may be substantially increased, but very high values are exceptional. The level of elevation remains nearly constant as the disease progresses. In contrast, CK in Duchenne muscular dystrophy is initially very high, but later gradually declines. Muscle biopsies show group atrophy and fiber type grouping characteristic of a neurogenic disorder, but myopathic features also occur.

Electromyography commonly shows fibrillation potentials and positive sharp waves, with an overall incidence of 20 to 40 percent in one series,[56] 64 percent in another,[73] and even higher in a group of more severely affected patients.[89] However, they are distributed less widely and detected less frequently than in the Werdnig-Hoffmann disease. Fasciculation potentials were common in one series,[45] but not in another.[73] Complex repetitive discharges are rare but, if present at a late stage, resemble myotonic volleys. Spontaneous activity is more prominent in the lower than upper extremities and in proximal as compared with distal muscles.[56] In contrast, patients with Werdnig-Hoffmann disease show a more diffuse involvement.

Individual motor unit potentials are increased in amplitude and duration, whereas the number of potentials recruited at maximal voluntary contraction is reduced.[15] The territory of a motor unit potential is enlarged, and late components are common, indicating the presence of slow conducting regenerating axons. The percentages of long duration and high amplitude potentials increase with duration of the disease.[56] In advanced cases, small polyphasic motor unit potentials appear, suggesting secondary myopathic changes of atrophic muscles. These low amplitude, short duration potentials are constant in configuration, unlike the varying waveforms seen in the more rapidly progressive infantile cases.[73]

Motor and sensory nerve conduction studies are normal.[84, 107] Compound muscle action potentials may be slightly to moderately reduced in amplitude, although they are better preserved than in Werdnig-Hoffmann disease. There is a strong correlation between the amplitude of the muscle potential and the patient's functional capacity; in one series,[73] 54 percent of those with the amplitude of the compound muscle action potential less than half of normal were bedridden. In contrast, bedridden patients constituted only 7 percent of the remainder.

## Juvenile progressive bulbar palsy

The juvenile type of slowly progressive bulbar palsy of Fazio-Londe is a very rare disorder which is inherited as an autosomal recessive trait.[2, 24, 80] The clinical features consist of ophthalmoplegia, facial diplegia, laryngeal palsy, and other progressive cranial nerve pareses with onset in early childhood. Differential diagnosis includes infantile myotonic dystrophy, infantile facioscapulohumeral dystrophy, and Möbius syndrome. Facial diplegia in these other conditions is, however, present at birth, a feature not seen in juvenile progressive bulbar palsy.[14] Progressive ophthalmoplegia and dysphagia may also develop in some cases of juvenile spinal muscular atrophy as late manifestations, but not as presenting features. Electromyographic abnormalities, prominent in bulbar and pontine musculature, consist of fibrillation potentials, positive sharp waves, and impaired recruitment of motor unit potentials.

## Scapuloperoneal spinal muscular atrophy

As indicated by the name, a unique pattern of muscular weakness distinguishes this type of spinal muscular atrophy from the others.[35, 37, 42, 64] The same distribution of weakness is seen in a form of muscular dystrophy. The term scapuloperoneal syndrome is preferred by some to include both neurogenic and myogenic forms, which are often difficult to differentiate. This is a slowly progressive disorder with atrophy and weakness primarily involving the anterior tibial and peroneal muscles. The musculature of the pectoral girdle is affected later, producing winging of the scapulae. The onset is usually in early adulthood with the suggested mode of inheritance being autosomal dominant. Sporadic cases have also been described. Muscle biopsies show mixed patterns of neuropathic and myopathic changes in most cases. Electromyographic studies also demonstrate changes consistent with myopathy, as well as fibrillation potentials and positive sharp waves. Motor and sensory nerve conduction studies are normal.

## Facioscapulohumeral spinal muscular atrophy

This condition is similar to the scapuloperoneal atrophy in having a unique distribution of weakness and a similar counterpart among the muscular dystrophies.[38] The muscles of the face and pectoral girdle musculature are primarily affected. The weakness begins in early adult life and takes a slowly progressive course. When inherited, it follows an autosomal dominant pattern. Clinical features resemble those of facioscapulohumeral muscular dystrophy. If the distinction between neurogenic and myogenic forms is not possible, the descriptive term facioscapulohumeral syndrome may be more appropriate.

## Arthrogryposis multiplex congenita

Arthrogryposis multiplex congenita may be defined as congenital contractures of at least two different joints in conjunction with significant muscle wasting in the absence of a progressive neurologic disorder.[40] The exact etiology has not been established, but the condition may result from a number of different neuromuscular and bony disorders causing immobilization of the limbs at the time of the embryonic formation of joints.[25] Both myogenic and neurogenic origins have been postulated, but disorders of the motor neuron are probably most common.[7, 8, 71] Electromyography may show fibrillation potentials. Motor unit potentials are reduced in number and recruit poorly. The nerve conduction studies reported in a few cases have been normal.

## Other disorders

Occasionally patients have been reported from Japan with juvenile onset, distal and segmental muscular atrophy of the upper extremities.[110] The clinical features include male preponderance, localized atrophy uniquely affecting the hand and forearm, sparing of the lower extremities and cranial nerves, and rapid progression at first, followed by a slower clinical course. The etiology is unknown, but the disease is distinguished from spinal muscular atrophy by the age of onset, distribution of atrophy, and slowly progressive benign course.[53] Electromyography shows large amplitude motor unit potentials with impaired recruitment. Nerve conduction velocities are normal, but compound muscle potentials are of reduced amplitude.

When only part of the body is involved, the diagnosis of focal motor neuron disease should be entertained with extreme caution. Alternative possibilities such as spinal cord tumors, radiculopathy, plexopathy, and mononeuropathy have more favorable prognoses. Sensory abnormalities, if present, are helpful in distinguishing these conditions from focal motor neuron disease.

# JAKOB-CREUTZFELDT DISEASE

Although this disease was described years ago,[20, 62] its transmissibility was only recently demonstrated in the chimpanzee.[48] Subsequently, evidence of transmission from man to man has been documented. Accidental inoculation occurred after a corneal transplant in one patient,[29] and following a surgical procedure using contaminated stereotactic electrodes in two other patients.[6] The organism has not been isolated, but brain tissue from persons dying of Jakob-Creutzfeldt disease causes scrapielike encephalopathy in goats.[50] The pathologic features resemble those of kuru, a transmissible disease seen in New Guinea,[47] and consist of widespread spongiform degeneration with loss of nerve cells in the cortex, basal ganglia, and spinal cord.

The disease occurs sporadically or familially. It affects both sexes equally with onset in middle age or later. Following vague prodromal symptoms, the patient develops mental deterioration, anxiety, depression, memory loss, and confusion. A variety of neurologic disturbances indicate cortical degeneration and upper and lower motor neuron involvement. The most commonly encountered symptoms are weakness, rigidity, spasticity with hyperreflexia, muscular atrophy, incoordination, tremor, and visual loss. Wasting of the muscles occurs late in the disease and is often associated with fasciculations, giving the typical appearance of motor neuron disease. Spontaneous myoclonus is characteristic, but generalized seizures may also occur. The disease normally follows a rapidly progressive course, leading to severe dementia, blindness, obtundation, and eventually coma. Myoclonus and rigidity may become less prominent in the advanced stages. Death occurs within a year after onset.

Electroencephalography reveals a characteristic abnormality in 90 percent of cases, with localized or diffuse bursts of high voltage sharp or slow waves. Electromyographic studies show evidence of denervation when muscular atrophy is present with involvement of motor cells in the medulla or spinal cord. Motor and sensory nerve conductions are normal, although compressive or diffuse nutritional neuropathy may occur in chronic stages.

There is increasing concern among electromyographers about the risks involved in examining patients with Jakob-Creutzfeldt disease. Exposure to breath, saliva, nasopharyngeal secretions, urine, or feces of the patient should not be cause for special concern according to Gajdusek and associates.[43] These authors recommend, however, thorough washing of hands or other exposed body parts with hospital detergent or ordinary soap. Needle electrodes used for electromyography should be incinerated and discarded as was discussed in Chapter 3.

# POLIOMYELITIS

Poliomyelitis is most commonly caused by Type I virus, but it may be caused by Type II or III. The intestinal and respiratory tracts are initially infected by the virus, which subsequently invades the nervous system via the bloodstream. Previously, epidemics usually occurred during the summer, but sporadic cases were seen during the year. Anterior horn cells invaded by the virus undergo degenerative changes. Motor cells are also affected in the brain stem. In addition, there is an inflammatory reaction of the meninges. Poliomyelitis virus can be isolated in about 90 percent of patients with paralytic illness.

The clinical features of systematic infection are nonspecific, consisting of flulike symptoms such as fever, general malaise, diarrhea, and loss of appetite. Only a small percentage of these patients develop meningeal involvement and complain of headache, stiff neck, and vomiting. This is followed in some cases by paralytic illness, which progresses over a period of several days to a week. Paralysis may involve only one extremity or may become generalized. Bulbar involvement occurs in a small number of children. Respiration may be shallow as the diaphragm and intercostal and abdominal muscles are weakened. Advanced cases require respiratory assistance. The stretch reflexes are diminished or absent in the affected limbs. Sensory examination is entirely normal. The spinal fluid examination reveals a mild pleocytosis.

Considerable recovery takes place, even if severe generalized weakness develops. However, late deterioration of function occurs in some survivors.[4, 87] A few studies have shown a statistically significant association between poliomyelitis and motor neuron disease.[66, 101] If the motor neurons are already depleted by poliomyelitis, minor damage to the surviving lower motor neurons during advancing age might result in exaggerated clinical signs. The diseased neurons may also be more susceptible to senile degeneration. A latent virus infection has been suggested, but histopathologic and virologic studies in one patient with amyotrophic lateral sclerosis and antecedent poliomyelitis provided no evidence of the continuing presence of poliovirus.[104] A long-term follow-up study of poliomyelitis patients with apparent late progression has shown a relatively benign course with the development of few upper motor neuron signs.[87]

The first electromyographic abnormality observed during the acute phase of poliomyelitis is a reduced recruitment pattern. Fibrillation potentials develop as the motor axons degenerate. Reinnervation is associated with diminution of spontaneous discharges and the appearance of large amplitude, long duration motor unit potentials. Weak muscles may have only a few motor unit potentials, which may be extremely large. In a prospective study of 24 patients with a history of paralytic poliomyelitis,[58] electromyographic evidence of chronic partial denervation was more widespread than clinically suspected. In these patients, mean interference amplitude was substantially increased, not only in weak muscles but also in apparently unaffected muscles, most commonly contralateral to the spinal segments clinically involved. Nerve conduction velocities were normal, but compound muscle action potentials were reduced in amplitude approximately in proportion to the degree of muscle atrophy.[63]

In the absence of adequate reinnervation, fibrillation potentials may persist many years after the acute episode. In these cases the spontaneous discharges are normally of very low amplitude, since they presumably originate from small atrophic muscle fibers. Even if reinnervation has taken place, diseased anterior horn cells may degenerate prematurely and cause the reappearance of spontaneous discharges. Alternatively, a recurring drop-out of muscle fibers may occur, because the motor neuron cannot meet the increased metabolic demand of an enlarged motor unit. In survivors of poliomyelitis, Wiechers and Hubbell[122] have shown a significant increase in jitter and fiber density without neurogenic blocking. These findings are consistent with defective neuromuscular transmission in reinnervated motor units.

Occasional cases of a poliomyelitislike syndrome have been reported in association with asthma.[21, 60, 61, 121] The disease occurs predominantly in boys 10 years old or younger. Acute flaccid monoplegia involving a single upper or lower limb without sensory deficits occurs. Marked atrophy develops in the involved extremity, which shows poor recovery. The cerebrospinal fluid examination reveals a pleocytosis and slight protein elevation but no significant rise in poliovirus antibody titers. The lesion appears to lie in the posterior cord of the brachial plexus, the motor root,[21, 27] or in the anterior horns of the spinal cord.[121] The absence of clinical or electrophysiologic sensory abnormalities seems to favor the latter as the locus of disease, although pathologic confirmation is not available. This syndrome can be confused with poliomyelitis, but the virus has never been cultured, and the disease occurs in children who have previously received poliovirus vaccination. Electromyographic features in affected muscles are very similar to those seen in poliomyelitis. Wheeler and Ochoa[121] have demonstrated electrophysiologic evidence of C-5 root synkinesis involving the biceps and inspiratory muscles, presumably resulting from aberrant regeneration.[67]

# SYRINGOMYELIA

Syringomyelia is characterized by cavitation and gliosis of the spinal cord and medulla. The disease can occur at any age, but most often symptoms appear in the third or fourth decade. Occasionally, syringomyelia may be familial affecting both sexes equally, but no clear genetic factors have been identified. Although the pathogenesis is unknown, it is frequently associated with other congenital defects such as spina bifida or Arnold-Chiari malformation. Scoliosis is very common, and trophic changes are regularly present. Intramedullary tumors have also been found in conjunction with a syrinx. Secondary cavitation may develop after traumatic, vascular, or infectious lesions of the spinal cord. Progression is generally prolonged over a period of many years. Damage to medullary nuclei, however, may lead to a rapid demise. The differential diagnoses include motor neuron disease, multiple sclerosis, spinal cord tumor, anomalies of the cervical spine, and posterior fossa lesions.

The location of the cavities and their longitudinal extent are variable, but the cervical cord region is most commonly affected. The cord may be distended by the fluid in the cavity or, conversely, appear flattened. The gliosis and cavities are irregular in shape and may involve the entire white and gray matter of the cord. Commonly they are located near the region of the central canal. Motor and sensory cells and various fiber tracts may be involved in any combination. The characteristic dissociation of sensory abnormalities described below is caused by damage to the anterior commissure of the spinal cord. Other common sites of involvement include the posterior and lateral funiculi with damage to the corticospinal tract.

Clinical symptoms and signs depend on the location and extent of the pathologic changes. With a syrinx in the cervical region, the most characteristic motor findings are atrophy and weakness of intrinsic hand muscles in one or both upper extremities. Dissociated loss of pain sensation with preservation of light touch is very characteristic in the lower cervical or upper thoracic dermatomes. Segmental loss of all modalities of cutaneous sensation may be seen with a syrinx involving the root entry zone. Vibratory sense may be lost with lesions of the posterior column. Other signs include spasticity, hyperreflexia, Babinski signs, ataxia of the lower extremities, and a neurogenic bladder. The lumbosacral region may be affected alone, or in association with lesions in the cervical region. The clinical features then include muscular atrophy and dissociated sensory loss of the lower extremities and paralysis of the bladder. Stretch reflexes may be absent if the reflex arc is interrupted at the root entry zone or if the anterior horn cells are damaged in the lumbar region.

If a syrinx is formed in the medulla, the condition is called syringobulbia. The descending nucleus of the fifth nerve and nuclei of the lower medulla are commonly involved, either unilaterally or bilaterally. Common features include atrophy of the tongue, loss of pain and temperature sensation in the face, abnormalities of extraocular muscles, and respiratory difficulties. Involvement of the spinal accessory nuclei causes atrophy of the trapezius and sternocleidomastoid. Spastic paraparesis is common in syringobulbia.

Electromyography reveals fibrillation potentials and positive sharp waves in the atrophic muscle. However, sparing of the lower limbs serves to distinguish syrinx from motor neuron disease. Motor nerve conduction velocities are normal, although the compound muscle action potentials may be reduced in amplitude. Sensory nerve conduction velocities and sensory nerve potentials are unaffected, despite clinical sensory loss,[39] as is characteristic of lesions located proximal to the sensory ganglion. In these instances, somatosensory evoked potentials may be helpful (see Fig. 19-3A). The electrically elicited blink reflex discloses a typical abnormality of R2 if the spinal tract and nucleus of the trigeminal nerve are involved (see Fig. 16-14).

# REFERENCE SOURCES

1.  ACHARI, AN AND ANDERSON, MS: *Myopathic changes in amyotrophic lateral sclerosis. Pathologic analysis of muscle biopsy changes in 111 cases.* Neurology (Minneap) 24:477, 1974.

2.  ALEXANDER, MP, EMERY, ES, III, AND KOERNER, FC: *Progressive bulbar paresis in childhood.* Arch Neurol 33:66, 1976.

3.  AMICK, LD, SMITH, HL, AND JOHNSON, WW: *An unusual spectrum of progressive spinal muscular atrophy.* Acta Neurologica Scand 42:275, 1966.

4. ANDERSON, AD, LEVINE, SA, AND GELLERT, H: *Loss of ambulatory ability in patients with old anterior poliomyelitis.* Lancet 2:1061, 1972.

5. BENJAMINS, D: *Progressive bulbar palsy of childhood in siblings.* Ann Neurol 8:203, 1980.

6. BERNOULLI, C, ET AL: *Danger of accidental person-to-person transmission of Creutzfeldt-Jakob disease by surgery.* Lancet 1:478, 1977.

7. BESSER, M AND BEHAR, A: *Arthrogryposis accompanying congenital spinal-type muscular atrophy.* Arch Dis Child 42:666, 1967.

8. BHARUCHA, EP, PANDYA, SS, AND DASTUR, DK: *Arthrogryposis multiplex congenita. Part 1: Clinical and electromyographic aspects.* J Neurol Neurosurg Psychiatry 35:425, 1972.

9. BOBOWICK, AR AND BRODY, JA: *Epidemiology of motor-neuron diseases.* N Engl J Med 288:1047, 1973.

10. BODDIE, HG AND STEWART-WYNNE, EG: *Quadriceps myopathy—Entity or syndrome?* Arch Neurol 31:60, 1974.

11. BOOTHBY, JA, DEJESUS, PV, AND ROWLAND, LP: *Reversible forms of motor neuron disease. Lead "neuritis".* Arch Neurol 31:18, 1974.

12. BRAIN, WR, CROFT, P, AND WILKINSON, M: *The course and outcome of motor neuron disease.* In NORRIS, FH, JR AND KURLAND, LT (EDS): *Motor Neuron Diseases: Research on Amyotrophic Lateral Sclerosis and Related Disorders.* Grune & Stratton, New York, 1969.

13. BRODY, JA AND CHEN, KM: *Changing epidemiologic patterns of amyotrophic lateral sclerosis and parkinsonism-dementia on Guam.* In NORRIS, FH, JR AND KURLAND, LT (EDS): *Motor Neuron Diseases: Research on Amyotrophic Lateral Sclerosis and Related Disorders.* Grune & Stratton, New York, 1969, pp 61–79.

14. BROOKE, MH: *A Clinician's View of Neuromuscular Diseases.* Williams & Wilkins, Baltimore, 1977.

15. BUCHTHAL, F AND OLSEN, PZ: *Electromyography and muscle biopsy in infantile spinal muscular atrophy.* Brain 93:15, 1970.

16. BUNDEY, S AND LOVELACE, RE: *A clinical and genetic study of chronic proximal spinal muscular atrophy.* Brain 98:455, 1975.

17. BUTLER, RC, ET AL: *Muscle biopsy in motor neurone disease.* In ROSE, FC (ED): *Motor Neurone Disease.* Grune & Stratton, New York, 1977, pp 79–93.

18. CARLETON, SA AND BROWN, WF: *Changes in motor unit populations in motor neurone disease.* J Neurol Neurosurg Psychiatry 42:42, 1979.

19. CARPENTER, S, ET AL: *Pathological involvement of primary sensory neurons in Werdnig-Hoffmann disease.* Acta Neuropathol 42:91, 1978.

20. CREUTZFELDT, HG: *Über eine eigenartige herdförmige Erkrankung des Zentralnervensystems.* In NISSL, F AND ALZHEIMER, A (EDS): *Histologische und Histopathologische.* Jena, G. Fisher, 1921, pp 1–48.

21. DANTA, G: *Electrophysiological study of amyotrophy associated with acute asthma (asthmatic amyotrophy).* J Neurol Neurosurg Psychiatry 38:1016, 1975.

22. DENYS, EH AND NORRIS, FH, JR: *Amyotrophic lateral sclerosis: Impairment of neuromuscular transmission.* Arch Neurol 36:202, 1979.

23. DESMEDT, JE AND BORENSTEIN, S: *Interpretation of electromyographical data in spinal muscular atrophy.* In ROSE, FC (ED): *Motor Neurone Disease.* Grune & Stratton, New York, 1977.

24. DOBKIN, BH AND VERITY, MA: *Familial progressive bulbar and spinal muscular atrophy. Juvenile onset and late morbidity with ragged-red fibers.* Neurology (Minneap) 26:754, 1976.

25. DODGE, PR: *Congenital neuromuscular disorders.* In ADAMS, RD, EATON, LM, AND SHY, GM (EDS): *Neuromuscular Disorders: (The Motor Unit and Its Disorders).* Research Publications, Association for Research In Nervous and Mental Disease, Vol 38. Williams & Wilkins, Baltimore, 1960.

26. DUBOWITZ, V: *Infantile muscular atrophy. A prospective study with particular reference to a slowly progressive variety.* Brain 87:707, 1964.

27. DUBOWITZ, V: *Muscle Disorders in Childhood.* In SCHAFFER, AJ AND MARKOWITZ, M (EDS): *Major Problems in Clinical Pediatrics,* Vol 16. WB Saunders, Philadelphia, 1978.

28. DUBOWITZ, V AND BROOKE, MH: *Muscle Biopsy: A Modern Approach.* WB Saunders, Philadelphia, 1973.

29. DUFFY, P, ET AL: *Possible person-to-person transmission of Creutzfeldt-Jakob disease.* N Engl J Med 290:692, 1974.

30. DYCK, PJ, ET AL: *Frequency of nerve fiber degeneration of peripheral motor and sensory neurons in amyotrophic lateral sclerosis. Morphometry of deep and superficial peroneal nerves.* Neurology (Minneap) 25:781, 1975.

31. EMERY, AEH: *The nosology of the spinal muscular atrophies.* J Med Genet 8:481, 1971.

32. EMERY, AEH, DAVIE, AM, AND SMITH, C: *Spinal muscular atrophy—resolution of heterogeneity.* In BRADLEY, WG, GARDNER-MEDWIN, D, AND WALTON, JN (EDS): *Recent Advances in Myology.* Excerpta Medica, Amsterdam, 1975, pp 557–565.

33. EMERY, AEH, ET AL: *International collaborative study of the spinal muscular atrophies. Part 2. Analysis of genetic data.* J Neurol Sci 30:375, 1976.

34. EMERY, AEH, ET AL: *International collaborative study of the spinal muscular atrophies. Part 1. Analysis of clinical and laboratory data.* J Neurol Sci 29:83, 1976.

35. EMERY, ES, FENICHEL, GM, AND ENG, G: *A spinal muscular atrophy with scapuloperoneal distribution.* Arch Neurol 18:129, 1968.

36. ERMINIO, F, BUCHTHAL, F, AND ROSENFALCK, P: *Motor unit territory and muscle fiber concentration in paresis due to peripheral nerve injury and anterior horn cell involvement.* Neurology (Minneap) 9:657, 1959.

37. FEIGENBAUM, JA AND MUNSAT, TL: *A neuromuscular syndrome of scapuloperoneal distribution.* Bull LA Neurol Soc 35:47, 1970.

38. FENICHEL, GM, EMERY, ES, AND HUNT, P: *Neurogenic atrophy simulating facioscapulohumeral dystrophy: A dominant form.* Arch Neurol 17:257, 1967.

39. FINCHAM, RW AND CAPE, CA: *Sensory nerve conduction in syringomyelia.* Neurology (Minneap) 18:200, 1968.

40. FISHER, RL, ET AL: *Arthrogryposis multiplex congenita: A clinical investigation.* J Pediatr 76:255, 1970.

41. FURUKAWA, T, AKAGAMI, N, AND MARUYAMA, S: *Chronic neurogenic quadriceps amyotrophy.* Ann Neurol 2:528, 1977.

42. FURUKAWA, T, ET AL: *Neurogenic muscular atrophy simulating facioscapulohumeral muscular dystrophy. With particular reference to the heterogeneity of Kugelberg-Welander disease.* J Neurol Sci 9:389, 1969.

43. GAJDUSEK, DC, ET AL: *Precautions in medical care of, and in handling materials from, patients with transmissible virus dementia (Creutzfeldt-Jakob Disease).* N Engl J Med 297:1253, 1977.

44. GARDNER-MEDWIN, D AND WALTON, JN: *A classification of the neuromuscular disorders and a note on the clinical examination of the voluntary muscles.* In WALTON, JN (ED): *Disorders of Voluntary Muscle,* ed 2. Little, Brown, & Co, Boston, 1969, pp 411–453.

45. GARDNER-MEDWIN, D, HUDGSON, P, AND WALTON, JN: *Benign spinal muscular atrophy arising in childhood and adolescence.* J Neurol Sci 5:121, 1967.

46. GARRUTO, RM, GAJDUSEK, C, AND CHEN, KM: *Amyotrophic lateral sclerosis among Chamorro migrants from Guam.* Ann Neurol 8:612, 1980.

47. GIBBS, CJ, JR AND GAJDUSEK, DC: *Kuru—A prototype subacute infectious disease of the nervous system as a model for the study of amyotrophic lateral sclerosis.* In NORRIS, FH, JR AND KURLAND, LT (EDS): *Motor Neuron Diseases: Research on Amyotrophic Lateral Sclerosis and Related Disorders.* Grune & Stratton, New York, 1969.

48. GIBBS, CJ, JR, ET AL: *Creutzfeldt-Jakob disease (spongiform encephalopathy): Transmission to the chimpanzee.* Science, 161:388, 1968.

49. GOMEZ, M, CLERMONT, V, AND BERNSTEIN, J: *Progressive bulbar paralysis in childhood (Fazio-Londe's disease).* Arch Neurol 6:317, 1962.

50. HADLOW, WJ, ET AL: *Brain tissue from persons dying of Creutzfeldt-Jakob disease causes scrapie-like encephalopathy in goats.* Ann Neurol 8:628, 1980.

51. HANSEN, S AND BALLANTYNE, JP: *A quantitative electrophysiological study of motor neurone disease.* J Neurol Neurosurg Psychiatry 41:773, 1978.

52. HARVEY, DG, TORACK, RM, AND ROSENBAUM, HE: *Amyotrophic lateral sclerosis with ophthalmoplegia. A clinicopathologic study.* Arch Neurol 36:615, 1979.

53. HASHIMOTO, O, ET AL: *Clinical observations of juvenile nonprogressive muscular atrophy localized in hand and forearm.* J Neurol 211:105, 1976.

54. HAUSMANOWA-PETRUSEWICZ, I: *Spinal Muscular Atrophy. Infantile and Juvenile Type.* US Department of Commerce, National Technical Information Service, Springfield, VA 22161, 1978.

55. HAUSMANOWA-PETRUSEWICZ, I, ET AL: *The possible mechanism of the motor conduction velocity changes in the anterior horn cells involvement (electrophysiological and histological studies).* In HAUSMANOWA-PETRUSEWICZ, I AND JEDRZEJOWSKA, H (EDS): *Structure and Function of Normal and Diseased Muscle and Peripheral Nerve.* Proceedings of the Symposium in Kazimierz upon Vistula, Poland, 1972.

56. HAUSMANOWA-PETRUSEWICZ, I, ET AL: *Is Kugelberg-Welander spinal muscular atrophy a fetal defect?* Muscle and Nerve 3:389, 1980.

57. HAUSMANOWA-PETRUSEWICZ, I, ET AL: *Infantile and juvenile spinal muscular atrophy.* J Neurol Sci 6:269, 1968.

58. HAYWARD, M AND SEATON, D: *Late sequelae of paralytic poliomyelitis: A clinical and electromyographic study.* J Neurol Neurosurg Psychiatry 42:117, 1979.

59. HOFFMANN, J: *Ueber chronische spinale Muskelatrophie im Kindesalter, auf familiärer Basis.* Deutsche Zeitschrift für Nervenheilkunde 3:427, 1893.

60. HOPKINS, IJ: *A new syndrome: Poliomyelitis-like illness associated with acute asthma in childhood.* Aust Paediatr J 10:273, 1974.

61. ILETT, SJ, PUGH, RJ, AND SMITHELLS, RW: *Poliomyelitis-like illness after acute asthma.* Arch Dis Child 52:738, 1977.

62. JAKOB, A: *Über eigenartige Erkrankungen des Zentralnervensystems mit bemerkenswertem anatomischen Befunde.* Z Neurol Psychiatr 64:147, 1921.

63. JOHNSON, EW, GUYTON, JD, AND OLSEN, KJ: *Motor nerve conduction velocity studies in poliomyelitis.* Arch Phys Med Rehabil 41:185, 1960.

64. KAESER, HE: *Scapuloperoneal muscular atrophy.* Brain 88:407, 1965.

65. KANTARJIAN, AD: *A syndrome clinically resembling amyotrophic lateral sclerosis following chronic mercurialism.* Neurology (Minneap) 11:639, 1961.

66. KAYSER-GATCHALIAN, MC: *Late muscular atrophy after poliomyelitis.* Eur Neurol 10:371, 1973.

67. KERR, FWL: *Structural and functional evidence of plasticity in the central nervous system.* Exp Neurol 48(No 3, Part 2):16, 1975.

68. KLOEPFER, HW AND EMERY, AEH: *Genetic aspects of neuromuscular disease.* In WALTON, JN (ED): *Disorders of Voluntary Muscle,* ed 3. Churchill Livingstone, Edinburgh, 1974.

69. KONDO, K, TSUBAKI, T, AND SAKAMOTO, F: *The Ryukyuan muscular atrophy. An obscure heritable neuromuscular disease found in the islands of southern Japan.* J Neurol Sci 11:359, 1970.

70. KOTT, E, ET AL: *Cell-mediated immunity to polio and HLA antigens in amyotrophic lateral sclerosis.* Neurology (New York) 29:1040, 1979.

71. KRUGLIAK, L, GADOTH, N, AND BEHAR, AJ: *Neuropathic form of arthrogryposis multiplex congenita. Report of 3 cases with complete necropsy, including the first reported case of agenesis of muscle spindles.* J Neurol Sci 37:179, 1978.

72. KUGELBERG, E AND WELANDER, L: *Heredofamilial juvenile muscular atrophy simulating muscular dystrophy.* Arch Neurol Psychiatry 75:500, 1956.

73. KUNTZ, NL, GOMEZ, MR, AND DAUBE, JR: *Prognosis in childhood proximal spinal muscular atrophy* (abstr). Neurology (New York) 30:378, 1980.

74. KURLAND, LT, CHOI, NW, AND SAYRE, GP: *Implications of incidence and geographic patterns on the classification of amyotrophic lateral sclerosis.* In NORRIS, FH, JR AND KURLAND, LT (EDS): *Motor Neuron Diseases: Research on Amyotrophic Lateral Sclerosis and Related Disorders.* Grune & Stratton, New York, 1969, pp 28–50.

75. KURLANDER, HM AND PATTEN, BM: *Metals in spinal cord tissue of patients dying of motor neuron disease.* Ann Neurol 6:21, 1979.

76. LAMBERT, EH: *Electromyography and electric stimulation of peripheral nerves and muscle.* In *Clinical Examinations in Neurology,* ed 2. Department of Neurology, Mayo Clinic, WB Saunders, Philadelphia, 1963, pp 311–341.

77. LAMBERT, EH: *Electromyography in amyotrophic lateral sclerosis.* In NORRIS, FH, JR AND KURLAND, LT (EDS): *Motor Neuron Diseases: Research on Amyotrophic Lateral Sclerosis and Related Disorders.* Grune & Stratton, New York, 1969, pp 135–153.

78. LAMBERT, EH AND MULDER, DW: *Electromyographic studies in amyotrophic lateral sclerosis.* Proc Staff Meet Mayo Clinic 32:441, 1957.

79. LIVERSEDGE, LA AND CAMPBELL, MJ: *Motor neurone diseases.* In WALTON, JN (ED): *Disorders of Voluntary Muscle,* ed 3. Churchill Livingstone, Edinburgh, 1974, pp 775–803.

80. MARKAND, ON AND DALY, DD: *Juvenile type of slowly progressive bulbar palsy: Report of a case.* Neurology (Minneap) 21:753, 1971.

81. MEADOWS, JC, MARSDEN, CD, AND HARRIMAN, DGF: *Chronic spinal muscular atrophy in adults. Part 1. The Kugelberg-Welander syndrome.* J Neurol Sci 9:527, 1969.

82. MEADOWS, JC, MARSDEN, CD, AND HARRIMAN, DGF: *Chronic spinal muscular atrophy in adults. Part 2. Other forms.* J Neurol Sci 9:551, 1969.

83. MILLER, JR, GUNTAKA, RV, AND MYERS, JC: *Amyotrophic lateral sclerosis: Search for poliovirus by nucleic acid hybridization.* Neurology (New York) 30:884, 1980.

84. MOOSA, A AND DUBOWITZ, V: *Motor nerve conduction velocity in spinal muscular atrophy of childhood.* Arch Dis Child 51:974, 1976.

85. MULDER, DW AND ESPINOSA, RE: *Amyotrophic lateral sclerosis: Comparison of the clinical syndrome in Guam and the United States.* In NORRIS, FH, JR AND KURLAND, LT (EDS): *Motor Neuron Diseases: Research on Amyotrophic Lateral Sclerosis and Related Disorders.* Grune & Stratton, New York, 1969, pp 12–19.

86. MULDER, DW, LAMBERT, EH, AND EATON, LM: *Myasthenic syndrome in patients with amyotrophic lateral sclerosis.* Neurology (Minneap) 9:627, 1959.

87. MULDER, DW, ROSENBAUM, RA, AND LAYTON, DD, JR: *Late progression of poliomyelitis or forme fruste amyotrophic lateral sclerosis.* Mayo Clin Proc 47:756, 1972.

88. MUNSAT, TL, ET AL: *Neurogenic muscular atrophy of infancy with prolonged survival. The variable course of Werdnig-Hoffmann disease.* Brain 92:9, 1969.

89. NAMBA, T, ABERFELD, DC, AND GROB, D: *Chronic proximal spinal muscular atrophy.* J Neurol Sci 11:401, 1970.

90. NELSON, JS AND PRENSKY, AL: *Sporadic juvenile amyotrophic lateral sclerosis. A clinico-pathological study of a case with neuronal cytoplasmic inclusions containing RNA.* Arch Neurol 27:300, 1972.

91. NORRIS, FH, JR: *Adult spinal motor neuron disease. Progressive muscular atrophy (Aran's disease) in relation to amyotrophic lateral sclerosis.* In VINKEN, PJ AND BRUYN, GW (EDS): *Handbook of Clinical Neurology,* Vol 22. System Disorders and Atrophies. North-Holland, Amsterdam, 1975, pp 1–56.

92. PARHAD, IM, ET AL: *Diaphragmatic paralysis in motor neuron disease. Report of 2 cases and a review of the literature.* Neurology (New York) 28:18, 1978.

93. PATTEN, BM, ZITO, G, AND HARATI, Y: *Histologic findings in motor neuron disease. Relation to clinically determined activity, duration and severity of disease.* Arch Neurol 36:560, 1979.

94. PEARN, JH: *The spinal muscular atrophies of childhood. A genetic and clinical study.* PHD Thesis, University of London, 1974.

95. PEARN, JH: *Autosomal dominant spinal muscular atrophy. A clinical and genetic study.* J Neurol Sci 38:263, 1978.

96. PEARN, JH AND WILSON, J: *Acute Werdnig-Hoffmann disease. Acute infantile spinal muscular atrophy.* Arch Dis Child 48:425, 1973.

97. PEARN, JH, CARTER, CO, AND WILSON, J: *The genetic identity of acute infantile spinal muscular atrophy.* Brain 96:463, 1973.

98. PEARN, JH, GARDNER-MEDWIN, D, AND WILSON, J: *A clinical study of chronic childhood spinal muscular atrophy. A review of 141 cases.* J Neurol Sci 38:23, 1978.

99. PEARN, JH, HUDGSON, P, AND WALTON, JN: *A clinical and genetic study of spinal muscular atrophy of adult onset. The autosomal recessive form as a discrete disease entity.* Brain 101:591, 1978.

100. PIERCE-RUHLAND, R AND PATTEN, BM: *Muscle metals in motor neuron disease.* Ann Neurol 8:193, 1980.

101. POSKANZER, DC, CANTOR, HM, AND KAPLAN, GS: The frequency of preceding poliomyelitis in amyotrophic lateral sclerosis. In NORRIS, FH, JR AND KURLAND, LT (EDS): Motor Neuron Diseases: Research on Amyotrophic Lateral Sclerosis and Related Disorders. Grune & Stratton, New York, 1969, pp 286–290.

102. RAIMBAULT, J AND LAGET, P: Electromyography in the diagnosis of infantile spinal amyotrophy of Werdnig-Hoffmann type. Path Biol 20:287, 1972.

103. RICHARDSON, AT AND BARWICK, DD: Clinical electromyography. In WALTON, JN (ED): Disorders of Voluntary Muscle, ed 3. Churchill Livingstone, Edinburgh, 1974.

104. ROOS, RP, ET AL: Amyotrophic lateral sclerosis with antecedent poliomyelitis. Arch Neurol 37:312, 1980.

105. ROSE, FC: Clinical aspects of motor neurone disease. In ROSE, FC (ED): Motor Neurone Disease. Grune & Stratton, New York, 1977, pp 1–13.

106. ROWLAND, LP, ET AL: Neurogenic muscular atrophies. In MILHORAT, AT (ED): Exploratory Concepts in Muscular Dystrophy and Related Disorders. International Congress, Excerpta Medica, Amsterdam, 1967, pp 41–45.

107. SCHWARTZ, MS AND MOOSA, A: Sensory nerve conduction in the spinal muscular atrophies. Dev Med Child Neurol 19:50, 1977.

108. SHIRAKI, H: The neuropathology of amyotrophic lateral sclerosis (ALS) in the Kii Peninsula and other areas of Japan. In NORRIS, FH, JR AND KURLAND, LT (EDS): Motor Neuron Diseases: Research on Amyotrophic Lateral Sclerosis and Related Disorders, Vol II. Grune & Stratton, New York, 1969, pp 80–84.

109. SIMPSON, JA: Disorders of neuromuscular transmission. Proc R Soc Med 59:993, 1966.

110. SOBUE, I, ET AL: Juvenile type of distal and segmental muscular atrophy of upper extremities. Ann Neurol 3:429, 1978.

111. STAAL, A AND WENT, LN: Juvenile amyotrophic lateral sclerosis—Dementia complex in a Dutch family. Neurology (Minneap) 18:800, 1968.

112. STÅLBERG, E, SCHWARTZ, MS, AND TRONTELJ, JV: Single fibre electromyography in various processes affecting the anterior horn cells. J Neurol Sci 24:403, 1975.

113. STEIMAN, GS, RORKE, LB, AND BROWN, MJ: Infantile neuronal degeneration masquerading as Werdnig-Hoffmann disease. Ann Neurol 8:317, 1980.

114. TELERMAN-TOPPET, N AND COËRS, C: Motor innervation and fiber type pattern in amyotrophic lateral sclerosis and in Charcot-Marie-Tooth disease. Muscle and Nerve 1:133, 1978.

115. TSUKAGOSHI, H, ET AL: Hereditary proximal neurogenic muscular atrophy in adult. Arch Neurol 12:597, 1965.

116. TYLER, HR: Double-blind study of modified neurotoxin in motor neuron disease. Neurology (New York) 29:77, 1979.

117. WALTON, JN: Two cases of myopathy limited to the quadriceps. J Neurol Neurosurg Psychiatry 19:106, 1956.

118. WALTON, JN (ED): Disorders of Voluntary Muscle, ed 3. Churchill Livingstone, Edinburgh and London, 1974.

119. WELCH, KMA AND GOLDBERG, DM: Serum creatine phosphokinase in motor neuron disease. Neurology (Minneap) 22:697, 1972.

120. WERDNIG, G: Zwei frühinfantile hereditäre Fälle von progressiver Muskelatrophie unter dem Bilde der Dystrophie, aber auf neurotischer Grundlage. Archiv Fur Psychiatrie und Nervenkrankheitnen 22:437, 1891.

121. WHEELER, SD AND OCHOA, J: Poliomyelitis-like syndrome associated with asthma. A case report and review of the literature. Arch Neurol 37:52, 1980.

122. WIECHERS, DO AND HUBBELL, SL: Late changes in the motor unit after acute poliomyelitis. Muscle and Nerve 4:524, 1981.

123. WOHLFART, G: Collateral regeneration from residual motor nerve fibers in amyotrophic lateral sclerosis. Neurology (Minneap) 7:124, 1957.

124. WOHLFART, G, FEX, J, AND ELIASSON, S: Hereditary proximal spinal muscular atrophy—A clinical entity simulating progressive muscular dystrophy. Acta Psychiatrica Neurologica 30:395, 1955.

125. ZELLWEGER, H, ET AL: Spinal muscular atrophy with autosomal dominant inheritance. Report of a new kindred. Neurology (Minneap) 22:957, 1972.

# 21
# DISEASES OF THE ROOT AND PLEXUS

A motor or sensory fiber may be affected proximally along its course at the level of the root or plexus. Regardless of the site of the lesion, clinical features are characterized by weakness and atrophy of the muscle, hyporeflexia, fatigue, cramps, and fasciculations. The motor signs are usually accompanied by sensory abnormalities which sometimes dominate the picture. Sensory symptoms range from mild distal paresthesias to complete loss of sensation. Paresthesias and dysesthesias are common and may be associated with severe pain. The differential diagnosis is relatively limited in radiculopathy and plexopathy, but peripheral lesions such as the carpal tunnel syndrome can mimic proximal abnormalities. Selective damage to these anatomic regions is most commonly caused by traumatic lesions or mechanical compression, although neoplastic or inflammatory processes may also occur.

The diagnosis of radicular or plexus injuries is based on clinical examination and electrophysiologic studies which help delineate the distribution of the affected muscles. Needle examination initially reveals reduced recruitment of motor unit potentials reflecting loss of axons. Subsequently, fibrillation potentials and positive sharp waves develop. Low amplitude, polyphasic unstable motor unit potentials suggest active reinnervation. High amplitude, motor unit potentials with stable configuration appear later with completion of reinnervation. For these proximal lesions, electromyography is generally more useful than nerve conduction studies. Needle studies, as an extension of the physical examination, help to further localize the level, extent, and chronicity of involvement.

## CERVICAL ROOTS

Diseases commonly affecting cervical roots include cervical spondylosis, herniated disc, and traumatic avulsions.[43] It is important to recognize that there are eight cervical roots and only seven cervical vertebrae. Thus, C-1 through C-7 roots emerge above their respective vertebrae but the C-8 root exits between the C-7 and T-1 vertebrae.

Compression of the C-5 root usually causes pain in the interscapular region. The pain radiates over the lateral aspect of the arm but does not extend below the elbow. With involvement of the C-6 root, pain extends over the shoulder to the lateral aspect of the arm and forearm and first digit. Pain induced by C-7 root irritation typically involves the entire arm and forearm with radiation into the second through fourth digits, but it particularly involves the third digit. Less commonly encountered are C-8 root pain radiating to the fourth and fifth digits, and T-1 root pain localized deep in the shoulder, axilla, and medial aspect of the arm. Although sensory symptoms are helpful in the evaluation of radiculopathy, they often fail to provide exact localization because of the overlapping and variable sensory dermatomes.

More reliable information may be derived from motor deficits and changes in the stretch reflexes. Clinical assessment of radiculopathy depends on testing movements of the arm that are controlled almost exclusively by single roots. Recommended maneuvers include shoulder abduction to 180 degrees (C-5), elbow flexion in full and half supination (C-6), and adduction of the shoulder, extension of the elbow, and extension and flexion of the wrist (C-7).[69] A C-8 root lesion results in weakness of the long extensors and flexors of the fingers and to a lesser extent the intrinsic hand muscles, although the latter may be exclusively supplied by the T-1 root. An ulnar nerve lesion spares the median-innervated thenar muscles, whereas a T-1 root lesion affects all the small hand muscles. The muscle stretch reflexes useful in assessing root lesions include the biceps brachii (C-5 or C-6), supinator (C-6), triceps (C-7), and finger flexors (C-8).

Electrophysiologic studies objectively corroborate clinical localization of a radicular lesion (see Tables 1-1, 1-2, and 1-3). Electromyography of the affected muscles shows reduced recruitment and incomplete interference pattern early, and fibrillation potentials, positive sharp waves, and high amplitude, long duration motor unit potentials later in the course of the disease. Sensory nerve action potentials remain normal in amplitude and latency, but compound muscle action potentials may be reduced in amplitude consequent to axonal degeneration and muscle atrophy.

## Cervical spondylosis

This condition results from bony overgrowth of the vertebrae following degeneration of the intervertebral disc. A spondylotic bar, protruding posteriorly, compresses the cord or roots. The most commonly affected are C-5 and C-6 roots, but the C-7 root may also be involved. The other cervical and thoracic roots are infrequent sites of impingement. Pain in the appropriate dermatome is usually triggered by neck movement, but some bars are painless or produce pain not altered by clinical maneuvers. The biceps and supinator stretch reflexes are reduced or absent when C-5 and C-6 roots are involved. The triceps reflex may be diminished if the C-7 root is affected. Less frequently, it may be enhanced in the face of diminished biceps and supinator reflexes, presumably as a result of compressive cervical myelopathy just rostral to the origin of the C-7 root.

## Herniated cervical disc

Cervical disc problems are less common than lumbar disc lesions. Acute herniation is often historically attributable to neck trauma. Herniation usually occurs between C-5 and C-6, or C-6 and C-7 vertebrae and compresses C-6 or C-7 root, respectively. The initial symptom is pain in a typical root distribution, which is aggravated by movement of the neck or the arm. With compression of the ventral root, weakness develops in the muscles innervated by the affected root. Cervical disc lesions occurring in an otherwise normal subject are almost invariably unilateral. Injury to a spine with pre-existing cervical spondylosis may cause bilateral symptoms, multiple root involvement, or myelopathy secondary to compression of the spinal cord.

## Root avulsion

The Erb-Duchenne palsy results from avulsion of C-5 and C-6 roots.[2] This type of injury occurs with downward traction on the plexus, which increases the angle between the head and shoulder; for example, following a forceps delivery while the shoulder is fixed in position.

The palsy produces a characteristic posture with adduction and internal rotation of the arm and extension and pronation of the forearm. Function of the intrinsic hand muscles is preserved, but the patient cannot abduct the arm or supinate the forearm to bring the hand into a useful position. The muscles innervated by C-5 and C-6 roots atrophy. The sensory exam is often limited in infants, but sensory changes are in any event usually mild.

The Klumpke palsy occurs much less frequently. Avulsion of C-8 and T-1 roots results from upward traction on the plexus, which increases the angle between the arm and thorax; for example, attempting to grasp an overhead support during a fall. Degeneration of the ulnar nerve, the inner head of the median nerve, and a portion of the radial nerve leads to denervation of the intrinsic hand muscles and long flexors and extensors of the fingers. The muscles become atrophic, producing a partial clawhand, associated with anesthesia along the inner aspect of the hand, forearm, and arm. Horner's syndrome indicates damage of the cervical sympathetic fibers.

Myelography usually delineates the extent of root injury.[49] It does not provide an absolute criterion, however, since pseudomeningoceles with intact roots and root avulsion without meningoceles may occur.[44, 49] With root avulsion, the histamine response, or reflex skin reaction to intradermal histamine injection, is preserved, since the cell body of the dorsal root ganglia remains connected to the peripheral axon.[8] Similarly, despite sensory loss, the sensory nerve action potential remains normal.[20, 89] In contrast, the histamine response and sensory nerve potentials are lost with plexus lesions.

The deep posterior muscles of the neck are supplied by posterior rami that arise from the spinal nerves as they exit from the intervertebral foramina. Therefore, evidence of denervation in the neck muscles indicates an intraforaminal root lesion. Other muscles receiving innervation proximal to the brachial plexus include the rhomboids supplied by the dorsal scapular and the serratus anterior innervated by the long thoracic nerve. Spontaneous activity in these proximal muscles is another useful sign of root avulsion.

# BRACHIAL PLEXUS

In peacetime, brachial plexus lesions are infrequent causes of arm weakness.[24] Penetrating injuries inflicted by firearms are most common. Bullet wounds often involve the upper and lower trunks and posterior cord. Damage to the brachial plexus may also occur during difficult births or sudden traction applied to the arm or neck. In addition to direct injuries, indirect trauma from fractures of the humerus or dislocation of the shoulder may injure the brachial plexus. Plexopathy may develop after anesthesia when an unusual posture is assumed for a prolonged period. Patients with hemiplegia may sustain a plexus injury by being repeatedly lifted under the arms. Plexus injury has also occurred as a complication of axillary arteriography.[63]

The most common nontraumatic condition affecting the brachial plexus is idiopathic. Brachial plexopathy has also been described in association with Hodgkin's disease,[70] desensitizing injections,[93] Ehlers-Danlos syndrome,[47] systemic lupus erythematosus,[7] and familial pressure-sensitive neuropathy.[10] Chronic compressive lesions of the brachial plexus include primary nerve tumors, metastatic breast cancer, and lymphoma. Any portion of the plexus may be affected, but damage to the lower trunk and medial cord is most common in neoplastic invasion of the plexus because of the location of lymph nodes. Radiation therapy of the axillary region for carcinoma of the breast may cause plexopathy, which is difficult to distinguish from tumor recurrence.[81] Intermittent compression, as in some cases of the thoracic outlet syndrome, produces less well-defined neurologic syndromes with little or no electrophysiologic abnormality.[22]

The clinical features of brachial plexus involvement depend on the area of the plexus primarily affected by the pathologic process. The upper trunk of the right brachial plexus may be injured by firearm recoil, which forcefully retracts the clavicle and presumably compresses a portion of the plexus against the underlying scalene muscles.[87] A heavy backpack may also compress the upper trunk of the brachial plexus.[21] With damage to the upper trunk, the distribution of weakness is similar to that seen in Erb-Duchenne palsy; that is, weakness of the shoulder and upper arm, with sparing of hand function. The patient is unable to abduct the arm, internally or externally rotate the shoulder, flex the elbow, or extend the wrist radially. The biceps and supinator stretch reflexes are reduced or absent. The rhomboid and serratus anterior are spared, since the lesion is distal to the branches supplying these muscles. Sensory changes are found over the lateral aspect of the arm, forearm, and hand.

Isolated injury to the middle trunk is rare. It produces weakness in the general distribution of the radial nerve, although the triceps is only partially paralyzed and the brachioradialis is entirely spared.

The lower trunk of the plexus is a frequent site of metastatic disease, direct invasion by malignant neoplasms from the apex of the lung (Pancoast's tumor), and local trauma. Damage to C8 and T1 root distribution impairs hand function and causes Horner's syndrome. These clinical features are not unlike those seen in Klumpke's palsy. In addition to the intrinsic hand muscles, finger flexors and extensors are weak. Sensory changes occur along the medial aspect of the arm, forearm, and hand, including the fourth and fifth digits.

With involvement of the posterior cord, which may be seen in shoulder dislocations, the clinical picture is one of combined axillary and radial nerve palsies. The patient is unable to extend the elbow, wrist, or fingers. The deltoid is weak, with limited arm abduction after the first 30 degrees, which is subserved by the supraspinatus. Sensory changes are found over the lateral aspect of the shoulder and arm, posterior portion of the forearm, and dorsal aspects of the lateral half of the hand, including the first two digits. The medial cord is commonly affected by compression lesions in the thoracic outlet. Motor and sensory deficits develop in the median- and ulnar-innervated region that receives axons from the C-8 root. Isolated damage of the lateral cord is uncommon, but it can occur following local trauma, causing weakness in musculocutaneous and median-innervated muscles that receive axons from C-6 and C-7 roots.

The characteristic findings in nerve conduction studies of pressure palsies of the brachial plexus include:[82] (1) severe amplitude attenuation of motor and antidromic sensory nerve action potentials evoked with stimulation proximal to the site of nerve injury compared with those evoked at a more distal site; and (2) slowing of conduction across the site of injury. Based on these findings, Trojaborg[82] suggests that the palsies are the result of a local demyelinating block with or without axonal loss. In traumatic plexopathies, electromyography is more informative than nerve conduction studies in delineating the degree, distribution, and time course of the disease.[77] Needle studies are also of value in documenting abnormal associated movements that may develop after diseases of the brachial plexus. Arm-diaphragm synkinesis may occur after injury to the proximal portion of the brachial plexus or cervical nerve roots, as the result of misdirected regeneration of phrenic motor neurons.[79] Abnormal synkinesis and axon reflexes between different, sometimes antagonistic, muscles have also been reported in patients with brachial plexus injury at birth.[25]

## Idiopathic brachial neuritis

Idiopathic brachial neuritis,[75] also known as neuralgic amyotrophy,[68, 95] or brachial neuralgia, probably originates in the roots, although the exact site of lesion has not been clearly demonstrated.[11, 76, 83, 84] A majority of cases occur sporadically after the third decade. Both sexes are affected, but the incidence is more than twice as frequent in men. The condition was initially identified as a complication of vaccination procedures, especially with injection into the deltoid. Trauma, infection, or serum sickness may be temporally associated with the acute onset of pain and other symptoms of neuralgia. A majority of the cases present with unilateral symptoms, but the condition may occasionally occur bilaterally and in rare incidences, recurrently. Prognosis is generally good in a majority of the patients.[84] However, it may take a few years before maximal recovery is achieved, especially if no improvement is evident during the first few months after onset.

The clinical picture is variable,[11, 61, 68, 75, 76, 83, 85] but the disease typically begins with pain localized in the distribution of C5 and C6 dermatomes. An intense aching sensation may radiate along the arm. Relatively mild sensory impairment occurs in two thirds of the patients. Within a few days, the shoulder girdle musculature becomes weak and atrophic. The most severely affected are C-5 and C-6 myotomes, but the muscles innervated by the spinal accessory nerve and C-7 root may also be involved. Pain usually subsides with the onset of weakness but may last much longer. The arm is characteristically maintained in flexion at the elbow and adduction at the shoulder.[90] This rigid posture at the shoulder sometimes leads to a frozen shoulder syndrome.[48]

The paralysis may be limited to the distribution of a single root, trunk, or cord of the plexus, or a peripheral nerve.[23] Individual nerves that may be selectively affected include the radial, long thoracic, and phrenic nerves. Suprascapular and accessory nerves may also be the sites of painful mononeuropathy.[4, 18, 53, 66] Occasionally the initial presenting symptoms are those of an anterior interosseous nerve palsy.[50, 85] Concurrent involvement of the shoulder muscles in neuralgic amyotrophy suggests two possibilities:[71] (1) the involvement of the anterior interosseous nerve might occur in the forearm as spatial scatter of the underlying pathology; or (2) the same clinical deficit may arise from selective damage of the brachial plexus nerve bundle destined to form the anterior interosseous nerve. Such topographic grouping at the level of the cord has indeed been described by Sunderland.[78]

No pathologic description has documented the site and type of nerve lesion. Electromyographic evidence of muscle denervation and the course of clinical recovery suggest axonal interruption and wallerian degeneration. However, mild injury leading to pure demyelination may also occur in some cases showing a rapid recovery and electrophysiologic data incompatible with axonal degeneration.[71] Selective latency increase from Erb's point to individual muscles of the shoulder girdle suggests multiple mononeuropathies.[65] Slowing of conduction, however, is usually more conspicuous after reinnervation has begun. Widespread slowing of conduction velocities may occur, even in extremities not affected clinically.[91] Electromyography may reveal subtle abnormalities on the clinically asymptomatic side.[84]

Electromyography of involved muscles shows fibrillation potentials, positive sharp waves, high amplitude polyphasic motor unit potentials, and reduced interference pattern.[12] The latencies on stimulation at Erb's point are slightly to moderately increased in severely affected muscles.[55, 56, 65] However, a modest increase in latency in conjunction with reduced amplitude of the compound muscle potentials may also occur in myelopathy[59, 60] and does not necessarily implicate the plexus. F-wave study may show increased latency and slow conduction velocity in the segment above the axilla, but this is not a consistent finding, especially in the early stages of illness.[51] The most helpful localizing signs are amplitude abnormalities of median or ulnar sensory studies, slowed conduction of musculocutaneous motor fibers, and lack of paraspinal fibrillation potentials on needle examinations.[34] Abnormality of the sensory nerve action potentials in the distal segment suggests a lesion distal to the dorsal root ganglion.[9, 20] Normal paraspinal examination is more consistent with plexopathy but does not preclude radiculopathy.[52]

# Familial brachial plexopathy

Acute nontraumatic brachial plexus neuropathy may develop in association with lesions outside the plexus or on a familial basis.[10, 12, 28, 88, 92] Acute episodes may be indistinguishable from sporadic idiopathic neuralgic amyotrophy. The familial cases, however, occur in a younger age group and are often inherited as an autosomal dominant trait. The disease shows no preference for either sex, but may occasionally be associated with pregnancy.[42] Recurrence is more frequent[36] and pain is less severe[35, 73] in the familial, than in the sporadic, variety. The disease is not necessarily limited to the plexus but can present with additional signs, including Horner's syndrome and dysphonia.[36] Lesions outside the brachial plexus can also involve the lumbosacral plexus, cranial nerves, individual peripheral nerves, and autonomic nervous system.[35, 42, 80] Nerve conduction studies are either normal or show reduction in amplitude of the recorded response. Electromyography reveals fibrillation potentials, positive sharp waves, and reduced recruitment, suggesting axonal damage.[28]

Some patients with familial pressure-sensitive neuropathy may also present with acute attacks of brachial plexopathy, but the peripheral nerves are diffusely affected in this condition as discussed in Chapter 22.[6, 10, 29] The motor and sensory conduction velocities of the individual nerves may be slowed, with predilection for the common sites of compression.[12] Sural nerve biopsies have revealed bizarre focal thickenings of the myelin sheaths, mild reduction in the total myelinated fiber count, and an abnormal fiber diameter spectrum with loss of the normal bimodal distribution. This pathologic condition has been termed tomaculous neuropathy because of the sausage-shaped thickenings of the myelin sheaths.[12]

# Plexopathy secondary to radiation

Plexopathy may develop months to years after radiation treatment and take a progressive course.[81] Slowing of nerve conduction velocity is minimal, if any, but evoked potentials are reduced in amplitude, especially in sensory nerves. This is in contrast to the frequent slowing of conduction in cases of neoplastic infiltration of the plexus. Electromyography shows fibrillation potentials, positive sharp waves, and large, polyphasic motor unit potentials. In addition, myokymic discharges are commonly seen in radiation plexopathies.[3] In patients with cancer and brachial plexus signs, one must differentiate radiation injury from tumor infiltration. According to a recent study of 100 cases,[54] painless upper trunk lesions with lymphedema suggest radiation injury, and painful lower trunk lesions with the Horner syndrome imply tumor infiltration.

## Cervical rib and thoracic outlet syndrome

A variety of anomalous structures in the neck may affect the roots or trunks of the brachial plexus. A rudimentary cervical rib tends to compress the lower trunk of the brachial plexus as well as the subclavian or axillary artery. A compression syndrome may also result when a fibrous band or the first thoracic rib is pressed upwards by distortion of the thorax. The once publicized compression by the scalenus anticus muscle is not widely accepted at this time. The cervical rib syndrome is also rare, but unequivocal cases do occur with a higher incidence in women, perhaps because the shoulder girdle has a greater tendency to sag in this sex. The symptoms are usually unilateral, even if cervical ribs are present on both sides.

Vascular symptoms result from upward displacement of the axillary or subclavian artery by the cervical rib. Stenosis of the compressed artery may give rise to intermittent embolic phenomena of the brachial artery, causing ischemic changes in the fingers. The hand is cold and blue, with diminished or absent pulsations in the radial and ulnar arteries. Although scalenotomies for the disputed scalenus anticus syndrome are no longer popular, removal of the first rib is still widely practiced.[57, 86] However, the procedure may not be indicated for the majority of patients with the so-called thoracic outlet syndrome.[37] Whether surgical intervention has a beneficial effect in the management of arm pain is, at best, difficult to assess in the absence of objective tests. Nerve conduction studies of the ulnar nerve with stimulation at Erb's point were advocated for this purpose,[15, 26, 45, 62, 72, 86] but the results have not been confirmed.[22, 57]

Apart from the poorly defined condition described above, there is a rare but more clearly recognizable neurologic entity, sometimes called classic thoracic outlet syndrome. It usually affects females with a rudimentary cervical rib.[38, 39] The neural symptoms include local and referred pain secondary to pressure, paresthesias in the hand and forearm along the medial aspect, and weakness of the intrinsic hand muscles. Prominent atrophy of the abductor pollicis brevis may lead to erroneous diagnosis of the carpal tunnel syndrome. The thoracic outlet syndrome, however, gives rise to pain and sensory changes in the ulnar-innervated fingers.

Electrophysiologic abnormalities found in patients with clear neurologic deficit of the classic thoracic outlet syndrome[39] consist of reduced or absent sensory action potentials of the ulnar nerve and evidence of denervation in the intrinsic hand muscles, especially the abductor pollicis brevis. The F-wave is increased in latency on the affected side when compared with the normal side.[27, 94] Reduced amplitude of the ulnar sensory action potential indicates that the lesion is distal to the dorsal root ganglia.[39] Normal conduction velocities of the median and ulnar nerve help exclude the possibility of distal entrapment. These abnormalities are not seen in patients free of neurologic deficits even when vascular symptoms appear with postural maneuvers.[22, 51]

# LUMBOSACRAL ROOTS

Root injury most commonly takes place as the root exits through its foramen. However, damage can occur anywhere along the long subarachnoid pathway of the cauda equina within the spinal canal. This anatomic peculiarity makes clinical and electrophysiologic localization of radicular lesions more difficult in the lower than upper extremities. The lumbar roots exit the spinal canal below their respective vertebrae. This is in contrast to the anatomic relationship between the cervical roots and the intervertebral spaces described earlier.

In assessing root lesions in the upper extremities, motor signs are considered more reliable than sensory impairment. The reverse seems to be true in the lower extremities. The first three lumbar roots supply the skin of the anterior thigh. Radiculopathies involving these spinal roots are rare. With compression of the L-4 root, pain radiates from the knee to the medial malleolus along the medial aspect. The pain produced by L-5 root irritation originates in the buttock and radiates along the posterior lateral aspect of the thigh, lateral aspect of the leg, dorsum of the foot, and first four toes. The pain induced by S-1 root irritation radiates down the back of the thigh, leg, and lateral aspect of the foot. Irritation of S-2 through S-5 roots causes pain along the posteromedial aspect of the thigh, over the perianal area of the buttock, and in the genital region.

Since most muscles are innervated by multiple roots in the lower extremities, involvement of a single root does not necessarily cause prominent weakness or wasting. Despite multiplicity of root supply in most leg muscles, a single root primarily controls certain movements. These include hip flexion (L-2), knee extension and thigh adduction (L-3), inversion of the foot (L-4), toe extension (L-5), and eversion of the foot (S-1).[69] Plantarflexion (S-1 and S-2) and dorsiflexion (L-4 and L-5) of the foot are affected to a lesser extent by lesions of a single root. These considerations are important in assessing the patients either clinically or electrophysiologically. The muscle stretch reflex is depressed at the knee with a lesion of the L-4 root, whereas an S-1 root lesion affects the reflex at the ankle and its electrical counterpart, the H-reflex.

# Conus lesion

The conus medullaris may be the primary seat of a variety of tumors including ependymoma, dermoid cyst, and lipoma. Typically the sacral roots are affected from below, beginning with the S-5 root. Thus, the usual presenting features are a dull backache and sensory disturbances in the genital and perianal region which may be detected only by careful examination. Impotence and impaired sphincter control soon develop. Later, the muscle stretch reflex may be diminished bilaterally at the ankle as the lesion extends upward to involve the origin of the S-1 root. However, the lesion typically spares the knee reflex. Initial weakness may be unilateral, but it soon spreads to the other extremity, leading to relatively symmetric involvement.

Electromyography shows evidence of denervation in the affected muscles. Bilateral involvement of multiple roots can be demonstrated electrically, even if clinical signs are asymmetric. The anal sphincter also shows evidence of denervation and loss of tonus. The amplitude of sensory nerve action potentials remains normal. Motor nerve conduction studies may reveal reduced amplitude of the compound muscle action potentials reflecting axonal degeneration. Electrophysiologic studies are normal in the upper extremities.

# Cauda equina lesion

A mass lesion located in the spinal canal anywhere below the T-12 vertebral level may affect any one of the lumbar or sacral roots singly or in combination. With a laterally located lesion at the level of L-1, L-2, and L-3 vertebrae, pain typically radiates over the anterior thigh. The lesions responsible for the lateral cauda equina syndrome include meningioma, neurofibroma, and a herniated disc. If the L-4 root is affected, the quadricep muscle is weak and atrophic and the knee reflex is lost. The invertors of the foot are also affected. Although uncommon, the cord may be simultaneously compressed by a high, laterally located lesion, giving rise to a hyperactive ankle reflex and other upper motor neuron signs. One must distinguish this rare but confusing presentation from amyotrophic lateral sclerosis.

Midline or diffuse involvement of the cauda equina may occur by external invasion. Common causes include metastasis from prostate cancer, direct spread of malignant tumors in the pelvic floor, leukemic or lymphomatous infiltration, chondromas of the sacral bone, and spinal arachnoiditis.[67] The cauda equina may become seeded with medulloblastoma, pinealoma, or other malignant tumors of the nervous system. Clinical features resemble those of a conus medullaris lesion with bilateral involvement of the lumbar and sacral roots, but the signs and symptoms of a cauda equina lesion are typically more asymmetric. The patient suffers from severe pain, a feature not commonly seen with a conus lesion. The pain is characteristically present at rest and is not relieved by different positions of the lower extremities. The distribution of pain is often outside the dermatomes ordinarily involved with a herniated lumbar disc. Reduced muscle stretch reflexes both at the knee and ankle also help differentiate a cauda equina from a conus lesion.

Electrophysiologic findings are similar to these of a conus medullaris lesion except for the asymmetric distribution of abnormalities which tend to spread above the sacral myotomes. In particular, substantial differences in the amplitude of the compound muscle action potentials from one side to the other are very common with cauda equina lesions.

# Herniated lumbar disc

Herniation of a lumbar disc can theoretically occur at any level, but in a majority of cases it involves the interspace between L-4 and L-5 or L-5 and S-1 vertebrae. Much less frequently, disc lesions may appear at the L-3 to L-4 intervertebral space. The remaining higher or lower levels are so rarely affected that other diagnostic possibilities should seriously be considered before attributing the symptoms to an uncomplicated herniated disc. The lumbosacral roots are commonly compressed slightly above their respective exit foramina, where they are located most laterally and closest to the protruding disc. A herniated disc at the L-4 to L-5 intervertebral space, therefore, tends to compress the L-5 root which emerges under the L-5 vertebra. Similarly, the S-1 root passing to the interspace below is damaged by a disc protrusion at the L-5 to S-1 level. As mentioned earlier, cervical disc herniation at the C-6 to C-7 level compresses the C-7 root, which exits above the C-7 vertebra. Thus, in both the cervical and lumbar regions, the root most frequently subject to damage is the one that is numbered the same as the vertebra below the herniated disc. Clinical symptoms usually consist of pain in the appropriate dermatomes, aggravated by leg-raising or other maneuvers that stretch the root, and weakness of the affected muscles. However, pure sensory or pure motor root lesions can also occur.

Electromyographic examination often precisely identifies the damaged root (see Fig. 13-7 bottom left). Denervation of the paraspinal muscles accompanies involvement of limb muscles (see Figs. 13-10 and 13-11) and implies a lesion located proximal to the origin of the posterior ramus.[14] However, marked disparity of involvement between anterior and posterior rami innervated muscles also occurs; for example, in metastatic disease affecting the paraspinal muscle.[58] Further, the absence of denervation in these muscles does not necessarily exclude the possibility of root compression.[52] In patients who have undergone laminectomy spontaneous activity may persist indefinitely. In one study electromyographic abnormalities were considered significant if they appeared at least 3 cm lateral to the incision and 4 to 5 cm deep.[46] In our laboratory, the findings considered pertinent to diagnose an active radiculopathy in postlaminectomy patients include: (1) fibrillation potentials and positive sharp waves on the symptomatic side only; (2) a mixture of large and small fibrillation and positive sharp waves on the symptomatic side but only large or small sparse spontaneous discharges on the asymptomatic side; and (3) the appearance of new spontaneous activity on the symptomatic side with serial studies.

Although paraspinal examination is essential in differentiating radiculopathy from diseases of the plexus or peripheral nerve, the exact level of radicular involvement cannot be determined on this basis alone because of the overlap in myotomes. More precise localization is possible by carefully exploring the affected muscles in the lower limbs. Because of anatomic peculiarities, L-5 and S-1 roots may occasionally be compressed within the cauda equina by lesions located much higher than the ordinary disc protrusion; for example, tumor of a high lumbar root. In this instance clinical features and myelographic abnormalities are critical. Nerve conduction studies are used primarily to exclude a neuropathy, but amplitude asymmetry of compound nerve and muscle action potentials assists in detection of modest nerve damage. H-reflex studies are abnormal with S-1 but not with L-5 radiculopathy. An increase in F-wave latency reflects delayed conduction, but its clinical value for early detection of radiculopathy remains to be determined.[30, 31, 51]

# Root avulsion

In contrast to well-known cervical root avulsion, intradural avulsion of the lumbosacral nerve roots has only rarely been reported,[33] probably because this condition is frequently overlooked.[5] Lumbosacral root avulsions occur in patients with pelvic fractures[41] and sacroiliac dislocation. In these instances, the nerve roots are stretched intradurally secondary to tension in the lumbar and sacral plexuses.[5] Nerve root avulsion is usually delineated by myelography. Electromyography shows evidence of denervation in the appropriate myotomes, including the paraspinal muscles.

# LUMBOSACRAL PLEXUS

The lumbosacral plexus, often considered a single anatomic entity, can be divided into lumbar and sacral portions with a connection between them. The division is convenient, since clinical problems tend to affect each portion independently. Lumbar plexus lesions result in weakness of hip flexion, knee extension and adduction, diminution of the knee reflex, and sensory loss in L-2, L-3, and L-4 dermatomes. Clinical and electromyographic abnormalities of the obturator-innervated muscles differentiate this condition from isolated femoral neuropathy. A lesion of the sacral plexus supplied by L-5, S-1, and S-2 roots produces a clinical picture similar to that seen with a sciatic nerve lesion, but with additional involvement of the gluteal muscles. The anal sphincter may also be affected.

The lumbosacral plexus is most commonly invaded by neoplasms extending from the rectum, prostate, or cervix. Metastatic, leukemic, or lymphomatous infiltration may also occur. This condition is usually painful and slowly progressive. Traumatic injuries include those associated with fractures of the pelvis or inappropriate traction during orthopedic or other operative manipulations.[5, 19] Lumbar plexopathy has been reported in diabetics, but some of these cases may represent femoral neuropathy[16] or lumbar radiculopathy. Lumbosacral plexopathies also occur presumably secondary to immune or vascular etiologies, but much less frequently than brachial plexopathies.

The plexus may be compressed by hematomas in patients with hemophilia or other coagulopathies and in those receiving anticoagulation therapy.[74] Two anatomically distinct syndromes have been described:[17, 40] (1) involvement of the lumbar plexus by hematoma within the psoas muscle;[32] and (2) compression of the femoral nerve alone.[96] In the former, clinical weakness involves the thigh adductors as well as hip flexors and quadriceps, and sensory loss affects the entire anterior thigh, including the lateral femoral cutaneous nerve distribution. In the latter, the findings consist of weakness of the quadriceps and hip flexors only, and sensory deficits are limited to the anterior femoral cutaneous and saphenous nerve distributions.[32]

Needle examination plays a major role in distinguishing a plexopathy from radiculopathy. Proximal muscles innervated rostral to the plexus are spared and should be specifically examined. These include, in addition to the paraspinal muscle, gluteus maximus, medius, and minimus, and iliopsoas. Electromyographic changes include a reduced recruitment pattern initially, and later, fibrillation potentials and positive sharp waves in the myotomes supplied by multiple peripheral and spinal nerves. Root stimulation may reveal increased latency across the plexus in the appropriate distribution.[64] Distal nerve stimulation may show reduction in amplitude of the compound muscle or nerve action potentials on the affected side as compared with the normal side.[1, 13] F-wave latencies may be prolonged or normal (see Fig. 17-12). With involvement of the S-1 root, the H-reflex may be absent or show an increased latency.

# REFERENCE SOURCES

1.  ADELMAN, JU, GOLDBERG, GS, AND PUCKETT, JD: *Postpartum bilateral femoral neuropathy.* Obstet and Gynecol 42:845, 1973.

2.  ADLER, JB AND PATTERSON, RL, JR: *Erb's palsy. Long-term results of treatment in eighty-eight cases.* J Bone Joint Surg 49A:1052, 1967.

3.  ALBERS, JW, ET AL: *Limb myokymia.* Muscle and Nerve 4:494, 1981.

4.  AUGUSTIN, P, VERDURE, L, AND SAMSON, M: *Le syndrome du nerf sus-scapulaire a l'étroit.* Rev Neurol (Paris) 132:219, 1976.

5.  BARNETT, HG AND CONNOLLY, ES: *Lumbosacral nerve root avulsion: Report of a case and review of the literature.* J Traum 15:532, 1975.

6.  BEHSE, F, ET AL: *Hereditary neuropathy with liability to pressure palsies. Electrophysiological and histopathological aspects.* Brain 95:777, 1972.

7. BLOCH, SL, ET AL: *Brachial plexus neuropathy as the initial presentation of systemic lupus erythematosus.* Neurology (New York) 29:1633, 1979.

8. BONNEY, G: *Prognosis in traction lesions of the brachial plexus.* J Bone Joint Surg 41B:4, 1959.

9. BONNEY, G AND GILLIATT, RW: *Sensory nerve conduction after traction lesion of the brachial plexus.* Proc R Soc Med 51:365, 1958.

10. BOSCH, EP, ET AL: *Brachial plexus involvement in familial pressure-sensitive neuropathy: Electrophysiological and morphological findings.* Ann Neurol 8:620, 1980.

11. BRADLEY, WG: *Disorders of Peripheral Nerves.* Blackwell Scientific Publications, Oxford, 1974.

12. BRADLEY, WG, ET AL: *Recurrent brachial plexus neuropathy.* Brain 98:381, 1975.

13. BUCHTHAL, A: *Femoralisparesen als Komplikation gynäkologischer Operationen.* Dtsch Med Wschr 98:2024, 1973.

14. BUFALINI, C AND PESCATORI, G: *Posterior cervical electromyography in the diagnosis and prognosis of brachial plexus injuries.* J Bone Joint Surg 51B:627, 1969.

15. CALDWELL, JW, CRANE, CR, AND KRUSEN, EM: *Nerve conduction studies: An aid in the diagnosis of the thoracic outlet syndrome.* South Med J 64:210, 1971.

16. CALVERLEY, JR AND MULDER, DW: *Femoral neuropathy.* Neurology (Minneap) 10:963, 1960.

17. CHIU, WS: *The syndrome of retroperitoneal hemorrhage and lumbar plexus neuropathy during anticoagulant therapy.* South Med J 69:595, 1976.

18. CLEIN, LJ: *Suprascapular entrapment neuropathy.* J Neurosurg 43:337, 1975.

19. COLES, CC AND MILLER, KD, JR: *Traumatic avulsion of the lumbar nerve roots.* South Med J 71:334, 1978.

20. CONRAD, B AND BENECKE, R: *How valid is the distal sensory nerve action potential for differentiating between radicular and non-radicular nerve lesions?* (abstr) Acta Neurol Scand (Suppl 73)60:122, 1979.

21. DAUBE, JR: *Rucksack paralysis.* JAMA 208:2447, 1969.

22. DAUBE, JR: *Nerve conduction studies in the thoracic outlet syndrome.* Neurology (Minneap) 25:347, 1975.

23. DAUBE, JR: *An electromyographer's view of plexopathy.* In Neuromuscular Diseases as Seen by the Electromyographer. Second Annual Continuing Education Course, American Association of Electromyography and Electrodiagnosis, October 4, 1979.

24. DAVIS, DH, ONOFRIO, BM, AND MACCARTY, CS: *Brachial plexus injuries.* Mayo Clin Proc 53:799, 1978.

25. DE GRANDIS, D, ET AL: *Anomalous reinnervation as a sequel to obstetric brachial plexus palsy.* J Neurol Sci 43:127, 1979.

26. DI BENEDETTO, M: *Thoracic outlet slowing. (A critical evaluation of established criteria for the diagnosis of outlet syndrome by nerve conduction studies.)* Electromyogr Clin Neurophysiol 17:191, 1977.

27. DORFMAN, LJ: *F-wave latency in the cervical-rib-and-band syndrome.* Letter to the editor. Muscle and Nerve 2:158, 1979.

28. DUNN, HG, DAUBE, JR, AND GOMEZ, MR: *Heredofamilial brachial plexus neuropathy (hereditary neuralgic amyotrophy with brachial predilection) in childhood.* Dev Med Child Neurol 20:28, 1978.

29. EARL, CJ, ET AL: *Hereditary neuropathy, with liability to pressure palsies.* Q J Med 33:481, 1964.

30. EISEN, A, SCHOMER, D, AND MELMED, C: *The application of F-wave measurements in the differentiation of proximal and distal upper limb entrapments.* Neurology (Minneap) 27:662, 1977.

31. EISEN, A, SCHOMER, D, AND MELMED, C: *An electrophysiological method for examining lumbosacral root compression.* J Canad des Sciences Neurol 4:117, 1977.

32. EMERY, S AND OCHOA, J: *Lumbar plexus neuropathy resulting from retroperitoneal hemorrhage.* Muscle and Nerve 1:330, 1978.

33.  FINNEY, LA AND WULFMAN, WA: *Traumatic intradural lumbar nerve root avulsion with associated traction injury to the common peroneal nerve.* Am J Roentgenol Rad Ther 84:952, 1960.

34.  FLAGGMAN, PD AND KELLY, JJ, JR: *Brachial plexus neuropathy. An electrophysiologic evaluation.* Arch Neurol 37:160, 1980.

35.  GARDNER, JH AND MALONEY, W: *Hereditary brachial and cranial neuritis genetically linked with ocular hypotelorism and syndactyly.* Neurology (Minneap) 18:278, 1968.

36.  GEIGER, LR, ET AL: *Familial neuralgic amyotrophy. Report of three families with review of the literature.* Brain 97:87, 1974.

37.  GILLIATT, RW: *Thoracic outlet compression syndrome.* Br Med J 1:1274, 1976.

38.  GILLIATT, RW, ET AL: *Wasting of the hand associated with a cervical rib or band.* J Neurol Neurosurg Psychiatry 33:615, 1970.

39.  GILLIATT, RW, ET AL: *Peripheral nerve conduction in patients with a cervical rib and band.* Ann Neurol 4:124, 1978.

40.  GOODFELLOW, J, FEARN, CBd'A, AND MATTHEWS, JM: *Iliacus haematoma. A common complication of haemophilia.* J Bone Joint Surg 49B:748, 1967.

41.  HARRIS, WR, ET AL: *Avulsion of lumbar roots complicating fracture of the pelvis.* J Bone Joint Surg 55A:1436, 1973.

42.  JACOB, JC, ANDERMANN, F, AND ROBB, JP: *Heredofamilial neuritis with brachial predilection.* Neurology (Minneap) 11:1025, 1961.

43.  JAEGER, R AND WHITELEY, WH: *Avulsion of the brachial plexus. Report of six cases.* JAMA 153:633, 1953.

44.  JELASIC, F AND PIEPGRAS, U: *Functional restitution after cervical avulsion injury with 'typical' myelographic findings.* Eur Neurol 11:158, 1974.

45.  JOHNSON, CR: *Treatment of thoracic outlet syndrome by removal of first rib and related entrapments through posterolateral approach. A 22 year experience.* J Thorac Cardiovasc Surg 68:536, 1974.

46.  JOHNSON, EW, BURKHART, JA, AND EARL, WC: *Electromyography in postlaminectomy patients.* Arch Phys Med Rehabil 53:407, 1972.

47.  KAYED, K AND KÅSS, B: *Acute multiple brachial neuropathy and Ehlers-Danlos syndrome.* Neurology (New York) 29:1620, 1979.

48.  KENNEDY, WR AND RESCH, JA: *Paralytic brachial neuritis.* Lancet 86:459, 1966.

49.  KEWALRAMANI, LS AND TAYLOR, RG: *Brachial plexus root avulsion: Role of myelography. Review of diagnostic procedures.* J Trauma 15:603, 1975.

50.  KILOH, LG AND NEVIN, S: *Isolated neuritis of the anterior interosseous nerve.* Br Med J 1:850, 1952.

51.  KIMURA, J: *A comment. Letter to the editor.* Muscle and Nerve 1:250, 1978.

52.  KNUTSSON, B: *Comparative value of electromyographic, myelographic and clinical-neurological examinations in diagnosis of lumbar root compression syndrome.* Acta Orthop Scand Suppl 49:1, 1961.

53.  KÓMÁR, J: *Eine wichtige Ursache des Schulterschmerzes: Incisura-scapulae-Syndrom.* Fortschr Neurol Psychiatr 44:644, 1976.

54.  KORI, SH, FOLEY, KM, AND POSNER, JB: *Brachial plexus lesions in patients with cancer: 100 cases.* Neurology (New York) 31:45, 1981.

55.  KRAFT, GH: *Multiple distal neuritis of the shoulder girdle: An electromyographic clarification of "paralytic brachial neuritis".* Electroenceph Clin Neurophysiol 27:722, 1969.

56.  KRAFT, GH: *Axillary, musculocutaneous and suprascapular nerve latency studies.* Arch Phys Med Rehabil 53:383, 1972.

57.  KREMER, RM AND AHLQUIST, RE, JR: *Thoracic outlet compression syndrome.* Am J Surg 130:612, 1975.

58.  LABAN, MM, ET AL: *Metastatic disease of the paraspinal muscles: Electromyographic and histopathologic correlation in early detection.* Arch Phys Med Rehabil 59:34, 1978.

59.  LAMBERT, EH: *Neurophysiological techniques useful in the study of neuromuscular disorders.* In ADAMS, R, EATON, L, AND SHY, G (EDS): *Neuromuscular Disorders.* Williams & Wilkins, Baltimore, 1960, pp 247–273.

60. LAMBERT, EH: *Diagnostic value of electrical stimulation of motor nerves*. Electroenceph Clin Neurophysiol (suppl 22): 9, 1962.

61. LISHMAN, WA AND RUSSELL, WR: *The brachial neuropathies*. Lancet 2:941, 1961.

62. LONDON, GW: *Normal ulnar nerve conduction velocity across the thoracic outlet: Comparison of two measuring techniques*. J Neurol Neurosurg Psychiatry 38:756, 1975.

63. LYON, BB, HANSEN, BA, AND MYGIND, T: *Peripheral nerve injury as a complication of axillary arteriography*. Acta Neurol Scand 51:29, 1975.

64. MACLEAN, I: *Nerve root stimulation to evaluate conduction across the lumbosacral plexus*. Acta Neurol Scand (Suppl 73)60:270, 1979.

65. MARTIN, WA AND KRAFT, GH: *Shoulder girdle neuritis: A clinical and electrophysiological evaluation*. Milt Med 139:21, 1974.

66. OLARTE, M AND ADAMS, D: *Accessory nerve palsy*. J Neurol Neurosurg Psychiatry 40:1113, 1977.

67. PARKER, KR, ET AL: *Electromyographic changes reviewed in chronic spinal arachnoiditis*. Arch Phys Med Rehabil 60:320, 1979.

68. PARSONAGE, MJ AND TURNER, JWA: *Neuralgic amyotrophy. The shoulder-girdle syndrome*. Lancet 1:973, 1948.

69. PATTEN, J: *Neurological Differential Diagnosis*. Springer-Verlag, New York, 1977.

70. PEZZIMENTI, JF, BRUCKNER, HW, AND DECONTI, RC: *Paralytic brachial neuritis in Hodgkin's disease*. Cancer 31:626, 1973.

71. RENNELS, GD AND OCHOA, J: *Neuralgic amyotrophy manifesting as anterior interosseous nerve palsy*. Muscle and Nerve 3:160, 1980.

72. SADLER, TR, JR, RAINER, WG, AND TWOMBLEY, G: *Thoracic outlet compression. Application of positional arteriographic and nerve conduction studies*. Am J Surg 130:704, 1975.

73. SMITH, BH, RAMAKRISHNA, T, AND SCHLAGENHAUFF, RE: *Familial brachial neuropathy. Two case reports with discussion*. Neurology (Minneap) 21:941, 1971.

74. SPIEGEL, PG AND MELTZER, JL: *Femoral-nerve neuropathy secondary to anticoagulation. Report of a case*. J Bone Joint Surg 56A:425, 1974.

75. SPILLANE, JD: *Localized neuritis of the shoulder girdle. A report of 46 cases in the MEF*. Lancet 2:532, 1943.

76. SPILLANE, JD: *An Atlas of Clinical Neurology*, ed 2. Oxford University Press, London, 1975.

77. STANWOOD, JE AND KRAFT, GH: *Diagnosis and management of brachial plexus injuries*. Arch Phys Med Rehabil 52:52, 1971.

78. SUNDERLAND, S: *The intraneural topography of the radial, median, and ulnar nerves*. Brain 68:243, 1945.

79. SWIFT, TR, LESHNER, RT, AND GROSS, JA: *Arm-diaphragm synkinesis: Electrodiagnostic studies of aberrant regeneration of phrenic motor neurons*. Neurology (New York) 30:339, 1980.

80. TAYLOR, RA: *Heredofamilial mononeuritis multiplex with brachial predilection*. Brain 83:113, 1960.

81. THOMAS, JE AND COLBY, MY, JR: *Radiation-induced or metastatic brachial plexopathy? A diagnostic dilemma*. JAMA 222:1392, 1972.

82. TROJABORG, W: *Electrophysiological findings in pressure palsy of the brachial plexus*. J Neurol Neurosurg Psychiatry 40:1160, 1977.

83. TSAIRIS, P: *Brachial plexus neuropathies*. In DYCK, PJ, THOMAS, PK, AND LAMBERT, EH (EDS): *Peripheral Neuropathy*, Vol 1. WB Saunders, Philadelphia, 1975.

84. TSAIRIS, P, DYCK, PJ, AND MULDER, DW: *Natural history of brachial plexus neuropathy. Report on 99 patients*. Arch Neurol 27:109, 1972.

85. TURNER, JWA AND PARSONAGE, MJ: *Neuralgic amyotrophy (paralytic brachial neuritis) with special reference to prognosis*. Lancet 2:209, 1957.

86. URSCHEL, HC, JR, ET AL: *Objective diagnosis (ulnar nerve conduction velocity) and current therapy of the thoracic outlet syndrome*. Ann Thorac Surg 12:608, 1971.

87. WANAMAKER, WM: *Firearm recoil palsy*. Arch Neurol 31:208, 1974.

88.  WAROT, P, ET AL: *Névrites amyotrophiantes brachiales familiales. Étude de deux familles.* Rev Neurol (Paris) 128:281, 1973.

89.  WARREN, J, ET AL: *Electromyographic changes of brachial plexus root avulsion.* J Neurosurg 31:137, 1969.

90.  WAXMAN, SG: *The flexion-adduction sign in neuralgic amyotrophy.* Neurology (Minneap) 29:1301, 1979.

91.  WEIKERS, NJ AND MATTSON, RH: *Acute paralytic brachial neuritis. A clinical and electrodiagnostic study.* Neurology (Minneap) 19:1153, 1969.

92.  WIEDERHOLT, WC: *Hereditary brachial neuropathy. Report of two families.* Arch Neurol 30:252, 1974.

93.  WOLPOW, ER: *Brachial plexus neuropathy. Association with desensitizing antiallergy injections.* JAMA 234:620, 1975.

94.  WULFF, CH AND GILLIATT, RW: *F waves in patients with hand wasting caused by a cervical rib and band.* Muscle and Nerve 2:452, 1979.

95.  WURMSER, P AND KAESER, HE: *Zur neuralgischen Amyotrophie.* Schweiz Med Wochr 93:1393, 1963.

96.  YOUNG, MR AND NORRIS, JW: *Femoral neuropathy during anticoagulant therapy.* Neurology (Minneap) 26:1173, 1976.

# 22
# POLYNEUROPATHIES

The triad of polyneuropathy consists of sensory changes in a glove and stocking distribution, distal weakness, and hyporeflexia. In certain types of neuropathy, sensory symptoms may be widespread and weakness may be more prominent proximally. In general, normal muscle stretch reflexes speak against peripheral neuropathy, but this is not an absolute rule. Anatomic diagnosis depends on clinical and electrodiagnostic evaluation, but no specific pattern of peripheral nerve involvement is characteristic of a given disorder. In many patients with an unequivocal diagnosis of polyneuropathy, the exact etiology remains obscure despite an extensive search.

A detailed history often uncovers general medical conditions known to be associated with diffuse damage to peripheral nerves, such as diabetes, alcoholism, renal disease, malignancies, amyloidosis, and polyarteritis nodosa. Infectious or postinfectious category includes diphtheria, leprosy, and the Guillain-Barré syndrome. Metabolic neuropathies result from nutritional deficiencies or the toxic effects of drugs or chemicals. Knowledge of the family history is essential for a number of inherited conditions associated with polyneuropathy. Sometimes even a patient's account is not always reliable, and it is often helpful to examine family members.

As discussed in Chapter 4, nerve conduction studies and electromyography play an important role in differentiating two major pathologic changes in the nerve fibers: axonal degeneration and demyelination. However, electrical studies are of limited value in distinguishing different types of neuropathies or establishing the exact etiology in a given case. The specific diagnosis of polyneuropathy, therefore, depends heavily on clinical and histologic assessments, even though electrophysiologic evaluations may delineate the extent and distribution of the lesion. This chapter will deal with the clinical and pathologic aspects of peripheral neuropathies as they relate to the electrophysiologic abnormalities. Only the essential characteristics will be described. Excellent comprehensive reviews are available elsewhere.[2, 9, 27, 40, 74]

## NEUROPATHIES ASSOCIATED WITH GENERAL MEDICAL CONDITIONS

This category includes some of the most commonly encountered polyneuropathies. Despite their clear association with a general medical condition, the exact cause of neuropathy remains uncertain.

# Diabetic neuropathy

Diabetes is one of the most common causes of neuropathy in the United States. The symmetric polyneuropathy likely has a metabolic basis, but its nature remains elusive. One attractive hypothesis postulates an increased amount of sorbitol in diabetic neural tissue.[92] In hyperglycemia, glucose is shunted through the sorbitol pathway, and the accumulation of sorbitol in Schwann cells may cause osmotic damage with segmental demyelination. Other factors considered important in the pathogenesis include insulin deficiency and altered myoinositol metabolism.[226] An alternative theory suggests that the peripheral nerves are probably affected by small vessel disease[181] and that all the asymmetric types of diabetic neuropathy and diabetic cranial mononeuropathies are caused by infarcts within the nerve. Ischemic changes in the nerve presumably result from proliferation of the endothelium in blood vessels and abnormalities of the capillaries, but neuropathologic studies have not shown occlusive arterial disease to be an obvious cause of peripheral nerve involvement.

A wide spectrum of neuropathic processes are seen in diabetics. The most commonly used clinical classification is that of Asbury and Johnson:[9] (1) distal symmetric primary sensory neuropathy; (2) autonomic neuropathy; (3) proximal asymmetric painful motor neuropathy; and (4) cranial mononeuropathies. Pathologic classification of the diabetic neuropathies separates them into two groups: predominantly large fiber and predominantly small fiber diseases. In the large fiber type,[18, 51] segmental demyelination and remyelination are more prominent features than axonal loss.[74] As a result, the linear relationship between internodal length and fiber diameter is disturbed.[50] In the small fiber type, the primary impact of the disease is axonal, and demyelination is secondary to the axonal involvement.[31, 74] A mixture of the large and small fiber types is common. Loss of both myelinated and unmyelinated fibers may occur with Schwann cell damage and axonal degeneration proceeding independently.[18] With distal axonopathy in experimental diabetes mellitus of the rat, fiber breakdown appears first in the terminal portions of the susceptible nerves.[32] In diabetics with autonomic neuropathy, abnormalities in the autonomic nervous system closely parallel changes in the peripheral nervous system.[82] The prominent histologic changes include active axonal degeneration, affecting mainly unmyelinated and small myelinated fibers.[147]

The clinical presentation depends on varying combinations of the two basic types. On the whole, the large fiber type is more prevalent in adult-onset diabetics. The symptoms are mild and consist of distal paresthesias and peripheral weakness. The patients tend to show dissociated loss of vibratory and position sense as well as two-point discrimination, with relative sparing of pain and temperature sense. Since the nerves are more vulnerable at the common sites of compression, the patient often presents with multiple pressure palsies. The small fiber type characteristically occurs in insulin dependent juvenile diabetics. Dysautonomia and pain are prominent features, as suggested by the name autonomic or painful diabetic neuropathy. The patient often awakens at night with painful dysesthesias. Charcot joints may develop in patients with severe loss of pain sensation. Perforating ulcers and other trophic changes of the feet are common. Impotence and postural hypotension result from involvement of the autonomic nerves.

In addition to symmetric polyneuropathy, mononeuropathies are commonly seen. The femoral nerve and lumbosacral plexus are sites of predilection, but sciatic, common peroneal, median, ulnar, and cranial nerves may also be affected.[207] Diabetic polyradiculoneuropathy and truncal mononeuropathy have also been described.[79] These entities, usually seen in association with advanced distal polyneuropathy, must be distinguished from a myelopathy.[223] Pressure neuropathy also affects the lateral cutaneous nerve of the calf.[85] Involvement of a major proximal nerve trunk may be heralded by the sudden onset of pain. Unilateral femoral neuropathy is a common complication in the elderly man with poorly controlled diabetes. Thigh pain precedes wasting of the quadriceps and other proximal muscles of the anterior thigh. Unlike the distal symptoms of diffuse polyneuropathy, the proximal weakness tends to improve with adequate control of the diabetes. This condition, although generally referred to as diabetic amyotrophy, may not constitute a separate entity[7, 49] and may represent a form of diabetic mononeuropathy.

Electrophysiologic studies in diabetics have revealed a number of different abnormalities.[172, 173, 174] Nerve conduction velocities are slower in diabetics with signs of neuropathy than those without clinical signs, and the evoked potential is reduced in size early.[97, 101, 113] Studies show a close correlation between clinical signs of neuropathy and the degree of slowing in conduction of the peroneal nerves.[100, 139, 165] In juvenile diabetics, patients with the longest duration of disease have the highest incidence of conduction abnormalities.[81] The nerves are diffusely affected, but more in distal than in proximal segments (see Fig. 17-11).[54, 126] Tibial and peroneal nerves show more abnormalities than median and ulnar nerves. Electromyography may show fibrillation potentials and positive sharp waves if axonal degeneration is a prominent feature, but this is not a constant finding. Diabetics have abnormal persistence of the sensory evoked potential during induced ischemia. This may be a sensitive indicator of neural dysfunction occurring even before the appearance of other electrophysiologic abnormalities.[110] According to estimates of motor unit numbers by a quantitative electrophysiologic technique, axonal dysfunction parallels the severity of the demyelinative process.[103]

## Alcoholic neuropathy

Alcohol is probably the most common cause of peripheral neuropathy in the United States. Clinical symptoms usually appear in those using a large quantity of alcoholic beverages for a number of years. In addition to a possible toxic effect of the alcohol itself, dietary insufficiency and impaired absorption may play important roles. Indeed, vitamin $B_1$ or thiamine deficiency alone is known to cause similar clinical findings. The pathologic changes in alcoholic neuropathy include a reduction in density of large and small myelinated fibers with evidence of some acute axonal degeneration and regeneration.[16, 222] Secondary paranodal demyelination may occur in the most distal segment.[153]

Clinical symptoms usually appear insidiously over weeks or months, but acute onset over a period of a few days is also seen. The initial sensory symptoms consist of distal pain, paresthesias, and dysesthesias, first in the legs and later in the arms. Painful burning sensations in the extremities are similar to those seen in the neuropathy of diabetes. Trophic changes such as plantar ulcers may occur in patients who have lost pain sensation. These patients often have preserved muscle power and subject insensitive tissues to usual amounts of trauma.[187] In more advanced cases, bilateral footdrop may develop. Muscular atrophy is more prominent distally, involving the extensors more than the flexors. Sensory symptoms may respond to daily administration of vitamin $B_1$, but the course of recovery is slow if muscular atrophy has already developed.

A number of electrophysiologic studies demonstrated impaired function in small caliber motor fibers and in distal large cutaneous sensory nerve fibers in alcoholic patients with or without clinical evidence of peripheral nerve disease.[20] Initially, nerve conduction velocities are either normal or only slightly reduced in most patients.[16, 42, 43, 222] As in other axonal neuropathies, slowing of conduction velocity occurs as a late finding and is proportional to the loss of evoked sensory and motor responses. Sensory nerve conduction may be more affected than motor conduction, and the degree of slowing in conduction velocity relates to the severity of the polyneuropathy.[151] Unfortunately, earlier evaluations tended to overemphasize the role of conduction velocity. However, other parameters of the conduction studies are equally important in patients with axonal lesions. In fact, early abnormalities of alcoholic neuropathy consist of decreased amplitude of both sensory nerve and compound muscle action potentials. Electromyography reveals fibrillation potentials and other neuropathic changes. Usually abnormal findings occur earlier and more prominently in the lower extremities.

## Uremic neuropathy

Peripheral neuropathy is a common complication of chronic renal failure. This may be a manifestation of still unidentified uremic toxins, including parathyroid hormone. Myoinosital and middle molecules with molecular weights of 300 to 2000 are elevated in uremia, but their effects on the peripheral nervous system remain to be determined.[21] Uremic neuropathy often develops in patients with severe chronic renal failure or in patients undergoing chronic hemodialysis. The use of neurotoxic drugs such as nitrofurantoin can contribute to the nerve damage. Histologic findings vary, but the most consistent abnormality is axonal degeneration with secondary segmental demyelination and, less frequently, segmental remyelination.[11, 76, 104, 208]

Clinical symptoms of neuropathy usually develop abruptly. A sudden rise in vibratory threshold is one of the early signs.[169] The lower extremities tend to show earlier and more prominent disturbances than the upper extremities. Restless legs is one symptom.[208] After successful treatment with hemodialysis, vibratory perception returns towards normal followed by improvement in other clinical findings. A distal ischemic neuropathy has developed in patients following placement of bovine arteriovenous shunts for chronic hemodialysis.[22] Proximal muscle weakness may also appear in uremic patients receiving hemodialysis.[141]

Electrophysiologic findings generally, but not always, correlate with the clinical signs, levels of serum creatinine, and pathologic changes of the peripheral nerve.[218, 224] Mild electric abnormalities may appear before clinical manifestations. Conduction velocities decrease with clinical deterioration and increase with improvement after dialysis or kidney transplant.[38, 169, 170, 177] Both motor and sensory conductions are abnormal in the upper and lower extremities in patients with severe renal insufficiency, but the peroneal nerve is more affected than the median nerve.[168] However, in one study with primary end-stage renal disease,[161] facial nerve latency was the most sensitive indicator of neuropathy, when compared with conduction velocities of the peroneal, median, and ulnar nerves. Studies of late responses and sural nerve conduction are of diagnostic value in patients with chronic renal failure.[1] A marked reversible reduction in amplitude of the muscle potential, considered characteristic of acute renal failure, is probably secondary to conduction block.[35] However, axonal degeneration is the most common abnormality associated with chronic renal failure. In this instance, diminution of the compound muscle action and sensory nerve potentials is accompanied by fibrillation potentials and positive sharp waves in electromyography.

## Neuropathies in malignant conditions

The peripheral nerve may be affected directly or remotely by a malignant process. Malignant lymphomas and leukemias may invade or infiltrate the peripheral nerve through hematogenous spread. Occasionally a metastasis may involve the dorsal root ganglia.[114] Nonlymphomatous solid tumors may cause external compression but seldom invade the nerve itself. Neuropathies may result from remote effects of cancer, most commonly with malignant lymphoma[190] and bronchogenic carcinoma.[108, 205] However, they are also seen with malignant tumors of the ovary, testes, penis, stomach, and oral cavity.[179] Neuropathic effects can include: (1) neuronal degenerations with secondary peripheral or central axonal changes; (2) demyelination which can mimic acute or chronic idiopathic polyneuritis;[145] (3) microvasculitis with active wallerian degeneration, clinically resembling mononeuritis multiplex;[115] and possibly (4) opportunistic neuropathic infection, although attempts at virus isolation have as yet been unsuccessful.[190] Changes are most commonly seen in dorsal root ganglia, but occasionally anterior horn cell lesions occur.

Clinically, neuropathies caused by remote effects of malignancies may be sensory, motor, or mixed in type. However, a purely motor neuropathy is rare, and such a syndrome must be distinguished from the myasthenic syndrome and a polyradiculopathy related to meningeal carcinomatosis. A mixed sensory and motor neuropathy is most common, but it is poorly characterized, because it probably represents a group of heterogenous conditions with overlapping clinical and histologic features.[9] One type of sensory neuropathy associated with oat cell carcinoma follows a subacute course and may result in severe sensory loss secondary to dorsal root ganglionitis.[111]

Electrophysiologic abnormalities develop in approximately one third of patients with malignancies[163, 179] and allow detection of clinically latent paraneoplastic neuropathies.[179] The incidence is slightly higher in patients with lung cancer.[39, 206] In the majority of patients, conduction velocity is only mildly slowed, affecting either sensory fibers,[156] motor fibers,[214] or both.[39, 163] However, conduction studies commonly show reduced amplitude of sensory nerve and muscle action potentials. Fibrillation potentials are regularly present in atrophic muscles.[179] Proximal muscles with wasting may show small, short duration polyphasic motor unit potentials,[196] probably on the basis of neuropathic abnormalities in the intramuscular axonal segments.[15]

## Amyloid neuropathy

Amyloidosis is characterized by the deposition of amyloid around blood vessels and connective tissue in multiple organ systems. Clinical features depend on the organs involved, which commonly include the peripheral nerve, heart, tongue, gastrointestinal tract, skeletal muscles, and kidney. Amyloid deposits in the flexor retinaculum may cause the carpal tunnel syndrome in about one quarter of the patients. Neurologic symptoms are rare in secondary amyloidosis seen in chronic debilitating inflammatory processes.

Familial amyloid neuropathies differ clinically from an increasing number of primary or secondary nonfamilial amyloid neuropathies. A form of autosomal dominant amyloidosis prevalent in northern Portugal produces progressive neuropathy of the legs in young adults. Another, milder form of autosomal dominant amyloidosis with neuropathy of the upper extremities primarily affects Swiss families and occurs later in life.

In nonfamilial cases, neuropathy is associated with plasma cell dyscrasias and amyloidogenic immunoglobulins.[87, 98, 215] Diffuse peripheral neuropathy may occur in about 15 percent of patients with primary systemic amyloidosis,[53, 134] possibly on the basis of metabolic or ischemic changes, or resulting from direct infiltration by amyloid, but the exact cause is not known. A painful sensory and motor neuropathy with prominent autonomic features may be the presenting manifestation of this multisystem illness. Axonal degeneration predominates in small myelinated and unmyelinated fibers.[210] This explains the typical dissociated sensory loss with predilection for pain and temperature sense and relative sparing of vibratory and position sense; that is, the reverse of the findings seen in large fiber type diabetic neuropathy.

Electrophysiologic features include slightly reduced motor nerve conduction velocity with mild reduction in amplitude of the compound muscle action potential and absence of the sensory nerve action potential with distal stimulation of the ulnar, median, and sural nerves. Evidence of denervation is present diffusely, but more conspicuously, in the distal muscles of the leg.[119] An in vitro study of sural nerve compound action potentials has shown a selective reduction of A delta and C potentials in familial amyloid neuropathy.[70] These findings support the view that familial amyloid neuropathy predominantly causes distal axonal damage first in the sensory and then in the motor fibers.[188]

# Periarteritis nodosa

This is an inflammatory arteritis of unknown cause, although probably related to auto-immune hypersensitivity. The small and medium-sized arteries are affected in multiple organ systems, including thoracic and abdominal viscera, joints, muscle, and the nervous system. Necrosis of the media gives rise to small aneurysms and thrombosis of the vessels. Characteristic nodules may be palpable along the affected arteries.

The clinical symptoms and signs may appear either abruptly or insidiously with malaise, fever, sweating, tachycardia, and abdominal and joint pain. Approximately one half of the patients develop neuronal disturbances such as diffuse polyneuropathy and mononeuritis multiplex. Ischemia is the likely cause of the neuropathy, since nutrient arteries are heavily infiltrated with inflammatory cells and are often thrombosed. Spontaneous remission may occur, but the prognosis is generally poor with survival of only a few months to a few years after the onset of clinical symptoms. Electrophysiologic studies show slowing of the conduction velocity of affected nerves and the presence of spontaneous activities in atrophic muscles.

## Sarcoid neuropathy

Polyneuropathy is a rare complication of sarcoidosis.[62, 80, 131] The clinical features are those of a sensory-motor polyneuropathy with distal predominance. Granulomata or inflammatory changes found in the epineural and perineural spaces give rise to perian-gitis, panangitis, and axonal degeneration.[175] Electrophysiologic findings also suggest axonal degeneration with prominent fibrillations and positive sharp waves.

The distal nerve segment may be inexcitable. The amplitude of the compound muscle action potential may be reduced, and mild slowing of nerve conduction velocities may be present.[80, 131, 175]

## Neuropathies associated with paraproteinemia

The neuropathy associated with multiple myeloma and macroglobulinemia may be a feature of the underlying disorder and may not be directly caused by parapro-teins.[157, 182, 203, 217, 219, 221] Neuropathies have been reported in monoclonal[221] and polyclonal gammopathies,[157] as well as in angioimmunoblastic lymphadenopathy with dysprotein-emia.[213] Electrophysiologic findings suggest diffuse demyelination with prominent slowing of nerve conduction in the extremities as well as in the face (see Fig. 16-10b and c).

# INFECTIVE AND POSTINFECTIVE NEUROPATHIES

The most common disorder in this category is the Guillain-Barré syndrome. It will be discussed in some detail, since nerve conduction studies often help establish the diagnosis. Other infectious polyneuropathies include those associated with diphtheria and leprosy, which are now seldom seen in the United States.

## Guillain-Barré syndrome

This is a very common form of inflammatory polyneuropathy of unknown etiology. Many of its clinical and pathologic features resemble experimental allergic neuropathy caused by the injection of Freund adjuvant with extracts of peripheral nerve. Since infective agents have never been isolated, an autoimmune pathogenesis is suspected, rather than direct invasion of the nerve by infectious agents. Pathologically, the common denominator is an inflammatory demyelinative neuritis affecting all levels of the peripheral nervous system, occasionally with retrograde degeneration in the motor cells of the spinal cord or brain stem. Pathologic changes may be very mild, consisting only of slight edema of the nerves or roots. The segment of maximal involvement varies from one patient to the next.[10] This helps to explain the diversity of clinical findings and also the various patterns of conduction abnormalities in different patients.

The clinical findings vary, but certain diagnostic criteria for the Guillain-Barré syndrome have been established.[12] In about two thirds of the cases, neurologic symptoms are preceded by a mild, transient infectious process of either the respiratory or, less commonly, of the gastrointestinal system. The first symptoms of neuropathy usually appear in about one to two weeks, when the infection is no longer present. Weakness initially appears in the lower extremities, but may rapidly progress to involve the upper extremities and cranial nerves within a few days. Unlike the distal weakness seen in other forms of neuropathy, paralysis of proximal muscles is common. Facial diplegia is characteristic. The muscle stretch reflexes are diminished or lost early in the course. Despite early painful distal paresthesias, definite sensory loss may not be present. However, careful testing usually reveals some deficiency in vibratory sense, two-point discrimination, and pain perception. Respiratory problems develop in approximately one quarter of the patients. Examination of the spinal fluid typically shows high protein with no cells, although some lymphocytes may be present. Dramatic improvement has been observed in some patients following corticosteroid therapy.[176] The therapeutic role of plasma exchange[88, 194] remains to be determined.[13] After treatment, nerve conduction velocities may or may not revert toward normal values.[194, 212]

An acute or subacute course is common with usual progression up to six weeks after onset. The symptoms and signs then plateau for a variable period of time before showing gradual improvement. The time course of recovery depends on the extent of demyelination and, perhaps more importantly, of axonal degeneration. Some patients with severe axonal loss may not regain motor function for one to two years. Apart from the chronicity as a result of axonal changes, the disease may continue to progress beyond six weeks with persistent evidence of ongoing demyelination in some patients. This variety, referred to as chronic inflammatory polyradiculopathy, may even progress with severe disability over several years.[74, 180] Immunoglobulin and complement deposits have been found in nerves of patients with this syndrome, also referred to as chronic relapsing polyneuropathy.[58] A variant of the Guillain-Barré syndrome originally described by Fisher[86] consists of ataxia of gait, absence of the muscle stretch reflexes, and ophthalmoplegia. A different form of the Guillain-Barré syndrome with abnormal pupils and normal eye movements has also been reported.[225]

Nerve conduction velocities are usually reduced by more than 30 to 40 percent in patients with the Guillain-Barré syndrome.[47, 112] The compound muscle action potential is commonly very polyphasic with increased temporal dispersion (see Fig. 5-6A and B). In milder forms of the syndrome, however, less dramatic changes may be present, since initial weakness is commonly associated with proximal conduction block without distal axonal loss. Indeed, in 15 to 20 percent of cases, motor nerve conduction tested conventionally may not be affected during the first three to four weeks.[77, 124] This fact, although clearly verified, has not been widely appreciated, perhaps because most conduction studies are done late.[117, 138] In the early stages of this primary demyelinating disorder, electromyography is often unremarkable except for a reduced interference pattern reflecting neuropraxia of some motor fibers.

In patients showing conduction abnormalities, initial slowing may occur at common sites of nerve compression.[138] Our experience also suggests a tendency towards involvement of both the terminal and the most proximal, possibly radicular, portions of the motor fibers, whereas the main nerve trunk is less affected.[123] The terminal segment may be peculiarly vulnerable because of its distance from the cell body. In some mild cases, the pathologic process may be confined to the central nerve segment, including the radicular portion, as suggested by the absence of F-waves initially and increased F-wave latencies later in conjunction with normal distal conduction velocity (see Figs. 17-

6 and 17-10 and Table 17-4).[124, 127] However, it has not been conclusively shown whether the radicular segment is generally more vulnerable than the remaining distal segments. Conduction of the facial nerve is usually slow, and the blink reflex is commonly abnormal, reflecting clinical facial palsy (see Figs. 16-10A and 16-12 and Tables 16-1 and 16-3). When a diagnosis of the Guillain-Barré syndrome is considered, the entire length of several nerves should be examined. In addition to the motor fibers, sensory fibers should be tested. Interestingly, the sural nerve sensory action potential, often regarded as one of the most sensitive indices, may be entirely normal, even when median or ulnar sensory action potentials are abnormal.[166]

Sequential conduction studies show great variability among different patients and even from one nerve to another in the same patient.[125] The nerve conduction velocity may become slower, even after the beginning of clinical improvement, demonstrating again the lack of strong correlation between clinical symptoms and conduction velocities.[106] The amplitude of compound nerve and muscle action potentials and electromyography show better correlations with the clinical status. Electrophysiologic findings at about the fourth week after onset usually provide a reasonable estimate for the clinical course. Persistent evoked responses with distal stimulation and paucity of fibrillation potentials and positive sharp waves suggest good prognosis, as they indicate proximal conduction block rather than axonotmesis. In contrast, loss of distal nerve excitability and the presence of profuse fibrillation are bad prognostic signs, since functional recovery depends on axonal regeneration, which takes considerably longer than remyelination.

## Diphtheric neuropathy

Prophylactic immunization and early use of immune sera and antibiotics in infected cases have drastically lowered the incidence of diphtheric polyneuropathy in the United States, but rare outbreaks still occur. The exotoxin of *Corynebacterium diphtheriae* becomes fixed to the nerve and produces segmental demyelination after several weeks. Local paralysis of the palatal muscles may occur early following an infection of the throat. Neuropathy may also develop in adults after contracting cutaneous diphtheria, common in the tropics.

The clinical symptoms, which typically develop two to four weeks after the initial infection, are characterized by a high incidence of lower cranial nerve dysfunction, causing palatal and pharyngeal weakness. Blurring of vision is common as a result of paralysis of accommodation. The sensory and motor nerves of the extremities are also affected, causing paresthesias and weakness of the affected limbs. The clinical signs are similar to those seen in the Guillain-Barré syndrome, and distinction between the two is sometimes difficult. A rapidly descending paralysis may occur, leading to respiratory problems. Since the primary pathologic change is segmental demyelination, slowing of sensory and motor conduction velocities is a common electrophysiologic finding. Decreased conduction velocity and increased distal motor latency may not be present before two weeks after the onset of neurologic symptoms, and maximal electrophysiologic abnormalities may be found after clinical recovery has begun.[132]

## Leprosy

This is a chronic infectious disease caused by an acid-fast bacillus, *Mycobacterium leprae*. The disease is transmitted by close and prolonged contact. Although rare in the United States, it is still prevalent in Africa, India, and South and Central America. There are two clinical forms. In the lepromatous type, granulomatous infiltration of the skin causes characteristic disfiguration. Diffuse sensory neuropathy occurs in this variety. The perineurium is directly involved by the bacillus. Nerve trunks are thickened by an overgrowth of connective tissue that compresses the myelin sheath and the axons.

The tuberculoid form is characterized by patches of depigmented, maculoanesthetic areas of the skin and some swelling of the nerves associated with mononeuritis multiplex. The organisms are not commonly found in the nerve. Most frequently affected are the great auricular, ulnar, radial, peroneal, facial, and trigeminal nerves. The two types of clinical presentation cannot always be clearly separated, since intermediate or mixed forms are common.

Clinical symptoms are those of mononeuritis multiplex and slowly progressive diffuse polyneuropathy. The initial sign of neural leprosy is an erythematous macule, which enlarges, forming anesthetic depigmented areas. Pain and temperature sensation are affected, resulting in ulcerated necrosis of the skin. The infective granulomatous process may give rise to characteristic fusiform swelling of the peripheral nerves, which may be palpable. The muscle innervated by the affected nerve becomes atrophic and paretic with histopathologic findings of fascicular atrophy and inflammatory nodules.[192] Common manifestations include facial palsy involving the upper half of the face, and wristdrop, footdrop, and clawhands. Moderate to marked slowing of the motor and sensory conduction velocities has been reported in enlarged segments,[150, 204] as well as in apparently normal nerves.[158] In one study, sensory nerve conduction studies of the radial nerve best correlated with the clinical findings and proved to be the most reliable diagnostic test.[191] Electromyography shows evidence of denervation in the atrophic muscles.[6, 192, 193]

# METABOLIC NEUROPATHIES

Metabolic neuropathies may be divided into two groups, those associated with nutritional disturbances and those resulting from toxic causes. Neuropathies attributable to a specific nutritional deficiency include beriberi, pellagra, and pernicious anemia. Toxic neuropathies are caused by administration of various drugs or by exposure to known chemical substances such as lead or arsenic. Many neuropathies associated with general medical conditions also belong to this broad category as mentioned earlier. No specific metabolic disturbances have been uncovered in these entities, however.

## Nutritional neuropathies

Diets deficient in vitamins and other nutritional factors are generally held responsible for the polyneuropathy seen in beriberi, pellagra, pernicious anemia, dysentery, and cachexia. Alcoholic and paraneoplastic neuropathies may be, at least in part, caused by inadequate food and vitamin intake or some toxin which interferes with the metabolism of the nerves. The sensory neuropathy associated with primary biliary cirrhosis may be nutritional in nature, although xanthomatous infiltrates or immunologic mechanisms have also been postulated.[48]

The symptoms and signs of beriberi are believed to be secondary to Vitamin $B_1$ or thiamine deficiency. The neuropathy associated with beriberi is very similar to the more common alcoholic polyneuropathy and consists of distal pain, paresthesias, sensory loss, distal leg weakness, and absence of the stretch reflexes. Pathologically, both the axon and myelin sheath are affected, although axonal damage is more conspicuous than demyelination.

Pellagra is another deficiency disease involving the vitamin $B_1$ complex. The condition may be seen with malnutrition or in association with chronic alcoholism. The clinical features consist of gastrointestinal symptoms, skin eruptions, and disorders of the peripheral and central nervous systems. Peripheral neuropathy is common and presents with paresthesias, loss of distal sensation, tenderness of the nerve trunks, and hyporeflexia. Paralysis, if present, is usually mild.

Pernicious anemia results from deficiency of intrinsic factors that are required in gastrointestinal secretions for the absorption of vitamin $B_{12}$. As indicated by its alternative name, combined system disease, pathologic changes are most intense in the dorsal and lateral funiculi of the spinal cord. The peripheral nerves, however, are also affected with fragmentation of myelin sheaths and degeneration of axons. The presenting clinical symptoms are mostly sensory and consist of paresthesias, dysesthesias, and loss of vibration and position sense. Flaccid or spastic paralysis of the lower extremities is common. Stretch reflexes may be increased during the early stages, but become diminished with progress of the disease. Peripheral nerve dysfunction with reduced conduction velocity is frequent in untreated patients, and thiamine deficiency is also present in the majority of cases.[55]

# Toxic neuropathies

Based on the presumed site of cellular involvement, toxic neuropathies may be divided into three groups: (1) neuronopathy affecting the cell body, especially those of dorsal root ganglion; (2) myelinopathy or schwannopathy with primary segmental demyelination; and (3) distal axonopathy causing dying-back axonal degeneration. Of these, the first two types are very rare. They include acute sensory neuronopathy following antibiotic treatment,[201] and myelinopathy by diphtheria toxin,[154] or following chronic exposure to lead in experimental animals. Distal axonopathy described below is the most common form of toxic neuropathy.

A variety of drugs and industrial chemicals causes distal axonopathy.[99] The drugs known to be neurotoxic include vincristine,[30, 44] disulfiram,[94, 178] metronidazol,[28] chloramphenicol, nitrofurantoin, diphenylhydantoin,[78] dapsone,[130] lithium,[34] perhexiline maleate,[26, 186] isoniazid, thalidomide,[91] and nitrous oxide.[140, 185] Industrial chemicals causing toxic axonal neuropathy include acrylamide,[164] methyl n-butyl ketone,[4, 199] carbon disulfide, organophosphates, and triorthocresyl phosphate.[220] In toxic axonal neuropathy, large diameter fibers are initially affected in the distal segments with involvement progressing proximally towards the cell body. The pathologic process then spreads to small diameter axons.

The onset of clinical symptoms in distal axonopathy reflects the acuteness of intoxication. The disease often develops rather insidiously from a chronic low-level exposure to the toxin. The nerves of the lower extremities are initially affected because the longer axons are more vulnerable. Weakness is more prominent distally. Hypesthesia and paresthesia occur in a glove and stocking distribution. Ankle stretch reflexes are lost early. Removal of the neurotoxin leads to gradual recovery. However, axonal regeneration takes place slowly, over months to years, and return of function may be incomplete. Selection of the proper electrophysiologic test depends largely on the nature of the condition being studied.[142, 143] In the absence of demyelination, nerve conduction velocities may be normal, but axonal loss results in reduced amplitude of the compound nerve and muscle action potentials. Substantial degeneration of large fast conducting fibers gives rise to increased distal latency initially and moderate slowing of conduction velocity later. Electromyography often shows fibrillation potentials and positive sharp waves.

Lead and arsenic, two specific agents in distal axonal neuropathies, merit further attention. The general features of lead poisoning include abdominal cramps, encephalopathy, and the occasional appearance of a blue lead line along the gingival border. The diagnosis should be suspected in the presence of basophilic stippling of erythrocytes and confirmed by elevated lead levels. Neuropathy occurs primarily in adults occupationally exposed to lead or following accidental ingestion of contaminated food, but may also be seen in children with known plumbism or pica.[83] Motor fibers are predominantly affected. The extensor muscles of the upper extremities are most vulnerable, producing bilateral radial nerve palsies. Sensory fibers are usually spared. Following removal of the toxin, recovery takes place over a period of several months. Lead produces segmental demyelination in some animal species, possibly because extravasated lead in the interstitial fluid causes direct injury to Schwann cells[167] but does not usually produce this type of pathologic change in man.[37] In a group of workers exposed to lead, temporally dispersed compound muscle action potentials were detected, indicating a minimal conduction defect, but the maximal conduction velocity remained normal.[45]

Arsenic poisoning is usually the result of accidental ingestion of rat poison or exposure to industrial sprays.[84] Polyneuropathy develops several weeks after acute poisoning or more slowly with chronic low-level exposure. Arsenic is found in the urine during acute exposure and may be detected in the hair and nails later. Early symptoms consist of pain and paresthesias of the lower extremities. Sensory loss is common in a glove and stocking distribution. Flaccid paralysis may develop later, beginning in the lower extremities, but eventually affecting the upper extremities. The stretch reflexes are lost or diminished. These clinical features are very similar to those of alcoholic neuropathy. Nerve conduction velocities are either normal or only slightly reduced, but there is evidence of denervation by electromyography. Nearly complete recovery may be expected if the toxin is removed in time.

# INHERITED NEUROPATHIES

Dyck has described seven types of hereditary motor and sensory neuropathy (HMSN). Of these, HMSN Types I and II correspond to the hypertrophic and neuronal varieties of Charcot-Marie-Tooth disease; Type III, Dejerine-Sottas disease; Type IV, Refsum disease; and Type V, spinocerebellar degeneration with neuropathy. Types VI and VII are accompanied by optic atrophy and retinitis pigmentosa, respectively. A number of other inherited polyneuropathies, which are sometimes associated with electrophysiologic abnormalities,[93] will be dealt with only briefly.

## Charcot-Marie-Tooth disease

This is the common form of inherited neuropathy. Males tend to be more severely affected, and formes frustes occur more commonly in the female.[105] Although long regarded as a single entity, two different varieties, hypertrophic and neuronal, may exist in the general category of Charcot-Marie-Tooth disease.[17, 36, 68, 69, 105] It has been demonstrated that these two types can be genetically separated. The bimodal distribution of nerve conduction velocities in a large group of patients clinically diagnosed as having Charcot-Marie-Tooth disease also supports the contention of two distinct entities.[105, 209, 211] At variance with this hypothesis is a kinship in which both the neuronal and hypertrophic types were found.[5] Based on available information the division seems appropriate; but the existence of an intermediate type has also been proposed.[29, 33, 149]

In the first type, called HMSN Type I, or hypertrophic, variety, the disease is usually inherited as an autosomal dominant, but sporadic cases have also been reported. It occurs more frequently in the male than female, although it is transmitted by either sex. It is characterized by enlargement of the peripheral nerves and segmental demyelination and remyelination. A primary Schwann cell disorder is suggested by clustered areas of segmental demyelination and remyelination and onion-bulb formation in the distal segments of peripheral nerves. However, certain features such as axonal atrophy and abnormalities in axonal transport of dopamine beta-hydroxylase suggest a neuronal disturbance.[66] In a kindred displaying a dominant inheritance, marriage between two heterozygotes resulted in two homozygous offspring.[120] Clinical features of the homozygotes were similar to the classic description of HMSN Type III or Dejerine-Sottas disease.

The clinical features of HMSN Type I may be summarized as follows. The onset is insidious within the first two decades. Some deformity of the feet is noted initially. The foot often has a high arch, and club feet are common. The peroneal musculature becomes atrophic. In advanced cases, the thigh and the upper extremities become involved, but the trunk and girdle musculature are seldom affected. The classic stork leg configuration is uncommon in this type. Bilateral footdrop causes characteristic gait difficulty. Paresthesias and dysesthesias are uncommon despite objective evidence of sensory loss. Patients often complain of muscle pain owing to foot deformity. Vibratory and position senses are lost and cutaneous sensations are reduced. The stretch reflexes are diminished early at the ankle, and later diffusely. Hypertrophic nerves may be palpable in some cases. The disease progresses very slowly over many decades, at times showing spontaneous arrest. Some patients become incapacitated by muscle atrophy and weakness, but this is the exception rather than the rule. Roussey-Levy syndrome with a static tremor of the hands may be a variant of this type.

Slow nerve conduction velocity is a hallmark of the HMSN Type I.[96, 105, 137, 171] The motor conduction velocities in affected family members average less than half those of normal individuals, varying from 9 to 41 m/s and averaging 25 m/s.[72] More severe slowing is seen in the terminal segments of the nerve, as demonstrated by the prolonged terminal latencies. Sensory fibers are also affected, and sensory potentials, if recordable, are of decreased amplitude and prolonged latency. Despite marked slowing, recorded potentials show minimal or no increase in temporal dispersion, indicating that different nerve fibers are affected equally. The degree of conduction abnormality is similar from one nerve to another in the same patient and also among different members in the same family. Uniform involvement of all nerves and all fibers in each nerve differentiates this entity from acute inflammatory polyneuropathy. Slow conduction velocities in patients with an otherwise normal clinical examination indicate early or subclinical involvement and constitute evidence of neuropathy.

F-waves are often absent, especially in the lower extremities.[125] When the response is elicitable, slowing of the F-wave velocity in the central segment is comparable with that of the motor nerve conduction distally (see Figs. 17-7 and 17-10 and Table 17-3).[122] Blink reflex latencies are frequently increased despite relatively normal strength of the facial muscles (see Figs. 16-10A and 16-12 and Tables 16-1 and 16-3).[121]

In the second type, labelled HMSN Type II, or neuronal, variety, nerve enlargement is not present and segmental demyelination is less prominent. It is also inherited as an autosomal dominant, but clinical symptoms and signs appear in early adult life or later. The clinical features are similar to those in the HMSN Type I but are much less generalized. The involvement of the upper extremities is less conspicuous and sensory disturbances are minimal. Weakness of the plantarflexors is more severe. As the name peroneal muscular atrophy indicates, the disease is characterized by rather selective muscular wasting of the legs in early states. An almost total loss of muscle bulk below the knee gives rise to a stork leg appearance. Despite footdrop and clubfeet, the patients are often able to walk fairly well and rarely are totally incapacitated. Tremors may be present in the upper extremities, but much less commonly than in HMSN Type I. In contrast to the hypertrophic form, the neuronal form is associated with only mild to moderate slowing of the nerve conduction velocities.[95, 105] Conduction studies, however, often reveal reduction in amplitude of the compound sensory nerve and muscle action potentials. Electromyography typically shows large motor unit potentials, fasciculation potentials, fibrillation potentials, and positive sharp waves.[69]

A third type of Charcot-Marie-Tooth disease designated as the spinal form is possibly a variant of the neuronal type or distal spinal muscular atrophy. The clinical features resemble Charcot-Marie-Tooth disease, but sensory changes are entirely absent and the nerve is not hypertrophic.

## Generalized or focal hypertrophic polyneuropathy

The most severe generalized form of sensory-motor neuropathy, HMSN Type III, was described by Dejerine[60] and Dejerine and Sottas[61] at the turn of the century.[189] It is inherited as an autosomal recessive. Marked thickening of the affected nerves is associated with onion-bulb formation, segmental demyelination, and thinning of the myelin surrounding the nerve.[67] Symptoms appear in infancy with delayed development of motor skills, especially walking. Clinical features consist of pes cavus, muscle cramps, incoordination, kyphoscoliosis, weakness, sensory loss, and abducens and facial nerve palsies. Adult patients are often wheelchair-bound by paraparesis and severe truncal ataxia. Nerve conduction velocities are markedly reduced.

In contrast to the generalized form, localized hypertrophic neuropathy is a rare condition consisting of isolated mononeuropathy with focal nerve enlargement.[107, 136, 198] This entity has been thought to represent either a localized form of Dejerine-Sottas disease, entrapment neuropathy, or intraneural neurofibroma. In some patients morphologic findings in the localized areas of enlarged nerves differed from all those seen in the above conditions and consisted of primary perineural cell hyperplasia or perineurinoma.[160] Nerve conduction studies in these patients suggested severe motor and sensory axonal loss with no evidence of slowed conduction velocity. Electromyography was also consistent with focal motor and sensory axonal loss, with evidence of severe active denervation limited to the territory of the affected nerve.

## Hereditary ataxic neuropathy of Refsum

The HMSN Type IV, a rare disorder transmitted by a recessive gene, is characterized pathologically by changes in the olivocerebellar tracts, anterior horn cells, and the peripheral nerves. Clinical features include deafness, anosmia, night blindness with retinitis pigmentosa, ichthyosislike skin, cerebellar signs, and nystagmus. Involvement of the peripheral nerve is indicated by lightning pain in the legs, wasting of muscles, hyporeflexia, hypotonia, and diminished vibration and position sense. The level of serum phytanic acid is elevated as a result of a metabolic defect of branched chain fatty acid oxidation. However, it is not clear how the metabolic defect leads to a hypertrophic neuropathy. Dietary restriction of phytol results in considerable improvement of symptoms. This neuropathy has not been adequately characterized electrophysiologically.

## Friedreich's ataxia

This autosomal recessive disorder primarily affects the spinal cord with involvement of the spinocerebellar tracts, corticospinal tracts, and posterior columns. In advanced cases, the degeneration also affects the dorsal roots and peripheral nerves with a severe loss of large myelinated fibers; unmyelinated C-fibers are preserved and conduct normally.[73] Clinical features of HMSN Type V include kyphosis or scoliosis, pes cavus, ataxia, loss of position and vibration sense, and hyporeflexia. Sensory nerve potentials are commonly absent or considerably reduced in amplitude.[155] Somatosensory evoked potentials may reveal abnormal peripheral as well as central conduction.[63]

## Acute intermittent porphyria

The porphyrias are rare hereditary disorders that belong to the large group of diseases referred to as inborn errors of metabolism. The acute intermittent form is the most common. In this form, a partial defect in hepatic heme synthesis at the level of uroporphyrinogen synthetase results in overproduction of delta aminolevulinic acid and porphobilinogen by negative feedback depression.[216] Its inheritance is autosomal dominant with higher incidence in females and variable degrees of expression.

Clinical features include abdominal pain, vomiting, peripheral neuropathy, neurogenic bladder, seizures, and mental status changes. Skin photosensitivity does not occur. The patient excretes excessive quantities of porphyrin intermediates in the urine and exposure to light may impart a deep red color to the urine as polypyrrols are formed from porphobilinogen. Although acute attacks may occur spontaneously, they are commonly triggered by the inadvertent administration of barbiturates, sulfonamides, or certain other drugs. If the neuropathy progresses rapidly, the proximal muscles may become weaker than distal muscles. The sensory loss may also occur more proximally than distally.[183]

The neuropathy of porphyria affects motor fibers regularly and sensory fibers in about 50 percent of patients. Sensory complaints, if present, are relatively mild. Weakness is often seen in proximal muscles, but distal muscles are not necessarily spared. Nerve conduction studies show low amplitude compound action potentials. Conduction velocities are normal. Fibrillation potentials and positive sharp waves are prominent in proximal muscles one to two weeks after onset.[3, 25] The time course of these findings suggests that this disorder is an acute axonal neuropathy.

## Pressure-sensitive hereditary neuropathy

In this familial disorder, slight traction or compression leads to motor and sensory symptoms of peripheral neuropathy in an otherwise asymptomatic patient.[152] The histopathologic changes include focal, sausagelike thickening of the myelin sheaths together with segmental demyelination and remyelination.[19, 148] Pressure induced, reversible motor weakness is the most prominent feature of the disease, but sensory symptoms also appear.[64] The ulnar, radial, and peroneal nerves are most susceptible to compression palsy, but plexopathy may also develop, as described in Chapter 21. Recovery from motor or sensory deficit is slow over weeks and months and may be incomplete.

The motor and sensory conduction velocities are generally slowed in paretic limbs. Electrophysiologic abnormalities of clinically normal nerves are found in approximately one half of the patients and some asymptomatic relatives.[57] Sensory and mixed nerve potentials may be affected more than motor conduction. The slowing of conduction has been attributed to an abnormally thick myelin sheath, although segmental demyelination may also be present.[24]

## Cerebral lipidosis

Polyneuropathy is a clinical feature of at least two types of cerebral lipidosis: Krabbe's disease and metachromatic leukodystrophy. In both types of cerebral lipidosis, marked slowing of nerve conduction helps establish the clinical diagnosis, although confirmation must depend on nerve or cerebral biopsy.[59, 90, 93, 227]

Krabbe's globoid cell leukodystrophy is characterized by diffuse loss of myelin throughout the cerebral white matter and peripheral nerves. Prominent perivascular cuffs of greatly enlarged cells appear with accumulation of cerebroside. The affected infants are normal at birth but, within the first few months of life, develop severe neurologic disturbances, including rigidity, head retraction, optic atrophy, bulbar paralysis, and a decorticate posture, which lead to death before the end of the first year. Neuropathy usually occurs late in the course of the disease,[65, 109, 135] but it can be the initial manifestation.[56, 144]

Metachromatic leukodystrophy is associated with abnormal breakdown of myelin resulting from a deficiency of arylsulfatase. A cerebroside sulfate that accumulates in the nervous tissue is responsible for the metachromatic staining properties. The neurologic signs include spasticity, ataxia, dementia, and neuropathy. Although generally considered a disease of infants, rare juvenile[52, 102] and adult varieties[23] have also been reported.

# Hereditary sensory neuropathy

Dyck and Ohta[71] have classified hereditary sensory neuropathy into four distinct entities. Type I is an autosomal dominant condition characterized by degeneration of the dorsal root ganglions, possibly preceded by more distal peripheral nerve degeneration. Clinical findings include loss of pain and temperature sensation, loss of stretch reflexes, and development of ulcers in the lower extremities with almost complete sparing of the upper extremities. The disease tends to be slowly progressive after its onset in the second decade of life, and deafness, diarrhea, or ataxia occasionally develop in affected individuals. Type II is autosomal recessive with onset in infancy or early childhood.[116] It tends to be more severe than Type I, affecting upper and lower extremities equally, with a higher incidence of chronic ulceration.[46] Sensory nerve action potentials are absent in this condition, with borderline slow motor nerve conduction velocities. Type III is more commonly known as familial dysautonomia or the Riley-Day syndrome;[184, 207] and Type IV is a rare congenital loss of C-fibers with complete insensitivity to pain.[146, 202]

# Lipoprotein neuropathies

Two types of lipoprotein disorders are associated with neuropathies. Bassen-Kornzweig syndrome, seen mostly in Jewish children, consists of malabsorption, cerebellar signs, retinitis pigmentosa, acanthocytosis, and virtual absence of beta-lipoprotein from the serum. Hence, the name a-beta-lipoproteinemia. The stretch reflexes and position and vibratory senses are diminished. The neurologic signs are very similar to those of Friedreich's ataxia and Refsum's syndrome. Bassen-Kornzweig disease has rarely been studied electrophysiologically, but the electromyographic findings in three patients[159] included signs of chronic partial denervation in distal limb muscles, myotonic discharges, large amplitude, long duration motor unit potentials, and reduced interference pattern. The nerve stimulation technique showed reduced amplitude of compound sensory nerve and muscle action potentials with normal conduction velocities. The fiber diameter spectrum of the sural nerve indicated loss of fibers in the 8 to 12 $\mu$ diameter range.

Tangier disease is associated with a low level of high density lipoprotein and cholesterol in the serum. The tonsils are enlarged and bright orange, reflecting deposition of cholesterol esters. The skin and rectal mucosa show similar changes. Both myelinated and unmyelinated fibers are affected.[129] Loss of pain and temperature sensation may be caused by a selective involvement of small fibers.[75] Conduction velocities may be abnormal in some cases of Tangier disease.[93]

# Giant axonal neuropathy

This is a progressive peripheral neuropathy with onset in childhood.[8, 14, 41] The condition is usually combined with minor central nervous system involvement and sometimes intellectual dysfunction.[162] Axons accumulate neurofilamentous material, which leads to ballooning and degeneration, often more prominent in motor than sensory fibers. Patients characteristically have tightly curled, reddish hair, which should be distinguished from the sparse hair in Menke's kinky hair disease. No adequate data are available at present to characterize the electrophysiologic abnormalities.

# Fabry's disease

This is a rare inborn error of glycosphingolipid metabolism with accumulation of ceramide trihexose in various tissues. The enzymatic defect of ceramide trihexosidase is transmitted as a sex-linked recessive trait. The disease affects multiple systems including skin, blood vessels, and cornea, and the cell bodies of the dorsal ganglia and spinal roots.[118] The central and peripheral nervous systems are affected as the result of accumulation of lipid in endothelial and perithelial cells of the vessel walls or secondary to perikaryal deposition of lipid.[197] Pathologic changes of axonal degeneration primarily occur in small myelinated and unmyelinated fibers. The presenting clinical features include severe burning sensations of the hands and feet. Nerve conduction velocities are frequently slowed in affected males and occasionally in female carriers.[89, 128, 195]

## Others

Other rare inherited systemic disorders that may be associated with peripheral neuropathy include sialidosis Type I or the cherry-red spot myoclonus syndrome[200] and cerebrotendinous xanthomatosis.[133]

# REFERENCE SOURCES

1. ACKIL, AA, ET AL: Late response and sural conduction studies: Usefulness in patients with chronic renal failure. Arch Neurol 38:482, 1981.

2. AGUAYO, AJ AND KARPATI, G (EDS): Current Topics in Nerve and Muscle Research. Excerpta Medica, Amsterdam, 1979.

3. ALBERS, JW, ROBERTSON, WC, AND DAUBE, JR: Electrodiagnostic findings in acute porphyric neuropathy. Muscle and Nerve 1:292, 1978.

4. ALLEN, N, ET AL: Toxic polyneuropathy due to methyl n-butyl ketone. Arch Neurol 32:209, 1975.

5. AMICK, LD AND LEMMI, H: Electromyographic studies in peroneal muscular atrophy. Charcot-Marie-Tooth disease. Arch Neurol 9:273, 1963.

6. ANTIA, NH, PANDYA, SS, AND DASTUR, DK: Nerves in the arm in leprosy. I. Clinical, electrodiagnostic and operative aspects. Int J Leprosy 38:12, 1970.

7. ASBURY, AK: Proximal diabetic neuropathy (editorial). Ann Neurol 2:179, 1977.

8. ASBURY, AK: Neuropathies with filamentous abnormalities. In AGUAYO, AJ AND KARPATI, G (EDS): Current Topics in Nerve and Muscle Research. Excerpta Medica, Amsterdam, 1979.

9. ASBURY, AK AND JOHNSON, PC: Pathology of Peripheral Nerve. WB Saunders, Philadelphia, 1978.

10. ASBURY, AK, ARNASON, BG, AND ADAMS, RD: The inflammatory lesion in idiopathic polyneuritis. Its role in pathogenesis. Medicine 48:173, 1969.

11. ASBURY, AK, VICTOR, M, AND ADAMS, RD: Uremic polyneuropathy. Trans Am Neurol Assn 87:100, 1962.

12. ASBURY, AK, ET AL: Criteria for diagnosis of Guillain-Barré syndrome. Ann Neurol 3:565, 1978.

13. ASBURY, AK, ET AL: Guillain-Barré syndrome: Is there a role for plasmapheresis? Neurology (New York) 30:1112, 1980.

14. ASBURY, AK, ET AL: Giant axonal neuropathy—A unique case with segmental neurofilamentous masses. Acta Neuropathol (Berl) 20:237, 1972.

15. BARRON, SA AND HEFFNER, RR, JR: Weakness in malignancy: Evidence for a remote effect of tumor on distal axons. Ann Neurol 4:268, 1978.

16. BEHSE, F AND BUCHTHAL, F: Alcoholic neuropathy: Clinical, electrophysiological, and biopsy findings. Ann Neurol 2:95, 1977.

17. BEHSE, F AND BUCHTHAL, F: Peroneal muscular atrophy (PMA) and related disorders. II. Histological findings in sural nerves. Brain 100:67, 1977.

18. BEHSE, F, BUCHTHAL, F, AND CARLSEN, F: Nerve biopsy and conduction studies in diabetic neuropathy. J Neurol Neurosurg Psychiatry 40:1072, 1977.

19. BEHSE, F, ET AL: *Conduction and histopathology of the sural nerve in hereditary neuropathy with liability to pressure palsies.* In DESMEDT, JE (ED): *New Developments in Electromyography and Clinical Neurophysiology,* Vol 2. Karger, Basel, 1973.

20. BLACKSTOCK, E, RUSHWORTH, G, AND GATH, D: *Electrophysiological studies in alcoholism.* J Neurol Neurosurg Psychiatry 35:326, 1972.

21. BOLTON, CF: *Peripheral neuropathies associated with chronic renal failure.* Can J Neurol Sci 7:89, 1980.

22. BOLTON, CF, DRIEDGER, AA, AND LINDSAY, RM: *Ischaemic neuropathy in uraemic patients caused by bovine arteriovenous shunt.* J Neurol Neurosurg Psychiatry 42:810, 1979.

23. BOSCH, EP AND HART, MN: *Late adult-onset metachromatic leukodystrophy. Dementia and polyneuropathy in a 63-year-old man.* Arch Neurol 35:475, 1978.

24. BOSCH, EP, ET AL: *Brachial plexus involvement in familial pressure sensitive neuropathy: Electrophysiologic and morphologic findings.* Ann Neurol 8:620, 1980.

25. BOSCH, EP, ET AL: *Effect of hematin in porphyric neuropathy.* Neurology (New York) 27:1053, 1977.

26. BOUCHE, P, ET AL: *Perhexiline maleate and peripheral neuropathy.* Neurology (New York) 29:739, 1979.

27. BRADLEY, WG: *Disorders of Peripheral Nerves.* Blackwell Scientific Publishers, Oxford, 1974.

28. BRADLEY, WG, KARLSSON, IJ, AND RASSOL, CG: *Metronidazole neuropathy.* Br Med J 2:610, 1977.

29. BRADLEY, WG, MADRID, R, AND DAVIS, CJF: *The peroneal muscular atrophy syndrome. Clinical, genetic, electrophysiological and nerve biopsy studies. Part 30—Clinical, electrophysiological and pathological correlations.* J Neurol Sci 32:123, 1977.

30. BRADLEY, WG, ET AL: *The neuromyopathy of vincristine in man. Clinical, electrophysiological and pathological studies.* J Neurol Sci 10:107, 1970.

31. BROWN, MJ, MARTIN, JR, AND ASBURY, AK: *Painful diabetic neuropathy. A morphometric study.* Arch Neurol 33:164, 1976.

32. BROWN, MJ, ET AL: *Distal neuropathy in experimental diabetes mellitus.* Ann Neurol 8:168, 1980.

33. BRUST, J, LOVELACE, R, AND DEVI, S: *Classification of Charcot-Marie-Tooth disorder by electrophysiological studies.* Fifth International Congress of Electromyography, Abstracts of Communications, Rochester, Minnesota, 1975.

34. BRUST, JCM, ET AL: *Acute generalized polyneuropathy accompanying lithium poisoning.* Ann Neurol 6:360, 1979.

35. BUCHTHAL, F: *Electrophysiological abnormalities in metabolic myopathies and neuropathies.* Acta Neurol Scand (suppl 43)46:129, 1970.

36. BUCHTHAL, F AND BEHSE, F: *Peroneal muscular atrophy (PMA) and related disorders. I. Clinical manifestations as related to biopsy findings, nerve conduction and electromyography.* Brain 100:41, 1977.

37. BUCHTHAL, F AND BEHSE, F: *Electrophysiology and nerve biopsy in men exposed to lead.* Br J Indust Med 36:135, 1979.

38. CADILHAC, J, ET AL: *Follow-up study of motor conduction velocity in uraemic patients treated by hemodialysis.* In DESMEDT, JE (ED): *New Developments in Electromyography and Clinical Neurophysiology,* Vol 2. Karger, Basel, 1973, pp 372–380.

39. CAMPBELL, MJ AND PATY, DW: *Carcinomatous neuromyopathy: 1. Electrophysiological studies. An electrophysiological and immunological study of patients with carcinoma of the lung.* J Neurol Neurosurg Psychiatry 37:131, 1974.

40. CANAL, N AND POZZA, G (EDS): *Peripheral Neuropathies. Developments in Neurology,* Vol 1. Elsevier/North-Holland Biomedical Press, Amsterdam, 1978.

41. CARPENTER, S, ET AL: *Giant axonal neuropathy. A clinically and morphologically distinct neurological disease.* Arch Neurol 31:312, 1974.

42. CASEY, EB AND LE QUESNE, PM: *Electrophysiological evidence for a distal lesion in alcoholic neuropathy.* J Neurol Neurosurg Psychiatry 35:624, 1972.

43. CASEY, EB AND LE QUESNE, PM: *Alcoholic neuropathy.* In DESMEDT, JE (ED): *New Developments in Electromyography and Clinical Neurophysiology,* Vol 2. Karger, Basel, 1973.

44. CASEY, EB, ET AL: *Vincristine neuropathy. Clinical and electrophysiological observations.* Brain 96:69, 1973.

45. CATTON, MJ, ET AL: *Subclinical neuropathy in lead workers.* Br Med J 2:80, 1970.

46. CAVANAGH, NPC, ET AL: *Hereditary sensory neuropathy with spastic paraplegia.* Brain 102:79, 1979.

47. CERRA, D AND JOHNSON, EW: *Motor nerve conduction velocity in "idiopathic" polyneuritis.* Arch Phys Med Rehabil 42:159, 1961.

48. CHARRON, L, PEYRONNARD, JM, AND MARCHAND, L: *Sensory neuropathy associated with primary biliary cirrhosis.* Arch Neurol 37:84, 1980.

49. CHOKROVERTY, S, ET AL: *The syndrome of diabetic amyotrophy.* Ann Neurol 2:181, 1977.

50. CHOPRA, JS, HURWITZ, LJ, AND MONTGOMERY, DAD: *The pathogenesis of sural nerve changes in diabetes mellitus.* Brain 92:391, 1969.

51. CHOPRA, JS, SAWHNEY, BB, AND CHAKRAVORTY, RN: *Pathology and time relationship of peripheral nerve changes in experimental diabetes.* J Neurol Sci 32:53, 1977.

52. CLARK, JR, MILLER, RG, AND VIDGOFF, JM: *Juvenile-onset metachromatic leukodystrophy: Biochemical and electrophysiologic studies.* Neurology (New York) 29:346, 1979.

53. COHEN, AS AND BENSON, MD: *Amyloid neuropathy.* In DYCK, PJ, THOMAS, PK, AND LAMBERT, EH (EDS): *Peripheral Neuropathy,* Vol II. WB Saunders, Philadelphia, 1975.

54. CONRAD, B, ASCHOFF, JC, AND FISCHLER, M: *Der diagnostische Wert der F-Wellen-Latenz.* J Neurol 210:151, 1975.

55. COX-KLAZINGA, M AND ENDTZ, LJ: *Peripheral nerve involvement in pernicious anaemia.* J Neurol Sci 45:367, 1980.

56. CRUZ MARTINEZ, A, ET AL: *Peripheral neuropathy detected on electrophysiological study as first manifestation of metachromatic leucodystrophy in infancy.* J Neurol Neurosurg Psychiatry 38:169, 1975.

57. CRUZ MARTINEZ, A, ET AL: *Recurrent familiar polyneuropathy with liability to pressure palsies. Special regards to electrophysiological aspects of twenty-five members from seven families.* Electromyogr Clin Neurophysiol 17:101, 1977.

58. DALAKAS, MC AND ENGEL, WK: *Immunoglobulin and complement deposits in nerves of patients with chronic relapsing polyneuropathy.* Arch Neurol 37:637, 1980.

59. DAYAN, AD: *Peripheral neuropathy of metachromatic leucodystrophy: Observations on segmental demyelination and remyelination and the intracellular distribution of sulphatide.* J Neurol Neurosurg Psychiatry 30:311, 1967.

60. DEJERINE, J: *Sur une forme particulière de maladie de Friedreich avec atrophie musculaire et troubles de la senibilité.* C R Soc Biol (Memoires) 42:43, 1890.

61. DEJERINE, J AND SOTTAS, J: *Sur la névrite interstitielle, hypertrophique et progressive de l'enfance.* C R Soc Biol 45:63, 1893.

62. DELANEY, P: *Neurologic manifestations in sarcoidosis. Review of the literature, with a report of 23 cases.* Ann Intern Med 87:336, 1977.

63. DESMEDT, JE AND NOËL, P: *Average cerebral evoked potentials in the evaluation of lesions in the sensory nerves and of the central somatosensory pathway.* In DESMEDT, JE (ED): *New Developments in Electromyography and Clinical Neurophysiology,* Vol 2. Karger, Basel, 1973, pp 352–871.

64. DUBI, J, ET AL: *Recurrent familial neuropathy with liability to pressure palsies. Reports of two cases and ultrastructural nerve study.* J Neurol 220:43, 1979.

65. DUNN, HG, ET AL: *The neuropathy of Krabbe's infantile cerebral sclerosis (globoid cell leucodystrophy).* Brain 92:329, 1969.

66. DYCK, PJ: *Inherited neuronal degeneration and atrophy affecting peripheral motor, sensory, and autonomic neurons.* In DYCK, PJ, THOMAS, PK, AND LAMBERT, EH (EDS): *Peripheral Neuropathy,* Vol 2. WB Saunders, Philadelphia, 1975, pp 825–867.

67. DYCK, PJ AND GOMEZ, MR: *Segmental demyelination in Dejerine-Sottas disease: Light, phase-contrast, and electron microscopic studies.* Mayo Clin Proc 43:280, 1968.

68. DYCK, PJ AND LAMBERT, EH: *Lower motor and primary sensory neuron diseases with peroneal muscular atrophy. I. Neurologic, genetic, and electrophysiolgic findings in hereditary polyneuropathies.* Arch Neurol 18:603, 1968.

69. DYCK, PJ AND LAMBERT, EH: *Lower motor and primary sensory neuron diseases with peroneal muscular atrophy. II. Neurologic, genetic, and electrophysiologic findings in various neuronal degenerations.* Arch Neurol 18:619, 1968.

70. DYCK, PJ AND LAMBERT, EH: *Dissociated sensation in amyloidosis. Compound action potential, quantitative histologic and teased-fiber, and electron microscopic studies of sural nerve biopsies.* Arch Neurol 20:490, 1969.

71. DYCK, PJ AND OHTA, M: *Neuronal atrophy and degeneration predominantly affecting peripheral sensory neurons.* In DYCK, PJ, THOMAS, PK, AND LAMBERT, EH (EDS): *Peripheral Neuropathy,* Vol 2. WB Saunders, Philadelphia, 1975, pp 791–824.

72. DYCK, PJ, LAMBERT, EH, AND MULDER, DW: *Charcot-Marie-Tooth disease: Nerve conduction and clinical studies of a large kinship.* Neurology (Minneap) 13:1, 1963.

73. DYCK, PJ, LAMBERT, EH, AND NICHOLS, PC: *Quantitative measurement of sensation related to compound action potential and number and sizes of myelinated and unmyelinated fibers of sural nerve in health, Friedreich's ataxia, hereditary sensory neuropathy, and tabes dorsalis.* In RÉMOND, A (ED): *Handbook of Electroencephalography and Clinical Neurophysiology,* Vol 9. Elsevier, Amsterdam, 1971, pp 83–118.

74. DYCK, PJ, THOMAS, PK, AND LAMBERT, EH (EDS): *Peripheral Neuropathy.* WB Saunders, Philadelphia, 1975.

75. DYCK, PJ, ET AL: *Adult-onset of Tangier disease: 1. Morphometric and pathologic studies suggesting delayed degradation of neutral lipids after fiber degeneration.* J Neuropathol Exp Neurol 37:119, 1978.

76. DYCK, PJ, ET AL: *Segmental demyelination secondary to axonal·degeneration in uremic neuropathy.* Mayo Clin Proc 46:400, 1971.

77. EISEN, A AND HUMPHREYS, P: *The Guillain-Barré syndrome. A clinical and electrodiagnostic study of 25 cases.* Arch Neurol 30:438, 1974.

78. EISEN, AA, WOODS, JF, AND SHERWIN, AL: *Peripheral nerve function in long-term therapy with diphenylhydantoin. A clinical and electrophysiologic correlation.* Neurology (Minneap) 24:411, 1974.

79. ELLENBERG, M: *Diabetic truncal mononeuropathy—A new clinical syndrome.* Diabetes Care 1:10, 1978.

80. EMERY, JP, LASSERRE, PP, AND DRYLL, A: *Les manifestations neurologiques périphériques de la sarcoïdose.* Sem Hop Paris 48:3039, 1972.

81. ENG, GD, ET AL: *Nerve conduction velocity determinations in juvenile diabetes: Continuing study of 190 patients.* Arch Phys Med Rehabil 57:1, 1976.

82. EWING, DJ, ET AL: *Peripheral motor nerve function in diabetic autonomic neuropathy.* J Neurol Neurosurg Psychiatry 39:453, 1976.

83. FELDMAN, RG, HADDOW, J, AND CHISOLM, JJ: *Chronic lead intoxication in urban children. Motor nerve conduction velocity studies.* In DESMEDT, JE (ED): *New Developments in Electromyography and Clinical Neurophysiology,* Vol 2. Karger, Basel, 1973.

84. FELDMAN, RG, ET AL: *Peripheral neuropathy in arsenic smelter workers.* Neurology (New York) 29:939, 1979.

85. FINELLI, PF AND DIBENEDETTO, M: *Bilateral involvement of the lateral cutaneous nerve of the calf in a diabetic.* Ann Neurol 4:480, 1978.

86. FISHER, M: *An unusual variant of acute idiopathic polyneuritis (syndrome of ophthalmoplegia, ataxia, and areflexia).* N Engl J Med 255:57, 1956.

87. FITTING, JW, ET AL: *Neuropathy, amyloidosis, and monoclonal gammopathy.* J Neurol Neurosurg Psychiatry 42:193, 1979.

88. FOWLER, H, ET AL: *Recovery from chronic progressive polyneuropathy after treatment with plasma exchange and cyclophosphamide.* Lancet 2:1193, 1979.

89. FUKUHARA, N, ET AL: *Fabry's disease on the mechanism of the peripheral nerve involvement.* Acta Neuropathol (Berl) 33:9, 1975.

90.  FULLERTON, PM: *Peripheral nerve conduction in metachromatic leucodystrophy (sulphatide lipidosis).* J Neurol Neurosurg Psychiatry 27:100, 1964.

91.  FULLERTON, PM AND O'SULLIVAN, DJ: *Thalidomide neuropathy: A clinical, electrophysiological, and histological follow-up study.* J Neurol Neurosurg Psychiatry 31:543, 1968.

92.  GABBAY, KH: *The sorbitol pathway and the complications of diabetes.* N Engl J Med 288:831, 1973.

93.  GAMSTORP, I: *Involvement of peripheral nerves in disorders causing progressive cerebral symptoms and signs in infancy and childhood.* In DESMEDT, JE (ED): *New Developments in Electromyography and Clinical Neurophysiology,* Vol 2. Karger, Basel, 1973.

94.  GARDNER-THORPE, C AND BENJAMIN, S: *Peripheral neuropathy after disulfiram administration.* J Neurol Neurosurg Psychiatry 34:253, 1971.

95.  GILLIATT, RW: *Peripheral nerve conduction in neurological patients (abstr).* J Neurol Neurosurg Psychiatry 22:344, 1959.

96.  GILLIATT, RW AND THOMAS, PK: *Extreme slowing of nerve conduction in peroneal muscular atrophy.* Ann Phys Med 4:104, 1957.

97.  GILLIATT, RW AND WILLISON, RG: *Peripheral nerve conduction in diabetic neuropathy.* J Neurol Neurosurg Psychiatry 25:11, 1962.

98.  GLENNER, GG: *Amyloid deposits and amyloidosis. The β-fibrilloses.* (First of two parts) N Engl J Med 302:1283, 1980.

99.  GOLDSTEIN, NP, MCCALL, JT, AND DYCK, PJ: *Metal neuropathy.* In DYCK, PJ, THOMAS, PK, AND LAMBERT, EH (EDS): *Peripheral Neuropathy,* Vol 2. WB Saunders, Philadelphia, 1975.

100.  GRAF, RJ, ET AL: *Nerve conduction abnormalities in untreated maturity-onset diabetes: Relation to levels of fasting plasma glucose and glycosylated hemoglobin.* Ann Int Med 90:298, 1979.

101.  GREGERSEN, G: *Diabetic neuropathy: Influence of age, sex, metabolic control, and duration of diabetes on motor conduction velocity.* Neurology (Minneap) 17:972, 1967.

102.  HALTIA, T, ET AL: *Juvenile metachromatic leukodystrophy. Clinical, biochemical, and neuropathologic studies in nine new cases.* Arch Neurol 37:42, 1980.

103.  HANSEN, S AND BALLANTYNE, JP: *Axonal dysfunction in the neuropathy of diabetes mellitus: A quantitative electrophysiological study.* J Neurol Neurosurg Psychiatry 40:555, 1977.

104.  HANSEN, S AND BALLANTYNE, JP: *A quantitative electrophysiological study of uraemic neuropathy. Diabetic and renal neuropathies compared.* J Neurol Neurosurg Psychiatry 41:128, 1978.

105.  HARDING, AE AND THOMAS, PK: *The clinical features of hereditary motor and sensory neuropathy types I and II.* Brain 103:259, 1980.

106.  HAUSMANOWA-PETRUSEWICZ, I, ET AL: *Nerve conduction in the Guillain-Barré-Strohl syndrome.* J Neurol 220:169, 1979.

107.  HAWKES, CH, ET AL: *Hypertrophic mononeuropathy.* J Neurol Neurosurg Psychiatry 37:76, 1974.

108.  HAWLEY, RJ, ET AL: *The carcinomatous neuromyopathy of oat cell lung cancer.* Ann Neurol 7:65, 1980.

109.  HOGAN, GR, GUTMANN, L, AND CHOU, SM: *The peripheral neuropathy of Krabbe's (globoid) leukodystrophy.* Neurology (Minneap) 19:1094, 1969.

110.  HOROWITZ, SH AND GINSBERG-FELLNER, F: *Ischemia and sensory nerve conduction in diabetes mellitus.* Neurology (New York) 29:695, 1979.

111.  HORWICH, MS, ET AL: *Subacute sensory neuropathy: A remote effect of carcinoma.* Ann Neurol 2:7, 1977.

112.  ISCH, F, ET AL: *Measurement of conduction velocity of motor nerve fibres in polyneuritis and polyradiculoneuritis.* Electroenceph Clin Neurophysiol 16:416, 1964.

113.  JOHNSON, EW AND WAYLONIS, GW: *Facial nerve conduction delay in patients with diabetes mellitus.* Arch Phys Med Rehabil 45:131, 1964.

114.  JOHNSON, PC: *Hematogenous metastases of carcinoma to dorsal root ganglia.* Acta Neuropathol (Berl) 38:171, 1977.

115. JOHNSON, PC, ET AL: *Paraneoplastic vasculitis of nerve: A remote effect of cancer.* Ann Neurol 5:437, 1979.

116. JOHNSON, RH AND SPALDING, JMK: *Progressive sensory neuropathy in children.* J Neurol Neurosurg Psychiatry 27:125, 1964.

117. KAESER, HE: *Klinische und elektromyographische Verlaufsuntersuchungen beim Guillain-Barré-syndrom.* Schweiz Arch Neurol Neurochir Psychiatr 94:278, 1964.

118. KAHN, P: *Anderson-Fabry disease: A histopathological study of three cases with observations on the mechanism of production of pain.* J Neurol Neurosurg Psychiatry 36:1053, 1973.

119. KELLY, JJ, JR, ET AL: *The natural history of peripheral neuropathy in primary systemic amyloidosis.* Ann Neurol 6:1, 1979.

120. KILLIAN, JM AND KLOEPFER, HW: *Homozygous expression of a dominant gene for Charcot-Marie-Tooth neuropathy.* Ann Neurol 5:515, 1979.

121. KIMURA, J: *An evaluation of the facial and trigeminal nerves in polyneuropathy: Electrodiagnostic study in Charcot-Marie-Tooth disease, Guillain-Barré syndrome, and diabetic neuropathy.* Neurology (Minneap) 21:745, 1971.

122. KIMURA, J: *F-wave velocity in the central segment of the median and ulnar nerves. A study in normal subjects and in patients with Charcot-Marie-Tooth disease.* Neurology (Minneap) 24:539, 1974.

123. KIMURA, J: *Proximal versus distal slowing of motor nerve conduction velocity in the Guillain-Barré syndrome.* Ann Neurol 3:344, 1978.

124. KIMURA, J AND BUTZER, JF: *F-wave conduction velocity in Guillain-Barré syndrome. Assessment of nerve segment between axilla and spinal cord.* Arch Neurol 32:524, 1975.

125. KIMURA, J, BOSCH, P, AND LINDSAY, GM: *F-wave conduction velocity in the central segment of the peroneal and tibial nerves.* Arch Phys Med Rehabil 56:492, 1975.

126. KIMURA, J, YAMADA, T, AND STEVLAND, NP: *Distal slowing of motor nerve conduction velocity in diabetic polyneuropathy.* J Neurol Sci 42:291, 1979.

127. KING, D AND ASHBY, P: *Conduction velocity in the proximal segments of a motor nerve in the Guillain-Barré syndrome.* J Neurol Neurosurg Psychiatry 39:538, 1976.

128. KOCEN, RS AND THOMAS, PK: *Peripheral nerve involvement in Fabry's disease.* Arch Neurol 22:81, 1970.

129. KOCEN, RS, ET AL: *Nerve biopsy findings in two cases of Tangier disease.* Acta Neuropathol (Berl) 26:317, 1973.

130. KOLLER, WC, ET AL: *Dapsone-induced peripheral neuropathy.* Arch Neurol 34:644, 1977.

131. KÖMPF, D, ET AL: *Mononeuritis multiplex bei Boeckscher Sarkoidose.* Nervenarzt 47:687, 1976.

132. KURDI, A AND ABDUL-KADER, M: *Clinical and electrophysiological studies of diphtheritic neuritis in Jordan.* J Neurol Sci 42:243, 1979.

133. KURITZKY, A, BERGINER, VM, AND KORCZYN, AD: *Peripheral neuropathy in cerebrotendinous xanthomatosis.* Neurology (New York) 29:880, 1979.

134. KYLE, RA AND BAYRD, ED: *Amyloidosis: Review of 236 cases.* Medicine (Baltimore) 54:271, 1975.

135. LAKE, BD: *Segmental demyelination of peripheral nerves in Krabbe's disease.* Nature 217:171, 1968.

136. LALLEMAND, RC AND WELLER, RO: *Intraneural neurofibromas involving the posterior interosseous nerve.* J Neurol Neurosurg Psychiatry 36:991, 1973.

137. LAMBERT, EH: *Electromyography and electric stimulation of peripheral nerves and muscle.* In *Clinical Examinations in Neurology.* By Depts of Neurology, Physiology, and Biophysics, Mayo Clinic and Mayo Foundation, ed 4, Chap 16, pp 298–329, WB Saunders, Philadelphia, 1976.

138. LAMBERT, EH AND MULDER, DW: *Nerve conduction in the Guillain-Barré syndrome.* Electroenceph Clin Neurophysiol 17:86, 1964.

139. LAMONTAGNE, A AND BUCHTHAL, F: *Electrophysiological studies in diabetic neuropathy.* J Neurol Neurosurg Psychiatry 33:442, 1970.

140. LAYZER, RB, FISHMAN, RA, AND SCHAFER, JA: *Neuropathy following abuse of nitrous oxide.* Neurology (New York) 28:504, 1978.

141. LAZARO, RP AND KIRSHNER, HS: *Proximal muscle weakness in uremia. Case reports and review of the literature.* Arch Neurol 37:555, 1980.

142. LE QUESNE, PM: *Neuropathy due to drugs.* In DYCK, PJ, THOMAS, PK, AND LAMBERT, EH (EDS): *Peripheral Neuropathy.* WB Saunders, Philadelphia, 1975.

143. LE QUESNE, PM: *Neurophysiological investigation of subclinical and minimal toxic neuropathies.* Muscle and Nerve 1:392, 1978.

144. LIEBERMAN, JS, ET AL: *Perinatal neuropathy as an early manifestation of Krabbe's disease.* Arch Neurol 37:446, 1980.

145. LISAK, RP, ET AL: *Guillain-Barré syndrome and Hodgkin's disease: Three cases with immunological studies.* Ann Neurol 1:72, 1977.

146. LOW, PA, BURKE, WJ, AND MCLEOD, JG: *Congenital sensory neuropathy with selective loss of small myelinated fibers.* Ann Neurol 3:179, 1978.

147. LOW, PA, ET AL: *The sympathetic nervous system in diabetic neuropathy. A clinical and pathological study.* Brain 98:341, 1975.

148. MADRID, R AND BRADLEY, WG: *The pathology of neuropathies with focal thickening of the myelin sheath (tomaculous neuropathy). Studies on the formation of the abnormal myelin sheath.* J Neurol Sci 25:415, 1975.

149. MADRID, R, BRADLEY, WG, AND DAVIS, CJF: *The peroneal muscular atrophy syndrome. Part 2—Observations on pathological changes in sural nerve biopsies.* J Neurol Sci 32:91, 1977.

150. MAGORA, A, ET AL: *The condition of the peripheral nerve in leprosy under various forms of treatment. Conduction velocity studies in long-term follow-up.* Int J Leprosy 39:639, 1971.

151. MAWDSLEY, C AND MAYER, RF: *Nerve conduction in alcoholic polyneuropathy.* Brain 88:335, 1965.

152. MAYER, RF: *Hereditary neuropathy manifested by recurring nerve palsies.* In VINKEN, PJ AND BRUYN, GW (EDS): *Handbook of Clinical Neurology, Vol 21.* American Elsevier, New York, 1975, pp 87–105.

153. MAYER, RF AND DENNY-BROWN, D: *Conduction velocity in peripheral nerve during experimental demyelination in the cat.* Neurology (Minneap) 14:714, 1964.

154. MCDONALD, WI: *Experimental neuropathy. The use of diphtheria toxin.* In DESMEDT, JE (ED): *New Developments in Electromyography and Clinical Neurophysiology, Vol 2.* Karger, Basel, 1973, pp 128–144.

155. MCLEOD, JG: *An electrophysiological and pathological study of peripheral nerves in Friedreich's ataxia.* J Neurol Sci 12:333, 1971.

156. MCLEOD, JG: *Carcinomatous neuropathy.* In DYCK, PJ, THOMAS, PK, AND LAMBERT, EH (EDS): *Peripheral Neuropathy, Vol 2.* WB Saunders, Philadelphia, 1975.

157. MCLEOD, JG AND WALSH, JC: *Neuropathies associated with paraproteinemias and dysproteinemias.* In DYCK, PJ, THOMAS, PK, AND LAMBERT, EH (EDS): *Peripheral Neuropathy, Vol 2.* WB Saunders, Philadelphia, 1975, pp 1012–1029.

158. MCLEOD, JG, ET AL: *Nerve conduction studies in leprosy.* Int J Leprosy 43:21, 1975.

159. MILLER, RG, ET AL: *The neuropathy of abetalipoproteinemia.* Neurology (New York) 30:1286, 1980.

160. MITSUMOTO, H, WILBOURN, AJ, AND GOREN, H: *Perineurioma as the cause of localized hypertrophic neuropathy.* Muscle and Nerve 3:403, 1980.

161. MITZ, M, ET AL: *Motor nerve conduction indicators in uremic neuropathy.* Arch Phys Med Rehabil 61:45, 1980.

162. MIZUNO, Y, ET AL: *Giant axonal neuropathy. Combined central and peripheral nervous system disease.* Arch Neurol 36:107, 1979.

163. MOODY, JF: *Electrophysiological investigations into the neurological complications of carcinoma.* Brain 88:1023, 1965.

164. MORGAN-HUGHES, JA, SINCLAIR, S, AND DURSTON, JHJ: *The pattern of peripheral nerve regeneration induced by crush in rats with severe acrylamide neuropathy.* Brain 97:235, 1974.

165. MULDER, DW, ET AL: *The neuropathies associated with diabetes mellitus. A clinical and electromyographic study of 103 unselected diabetic patients.* Neurology (Minneap) 11:275, 1961.

166. MURRAY, NMF AND WADE, DT: *The sural sensory action potential in Guillain-Barré syndrome.* Muscle and Nerve 3:444, 1980.

167. MYERS, RR, ET AL: *Changes in endoneurial fluid pressure, permeability, and peripheral nerve ultrastructure in experimental lead neuropathy.* Ann Neurol 8:392, 1980.

168. NIELSEN, VK: *The peripheral nerve function in chronic renal failure. V. Sensory and motor conduction velocity.* Acta Med Scand 194:445, 1973.

169. NIELSEN, VK: *The peripheral nerve function in chronic renal failure. VII. Longitudinal course during terminal renal failure and regular hemodialysis.* Acta Med Scand 195:155, 1974.

170. NIELSEN, VK: *The peripheral nerve function in chronic renal failure. IX. Recovery after renal transplantation. Electrophysiological aspects (sensory and motor nerve conduction).* Acta Med Scand 195:171, 1974.

171. NIELSEN, VK AND PILGAARD, S: *On the pathogenesis of Charcot-Marie-Tooth disease. A study of the sensory and motor conduction velocity in the median nerve.* Acta Orthop Scand 43:4, 1972.

172. NOËL, P: *Diabetic neuropathy.* In DESMEDT, JE (ED): *New Developments in Electromyography and Clinical Neurophysiology,* Vol 2. Karger, Basel, 1973, pp 318–332.

173. NOËL, P: *Sensory nerve conduction in the upper limbs at various stages of diabetic neuropathy.* J Neurol Neurosurg Psychiatry 36:786, 1973.

174. NOËL, P, LAUVAUX, JP, AND PIRART, J: *Upper limbs diabetic neuropathy: A clinical and electrophysiological study.* Horm Metab Res 3:386, 1971.

175. OH, SJ: *Sarcoid polyneuropathy: A histologically proved case.* Ann Neurol 7:178, 1980.

176. OH, SJ: *Subacute demyelinating polyneuropathy responding to corticosteroid treatment.* Arch Neurol 35:509, 1978.

177. OH, SJ, ET AL: *Rapid improvement in nerve conduction velocity following renal transplantation.* Ann Neurol 4:369, 1978.

178. OLNEY, RK AND MILLER, RG: *Peripheral neuropathy associated with disulfiram administration.* Muscle and Nerve 3:172, 1980.

179. PAUL, T, ET AL: *Carcinomatous neuromuscular syndromes. A clinical and quantitative electrophysiological study.* Brain 101:53, 1978.

180. PRINEAS, JW AND MCLEOD, JG: *Chronic relapsing polyneuritis.* J Neurol Sci 27:427, 1976.

181. RAFF, MC AND ASBURY, AK: *Ischemic mononeuropathy and mononeuropathy multiplex in diabetes mellitus.* N Engl J Med 279:17, 1968.

182. READ, DJ, VANHEGAN, RI, AND MATTHEWS, WB: *Peripheral neuropathy and benign IgG paraproteinaemia.* J Neurol Neurosurg Psychiatry 41:215, 1978.

183. RIDLEY, A: *The neuropathy of acute intermittent porphyria.* Q J Med 38:307, 1969.

184. RILEY, CM, ET AL: *Central autonomic dysfunction with defective lacrimation. I. Report of 5 cases.* Paediatrics 3:468, 1949.

185. SAHENK, Z, ET AL: *Polyneuropathy from inhalation of $N_2O$ cartridges through a whipped-cream dispenser.* Neurology (New York) 28:485, 1978.

186. SAID, G: *Perhexiline neuropathy: A clinicopathological study.* Ann Neurol 3:259, 1978.

187. SAID, G: *A clinicopathologic study of acrodystrophic neuropathies.* Muscle and Nerve 3:491, 1980.

188. SALES LUÍS, ML: *Electroneurophysiological studies in familial amyloid polyneuropathy— Portuguese type.* J Neurol Neurosurg Psychiatry 41:847, 1978.

189. SATRAN, R: *Dejerine-Sottas disease revisited.* Arch Neurol 37:67, 1980.

190. SCHOLD, SC, ET AL: *Subacute motor neuronopathy: A remote effect of lymphoma.* Ann Neurol 5:271, 1979.

191. SEBILLE, A: *Respective importance of different nerve conduction velocities in leprosy.* J Neurol Sci 38:89, 1978.

192. SEBILLE, A AND GRAY, F: *Electromyographic recording and muscle biopsy in lepromatous leprosy.* J Neurol Sci 40:3, 1979.

193. DE SENA, PG: *Aspectos neurologicos e electromyographicos da Hanseniase.* Arq Neuro-Psiquiat 34:1, 1976.

194. SERVER, AC, ET AL: *Treatment of chronic relapsing inflammatory polyradiculoneuropathy by plasma exchange.* Ann Neurol 6:258, 1979.

195. SHETH, KJ AND SWICK, HM: *Peripheral nerve conduction in Fabry disease.* Ann Neurol 7:319, 1980.

196. SHY, GM AND SILVERSTEIN, I: *A study of the effects upon the motor unit by remote malignancy.* Brain 88:515, 1965.

197. SIMA, AAF AND ROBERTSON, DM: *Involvement of peripheral nerve and muscle in Fabry's disease. Histologic, ultrastructural, and morphometric studies.* Arch Neurol 35:291, 1978.

198. SNYDER, M, CANCILLA, PA, AND BATZDORF, U: *Hypertrophic neuropathy simulating a neoplasm of the brachial plexus.* Surg Neurol 7:131, 1977.

199. SPENCER, PS, ET AL: *Nervous system degeneration produced by the industrial solvent methyl n-butyl ketone.* Arch Neurol 32:219, 1975.

200. STEINMAN, L, ET AL: *Peripheral neuropathy in the cherry-red spot-myoclonus syndrome (sialidosis type I).* Ann Neurol 7:450, 1980.

201. STERMAN, AB, SCHAUMBURG, HH, AND ASBURY, AK: *The acute sensory neuronopathy syndrome: A distinct clinical entity.* Ann Neurol 7:354, 1980.

202. SWANSON, AG: *Congenital insensitivity to pain with anhydrosis. A unique syndrome in two male siblings.* Arch Neurol 8:299, 1963.

203. SWASH, M, PERRIN, J, AND SCHWARTZ, MS: *Significance of immunoglobulin deposition in peripheral nerve in neuropathies associated with paraproteinaemia.* J Neurol Neurosurg Psychiatry 42:179, 1979.

204. SWIFT, TR, ET AL: *The peroneal and tibial nerves in lepromatous leprosy. Clinical and electrophysiologic observations.* Int J Leprosy 41:25, 1973.

205. TERÄVÄINEN, H AND LARSEN, A: *Some features of the neuromuscular complications of pulmonary carcinoma.* Ann Neurol 2:495, 1977.

206. THAGE, O, TROJABORG, W, AND BUCHTHAL, F: *Electromyographic findings in polyneuropathy.* Neurology (Minneap) 13:273, 1963.

207. THOMAS, PK: *Peripheral neuropathy.* In MATTHEWS, WB (ED): *Recent Advances in Clinical Neurology.* Churchill Livingstone, Edinburgh, 1975, pp 253–283.

208. THOMAS, PK: *Screening for peripheral neuropathy in patients treated by chronic hemodialysis.* Muscle and Nerve 1:396, 1978.

209. THOMAS, PK AND CALNE, DB: *Motor nerve conduction velocity in peroneal muscular atrophy: Evidence for genetic heterogeneity.* J Neurol Neurosurg Psychiatry 37:68, 1974.

210. THOMAS, PK AND KING, RHM: *Peripheral nerve changes in amyloid neuropathy.* Brain 97:395, 1974.

211. THOMAS, PK, CALNE, DB, AND STEWART, G: *Hereditary motor and sensory polyneuropathy (peroneal muscular atrophy).* Ann Hum Genet (Lond) 38:111, 1974.

212. TOYKA, KV, ET AL: *Plasma exchange in polyradiculoneuropathy.* Ann Neurol 8:205, 1980.

213. TREDICI, G, MINAZZI, M, AND LAMPUGNANI, E: *Peripheral neuropathy in angioimmunoblastic lymphadenopathy with dysproteinaemia.* J Neurol Neurosurg Psychiatry 42:519, 1979.

214. TROJABORG, W, FRANTZEN, E, AND ANDERSEN, I: *Peripheral neuropathy and myopathy associated with carcinoma of the lung.* Brain 92:71, 1969.

215. TROTTER, JL, ENGEL, WK, AND IGNACZAK, TF: *Amyloidosis with plasma cell dyscrasia. An overlooked cause of adult onset sensorimotor neuropathy.* Arch Neurol 34:209, 1977.

216. TSCHUDY, DP, VALSAMIS, M, AND MAGNUSSEN, CR: *Acute intermittent porphyria: Clinical and selected research aspects.* Ann Int Med 83:851, 1975.

217. VALLAT, JM, ET AL: *Cryoglobulinemic neuropathy: A pathological study.* Ann Neurol 8:179, 1980.

218. VAN DER MOST VAN SPIJK, D, HOOGLAND, RA, AND DIJKSTRA, S: *Conduction velocities compared and related to degrees of renal insufficiency.* In DESMEDT, JE (ED): *New Developments in Electromyography and Clinical Neurophysiology,* Vol 2. Karger, Basel, 1973, pp 381–389.

219. VAN LIS, JMJ AND JENNEKENS, FGI: *Plasma proteins in human peripheral nerve.* J Neurol Sci 34:329, 1977.

220. VASILESCU, C: *Motor nerve conduction velocity and electromyogram in triorthocresyl-phosphate poisoning.* Rev Roum Neurol 9:345, 1972.

221. WALSH, JC: *The neuropathy of multiple myeloma. An electrophysiological and histological study.* Arch Neurol 25:404, 1971.

222. WALSH, JC AND McLEOD, JG: *Alcoholic neuropathy. An electrophysiological and histological study.* J. Neurol Sci 10:457, 1970.

223. WAXMAN, SG AND SABIN, TD: *Diabetic truncal polyneuropathy.* Arch Neurol 38:46, 1981.

224. WILLIAMS, IR, ET AL: *Neuropathy in chronic renal failure.* In DESMEDT, JE (ED): *New Developments in Electromyography and Clinical Neurophysiology,* Vol 2. Karger, Basel, 1973, pp 390–399.

225. WILLIAMS, D ET AL: *Landry-Guillain-Barré syndrome with abnormal pupils and normal eye movements: A case report.* Neurology (New York) 29:1033, 1979.

226. WINEGRAD, AI AND GREENE, DA: *Diabetic polyneuropathy: The importance of insulin deficiency, hyperglycemia and alterations in myoinositol metabolism in its pathogenesis.* N Engl J Med 295:1416, 1976.

227. YUDELL, A, ET AL: *The neuropathy of sulfatide lipidosis (metachromatic leukodystrophy).* Neurology (Minneap) 17:103, 1967.

# MONONEUROPATHIES AND ENTRAPMENT SYNDROMES

Traumatic injury can occur anywhere in the peripheral nervous system, but certain individual nerves are particularly subject to isolated damage. These include the long thoracic, suprascapular, musculocutaneous and axillary nerves in the shoulder girdle, and lateral femoral cutaneous, femoral, and sciatic nerves in the pelvic girdle. More distally, entrapment syndromes develop at vulnerable segments, secondary to chronic or recurrent trauma.[2, 74, 108] The common sites of compression are well known for the radial, median, ulnar, common peroneal, and tibial nerves. The clinical pattern most useful in the diagnosis of a focal nerve lesion is weakness and atrophy of all muscles supplied by the nerve distal to the lesion. Sensory findings usually appear earlier but are less reliable than motor deficits as localizing signs. This is particulary true in the upper extremities, where sensory dermatomes overlap considerably.

Electrophysiologic studies are of great assistance in the differential diagnosis of mononeuropathies. Nerve conduction studies may detect evidence of demyelination which usually precedes axonal degeneration in a compression neuropathy. Determination of conduction abnormalities is particularly useful with stimulation above and below the suspected site of lesion. In addition to slowing of conduction velocity, changes in amplitude of the muscle or nerve action potential are valuable indices of conduction block. The pattern of conduction abnormalities helps to differentiate an entrapment syndrome from a diffuse neuropathy, although sometimes this distinction is difficult, since early polyneuropathies may only be manifest at the common sites of compression. Electromyographic examination, delineating the exact distribution of denervated muscles, helps to localize a focal nerve lesion. The test may show no evidence of denervation in the presence of advanced demyelination as long as the axon is preserved; however, the conduction block usually associated with demyelination results in a reduced recruitment pattern of motor unit potentials.

## CRANIAL NERVES

The facial and accessory nerves are the most common cranial nerves assessed in an electromyographic laboratory. They are both easy to stimulate electrically, and the muscles they innervate are readily accessible to needle examination.

# Facial nerve

One of the most common diseases affecting the facial nerve is Bell's palsy. The etiology remains unknown, but the intraosseous portion of the facial nerve is swollen and hyperemic during the acute stage. Paralysis of the upper and lower portions of the face develops suddenly and may be associated with pain behind the ear. Additional features may include loss of taste in the anterior two thirds of the tongue and hyperacusis on the affected side. Function returns in at least 80 percent of patients without specific therapy.[161] Recovery is complete if denervation does not occur, whereas the return of function is late and incomplete after total degeneration of the facial nerve. The development of synkinetic movements is the rule in the latter group (see Fig. 16-9).[66] Peripheral facial paresis secondary to herpes zoster infection carries a less favorable prognosis. Diabetic patients with facial palsy are much more likely to display complete paresis and evidence of denervation.[1] Sensory signs in the trigeminal distribution may occur in an otherwise typical case of Bell's palsy.[138]

Serial electrodiagnostic studies are helpful in following the course of the illness (see Fig. 16-3 and Tables 16-2 and 16-3). Normal nerve excitability and a normal direct response elicited by stimulation of the facial nerve after the fourth to fifth day is a sign of good prognosis, although late degeneration can still occur. If previously absent blink reflex responses, either R1 or R2, return while the direct response is normal, or nearly normal, recovery will almost certainly be complete (see Fig. 16-7). Thus, the return of R1 or R2 offers a reasonable assurance that the remaining axons will survive without undergoing further deterioration. Unfortunately, the initial recovery of the reflex rarely occurs during the first few days after onset. In a series of 56 patients who recovered from Bell's palsy without distal degeneration, the reflex on the affected side was elicitable in 57 percent during the latter half of the first week, in 67 percent during the second week, and in 89 percent during the third week.[66] Other signs for good prognosis include incomplete clinical paresis and the presence of voluntary motor unit potentials in electromyography.

In the absence of substantial nerve degeneration, the latency of the direct response remains unaltered throughout the course on the affected side. In these patients, however, the latency of R1 of the blink reflex, if present, is slightly prolonged during the first days, increases during the latter half of the first week, then remains essentially unchanged up to the fourth week. It then shows a notable recovery during the second month and becomes essentially normal during the third or fourth month (see Fig. 16-8). A marked delay of R1 in this group of patients suggests neurapraxia with demyelination of the facial nerve and implies that the commonly used term physiologic or functional block is inappropriate to describe most cases of the milder form of Bell's palsy, despite the absence of axonal degeneration. If the facial nerve is substantially degenerated, the ultimate recovery, of course, depends on the completeness of regeneration, which generally takes a few months to a few years.

Facial nerve involvement may be part of a more diffuse condition, such as the Guillain-Barré syndrome and hereditary motor and sensory neuropathy Type I or hypertrophic variety of Charcot-Marie-Tooth disease (see Figs. 16-10A and 16-12).[60] In the former, conduction abnormalities are characteristically associated with prominent facial paresis, whereas in the latter, weakness of the facial muscles, if any, is surprisingly subtle despite a marked delay in conduction. The apparent discrepancy presumably results in part from chronicity of the disease process. Weakness usually occurs as the consequence of conduction block that typically accompanies demyelination during acute, fulminating courses of the Guillain-Barré syndrome. In contrast, the insidious onset and slow progression in Charcot-Marie-Tooth disease allow considerable compensation of motor function to occur despite slowed nerve conduction.

Other entities commonly associated with facial nerve palsy include cerebellopontine angle tumors and multiple sclerosis. The electrically elicited blink reflex is abnormal in a majority of patients with acoustic neuroma (see Tables 16-2 and 16-3). The incidence of abnormality is very high, since the tumor, strategically located at the cerebellopontine angle, may compress the trigeminal nerve, facial nerve, or the pons; that is, the afferent, efferent, and central arcs of the reflex.[65, 67, 83] Multiple sclerosis is a cause of peripheral facial palsy in young adults (see Fig. 16-11B). Electromyographic examination may reveal myokymia as mentioned earlier. The R1 component of the blink reflex may be absent or delayed, indicating demyelination of the central reflex arc, which includes the intrapontine portion of the facial nerve.[59, 61, 62]

Selective involvement of the orbicularis oculi and frontalis, a typical feature of peripheral facial weakness, sometimes appears with central lesions. However, increased latency of electrically elicited R1 usually implies a lesion directly involving the reflex arc. The latency of R1 may increase during the acute stage of contralateral hemispheric lesions if elicited by the glabellar tap.[32] In doubtful cases, paired stimuli minimize the latency change secondary to reduced excitability and make the shortest latency of R1 a more accurate measure of conduction along the reflex arc itself. The excitability of R2 may be significantly altered with a supranuclear lesion and shows either an afferent or efferent pattern as discussed in Chapter 16 (see Fig. 16-17).

## Accessory nerve

A spinal accessory nerve injury may occur as a result of pressure by a tumor or from surgical procedures of the posterior triangle.[44, 112, 162] In trapezius palsies following injury of the accessory nerve, the upper vertebral border of the scapula moves away from the spinal vertebrae. Since the lower angle of the scapula is relatively fixed by muscles supplied by C-3 and C-4 roots through the cervical plexus, the whole scapula rotates and slips downward. This type of winging of the scapula tends to worsen by abduction of the arm to the horizontal plane. The paralysis of the sternocleidomastoid results in weakness in rotating the face toward the opposite shoulder. The muscle is easily palpated for assessment of the degree of atrophy. If the muscles are affected on both sides, flexion of the neck becomes difficult.

# NERVES OF THE SHOULDER GIRDLE

Certain peripheral nerves derived directly from the brachial plexus are subject to isolated injury by compression or stab wound. The most commonly injured are the long thoracic, dorsal scapular, suprascapular, musculocutaneous and axillary nerves.

## Long thoracic nerve

The long thoracic nerve lies superficially in the supraclavicular region, where it is subject to trauma. It is also vulnerable to stretch because of its straight course from origin to insertion. In addition to stab injury, the nerve may suffer direct pressure from a heavy shoulder bag or shoulder braces during surgery.[52] Radical mastectomy may also damage the nerve.

The serratus anterior, the only muscle innervated by the long thoracic nerve, functions as a stabilizer of the shoulder in abduction of the arm. It holds the scapula flat against the back by keeping its inner margin fixed to the thorax. When the muscle is paretic, the patient is unable to raise the arm up straight. Because of the unopposed action of the rhomboids and levator scapulae, the scapula rotates inwards with the lower angle moving medially closer to the spinal column. The vertebral border of the lower scapula projects backward, away from the thorax. This tendency, called scapular winging, worsens with the outstretched arm thrust forward. As mentioned earlier, winging of the scapula caused by trapezius weakness becomes more prominent with abduction of the arm laterally. Lesions of the long thoracic nerve give rise to isolated electromyographic abnormalities in the serratus anterior muscle.

## Dorsal scapular nerve

Entrapment of this nerve causes a tendency for the scapula to wing on wide abduction of the arm.[98] The patient may complain of pain in C-5 and C-6 distribution. The diagnosis depends on electromyographic demonstration of abnormalities restricted to the rhomboid major and minor, and levator scapulae.

## Suprascapular nerve

Suprascapular nerve injury may result from pressure on the shoulder or stab wounds above the scapula.[14, 27, 38, 71, 137] Downward displacement of the upper trunk may also stretch the nerve anchored at the notch, a mechanism in part responsible for Erb's palsy. Injury to this nerve results in atrophy of the supraspinatus with weakness in initiating abduction of the arm and external rotation of the glenohumeral joint. The infraspinatus is also weakened causing difficulty in external rotation of the arm at the shoulder, although partially compensated by the teres minor and deltoid supplied by the axillary nerve. The sensory component of the suprascapular nerve supplies the posterior capsule of the shoulder joint. Compressive lesions, therefore, often cause a poorly defined aching pain along the posterior and lateral aspect of the shoulder joint and the adjacent scapula.[117, 121, 122, 123] Electromyographic exploration often reveals evidence of denervation in the supraspinatus and infraspinatus, but in no other muscles supplied by C-5 and C-6 roots.

## Musculocutaneous nerve

Fractures or dislocations of the humerus, gunshot or stab wounds, compression of the arm, and heavy exercise can lead to injuries of the musculocutaneous nerve.[8] Isolated lesions of this nerve have also occurred as rare complications of surgery[23] or secondary to entrapment by the coracobrachialis muscle. Sensory examination reveals numbness along the lateral aspect of the forearm. Paralysis of the biceps results in weakness of elbow flexion, although this is partially compensated by the brachioradialis. The biceps stretch reflex is absent. In addition to electromyographic evidence of denervation in the biceps brachii, brachialis, and coracobrachialis, conduction studies of the musculocutaneous nerve are of value in corroborating the diagnosis.[152]

## Axillary nerve

Injury to this nerve commonly occurs as a part of brachial plexus neuritis or by a direct trauma sustained at the time of fracture or dislocation of the head of the humerus. Other causes include the pressure of crutches or hyperextension of the shoulder, as might occur in wrestling. A circumscribed area of numbness develops in the lateral aspect of the upper arm over the belly of the deltoid muscle. Atrophy of the deltoid produces obvious flattening of the shoulder. Abduction of the arm is weak after the first 30 degrees subserved by the supraspinatus. In contrast, a C-5 root lesion weakens all 180 degrees of shoulder abduction. Isolated weakness of the teres minor is difficult to assess clinically, since the infraspinatus also rotates the arm outward. Electromyography confirms involvement of the teres minor and deltoid.

# RADIAL NERVE

The most common site for a radial nerve lesion is at the spiral groove of the humerus. The nerve may be injured here by fracture of the humerus or by trauma. A local compression also may occur when an individual, often intoxicated, falls asleep leaning against some hard surface or with an arm draped over a bench (Saturday night palsy). The lesion at this level usually spares the triceps, but the remaining extensor muscles of the hand, wrist, and fingers, as well as the brachioradialis, are all weak. The sensory loss is variable but is most often present over the dorsum of the hand and first two digits. Nerve injury may occur at the axilla secondary to pressure from an incorrectly used crutch, which causes weakness of all the radial-innervated muscles, including the triceps. The triceps stretch reflex is abolished or reduced. More distally, fractures of the head of the radius may injure the nerve.

Compression of the recurrent epicondylar branch of the radial nerve gives rise to pain at the elbow usually with simultaneous entrapment of the deep branch. This syndrome is one of the many entities commonly known as tennis elbow, since repeated indirect trauma by forceful supination is the predisposing factor. Pain and tenderness localized to the lateral aspect of the elbow resemble the symptoms of lateral epicondylitis, another condition referred to by some as tennis elbow. However, in the entrapment syndrome, additional dysfunction indicates involvement of the deep radial branch as well. Subluxation of the head of the radius may produce a radial palsy. Superficial radial neuropathy may develop after wearing a tight watch band.[118] Handcuff-related compression injuries may involve the sensory fibers of both radial and median nerves at the wrist.[21, 89]

Conduction studies may reveal the absence of both motor and sensory potentials after a fracture of the humerus or slowing of conduction across the compression site at the spiral groove. Testing nerve excitability distal to the presumed site of lesion helps differentiate neurapraxia and axonotomesis, although these two types of injury coexist to a varying degree in a majority of cases. Pressure neuropathy of the radial nerve usually resolves in six to eight weeks, but the recovery may take considerably longer if a substantial number of axons degenerate. Electromyographic exploration is valuable in demonstrating the type and location of injury (see Figs. 13-13 and 13-16).[151]

## Posterior interosseous syndrome

The posterior interosseous nerve is the terminal motor branch of the radial nerve in the forearm. Injury commonly occurs as it penetrates the supinator muscle in its entrance to the forearm by trauma, fracture, and occasionally in rheumatoid arthritis by a compressive synovitis.[91] The compression usually involves the nerve at the arcade of Frohse between the two heads of the supinator.[105] A lesion at this level causes weakness in the extensors of the wrist and digits without sensory loss. The supinator, innervated proximal to the site of compression, is spared. The extensor carpi radialis longus and brevis also receive the innervation more proximally from the radial nerve proper. Sparing of these muscles in the face of a paralyzed extensor carpi ulnaris results in the characteristic radial deviation of the wrist on attempted dorsiflexion. The differential diagnosis includes rupture of the extensor tendons, especially if paralysis affects only the last three digits, with preservation of the first two. In the posterior interosseous nerve syndrome, integrity of the extensor tendons is demonstrated by passive palmar flexion of the wrist that results in the extension of the metacarpophalangeal joints.

# MEDIAN NERVE

The median nerve may be subject to compression at several points along its course. At the elbow, entrapment may occur between the two heads of the pronator teres. Distal to the elbow, the nerve injury may selectively affect the anterior interosseous branch. The most common compression neuropathy of the median nerve is the carpal tunnel syndrome with lesions at the distal edge of the transverse carpal ligament. Less commonly the nerve may be affected in the intermetacarpal tunnel.

# Pronator teres syndrome

In 83 percent of dissections, the median nerve pierces the two heads of the pronator teres before passing under it.[5] Trauma, fracture, muscle hypertrophy, or an anomalous fibrous band connecting the pronator teres to the tendinous arch of the flexor digitorum sublimis may injure the nerve at this point, giving rise to the pronator teres syndrome.[30, 70, 95] The clinical features include pain and tenderness over the pronator teres; weakness of flexor pollicis and abductor pollicis brevis; and preservation of forearm pronation. Sensory changes occur over the thenar eminence, which is innervated by a branch of the median nerve. This sensory branch, which passes superficially to the flexor retinaculum, is not involved in the carpal tunnel syndrome. The conduction velocity of the median nerve in the proximal forearm is usually slow, but the distal latency and sensory nerve action potentials at the wrist are normal.[95] Injection of corticosteroids into the pronator teres may relieve the pain and aid in diagnosis, but surgical decompression may be necessary for definitive treatment.[74]

The pronator teres syndrome is distinct from a similar entrapment of the median nerve by the ligament of Struthers, which is a fibrous band attached to an anomalous spur on the anteromedial aspect of the lower humerus.[88] This ligament may compress the median nerve together with the brachial artery above the elbow, proximal to the innervation to the pronator teres. Weakness and electromyographic abnormalities of this muscle thus serve to differentiate this condition from the pronator teres syndrome, which usually spares the muscle. Compression of the brachial artery with full extension of the forearm obliterates the radial pulse.

# Anterior interosseous syndrome

The anterior interosseous nerve branches off the median nerve just distal to the pronator passage. Selective injury by dislocation of the elbow produces the anterior interosseous syndrome of Kiloh and Nevin.[58] The common presenting symptoms include pain in the forearm or elbow[37, 79, 104] without distinct clinical or electrophysiologic sensory abnormalities. Asked to make an OK sign with the first two digits the patient will form a triangle instead of a circle—the so-called pinch sign. The syndrome may occur bilaterally.[100] Spontaneous recovery may take place from 6 weeks to 18 months. As discussed in Chapter 21, neuralgic amyotrophy with lesions in the brachial plexus may manifest as an anterior interosseous nerve palsy.[124] Ordinary nerve conduction studies of the median nerve are normal,[106] but slowed conduction velocities of the anterior interosseous nerve may be demonstrated by recording a compound muscle action potential from the pronator quadratus after stimulation of the nerve at the elbow.[100] Electromyographic explorations show evidence of denervation in the flexor pollicis longus, flexor digitorum profundus I and II, and pronator quadratus.

# Carpal tunnel syndrome

The carpal tunnel syndrome is the best known and most commonly encountered of all the entrapment neuropathies. The syndrome was also the first to be documented by nerve conduction studies.[135] Although the syndrome appears as an isolated entity in the majority of patients,[48] a generalized polyneuropathy or systemic illness may predispose to nerve entrapment.[6, 68, 155, 164] These include amyloidosis,[15] acromegaly,[109] hypothyroidism,[129] rheumatoid arthritis,[97, 156] lupus erythematosus,[134] and hyperparathyroidism.[154] The carpal tunnel syndrome may occur in association with degenerative cervical spine disease. This combination, called the double-crush syndrome by Upton and McComas,[153] may represent the chance occurrence of two very common entities. However, it is important to recognize that the presence of one condition does not preclude the other. Awareness of this possibility is essential for adequate clinical as well as electrophysiologic assessments of the median nerve.

Incidence of the carpal tunnel syndrome is highest in the fifth and sixth decades, affecting females more than males. In young women, symptoms may appear during pregnancy and resolve after delivery. Although entrapment frequently occurs bilaterally, the dominant hand is usually more severely involved. A majority of patients have occupations involving considerable use of their hands.[35] Painful paresthesias in the median nerve distribution frequently awaken the patient at night. This pain typically spares the part of the thenar eminence innervated by the palmar cutaneous branch, which arises proximal to the carpal tunnel. On the other hand, the pain is often referred to the elbow and not uncommonly to the shoulder. Numbness or paresthesia typically involve the first three digits and the radial half of the fourth digit. Sensory changes are variable and not entirely reliable, since the complaint of numbness outside the median nerve distribution is not rare. Compression may affect the peripheral vasomotor fibers.[3] Advanced cases show weakness and wasting of the abductor pollicis brevis and other median-innervated thenar muscles.

The symptoms may worsen after passive flexion of the affected hand at the wrist for more than one minute.[115] In some cases, hyperextension of the wrist has the same effect. Wrist flexion may also cause an increase in the motor or sensory latency.[130] Percussion of the median nerve at the wrist may induce paresthesia of the fingers (Tinel's sign), but this is not as specific to the carpal tunnel syndrome[143] as was once advocated. In fact, a percussion on the volar aspect of the wrist misses the compression site by 2 to 3 cm.[64] Parenthetically, Tinel[150] described a tingling sensation produced by tapping the proximal stump of an injured nerve and used it only to indicate axonal regeneration, and not to indicate entrapment neuropathy.[139, 159]

The median nerve of many patients with the carpal tunnel syndrome is abnormally susceptible to ischemia whether evaluated clinically[42] or electrophysiologically.[33] This susceptibility is related to the severity of pain and paresthesia but not to the duration of disease or degree of muscle wasting or weakness.[33] Thus, the clinical symptoms of this syndrome may in part result from rapidly reversible changes in the nerve fibers associated with ischemic attacks. However, mechanical factors are probably more important as suggested by sharply localized structural changes found under both distal and proximal edges in experimental acute and chronic compression neuropathy.[34, 107]

Pathologic studies suggest that the smallest cross-sectional area within the carpal tunnel is found 2.0 to 2.5 cm distal to the entrance, where the tunnel is rigidly bound on three sides by bony structures and roofed by a thickened transverse carpal ligament.[125] It is indeed under the retinaculum that a striking reduction in myelinated fiber size takes place.[148] Compression of the median nerve by the lateral border of the sublimis muscle may cause a similar syndrome.[36] Interestingly, even in normal subjects, the 1 cm segment with maximal conduction time was found 2 to 4 cm distal to the origin of the ligament.[64] Thus, mild involvement of the median nerve at this particular level may be present in clinically asymptomatic hands.[39] Neary, Ochoa, and Gilliatt[102] have shown such focal abnormalities in 5 of 12 median nerves at routine autopsy from patients without known disease of the median nerve. Retrograde changes may occur in the forearm when a severe compressive lesion is present at the wrist.[4, 144]

The carpal tunnel syndrome has been the subject of extensive electrophysiologic studies.[22, 40, 55, 80, 90, 115, 135, 149] Conduction abnormalities often appear selectively in the wrist-to-palm segment of the median nerve for both sensory[9, 10, 18, 63, 158] and motor fibers.[63, 126] The remaining distal segment, however, shows only mild or no abnormalities of sensory or motor conduction in the patients. In our series,[64] palmar stimulation documented mild slowing across the carpal tunnel in 36 (21 percent) sensory and 40 (23 percent) motor axons of 172 symptomatic hands when the conventional distal latencies were normal. Sensory or motor conduction was abnormal in all but 13 (8 percent) clinically affected hands. Without palmar stimulation, however, an additional 32 (20 percent) hands would have been regarded as normal. Palmar stimulation also provides a simple means to establish whether the slowing of sensory or motor conduction is attributable to compression by the transverse carpal ligament or to disease of the most terminal segment. This distinction is potentially important in differentiating the carpal tunnel syndrome from a distal neuropathy.[12]

With serial stimulation from midpalm to distal forearm in 1 cm increments, sensory axons normally showed a latency change of 0.16 to 0.21 ms per cm (see Fig. 6-3A and B). In about one half of the affected nerves, an abrupt latency increase occurred across a 1 cm segment, most commonly 2 to 4 cm distal to the origin of the transverse carpal ligament.[64] In these hands, the focal latency change across the affected 1 cm segment averaged more than four times that of the adjoining distal or proximal 1 cm segments (see Fig. 6-3C and D). In the remaining hands, the latency increased more evenly across the carpal tunnel. Comparable serial studies of the motor axons were difficult because of the recurrent course of the thenar nerve, which might be contained in a separate tunnel.[54]

Electromyographic studies may be normal or, in advanced cases, show fibrillation potentials and positive sharp waves in the median-innervated intrinsic hand muscles. Electrophysiologic evidence of an ulnar nerve lesion may occur in some patients with the carpal tunnel syndrome[131] but not in others.[10, 48]

### Digital nerve entrapment

The interdigital nerves supplying the skin of the second and third digits and half of the fourth digit are extensions of the median sensory fibers. These small sensory branches may be compressed against the edge of the deep transverse metacarpal ligament. Entrapment appears in association with trauma, tumor, phalangeal fracture, or inflammation of the metacarpophalangeal joint or tendon.[74] The presenting symptom is pain in one or two fingers exacerbated by lateral hyperextension of the affected digits. The palmar surfaces between the metacarpals are tender and dysesthetic or hypoesthetic. Local infiltration of steroid may relieve the symptoms and assist in diagnosis.[98]

# ULNAR NERVE

## Tardy ulnar palsy and cubital tunnel syndrome

Ulnar nerve injury commonly occurs at the elbow after repeated trauma, following immobilization of the upper limb during surgery, or as part of a more diffuse neuropathy. Originally, tardy ulnar palsy referred to nerve injury resulting from joint deformity or recurrent subluxation secondary to previous trauma. However, the term now implies entrapment of the ulnar nerve at the elbow, even without history of trauma. Ulnar nerve entrapment at the elbow may occur concomitantly with lower cervical spine disease involving C-8 and T-1 roots or with the thoracic outlet syndrome.[98] Nerve conduction studies and electromyography help explore this possibility in patients with radicular as well as entrapment symptoms.

Ulnar neuropathy at the elbow reveals a widely varying incidence of causes,[47, 82] but more recent reports suggest that the cubital tunnel syndrome is the most common.[29, 92] A number of factors may give rise to this condition,[74, 93, 140, 147] but in the majority of cases, nerve entrapment occurs unaccompanied by joint deformity or history of major trauma[28, 113] under the aponeurosis connecting the two heads of the flexor carpi ulnaris,[31] where the nerve is also largest.[13] The nerve is often palpably swollen in the ulnar groove and appears hyperemic at surgery.

The appearance of bilateral ulnar neuropathy in a large number of patients suggests a congenital predisposition to this syndrome.[92] In some patients with idiopathic ulnar neuropathy the asymptomatic contralateral ulnar nerve may show some involvement histologically.[101] Neary, Ochoa, and Gilliatt[102] have shown focal pathologic changes at the aponeurosis in 5 of 12 ulnar nerves at routine autopsy from patients without symptoms of ulnar neuropathy.

The symptoms tend to develop with frequent hand use in the elbow flexed position, which narrows the cubital tunnel.[31, 92] Earliest clinical features include impairment of sensation over the fifth digit and ulnar half of the fourth digit, and weakness with wasting of the first dorsal interosseous and other ulnar-innervated intrinsic hand muscles. Surgical transposition[49] or simple decompression[94, 160] may result in a reasonably functional recovery.[49, 78, 103, 114] However, once a moderate degree of motor deficit has occurred, 30 percent or more of patients still will be symptomatic after operative intervention.[29]

Nerve conduction studies show localized slowing of motor or sensory conduction velocity across the elbow as compared with the more proximal or distal segments.[135] The difference is significant only if it exceeds 10 m/s.[28] The segment distal to the presumed compression may also show mild slowing of conduction velocity.[41] In the presence of conduction block, the compound muscle action potentials are of reduced amplitude with stimulation of the nerve above the elbow. Similarly, sensory nerve action potentials recorded at the axilla are diminished if the nerve is stimulated below the elbow, but normal after nerve stimulation above the elbow.[41]

Eisen[28] and Odusote and Eisen[110] reported four electrodiagnostic features that were of particular value in the diagnosis of a mild ulnar lesion: (1) slowing of motor nerve conduction velocity across the elbow by 10 m/s or more, compared with the more proximal and distal segments; (2) absent sensory action potential at the wrist; (3) distal motor latency with stimulation above the elbow greater than 8.8 ms; and (4) terminal motor latency at the wrist greater than 3.4 ms. The last two criteria only apply for specified nerve lengths. More precise localization of the conduction abnormality may become evident by stimulating the nerve at multiple sites across the cubital tunnel.[92]

An electrophysiologic assessment of the cubital tunnel syndrome should include electromyography, which may further define the area of dysfunction by demonstrating denervation in selected groups of ulnar-innervated muscles. In contrast to the flexor carpi ulnaris, which is supplied by a branch derived from the ulnar nerve proximal to the cubital tunnel, the ulnar half of the flexor digitorum profundus receives the nerve supply distal to the aponeurosis. Thus, nerve compression in the cubital tunnel usually leads to electromyographic abnormalities in the latter muscle without affecting the former.

## Compression at Guyon's canal

Ulnar nerve injury occurs less commonly at the wrist as it enters the hand through Guyon's canal than at the elbow.[132] The clinical features are similar to those of tardy ulnar palsy. Sensory deficit is confined to the palm, since the dorsal cutaneous branch, which innervates the dorsum of the hand, arises proximal to the wrist. Entrapment in Guyon's canal is most commonly caused by a ganglion and less frequently by trauma or rheumatoid arthritis. The ulnar-innervated intrinsic hand muscles are all weak, with evidence of denervation by electromyography. However, function of the flexor carpi ulnaris and flexor digitorum profundus III and IV is preserved. Reduced or absent sensory action potentials of the fourth and fifth digits indicate involvement of the superficial sensory branch. The mixed nerve action potential between wrist and elbow remains normal.

## Involvement of the palmar branch

Further distally, the deep motor branch of the nerve may be subject to external trauma or compression by a ganglion arising from the carpal articulations.[16, 24, 51, 132] Repeated trauma to this branch occurs while using the heel of the hand against a crutch or in an attempt to shut or raise a window by striking the bottom edge with the palm. Symptomatic compression of the ulnar nerve at the wrist has also developed following prolonged bicycle riding.[26] Since the damage occurs distal to the origin of the superficial sensory branch, the patient has no sensory abnormality clinically or electrophysiologically. This lesion also spares the motor branches supplying the hypothenar muscles. Thus, conduction studies reveal a normal velocity between the elbow and wrist and a normal distal latency from the wrist to the abductor digiti minimi. The compound action potential recorded from the first dorsal interosseous, however, may show prolonged latency and reduced amplitude compared with the unaffected side. These findings indicate slowing or block of nerve conduction distal to the origin of the hypothenar branch.[25, 135]

### Digital nerve entrapment

The interdigital branch to the fifth digit receives fibers solely from the ulnar nerve, whereas branches supplying the third and fourth digits are formed by anastomosis between median and ulnar nerves. Clinical symptoms and signs are similar to the median digital nerve entrapments described earlier.

## NERVES OF THE PELVIC GIRDLE

Although the lumbar plexus is a rare site of traumatic injury because of the protection afforded by the pelvic bones, individual nerves derived from the plexus are subject to isolated damage by either chronic compression or acute injury.

### Ilioinguinal nerve

This nerve may be subject to accidental trauma or to injury during surgery. Patients with ilioinguinal neuropathy[75] complain of pain in the groin region, especially when standing. Pressure immediately medial to the anterior-superior iliac spine causes pain radiating into the crural region. Muscle weakness and increased intra-abdominal tension may lead to formation of a direct inguinal hernia.

### Genitofemoral nerve

Injury to this nerve may be due to trauma to the groin or surgical adhesions. Clinical features include pain in the inguinal region, sensory deficits over the femoral triangle, and the absence of the cremasteric reflex.

### Lateral femoral cutaneous nerve

A condition known as meralgia paresthetica arises as a result of lateral femoral cutaneous nerve entrapment at the anterior superior iliac spine as the nerve emerges from the lateral border of the psoas major. The nerve can be compressed as it penetrates the inguinal fascia by tight belts, corsets, or seatbelts, or without obvious cause. Damage to the nerve is most prominent in the region of the anterior superior iliac spine where the nerve sharply angulates over the inguinal ligament.[74] The syndrome consists of paresthesias, pain, and objective sensory loss over the anterolateral surface of the thigh.[73] Since the nerve is a purely sensory branch, no motor weakness develops. Pathologic changes include local demyelination and wallerian degeneration, particularly affecting the fibers with the largest diameters.[53]

Clinical diagnosis depends on the characteristic distribution of sensory loss. Sensory conduction study may be slowed across the compression site.[11, 128, 142] Patients with a herniated disc of the high lumbar spine may present with radiating pain along the lateral aspect of the thigh. However, objective sensory loss is usually lacking and motor deficits demonstrated clinically as well as electromyographically implicate the L-3 or L-4 innervated muscles.

## Femoral nerve

The intrapelvic portion of the femoral nerve is vulnerable to compression by tumors of the vertebrae, psoas abscesses, retroperitoneal lymphadenopathy, or hematoma.[17, 57, 76, 141, 163] Direct trauma may occur with fractures of the femur or cardiac catheterization. Diabetes and vascular disease are also common causes of femoral neuropathy. A complete lesion of the femoral nerve is characterized by three findings:[7] (1) inability to flex the thigh on the abdomen or to extend the leg at the knee; (2) reduced or absent knee stretch reflex; and (3) variable sensory loss. Electrophysiologic studies show an increase in femoral nerve latency with reduction in the amplitude of the compound muscle action potential and evidence of denervation in the appropriate muscles.

Apparent mononeuropathy of the femoral nerve is common in diabetics, with pain in the anterior aspect of the thigh followed by weakness and atrophy of the quadriceps. In these cases, however, careful clinical and electromyographic examination often reveals more widespread involvement in the territory of the L-2 through L-4 roots.

## Saphenous nerve

The saphenous nerve may be compressed at its exit from Hunter's subsartorial canal, through which it passes.[72] Hunter's canal also contains the femoral vessels, and obstructive vascular disease may entrap the saphenous nerve. The main clinical feature is pain localized to the medial aspect of the knee, often radiating distally to the medial side of the foot.[98] The pain worsens with any exercise but particularly with climbing stairs. Saphenous nerve conduction determined orthodromically[145] or antidromically[157] may be slowed.

## Obturator nerve

Selective damage of the obturator nerve commonly occurs during labor. Other causes of nerve injury include pressure from a gravid uterus, pelvic fracture, and surgical procedures for obturator hernia. In the last condition, nerve entrapment in the obturator canal results from increased intra-abdominal pressure. Injury to this nerve causes weakness of adduction and internal and external rotation of the thigh. Typically, the patient complains of pain in the groin radiating along the medial aspect of the thigh, as well as hypesthesia or dysesthesia over the medial aspect of the upper thigh. Electromyographic studies show evidence of denervation in the gracilis and adductor muscles.

## Superior and inferior gluteal nerves

These nerves, situated directly behind the hip joint, are subject to damage by fractures of the upper femur or by misdirected intramuscular injection. Anterior-superior tendinous fibers of the pyriformis may compress the superior gluteal nerve, causing buttock pain and tenderness to palpation in the area superolateral to the greater sciatic notch.[119] Neurogenic damage to the superior gluteal nerve gives rise to weakness and electromyographic evidence of denervation of gluteus medius and minimus, which adduct and rotate the thigh inward. A lesion of the inferior gluteal nerve results in weakness and denervation of the gluteus maximus, which extends, adducts, and rotates the thigh externally.

## Sciatic nerve

A number of conditions cause sciatic nerve injury in the pelvis. These include the direct spread of neoplasm originating from the genitourinary tract or rectum, neurinoma of the sciatic nerve itself, abscess of the pelvic floor, pressure from a gravid uterus, and fractures of the pelvis, hip, and femur. Penetrating injury, misdirected intramuscular injections, hip surgery, and insertion of a prosthesis may also damage the sciatic nerve. Although rare, entrapment of the sciatic nerve by the pyriformis muscle may occur where the nerve exits the pelvis through the greater sciatic notch.[74] The pyriformis syndrome, unlike more proximal conditions, spares the gluteus medius, gluteus minimus, tensor fasciae latae, and paraspinal muscles clinically and electromyographically.

During prolonged squatting, sciatic nerve compression may develop in the segment between the ischial tuberosity and trochanter major or between the adductor magnus and hamstring muscles.[136] The lower portion of the sciatic nerve may be entrapped above the popliteal fossa by Baker's popliteal cyst.[99] The cyst, formed by an effusion into the semimembranous bursa, produces a palpable enlargement, especially with the knee extended. It may compress the peroneal, tibial, or sural nerve in any combination. Nerve conduction studies and electromyography are useful in delineating the extent and distribution of abnormality.

For reasons not entirely clear, the peroneal component of the sciatic nerve is much more likely to be damaged than the tibial portion, even when trauma affects the nerve as a whole.[96, 146] Reaction to injuries may depend on funicular size and disposition of the nerves. The peroneal nerve trunk has less connective tissue and fewer but longer nerve bundles than the tibial nerve. The topical distribution of the nerve, with the peroneal component located laterally and posteriorly to the tibial component, may make the former more susceptible to an injection needle, which is usually placed laterally in the buttock.

Lesions affecting the peroneal nerve distally as it crosses the neck of the fibula or more proximal lesions of the sciatic nerve may cause footdrop. Careful electromyographic exploration of the hamstring muscles and the posterior compartment of the leg usually reveals evidence of denervation with the more proximal lesion. Commonly tested for this purpose are the short head of the biceps femoris, which is innervated by the peroneal component of the sciatic nerve above the knee, and the tibialis posterior supplied by the tibial nerve. Nerve conduction studies of the sciatic nerve by means of the H-reflex, F-wave, or direct needle stimulation at the radicular level and sciatic notch[85] may be of value.

# TIBIAL NERVE

The tibial nerve remains deep in the posterior compartment of the thigh and leg and is rarely subject to injury at this level. Most commonly the nerve is compressed by the flexor retinaculum as it passes behind the medial malleolus.[20, 43, 56, 86] This condition, known as the tarsal tunnel syndrome, may result from trauma, tenosynovitis, venous stasis of the posterior tibial vein, or, rarely, a ganglion arising from the subtalar joint.[84] The clinical features consist of painful dysesthesia in the toes and sole with some sensory deficits and weakness of the intrinsic foot muscles. Electromyographic exploration reveals evidence of denervation in tibial-innervated intrinsic foot muscles.

In the tarsal tunnel syndrome nerve conduction studies show increased motor latencies along the medial or lateral plantar nerve with stimulation of the tibial nerve slightly above the medial malleolus. Additional stimulation of the nerve slightly below the malleolus may document slowing of conduction velocity across the compression site. However, the calculated conduction velocity may not be accurate in view of the short distance between the two stimuli. Alternatively, serial stimulation in 1 cm increments along the course of the nerve may reveal a disproportionate latency increase at the compression site. The latencies and nerve conduction studies on the clinically unaffected side serve as a control.

The nerve is rarely compressed more proximally in the popliteal fossa, or more distally as it enters the abductor hallucis muscle. A lesion distal to the flexor retinaculum results in deficit of either medial or lateral plantar branches of the tibial nerve. The patient complains of pain and sensory changes in the plantar aspect of the foot but not in the heel. Useful diagnostic techniques include nerve conduction studies of the medial and lateral plantar nerves and electromyography of the intrinsic foot muscles.[46, 111]

The terminal digital branches, usually in the third and fourth interspace, are subject to trauma under the metatarsal heads, giving rise to a syndrome of painful toes called Morton's neuroma. The interdigital nerve syndrome also results from ligamentous mechanical irritation with hyperextension of the toes in high-heeled shoes, hallux valgus deformities, congenital malformation, rheumatoid arthritis, or any form of trauma.[98] Walking typically precipitates pain in the affected digits, but spontaneous nocturnal pain may also occur.

# COMMON PERONEAL NERVE

Following the separation into individual nerves in the lower thigh, the common peroneal nerve becomes superficial to reach the lateral aspect of the knee, where it is most susceptible to trauma.[2] Leg-crossing causes compression of the nerve against the head of the fibula.[133] Injury at this level most frequently affects the deep branch, and less commonly, the whole nerve. Selective involvement of the superficial branch is rare.[133, 147] A ganglion in the same location may damage the nerve. Common peroneal nerve palsy may also occur as a result of prolonged squatting, which compresses the nerve among the biceps tendon, lateral head of the gastrocnemius, and the head of the fibula.[69, 147]

With injury to the deep branch, the toe and foot dorsiflexors are weakened and show evidence of denervation by electromyography. The patient has sensory changes only over the web of skin between the first and second toe. Lesions of the superficial branch affect the evertors and cause sensory deficits over most of the dorsum of the foot. The ankle reflex and inversion of the foot remain normal and serve to distinguish a sciatic nerve or lumbosacral root lesion. The latter also presents with footdrop, but the ankle reflexes are typically absent. Electromyographic examination of the tibialis posterior, although somewhat difficult technically, is useful in differentiating between peroneal palsy and L-5 radiculopathy, since this muscle receives L-4 and L-5 innervation via the tibial nerve.[50]

A nerve conduction study across the fibular head helps to localize the site of lesion. Slowing in this segment is considered significant if it exceeds by 10 m/s that in the remaining distal segment below the knee. Conduction block at the compression site is likely if the compound muscle action potential is smaller with proximal than with distal stimulation. In contrast, in the presence of the accessory deep peroneal nerve, the evoked potential from the extensor digitorum brevis is smaller with distal stimulation at the ankle than proximally at the knee.[81] If the extensor digitorum brevis is very atrophic, compound action potentials from the tibialis anterior can be used to demonstrate slowing of conduction across the knee.[19, 120] The mixed nerve potential recorded above the head of the fibula with distal stimulation shows reduced amplitude and increased latency. In advanced cases, the response may be totally absent.

The deep peroneal nerve is susceptible to compression at the ankle. This rare entrapment, called the anterior tarsal tunnel syndrome,[87] gives rise to pain on the dorsum of the foot, sensory deficits in the small web area between the first and second toes, and atrophy of the extensor digitorum brevis. An incomplete form affects the motor or sensory fibers selectively after their division under the inferior extensor retinaculum.[77]

Nerve conduction studies show increased distal motor latency with stimulation of the deep peroneal nerve proximal to the inferior extensor retinaculum.[127] Electromyography reveals evidence of denervation in the extensor digitorum brevis and other appropriate muscles. Some fibrillation potentials, however, may be present in the intrinsic foot muscles as a result of chronic nerve damage caused by a tight shoe.

# SURAL NERVE

Isolated compression and traumatic neuropathy of the sural nerve are rare. Common causes include a ganglion,[116] Baker's cyst,[99] and stretch injury.[45] The sural nerve is frequently biopsied for diagnostic purposes because of its superficial location. The sensory innervation of this nerve is variable, since the relative contribution from the tibial and peroneal nerves differs from one subject to another. In general, sensory changes occur in the posterolateral aspects of the lower third of the leg and the lateral aspects of the dorsum of the foot. Nerve conduction testing usually delineates the lesion.[45]

# REFERENCE SOURCES

1. ADOUR, KK, BELL, DN, AND WINGERD, J: *Bell palsy. Dilemma of diabetes mellitus.* Arch Otolaryngol 99:114, 1974.

2. AGUAYO, AJ: *Neuropathy due to compression and entrapment.* In DYCK, PJ, THOMAS, PK, AND LAMBERT, EH (EDS): *Peripheral Neuropathy,* Vol 1. WB Saunders, Philadelphia, 1975.

3. AMINOFF, MJ: *Involvement of peripheral vasomotor fibres in carpal tunnel syndrome.* J Neurol Neurosurg Psychiatry 42:649, 1979.

4. ANDERSON, MH, ET AL: *Changes in the forearm associated with median nerve compression at the wrist in the guinea-pig.* J Neurol Neurosurg Psychiatry 33:70, 1970.

5. ANSON, BJ: *An Atlas of Human Anatomy,* ed 2. WB Saunders, Philadelphia, 1963.

6. BASTIAN, FO: *Amyloidosis and the carpal tunnel syndrome.* Am J Clin Pathol 61:711, 1974.

7. BIEMOND, A: *Femoral neuropathy.* In VINKEN, PJ AND BRUYN, GW (EDS): *Handbook of Clinical Neurology,* Vol 8. Diseases of the Nerves. American Elsevier, New York, 1970.

8. BRADDOM, RL AND WOLFE, C: *Musculocutaneous nerve injury after heavy exercise.* Arch Phys Med Rehabil 59:290, 1978.

9. BUCHTHAL, F AND ROSENFALCK, A: *Sensory conduction from digit to palm and from palm to wrist in the carpal tunnel syndrome.* J Neurol Neurosurg Psychiatry 34:243, 1971.

10. BUCHTHAL, F, ROSENFALCK, A, AND TROJABORG, W: *Electrophysiological findings in entrapment of the median nerve at wrist and elbow.* J Neurol Neurosurg Psychiatry 37:340, 1974.

11. BUTLER, ET, JOHNSON, EW, AND KAYE, ZA: *Normal conduction velocity in the lateral femoral cutaneous nerve.* Arch Phys Med Rehabil 55:31, 1974.

12. CASEY, EB AND LE QUESNE, PM: *Digital nerve action potentials in healthy subjects, and in carpal tunnel and diabetic patients.* J Neurol Neurosurg Psychiatry 35:612, 1972.

13. CHANG, KSF, ET AL: *Enlargement of the ulnar nerve behind the medial epicondyle.* Anat Rec 145:149, 1963.

14. CLEIN, LJ: *Suprascapular entrapment neuropathy.* J Neurosurg 43:337, 1975.

15. COHEN, AS: *Amyloidosis.* N Engl J Med 277:522, 1967.

16. COWEN, NJ: *Hypothenar mass and ulnar neuropathy. A case report.* Clin Orthop Rel Res 69:203, 1970.

17. CRANBERG, L: *Femoral neuropathy from iliac hematoma: Report of a case.* Neurology (New York) 29:1071, 1979.

18. DAUBE, JR: *Percutaneous palmar median nerve stimulation for carpal tunnel syndrome.* Electroenceph Clin Neurophysiol 43:139, 1977.

19. DEVI, S, LOVELACE, RE, AND DUARTE, N: *Proximal peroneal nerve conduction velocity: Recording from anterior tibial and peroneus brevis muscles.* Ann Neurol 2:116, 1977.

20. DI STEFANO, V, ET AL: *Tarsal-tunnel syndrome. Review of the literature and two case reports.* Clin Orthop Rel Res 88:76, 1972.

21. DORFMAN, LJ AND JAYARAM, AR: *Handcuff neuropathy.* JAMA 239:957, 1978.

22. DUENSING, F, ET AL: *Neurophysiologische Befunde beim Karpaltunnelsyndrom. Korrelationen zum klinischen Befund.* Z Neurol 206:267, 1974.

23. DUNDORE, DE AND DELISA, JA: *Musculocutaneous nerve palsy: An isolated complication of surgery.* Arch Phys Med Rehabil 60:130, 1979.

24. DUPONT, C, ET AL: *Ulnar-tunnel syndrome at the wrist. A report of four cases of ulnar-nerve compression at the wrist.* J Bone Joint Surg (Am) 47A:757, 1965.

25. EBELING, P, GILLIATT, RW, AND THOMAS, PK: *A clinical and electrical study of ulnar nerve lesions in the hand.* J Neurol Neurosurg Psychiatry 23:1, 1960.

26. ECKMAN, PB, PERLSTEIN, G, AND ALTROCCHI, PH: *Ulnar neuropathy in bicycle riders.* Arch Neurol 32:130, 1975.

27. EDELAND, HG AND ZACHRISSON, BE: *Fracture of the scapular notch associated with lesion of the suprascapular nerve.* Acta Orthop Scand 46:758, 1975.

28. EISEN, A: *Early diagnosis of ulnar nerve palsy. An electrophysiologic study.* Neurology (Minneap) 24:256, 1974.

29. EISEN, A AND DANON, J: *The mild cubital tunnel syndrome. Its natural history and indications for surgical intervention.* Neurology (Minneap) 24:608, 1974.

30. ESPOSITO, GM: *Peripheral entrapment neuropathies of upper extremity.* NY State J Med 72:717, 1972.

31. FEINDEL, W AND STRATFORD, J: *The role of the cubital tunnel in tardy ulnar palsy.* Canad J Surg 1:287, 1958.

32. FISHER, MA, SHAHANI, BT, AND YOUNG, RR: *Assessing segmental excitability after acute rostral lesions. II. The blink reflex.* Neurology (Minneap) 29:45, 1979.

33. FULLERTON, PM: *The effect of ischaemia on nerve conduction in the carpal tunnel syndrome.* J Neurol Neurosurg Psychiatry 26:385, 1963.

34. FULLERTON, PM AND GILLIATT, RW: *Median and ulnar neuropathy in the guinea-pig.* J Neurol Neurosurg Psychiatry 30:393, 1967.

35. GAINER, JV, JR AND NUGENT, GR: *Carpal tunnel syndrome. Report of 430 operations.* South Med J 70:325, 1977.

36. GARDNER, RC: *Confirmed case and diagnosis of pseudocarpal-tunnel (sublimis) syndrome.* N Engl J Med 282:858, 1970.

37. GARDNER-THORPE, C: *Anterior interosseous nerve palsy: Spontaneous recovery in two patients.* J Neurol Neurosurg Psychiatry 37:1146, 1974.

38. GELMERS, HJ AND BUYS, DA: *Suprascapular entrapment neuropathy.* Acta Neurochirurgica 38:121, 1977.

39. GILLIATT, RW: *Sensory conduction studies in the early recognition of nerve disorders.* Muscle and Nerve 1:352, 1978.

40. GILLIATT, RW AND SEARS, TA: *Sensory nerve action potentials in patients with peripheral nerve lesions.* J Neurol Neurosurg Psychiatry 21:109, 1958.

41. GILLIATT, RW AND THOMAS, PK: *Changes in nerve conduction with ulnar lesions at the elbow.* J Neurol Neurosurg Psychiatry 23:312, 1960.

42. GILLIATT, RW AND WILSON, TG: *Ischaemic sensory loss in patients with peripheral nerve lesions.* J Neurol Neurosurg Psychiatry 17:104, 1954.

43. GOODGOLD, J, KOPELL, HP, AND SPIELHOLZ, NI: *The tarsal-tunnel syndrome. Objective diagnostic criteria.* N Engl J Med 273:742, 1965.

44. GORDON, SL, ET AL: *Accessory nerve function after surgical procedures in the posterior triangle.* Arch Surg 112:264, 1977.

45. GROSS, JA, HAMILTON, WJ, AND SWIFT, TR: *Isolated mechanical lesions of the sural nerve.* Muscle and Nerve 3:248, 1980.

46. GUILOFF, RJ AND SHERRATT, RM: *Sensory conduction in medial plantar nerve. Normal values, clinical applications, and a comparison with the sural and upper limb sensory nerve action potentials in peripheral neuropathy.* J Neurol Neurosurg Psychiatry 40:1168, 1977.

47. HAGSTRÖM, P: *Ulnar nerve compression at the elbow. Results of surgery in 85 cases.* Scand J Plast Reconstr Surg 11:59, 1977.

48. HARRISON, MJG: *Lack of evidence of generalized sensory neuropathy in patients with carpal tunnel syndrome.* J Neurol Neurosurg Psychiatry 41:957, 1978.

49. HARRISON, MJG AND NURICK, S: *Results of anterior transposition of the ulnar nerve for ulnar neuritis.* Br Med J 1:27, 1970.

50. HEFFERNAN, LPM: *Electromyographic value of the tibialis posterior muscle.* Arch Phys Med Rehabil 60:170, 1979.

51. HUNT, JR: *Occupation neuritis of the deep palmar branch of the ulnar nerve.* J Nerv Ment Dis 35:673, 1908.

52. ILFELD, FW AND HOLDER, HG: *Winged scapula: Case occurring in soldier from knapsack.* JAMA 120:448, 1942.

53. JEFFERSON, D AND EAMES, RA: *Subclinical entrapment of the lateral femoral cutaneous nerve: An autopsy study.* Muscle and Nerve 2:145, 1979.

54. JOHNSON, RK AND SHREWSBURY, MM: *Anatomical course of the thenar branch of the median nerve—Usually in a separate tunnel through the transverse carpal ligament.* J Bone Joint Surg 52A:269, 1970.

55. KAESER, HE: *Diagnostische Probleme beim Karpaltunnelsyndrom.* Deutsche Zeitschrift Für Nervenheilkunde 185:453, 1963.

56. KECK, C: *The tarsal-tunnel syndrome.* J Bone Joint Surg 44A:180, 1962.

57. KHELLA, L: *Femoral nerve palsy: Compression by lymph glands in the inguinal region.* Arch Phys Med Rehabil 60:325, 1979.

58. KILOH, LG AND NEVIN, S: *Isolated neuritis of the anterior interosseous nerve.* Br Med J 1:850, 1952.

59. KIMURA, J: *Alteration of the orbicularis oculi reflex by pontine lesions. Study in multiple sclerosis.* Arch Neurol 22:156, 1970.

60. KIMURA, J: *An evaluation of the facial and trigeminal nerves in polyneuropathy: Electrodiagnostic study in Charcot-Marie-Tooth disease, Guillain-Barré syndrome, and diabetic neuropathy.* Neurology (Minneap) 21:745, 1971.

61. KIMURA, J: *The blink reflex as a test for brain-stem and higher central nervous system function.* In DESMEDT, JE (ED): New Developments in Electromyography and Clinical Neurophysiology, Vol 3. Karger, Basel, 1973, pp 682–691.

62. KIMURA, J: *Electrically elicited blink reflex in diagnosis of multiple sclerosis—Review of 260 patients over a seven-year period.* Brain 98:413, 1975.

63. KIMURA, J: *A method for determining median nerve conduction velocity across the carpal tunnel.* J Neurol Sci 38:1, 1978.

64. KIMURA, J: *The carpal tunnel syndrome. Localization of conduction abnormalities within the distal segment of the median nerve.* Brain 102:619, 1979.

65. KIMURA, J AND LYON, LW: *Alteration of orbicularis oculi reflex by posterior fossa tumors.* J Neurosurg 38:10, 1973.

66. KIMURA, J, GIRON, LT, JR, AND YOUNG, SM: *Electrophysiological study of Bell palsy. Electrically elicited blink reflex in assessment of prognosis.* Arch Otolaryngol 102:140, 1976.

67. KIMURA, J, RODNITZKY, RL, AND VAN ALLEN, MW: *Electrodiagnostic study of trigeminal nerve. Orbicularis oculi reflex and masseter reflex in trigeminal neuralgia, paratrigeminal syndrome, and other lesions of the trigeminal nerve.* Neurology (Minneap) 20:574, 1970.

68. KLOFKORN, RW AND STEIGERWALD, JC: *Carpal tunnel syndrome as the initial manifestation of tuberculosis.* Am J Med 60:583, 1976.

69. KOLLER, RL AND BLANK, NK: *Strawberry picker's palsy.* Arch Neurol 37:320, 1980.

70. KOPELL, HP AND THOMPSON, WAL: *Pronator syndrome. A confirmed case and its diagnosis.* N Engl J Med 259:713, 1958.

71. KOPELL, HP AND THOMPSON, WAL: *Pain and the frozen shoulder.* Surg Gynecol Obstet 109:92, 1959.

72. KOPELL, HP AND THOMPSON, WAL: *Knee pain due to saphenous nerve entrapment.* N Engl J Med 263:351, 1960.

73. KOPELL, HP AND THOMPSON, WAL: *Peripheral entrapment neuropathies of the lower extremity.* N Engl J Med 262:56, 1960.

74. KOPELL, HP AND THOMPSON, WAL: *Peripheral Entrapment Neuropathies,* ed 2. Robert E. Krieger, Huntington, NY, 1976.

75. KOPELL, HP, THOMPSON, WAL, AND POSTEL, AH: *Entrapment neuropathy of the ilioinguinal nerve.* N Engl J Med 266:16, 1962.

76. KOUNIS, NG, MACAULEY, MB, AND GHORBAL, MS: *Iliacus hematoma syndrome.* Canad Med Assoc J 112:872, 1975.

77. KRAUSE, KH, WITT, T, AND ROSS, A: *The anterior tarsal tunnel syndrome.* J Neurol 217:67, 1977.

78. LAHA, RK AND PANCHAL, PD: *Surgical treatment of ulnar neuropathy.* Surg Neurol 11:393, 1979.

79. LAKE, PA: *Anterior interosseous nerve syndrome.* J Neurosurg 41:306, 1974.

80. LAMBERT, EH: *Diagnostic value of electrical stimulation of motor nerves.* Electroenceph Clin Neurophysiol (suppl 22):9, 1962.

81. LAMBERT, EH: *The accessory deep peroneal nerve. A common variation in innervation of extensor digitorum brevis.* Neurology (Minneap) 19:1169, 1969.

82. LEVY, DM AND APFELBERG, DB: *Results of anterior transposition for ulnar neuropathy at the elbow.* Am J Surg 123:304, 1972.

83. LYON, LW AND VAN ALLEN, MW: *Alteration of the orbicularis oculi reflex by acoustic neuroma.* Arch Otolaryngol 95:100, 1972.

84. MACFARLANE, IJA AND DU TOIT, SN: *A ganglion causing tarsal tunnel syndrome.* S Afr Med J 48:2568, 1974.

85. MACLEAN, IC: *Spinal nerve and phrenic nerve studies.* Amer Acad Neurol Spec Course #16, 1979.

86. MANN, RA: *Tarsal tunnel syndrome.* Orthop Clin North Am 5:109, 1974.

87. MARINACCI, AA: *Neurological syndromes of the tarsal tunnels.* Bull LA Neurol Soc 33:90, 1968.

88. MARQUIS, JW, BRUWER, AJ, AND KEITH, HM: *Supracondyloid process of the humerus.* Proc Staff Meet Mayo Clin 32:691, 1957.

89. MASSEY, EW AND PLEET, AB: *Handcuffs and cheiralgia paresthetica.* Neurology (New York) 28:1312, 1978.

90. MELVIN, JL, SCHUCHMANN, JA, AND LANESE, RR: *Diagnostic specificity of motor and sensory nerve conduction variables in the carpal tunnel syndrome.* Arch Phys Med Rehabil 54:69, 1973.

91. MILLENDER, LH, NALEBUFF, EA, AND HOLDSWORTH, DE: *Posterior interosseous-nerve syndrome secondary to rheumatoid synovitis.* J Bone Joint Surg 55A:753, 1973.

92. MILLER, RG: *The cubital tunnel syndrome: Diagnosis and precise localization.* Ann Neurol 6:56, 1979.

93. MILLER, RG AND CAMP, PE: *Postoperative ulnar neuropathy.* JAMA 242:1636, 1979.

94. MILLER, RG AND HUMMEL, EE: *The cubital tunnel syndrome: Treatment with simple decompression.* Ann Neurol 7:567, 1980.

95. MORRIS, HH AND PETERS, BH: *Pronator syndrome: Clinical and electrophysiological features in seven cases.* J Neurol Neurosurg Psychiatry 39:461, 1976.

96. MUMENTHALER, M AND SCHLIACK, H (EDS): *Läsionen peripherer Nerven,* ed 3. Georg Thieme Verlag, Stuttgart, 1977.

97. NAKANO, KK: *The entrapment neuropathies of rheumatoid arthritis.* Orthop Clin North Am 6:837, 1975.

98. NAKANO, KK: *The entrapment neuropathies.* Muscle and Nerve 1:264, 1978.

99. NAKANO, KK: *Entrapment neuropathy from Baker's cyst.* JAMA 239:135, 1978.

100. NAKANO, KK, LUNDERGAN, C, AND OKIHIRO, MM: *Anterior interosseous nerve syndromes. Diagnostic methods and alternative treatments.* Arch Neurol 34:477, 1977.

101. NEARY, D AND EAMES, RA: *The pathology of ulnar nerve compression in man.* Neuropathol Appl Neurobiol 1:69, 1975.

102. NEARY, D, OCHOA, J, AND GILLIATT, RW: *Sub-clinical entrapment neuropathy in man.* J Neurol Sci 24:283, 1975.

103. NEBLETT, C AND EHNI, G: *Medial epicondylectomy for ulnar palsy.* J Neurosurg 32:55, 1970.

104. NEUNDÖRFER, B AND KRÖGER, M: *The anterior interosseous nerve syndrome.* J Neurol 213:347, 1976.

105. NIELSEN, HO: *Posterior interosseous nerve paralysis caused by fibrous band compression at the supinator muscle. A report of four cases.* Acta Orthop Scand 47:304, 1976.

106. O'BRIEN, MD AND UPTON, ARM: *Anterior interosseous nerve syndrome. A case report with neurophysiological investigation.* J Neurol Neurosurg Psychiatry 35:531, 1972.

107. OCHOA, J AND MAROTTE, L: *The nature of the nerve lesion caused by chronic entrapment in the guinea-pig.* J Neurol Sci 19:491, 1973.

108. OCHOA, J AND NEARY, D: *Localised hypertrophic neuropathy, intraneural tumour, or chronic nerve entrapment?* Lancet 1:632, 1975.

109. O'DUFFY, JD, RANDALL, RV, AND MACCARTY, CS: *Median neuropathy (carpal-tunnel syndrome) in acromegaly. A sign of endocrine overactivity.* Ann Intern Med 78:379, 1973.

110. ODUSOTE, K AND EISEN, A: *An electrophysiological quantitation of the cubital tunnel syndrome.* Canad J Neurol Sci 6:403, 1979.

111. OH, SJ, ET AL: *Tarsal tunnel syndrome: Electrophysiological study.* Ann Neurol 5:327, 1979.

112. OLARTE, M AND ADAMS, D: *Accessory nerve palsy.* J Neurol Neurosurg Psychiatry 40:1113, 1977.

113. PAYAN, J: *Electrophysiological localization of ulnar nerve lesions.* J Neurol Neurosurg Psychiatry 32:208, 1969.

114. PAYAN, J: *Anterior transposition of the ulnar nerve: An electrophysiological study.* J Neurol Neurosurg Psychiatry 33:157, 1970.

115. PHALEN, GS: *The carpal-tunnel syndrome. Seventeen years' experience in diagnosis and treatment of six hundred fifty-four hands.* J Bone Joint Surg 48A:211, 1966.

116. PRINGLE, RM, PROTHEROE, K, AND MUKHERJEE, SK: *Entrapment neuropathy of the sural nerve.* J Bone Joint Surg 56B:465, 1974.

117. RASK, MR: *Suprascapular nerve entrapment: A report of two cases treated with suprascapular notch resection.* Clin Orthop 123:73, 1977.

118. RASK, MR: *Watchband superficial radial neurapraxia.* JAMA 241:2702, 1979.

119. RASK, MR: *Superior gluteal nerve entrapment syndrome.* Muscle and Nerve 3:304, 1980.

120. REDFORD, JB: *Nerve conduction in motor fibers to the anterior tibial muscle in peroneal palsy.* Arch Phys Med Rehabil 45:500, 1964.

121. REID, AC AND HAZELTON, RA: *Suprascapular nerve entrapment in the differential diagnosis of shoulder pain.* Lancet 2:477, 1979.

122. RENGACHARY, SS, ET AL: *Suprascapular entrapment neuropathy: A clinical, anatomical, and comparative study. Part 1: Clinical study.* Neurosurgery 5:441, 1979.

123. RENGACHARY, SS, ET AL: *Suprascapular entrapment neuropathy: A clinical, anatomical, and comparative study. Part 2: Anatomical study.* Neurosurgery 5:447, 1979.

124. RENNELS, GD AND OCHOA, J: *Neuralgic amyotrophy manifesting as anterior interosseous nerve palsy.* Muscle and Nerve 3:160, 1980.

125. ROBBINS, H: *Anatomical study of the median nerve in the carpal tunnel and etiologies of the carpal-tunnel syndrome.* J Bone Joint Surg 45A:953, 1963.

126. ROTH, G: *Vitesse de conduction motrice du nerf médian dans le canal carpien.* Annales De Médecine Physique 13:117, 1970.

127. RUPRECHT, EO: *Befunde bei Neuropathien.* In HOPF, HC AND STRUPPLER, A (EDS): *Electromyographie.* George Thieme Verlag, Stuttgart, 1974, pp 37–65.

128. SARALA, PK, NISHIHARA, T, AND OH, SJ: *Meralgia paresthetica: Electrophysiologic study.* Arch Phys Med Rehabil 60:30, 1979.

129. SCARPALEZOS, S, ET AL: *Neural and muscular manifestations of hypothyroidism.* Arch Neurol 29:140, 1973.

130. SCHWARTZ, MS, GORDON, JA, AND SWASH, M: *Slowed nerve conduction with wrist flexion in carpal tunnel syndrome.* Ann Neurol 8:69, 1980.

131. SEDAL, L, MCLEOD, JG, AND WALSH, JC: *Ulnar nerve lesions associated with the carpal tunnel syndrome.* J Neurol Neurosurg Psychiatry 36:118, 1973.

132. SHEA, JD AND MCCLAIN, EJ: *Ulnar-nerve compression syndromes at and below the wrist.* J Bone Joint Surg 51A:1095, 1969.

133. SIDEY, JD: *Weak ankles. A study of common peroneal entrapment neuropathy.* Br Med J 3:623, 1969.

134. SIDIQ, M, KIRSNER, AB, AND SHEON, RP: *Carpal tunnel syndrome. First manifestation of systemic lupus erythematosus.* JAMA 222:1416, 1972.

135. SIMPSON, JA: *Electrical signs in the diagnosis of carpal tunnel and related syndromes.* J Neurol Neurosurg Psychiatry 19:275, 1956.

136. SINGH, A AND JOLLY, SS: *Wasted leg syndrome (a compression neuropathy of lower limbs).* J Assoc Physicians India 11:1031, 1963.

137. SOLHEIM, LF AND ROAAS, A: *Compression of the suprascapular nerve after fracture of the scapular notch.* Acta Orthop Scand 49:338, 1978.

138. SPECTOR, RH AND SCHWARTZMAN, RJ: *Benign trigeminal and facial neuropathy.* Arch Intern Med 135:992, 1975.

139. SPINNER, M: *Injuries to the Major Branches of Peripheral Nerves of the Forearm, ed 2.* WB Saunders, Philadelphia, 1978.

140. STAAL, A: *The entrapment neuropathies.* In VINKEN, PJ AND BRUYN, GW (EDS): *Handbook of Clinical Neurology.* North-Holland, Amsterdam, 1970, pp 285–325.

141. STERN, MB AND SPIEGEL, P: *Femoral neuropathy as a complication of heparin anticoagulation therapy.* Clin Orthop Rel Res 106:140, 1975.

142. STEVENS, A AND ROSSELLE, N: *Sensory nerve conduction velocity of N. cutaneous femoris lateralis.* Electromyography 10:397, 1970.

143. STEWART, JD AND EISEN, A: *Tinel's sign and the carpal tunnel syndrome.* Br Med J 2:1125, 1978.

144. STÖHR, M, ET AL: *Retrograde changes of nerve fibers with the carpal tunnel syndrome. An electroneurographic investigation.* J Neurol 218:287, 1978.

145. STÖHR, M, SCHUMM, F, AND BALLIER, R: *Normal sensory conduction in the saphenous nerve in man.* Electroenceph Clin Neurophysiol 44:172, 1978.

146. SUNDERLAND, S: *The relative susceptibility to injury of the medial and lateral popliteal divisions of the sciatic nerve.* Br J Surg 41:300, 1953.

147. SUNDERLAND, S: *Nerves and Nerve Injuries, ed 2.* Churchill Livingstone, Edinburgh, 1978.

148. THOMAS, PK AND FULLERTON, PM: *Nerve fibre size in the carpal tunnel syndrome.* J Neurol Neurosurg Psychiatry 26:520, 1963.

149. THOMAS, JE, LAMBERT, EH, AND CSEUZ, KA: *Electrodiagnostic aspects of the carpal tunnel syndrome.* Arch Neurol 16:635, 1967.

150. TINEL, J: *Le Signe du "Fourmillement" dans les Lésions des Nerfs Péripheriques.* Press Med 47:388, October, 1915. Translated into English by Dr. Emanuel B. Kaplan, J. Tinel's "Fourmillement" paper, The "Tingling" sign in peripheral nerve lesions. In SPINNER, M (ED): *Injuries to the Major Branches of Peripheral Nerves of the Forearm, ed 2.* WB Saunders, Philadelphia, 1978.

151. TROJABORG, W: *Rate of recovery in motor and sensory fibres of the radial nerve: Clinical and electrophysiological aspects.* J Neurol Neurosurg Psychiatry 33:625, 1970.

152. TROJABORG, W: *Motor and sensory conduction in the musculocutaneous nerve.* J Neurol Neurosurg Psychiatry 39:890, 1976.

153. UPTON, ARM AND MCCOMAS, AJ: *The double crush in nerve-entrapment syndromes.* Lancet 2:359, 1973.

154. VALENTA, LJ: *Hyperparathyroidism due to parathyroid adenoma and carpal tunnel syndrome.* Ann Intern Med 82:541, 1975.

155. VALLAT, JM AND DUNOYER, J: *Familial occurrence of entrapment neuropathies.* Arch Neurol 36:323, 1979.

156. VEMIREDDI, NK, REDFORD, JB, AND POMBEJARA, CN: *Serial nerve conduction studies in carpal tunnel syndrome secondary to rheumatoid arthritis: Preliminary study.* Arch Phys Med Rehabil 60:393, 1979.

157. WAINAPEL, SF, KIM, DJ, AND EBEL, A: *Conduction studies of the saphenous nerve in healthy subjects.* Arch Phys Med Rehabil 59:316, 1978.

158. WIEDERHOLT, WC: *Median nerve conduction velocity in sensory fibers through carpal tunnel.* Arch Phys Med Rehabil 51:328, 1970.

159. WILKINS, RH AND BRODY, IA: *Tinel's sign.* Arch Neurol 24:573, 1971.

160. WILSON, DH AND KROUT, R: *Surgery of ulnar neuropathy at the elbow: 16 cases treated by decompression without transposition. Technical note.* J Neurosurg 38:780, 1973.

161. WOLF, SM, ET AL: *Treatment of Bell palsy with prednisone: A prospective, randomized study.* Neurology (New York) 28:158, 1978.

162. WRIGHT, TA: *Accessory spinal nerve injury.* Clin Orthop 108:15, 1975.

163. YOUNG, MR AND NORRIS, JW: *Femoral neuropathy during anticoagulant therapy.* Neurology (Minneap) 26:1173, 1976.

164. YU, J, BENDLER, EM, AND MENTARI, A: *Neurological disorders associated with carpal tunnel syndrome.* Electromyogr Clin Neurophysiol 19:27, 1979.

# DISORDERS OF THE NEUROMUSCULAR JUNCTION, MYOPATHIES, AND ABNORMAL MUSCLE ACTIVITY

# MYASTHENIA GRAVIS AND OTHER DISORDERS OF NEUROMUSCULAR TRANSMISSION

Recent work has elucidated the pathophysiology and morphology underlying disorders of neuromuscular transmission (see Figs. 8-1 and 8-2). Morphologic abnormalities correlate with physiologic alterations in the kinetics of acetylcholine (ACh). Contrary to previous views, current evidence clearly indicts the postsynaptic ACh receptor as the site of pathology in myasthenia gravis. In contrast, presynaptic defects of ACh release are responsible for the weakness seen in the myasthenic syndrome and in botulism. Despite the dichotomy between presynaptic and postsynaptic pathologies, the exact physiologic or morphologic basis of these transmission defects remains unknown. It is plausible that different diseases of the neuromuscular junction affect the complex process of chemical transmission at different steps. For example, a congenital defect of acetylcholinesterase is the basis for a new myasthenic syndrome recently described by Engel, Lambert, and Gomez.[33]

    A possible defect of neuromuscular transmission should be considered in any patient presenting with unexplained weakness. Diagnostic possibilities include not only primary diseases of the neuromuscular junction, such as myasthenia gravis, myasthenic syndromes, and botulism, but also abnormalities of the nerve terminals seen in motor neuron disease and certain types of neuropathy. Electrodiagnostic studies are valuable in confirming abnormalities of neuromuscular transmission.

## MYASTHENIA GRAVIS

Myasthenia gravis is a common disease with an incidence of approximately 1 in 20,000 in the United States.[74] It is a disease of young females in their third decade and middle-aged males in their fifth and sixth decades. The overall average incidence is slightly higher in females by a ratio of 3:2. The disease usually occurs sporadically, but about 5 percent of the cases are familial. The symptoms and signs usually appear in the second to fourth decade. Children account for 11 percent of all patients with myasthenia gravis,[74] and often have some other systemic disease or a seizure disorder.[102]

### Etiologic considerations

Mounting evidence indicates that myasthenia gravis is an autoimmune disorder.[99] Its established relationship to thymoma and thymic hyperplasia, found in about 10 and 70 percent of patients with myasthenia gravis, respectively, provides strong support for the autoimmune hypothesis.[36] Further, myasthenia gravis is commonly associated with other potentially immunologic diseases such as thyroiditis, hyperthyroidism or hypothyroidism,[75, 85, 103] polymyositis, systemic lupus erythematosus, and rheumatoid arthritis. Although the autoimmune process in myasthenia gravis may originate within the thymus, immunization of rats with thymus extracts has failed to produce a myasthenia-like condition.[67]

Passive transfer of a certain serum fraction from patients with myasthenia gravis causes myasthenic features in mice histologically as well as electrophysiologically.[109] Similar passive transfer occurs as an experiment of nature, since 20 percent of infants born of myasthenic mothers have transient myasthenia because of transplacental transfer of antibody. Injection of nicotinic ACh receptor protein from the electric eel into the rabbit or monkey with Freund's adjuvant sensitizes the animal. After a second injection, given 15 days later, many animals develop myasthenic features that improve with administration of an anticholinesterase.[77, 108] Antireceptor antibodies are present in about 80 percent of patients with myasthenia gravis.[1, 4, 57] In addition to a circulating immunoglobulin, altered cellular immunity is certain to play a major role in this disease.

Considerable progress has been made during recent years in the understanding of myasthenia gravis.[78, 100, 101] Histometric studies of motor end-plate ultrastructure[31, 32, 34] have revealed a reduced size of the nerve terminal area and a simplified postsynaptic membrane with poorly developed folds and clefts. Myasthenic muscles contain IgG and complement bound to postsynaptic membranes, implicating an immunologic process in the destruction of the membrane architecture. In contrast, mean synaptic vesicle diameter and mean synaptic vesicle count per unit nerve terminal area remain unaltered. These observations implicate the ACh receptor in the pathogenesis of myasthenia gravis. Microphysiologic findings indicate reduced sensitivity of the postsynaptic membrane to iontophoretic application of ACh. Furthermore, a decreased number of functional ACh receptors has been demonstrated by reduced binding of alpha bungarotoxin to myasthenic motor end-plates.[37, 47, 110]

## Clinical signs and symptoms

Weakness and excessive fatigability of striated muscles are the main clinical features of myasthenia gravis.[71] Although usually of insidious onset, the disease may become clinically manifest after acute infection or following various surgical procedures, including a thymectomy.[52] Initial symptoms tend to appear towards the end of the day or after strenuous exercise. In an advanced stage symptoms are present more or less constantly. Symptoms may be generalized or confined to restricted groups of muscles.[82] Weakness initially affects the ocular muscles, causing diplopia in about half of the patients. Less frequently, bulbar weakness occurs as the presenting symptom. Paralysis of palatal and pharyngeal muscles, seen in about one third of the patients, results in nasal speech and difficulty in swallowing and chewing. Generalized weakness of the trunk and extremities is the least common initial symptom. In most patients, weakness worsens with elevation of body temperature.[7, 8, 42, 43]

Characteristic physical signs include a wide spectrum of ocular disturbance, ranging from nystagmus to complete ophthalmoplegia. Pupillary dysfunction can be seen;[58] this is an exception to the rule that signs of myasthenia gravis are restricted to striated muscles. Ptosis, if present as an early sign, is usually asymmetric and may alternate between sides. Involvement of ocular muscles is also variable from one examination to the next and is not confined to the disturbance of a single nerve. Weakness of the orbicularis oris and other muscles of the lower face produces a characteristic, expressionless myasthenic face. Because of weakness of the neck extensors, a patient may support his chin with his hand. This position also facilitates chewing and swallowing when the muscles of mastication tire, especially at the end of a meal. Speech may fatigue to a flaccid dysarthria. Involvement of the respiratory muscles is common in advanced cases and constitutes the major threat to life. Generalized or focal muscular atrophy is present in some cases.[72] The sensory examination is normal.

The clinical course is variable and often shows remission and exacerbation. Approximately one third of the patients improve spontaneously, some nearly completely, requiring no further medication. Some patients develop respiratory failure and pneumonia. Symptoms often fluctuate unpredictably but several circumstances are likely to exacerbate the disease. These include infection, exposure to heat, emotional stress, thyroid disease, and perhaps most importantly, overmedication. The effect of pregnancy is unpredictable, but early worsening and later improvement is common. Prognosis has improved with the advent of newer therapeutic regimens, including thymectomy, steroids, plasma exchange, and immunosuppressive drugs.[81] In the mildest form of the disease, weakness is limited to the muscles of the eye. This entity, designated ocular myasthenia, is distinguished by its benign course. If signs outside the eye have not appeared within one year, 90 percent of the patients initially diagnosed as having ocular myasthenia will develop no further progression of symptoms.[73, 82]

Differential diagnoses include all diseases characterized by weakness of ocular, bulbar, or extremity muscles. These include muscular dystrophy, motor neuron disease, progressive bulbar palsy, multiple sclerosis, ophthalmoplegia, pseudobulbar palsy, and psychoneurosis. In mild cases of myasthenia gravis, in which symptoms may appear only after exertion, patients are not uncommonly mistaken for hysterics. The diagnosis of myasthenia gravis depends on the characteristic distribution of weakness and excessive fatigability after exercise.

Fatigability may be demonstrated by ptosis with sustained upward gaze, grip dynamometry, serial vital capacity measurements, and prolonged arm abduction. Following the limb exercise with a pneumatic cuff inflated around the upper arm, myasthenic signs worsen in the rest of the body upon release of the cuff.[113] This phenomenon, originally taken to indicate the presence of a circulating toxic substance, may be related to a reduction in calcium secondary to the increased lactate produced during ischemic exercise.[79] Neuromuscular fatigue also occurs after repetitive electrical stimulation of a nerve. Myasthenic muscles characteristically show hypersensitivity to curare administered systemically.[91] Excess sensitivity is nonspecific, however, as it simply indicates defective neuromuscular transmission and may be seen in motor neuron disease,[65] ocular myopathy,[60, 90] and antibiotic toxicity.[84]

Intravenous administration of edrophonium (Tensilon) is a valuable clinical diagnostic test, since, in previously untreated cases, the strength of involved muscles improves almost uniformly. Usually a 2 mg test dose is given initially, followed by up to 10 mg total. The effect of edrophonium begins within 1 minute and is over in 5 to 10 minutes. For objective assessment, the test should include a control injection of normal saline, preferably in a double blind fashion. In some patients, especially those with ocular myasthenia, the effect of edrophonium is very brief and equivocal, giving rise to a false negative result. The administration of longer-acting neostigmine (Prostigmin) may improve the strength more appreciably. A hot bath may worsen symptoms, since a higher body temperature lowers the margin of safety of neuromuscular transmission.[7, 99] Distinction from multiple sclerosis may be difficult, especially if the patient presents with pseudo internuclear ophthalmoplegia.[59] Routine muscle biopsy is of little diagnostic value. Type II fiber atrophy is commonly seen but is not specific to myasthenia and can also result from disuse atrophy or corticosteroid treatment.

## Electrophysiologic tests

Electrophysiologic studies play an important role in establishing the diagnosis of myasthenia gravis. However, the reliability of obtaining a significant decremental response in myasthenic muscles is variable, with one laboratory reporting a positive test in 95 percent[76] and another in only 41 percent.[93] In general, 65 to 85 percent of patients show decremental responses if a number of distal and proximal muscles are tested. Movement artifact must be controlled to ensure accurate interpretation of these tests. Unfortunately, the muscles easiest to immobilize tend to be distal, whereas those most likely to be abnormal are proximal. However, the trapezius is an easily stabilized proximal muscle. For this reason, we proceed from the intrinsic hand muscles, to the trapezius and other shoulder girdle muscles, and finally to the facial muscles. Warming the muscle increases test sensitivity (see Fig. 9-1). When conventional studies are equivocal, nerve stimulation under ischemic conditions or following regional administration of curare[12] may be of diagnostic value.

The compound muscle action potential is normal or only slightly reduced in amplitude when elicited by a single nerve stimulus. However, the muscle action potentials characteristically show a decremental response to repetitive stimulation at low rates and to a lesser extent at higher rates. The most effective stimulus rate is 2 to 3 per second (see Figs. 8-6 and 8-8). According to generally accepted criteria, at least two muscles should show reproducible decrement of more than 10 percent between the first response and the smallest of the first five of a stimulation train. However, this is a conservative estimate. In our experience, any reproducible decrement is suspicious if the tracing is free of technical problems.

Brief voluntary exercise is of great help in differentiating abnormal neuromuscular transmission from technical problems such as submaximal stimulation or movement artifact (see Fig. 9-3). If repetitive stimulation at 2 to 3 per second demonstrates a small decrement, brief voluntary exercise for five seconds or intravenous administration of edrophonium will usually normalize the response partially or completely in myasthenic muscles. If the decrement persists, it may be attributable to technical factors and not to defective neuromuscular transmission. Compared with baseline response at rest, a bona fide decremental tendency also becomes less noticeable after a more sustained, 30 seconds to 1 minute, maximal voluntary exercise or tetanic stimulation, a phenomenon called post-tetanic potentiation. The decrement is greater than at rest two to four minutes after the exercise, during post-tetanic exhaustion. Again, an additional five seconds of exercise will partially correct the change.

Electromyography shows a characteristic variability in the successive configurations of a given motor unit potential. Although this variation is often random, the initial few motor unit potentials tend to show a progressive decrease in amplitude and duration. Fibrillation potentials and positive sharp waves may be present in severely affected muscles, possibly reflecting loss of innervation. Single fiber electromyography (SFEMG) is probably one of the most sensitive tests for myasthenia gravis. A pair of single fibers innervated by the same axon characteristically shows increased jitter in mildly affected muscles and blocking in later stages. Abnormalities may be detected in muscles that are clinically asymptomatic and show no decrement to repetitive nerve stimulation.

In occasional patients with myasthenia gravis, the electrophysiologic features are more typically associated with the myasthenic syndrome. These cases suggest the existence of an intermediate disorder characterized by defective ACh release as well as diminished numbers of ACh receptors.[23] However, microelectrode studies have provided no convincing evidence to support such contention. As described in Chapter 8, decremental ACh release and incremental ACh release at low and high rates of stimulation, respectively, are both normal physiologic phenomena that become clinically significant in the presence of defective neuromuscular transmission (see Fig. 8-8). The response pattern to repetitive stimulation is in part determined by the size of the first compound muscle potential, which varies among individuals with the same disease. An initially subnormal response may be followed by an incrementing rather than decrementing train during rapid repetitive stimulation, even in patients with myasthenia gravis (see Fig. 8-7). Indeed, in the same patient, some muscles may demonstrate a defect typical of myasthenia gravis, whereas others may show changes reminiscent of the myasthenic syndrome.

# MYASTHENIC SYNDROME

The myasthenic syndrome was first described by Eaton and Lambert[29] under the descriptive term myasthenic syndrome sometimes associated with small cell bronchogenic carcinoma. The disease is twice as common in men. The onset is usually after age 40, although the syndrome has appeared as early as 9 years of age.[18]

## Etiologic considerations

Small cell carcinoma of the bronchus is the most common tumor seen in conjunction with this syndrome, being detected in over 50 percent of the patients. Careful search reveals a malignant neoplasm of one kind or another in about 75 percent of men and 25 percent of women, although not necessarily at the time of initial neuromuscular symptoms. These include reticulum cell sarcoma,[89] rectal carcinoma,[16] renal carcinoma,[17] basal cell carcinoma of the skin,[106] leukemia,[98] and malignant thymoma.[56] Systemic disorders associated with the syndrome include thyrotoxicosis,[70] Sjögren's syndrome,[13] rheumatoid arthritis,[106] and other autoimmune disorders.[44] The malignancy may not become apparent for many months or, occasionally, for many years after the onset of the myasthenic syndrome. With adequate follow up, however, only 30 percent of the patients remain free of detectable cancer.[55] Despite the clear association between malignancy and the syndrome, the manner by which a tumor leads to defective release of acetylcholine (ACh) is not known. Perhaps biologically active polypeptides are produced which, like botlinum toxin or magnesium ($Mg^{++}$) ions, block ACh release from the motor terminals by interfering with the utilization of calcium ($Ca^{++}$).

Histometric studies of motor end-plate ultrastructure[31, 32] have shown overdevelopment and increased area of the postsynaptic membrane (see Fig. 8-2). The nerve terminal retains a normal mean synaptic vesicle diameter and mean synaptic vesicle density. Routine muscle biopsy shows only nonspecific findings with some Type II fiber atrophy and mild inflammatory reactions. Microelectrode studies of excised intercostal muscles show the miniature end-plate potential (MEPP) to be normal in amplitude, although low in frequency.[30] The mean quantum content of the end-plate potentials (EPP) following a single nerve impulse is abnormally low but increases with repetitive nerve impulses.[54] These findings are compatible with either a defect in the calcium-dependent release of ACh from the motor nerve terminals or with a decreased store of available ACh. Ultrastructural studies showing a normal synaptic vesicle number per unit nerve terminal area tend to discount the latter possibility. Thus, in contrast to myasthenia gravis, which is characterized by a reduced number of functional ACh receptors, weakness in the myasthenic syndrome is caused by presynaptic abnormalities that result in a reduced number of ACh quanta released per volley of nerve impulse. This is reminiscent of neuromuscular transmission block induced experimentally by high magnesium or low calcium ion concentrations.

## Clinical signs and symptoms

In striking contrast to myasthenia gravis, the myasthenic syndrome is characterized by greatest weakness at rest or right after awakening in the morning. Strength tends to transiently improve after brief exercise, but patients are unable to sustain prolonged effort. Weakness and fatigability in the myasthenic syndrome primarily affect the lower extremities, particularly the pelvic girdle and thigh muscles. Climbing stairs or, to a lesser degree, arising from a chair, are especially difficult. Shoulders and the four extremity muscles are also commonly weak. Characteristically spared are neck, bulbar, and extraocular musculature. This distribution of weakness contrasts with the typical patterns seen in myasthenia gravis. However, whereas ocular and bulbar symptoms are not as conspicuous as in myasthenia gravis, ptosis, diplopia, dysphagia, and dysarthria may occur. The patient often complains of dryness of the mouth, and less frequently, impotence, paresthesias, and dysautonomia. These symptoms suggest that the defect of ACh release may not be restricted to skeletal muscle but may affect the autonomic nervous system as well.[92] Peripheral neuropathy and subacute cerebellar degeneration have been reported in conjunction with the myasthenic syndrome, both of which are probably epiphenomena of a paraneoplastic syndrome.

Neurologic evaluation usually reveals marked weakness of proximal muscles of the lower limbs. Appreciable improvement occurs after exercise. With each successive effort the resistance needed to overcome the patient's strength increases, giving the examiner a sensation similar to drawing up water from a well with a hand pump.[11] Reduced muscle stretch reflexes and other signs of polyneuropathy may be present. The edrophonium (Tensilon) test is ordinarily negative or equivocal, but the patient is very sensitive to d-tubocurarine and decamethonium, which cause a depolarizing block at the neuromuscular junction. Guanidine partially corrects defective calcium-dependent ACh release and results in dramatic improvement in strength. The neuromuscular defect in the myasthenic syndrome can also be partially reversed experimentally by the injection of calcium and by the administration of 4-aminopyridine, aminophylline, or caffeine, which increases the cyclic adenosine monophosphate essential in calcium mobilization in cells.[107]

## Electrophysiologic tests

The electrical hallmark of the syndrome is a very small amplitude compound muscle action potential elicited by nerve stimulation (see Figs. 8-8 and 9-6). This contrasts strikingly with normal sensory evoked potentials. Progressive decline in muscle action potential amplitude with repetitive stimulation at low rates is similar to that seen in myasthenia gravis. In contrast, at high stimulation rates or with brief voluntary contraction, for up to 10 seconds, the muscle action potentials show a significant increment, usually exceeding 50 to 200 percent (see Figs. 9-4 and 9-5). Paired stimulation with interstimulus intervals of 5 to 10 ms causes the second response to increase rather than decrease as expected in normal muscles. Post-tetanic facilitation decays within 20 seconds and is followed in two to four minutes by post-tetanic exhaustion when the muscle potential falls below the resting level (see Figs. 9-8 and 9-9).

Nerve stimulation may reveal marked abnormalities even if clinical symptoms are mild. Interestingly, patients with a mild myasthenic syndrome may not be aware of their motor dysfunction, because, with post-tetanic facilitation, muscle strength may be nearly normal during voluntary contraction. Rested muscles, however, show an unequivocal defect of neuromuscular transmission. In myasthenia gravis the response pattern to repetitive stimulation varies greatly among patients. However, in the myasthenic syndrome, nearly all muscles show a mild decrement at low rates and prominent increment at high rates of stimulation. This is in contrast to myasthenia gravis, in which electrical abnormalities are usually limited to clinically symptomatic muscles. In a unique case, electrophysiologic studies revealed a marked depression to single nerve stimulation and facilitation at all rates from 1 to 200 per second.[53] This case may represent a separate entity or variation of the myasthenic syndrome.

Needle studies show varying configurations of repetitive motor unit potentials with an incrementing tendency. As expected, single fiber studies have revealed increased jitter and blocking which improve with high rates of stimulation and worsen following rest.[96]

# OTHER FORMS OF MYASTHENIA GRAVIS

## Neonatal myasthenia gravis

Neonatal myasthenia gravis is a self-limited state that occurs in approximately 15 percent of infants born to myasthenic mothers.[104, 111] This condition presumably results from transplacental transfer of anti-acetylcholine (ACh) receptor antibodies.[69] Clinical weakness remits as the serum concentration of ACh receptor antibodies declines.[51] A similar clinical syndrome develops in mice following injection of the IgG serum fraction from patients with myasthenia gravis.[109]

Symptoms occur during the first three days after birth and consist of hypotonia and difficulty in breathing and sucking. The neonates usually respond to anticholinesterase medication. Symptoms generally disappear when the infant's own immune system has developed in a few weeks,[68, 114] but they may occasionally persist beyond two months of age.[10] Desmedt and Borenstein[27] have found characteristic electrophysiologic abnormalities in distal muscles 30 days after clinical recovery. An elevated antibody titer against ACh receptor returns to the normal range over a three-month period.[51]

## Congenital myasthenia gravis

Distinct from transient neonatal myasthenia are several rare varieties of congenital myasthenia gravis with onset at birth or in childhood and a persistent clinical course.[9] One type, seen in infants or children born to normal mothers, primarily involves extraocular muscles without associated generalized weakness.[73] The symptoms are initially mild but often slowly progressive despite therapy.[63] A familial type shows respiratory depression at birth, and episodic weakness and apnea during the first two years.[22, 38, 41] This condition may improve with anticholinesterase medication.[88] Unlike infants with neonatal myasthenia gravis, patients with congenital myasthenia gravis have no anti-ACh receptor antibodies in the serum.[112] These and other syndromes of congenital myasthenia may represent separate pathologic, electrophysiologic, and clinical entities. In vitro intracellular microelectrode studies revealed a different mechanism of defective neuromuscular transmission in each of the following three recently described entities.

Engel, Lambert, and Gomez[33] described a 15-year-old boy with intermittent ptosis, delayed motor development, and generalized weakness. Edrophonium (Tensilon) and neostigmine (Prostigmin) tests were negative. A serum assay showed no antibodies to muscle ACh receptors. Nerve stimulation produced repetitive discharges following a single shock and a decremental response to a train of stimuli at 2 and 40 per second. Needle studies showed temporal variability in the configuration of the action potentials for a given motor unit during weak voluntary contraction. In vitro intracellular microelectrode studies showed the miniature end-plate potential (MEPP) to be normal in amplitude but low in frequency. A markedly reduced number of ACh quanta released per nerve stimulation presumably reflected a reduced store of immediately available ACh. The MEPP and end-plate potential (EPP) were of unusually long duration, which possibly explains the repetitive muscle action potential discharges following a single nerve impulse. Acetylcholinesterase was absent at the end-plates. Nerve terminals were abnormally small, being on the average one third to a quarter of the normal size.

A familial congenital myasthenic syndrome with prolonged EPP but normal muscle acetylcholinesterase occurred in one sporadic case and in four others from two different families.[35] The affected infants had ophthalmoparesis and weakness of neck muscles. Easy fatigability and weakness of shoulder girdle and forearm muscles developed later in the teens or in adulthood. Single stimuli to motor nerves elicited repetitive muscle action potentials in proximal and distal muscles tested. Since muscle acetylcholinesterase was normal, the cause of the prolonged EPP might be attributed to an abnormal ACh receptor with a prolonged open time, or an abnormal transmitter resistant to muscle acetylcholinesterase.

A third type, also a familial congenital myasthenic syndrome, is probably caused by deficient synthesis of ACh.[46] Affected infants had intermittent ptosis, feeding difficulties, dyspnea or apnea, and vomiting. Weakness worsened with febrile illness and during exercise. Symptoms gradually improved with age. Progressive weakness developed during prolonged nerve stimulation at 10 per second. However, no decrement of the action potential occurred with brief repetitive nerve stimulation. The temporal decline in EPP and MEPP amplitude during prolonged nerve stimulation resembled that produced in normal muscle by blocking ACh synthesis with hemicholinium.[26]

# BOTULISM

## Botulinum toxin

Poisoning by the exotoxin of *Clostridium botulinum* results in weakness of both striated and smooth muscles, because the toxin has a generalized effect on the neuromuscular junction. Of the six immunologic types of Bacillus botulinus, types A, B, and E are chiefly responsible for human poisoning. Since the toxin is heat sensitive, poisoning usually follows the ingestion of raw or inadequately cooked or canned vegetables, meat, or fish. An infected wound may occasionally harbor the toxins.[25] Types A and B are usually associated with contaminated canned vegetables and Type E with fish products. The mortality is considered higher in Types A or E than in Type B.[62]

The incidence of botulism appears to be greater at high altitudes, probably because of the lower temperature required to boil water.[19] The defect in neuromuscular transmission in botulism is similar to that found in the myasthenic syndrome, with marked impairment of acetylcholine (ACh) release from the nerve terminal.[49] The amplitude of the miniature end-plate potential (MEPP) is either normal or only slightly reduced, but its frequency is extremely low. A small quantum content per volley of nerve impulse results in a markedly decreased end-plate potential (EPP).

## Clinical signs and symptoms

Clinical symptoms appear within one to two days after eating contaminated food and in one to two weeks after wound inoculation, the time interval necessary for the elaboration of toxin. The initial symptoms may be diarrhea, nausea, or vomiting. Weakness normally manifests itself as external ophthalmoplegia and ptosis. Failure of convergence may be the first symptom. The pupils are fixed and dilated. Dysarthria, dysphagia, and weakness of muscles of mastication may follow. The muscles of the extremities and the trunk are usually affected later. The involvement of intestine and bladder causes constipation and urinary retention. Rapid development of cardiac or respiratory failure may be fatal with ingestion of a large amount of toxin. In less severe cases, mild symptoms abate and complete recovery is the rule. Commonly, several members of a family who have shared the same contaminated food develop similar symptoms. The diagnosis may be more difficult in isolated cases. Infant botulism, now recognized with increasing frequency, may be responsible for some cases of the sudden infant death syndrome.[48, 83]

On examination, the patient is flaccid and areflexic. Paralysis of the pupil is usually but not always present.[20] The extraocular muscles are involved. Widespread paralysis involves not only the extremities but also the muscles of respiration. Fatigability following exercise is not as prominent as in patients with myasthenia gravis. Unlike the weakness seen in the myasthenic syndrome, muscle strength does not improve with repeated efforts. Treatment with guanidine does not enhance recovery from botulism.[50] Diagnosis is corroborated by a positive mouse toxin neutralization test and confirmed by culture of the suspected food.

## Electrophysiologic tests

Sensory nerve action potentials are normal in amplitude and latency. The compound muscle action potential elicited by single stimuli to the nerve is small and declines with repetitive stimulation at a slow rate. Paired stimuli at interstimulus intervals of less than 10 ms characteristically potentiate the second response by summation of the two EPPs (see Fig. 9-2). This contrasts with the smaller second response produced in normal muscles at such short interstimulus intervals because of the refractory period. In botulism, as in the myasthenic syndrome, the refractory period plays a lesser role, since only a limited number of muscle fibers discharge in response to the first stimulus. Some facilitation of muscle response occurs during a fast train of stimuli or during post-tetanic potentiation, but to a considerably lesser degree when compared with the myasthenic syndrome (see Fig. 9-7). The presence of fibrillation potentials may indicate a functional denervation as a result of limited release of ACh.[39] Single fiber studies have shown increased jitter and blocking and some reduction in fiber density.[94]

# OTHER DISORDERS
## Tick paralysis

Available data suggest that neurotoxin of tick paralysis affects either the nerve terminal or the neuromuscular junction. The condition is rare but has been reported world wide. The disease is caused by the gravid female tick, *Dermacentor andersoni* (wood tick) or *Dermacentor paridulis* (dog tick) in the United States, and *Ixodes holocyclus* (scrub tick) in Australia.[80] Most cases of tick paralysis occur in spring or summer when ticks are active. A majority of cases involve young children, especially girls with long hair.[95] The symptoms and signs begin five to seven days after the tick has embedded. During this latent period, the organism, attached near the hairline, remains unnoticed.

Illness begins with general symptoms such as irritability and diarrhea. Weakness initially affects the legs and, within a day, the remaining voluntary muscles. Paralyses of the bulbar and respiratory musculature, although now rare, are always a threat until removal of the embedded tick. Other features include dysarthria, dysphagia, blurred vision, facial weakness, and reduced muscle stretch reflexes. Sensory abnormalities are rare, but occasionally patients complain of numbness and tingling of the extremities. Removal of the tick is usually followed by a rapid improvement. However, persistent weakness and the presence of fibrillation potentials in some cases suggest a structural lesion of distal motor axons.[28] To prevent local infection, it is best to first cause the tick to withdraw from the skin by applying heat or Vaseline or some other chemical substance, and then gently remove it in one piece with a forceps.

Electrophysiologic studies in a few confirmed cases have consistently shown reduced amplitude of the compound muscle action potential.[21, 45, 64, 80, 105] In one study,[105] muscle action potentials did not change significantly on repetitive stimulation even up to 50 per second. Motor and sensory nerve conduction times were mildly increased in the distal segments during the paralytic phase but returned to normal after clinical recovery. These findings suggest that the major effect of the toxin is to prevent depolarization in the terminal portions of motor nerves, which results in reduction in amplitude of the evoked muscle action potential. The toxin seems to increase distal latencies of the large myelinated motor and sensory axons by altering the ionic fluxes that mediate action potentials in the nerve terminals. Like other potent biotoxins such as tetrodotoxin and saxitoxin, tick toxin probably blocks the inward flux of sodium ions at sensory and motor nerve terminals and at internodes. Some evidence suggests that tick toxin may also interfere with release of acetylcholine (ACh) at the nerve terminal[21] but not with its synthesis and storage.[66] However, intracellular studies of hamsters paralyzed by tick toxin have shown normal size and frequency of miniature end-plate potentials (MEPP) and normal quantal content of end-plate potentials (EPP).[61]

## Drug-associated myasthenia

Administration of some antibiotics, notably kanamycin and neomycin and all other polypeptide aminoglycoside antibiotics, may cause abnormalities of neuromuscular transmission.[5] The muscle action potentials show a decremental response, reminiscent of myasthenia gravis, at low rates of repetitive stimulation. Facilitation after exercise, however, may be more prominent than in patients with myasthenia gravis. Experimental data in rats indicate that MEPPs are of small amplitude and that the mean quantum content of EPP is abnormally low.[24] These findings suggest combined pre- and postsynaptic effects. Another type of abnormality produced experimentally with hemicholinium impairs ACh synthesis.[26]

An increasing number of reports have described the onset of myasthenia gravis following penicillamine therapy for rheumatoid arthritis.[6, 14, 15, 97] In one carefully studied case clinical symptoms and electrodiagnostic parameters, including those of single-fiber studies, improved after discontinuing penicillamine.[2] The syndrome is clinically and electrophysiologically indistinguishable from idiopathic myasthenia gravis except for its temporal association with penicillamine therapy.

## Lower motor neuron disorders

Defects of neuromuscular transmission have also appeared in motor neuron disease and peripheral neuropathies.[65] Experimental studies suggest that the immediately available store of ACh is diminished during regeneration. Or, a defect may lie in the propagation of impulses along the terminal portion of the nerve, if the axonal refractory period is abnormally prolonged. In these cases, repetitive stimulation at low rates results in a progressive decrement of the muscle action potential. In a demyelinating neuropathy, this decrement is minimal at low rates but becomes progressively more prominent at faster rates of stimulation.[40] This contrasts the changes seen in myasthenia gravis. Such phenomena as post-tetanic potentiation and exhaustion may also occur. Thus, in the presence of peripheral neuropathy, a decremental response to repetitive stimulation does not necessarily imply abnormalities of neuromuscular transmission.

## Muscle diseases

A decrementing response may also result from increasing muscle membrane refractoriness associated with repetitive discharges in myotonia[3] and periodic paralysis.[87] In these disorders, a decrement occurs regardless of the rate of stimulation. The pattern of decrement differs from that in myasthenia gravis in that it is steadily progressive with no tendency for the amplitude to plateau or recover at the fifth or sixth stimulus. Immediately after exercise, the muscle action potential is much reduced, since many muscle fibers are refractory. The amplitude recovers to resting values in 15 to 30 seconds. Thus, the time course of exercise-induced muscle excitability change in myotonia is the converse of the post-tetanic potentiation and exhaustion seen in myasthenia gravis. Decremental response in myotonia may erroneously suggest defective neuromuscular transmission. Improper interpretation of such findings may be responsible for literature reports of patients with both myotonic dystrophy and myasthenia gravis.

In McArdle's syndrome, weakness increases with exertion, and associated muscle contractures are electrically silent (see Fig. 11-3). The compound muscle action potential progressively decreases in amplitude as contractures develop in response to rapid repetitive stimulation.[86]

# REFERENCE SOURCES

1. AHARONOV, A, ET AL: *Humoral antibodies to acetylcholine receptor in patients with myasthenia gravis.* Lancet 2:340, 1975.

2. ALBERS, JW, ET AL: *Penicillamine-associated myasthenia gravis.* Neurology (New York) 30:1246, 1980.

3. AMINOFF, MJ, ET AL: *The declining electrical response of muscle to repetitive nerve stimulation in myotonia.* Neurology (Minneap) 27:812, 1977.

4. APPEL, SH, ALMON, RR, AND LEVY, N: *Acetylcholine receptor antibodies in myasthenia gravis.* N Engl J Med 293:760, 1975.

5. ARGOV, Z AND MASTAGLIA, FL: *Disorders of neuromuscular transmission by drugs.* N Engl J Med 301:409, 1979.

6. ATCHESON, SG AND WARD, JR: *Ptosis and weakness after start of D-penicillamine therapy.* Ann Intern Med 89:939, 1978.

7. BORENSTEIN, S AND DESMEDT, JE: *Temperature and weather correlates of myasthenic fatigue.* Lancet 2:63, 1974.

8. BORENSTEIN, S AND DESMEDT, JE: *Local cooling in myasthenia. Improvement of neuromuscular failure.* Arch Neurol 32:152, 1975.

9. BOWMAN, JR: *Myasthenia gravis in young children. Report of three cases—One congenital.* Pediatrics 1:472, 1948.

10. BRANCH, CE, JR, SWIFT, TR, AND DYKEN, PR: *Prolonged neonatal myasthenia gravis: Electrophysiological studies.* Ann Neurol 3:416, 1978.

11. BROOKE, MH: *A Clinician's View of Neuromuscular Diseases.* Williams & Wilkins, Baltimore, 1977.

12. BROWN, JC, CHARLTON, JE, AND WHITE, DJK: *A regional technique for the study of sensitivity to curare in human muscle.* J Neurol Neurosurg Psychiatry 38:18, 1975.

13. BROWN, JW, NELSON, JR, AND HERRMANN, C, JR: *Sjögren's syndrome with myopathic and myasthenic features.* Bull LA Neurol Soc 33:9, 1968.

14. BUCKNALL, RC: *Myasthenia associated with D-penicillamine therapy in rheumatoid arthritis.* Proc R Soc Med 70 (suppl 3):114, 1977.

15. BUCKNALL, RC, ET AL: *Myasthenia gravis associated with penicillamine treatment for rheumatoid arthritis.* Br Med J 1:600, 1975.

16. CANAK, S, ET AL: *Zur Kenntnis der Neuromyopathia carcinomatosa mit myasthenischem Syndrom.* Der Anaesthesist 13:65, 1964.

17. CASTAIGNE, P, ET AL: *Le syndrome pseudo-myasthénique paranéoplasique de Lambert-Eaton.* Ann Med Intern (Paris) 120:313, 1969.

18. CHELMICKA-SCHORR, E, ET AL: *Eaton-Lambert syndrome in a 9-year-old girl.* Arch Neurol 36:572, 1979.

19. CHERINGTON, M: *Botulism: Clinical and therapeutic observations.* Rocky Mt Med J 69:55, 1972.

20. CHERINGTON, M: *Botulism: Ten-year experience.* Arch Neurol 30:432, 1974.

21. CHERINGTON, M AND SNYDER, RD: *Tick paralysis. Neurophysiologic studies.* N Engl J Med 278:95, 1968.

22. CONOMY, JP, LEVINSOHN, M, AND FANAROFF, A: *Familial infantile myasthenia gravis: A cause of sudden death in young children.* J Pediatr 87:428, 1975.

23. DAHL, DS AND SATO, S: *Unusual myasthenic state in a teen-age boy.* Neurology (Minneap) 24:897, 1974.

24. DAUBE, JR AND LAMBERT, EH: *Post-activation exhaustion in rat muscle.* In DESMEDT, JE (ED): *New Developments in Electromyography and Clinical Neurophysiology,* Vol 1. Karger, Basel, 1973, pp 343–349.

25. DE JESUS, PV, JR, ET AL: *Neuromuscular physiology of wound botulism.* Arch Neurol 29:425, 1973.

26. DESMEDT, JE: *The neuromuscular disorder in myasthenia gravis. II. Presynaptic cholinergic metabolism, myasthenia-like syndromes and a hypothesis.* In DESMEDT, JE (ED): *New Developments in Electromyography and Clinical Neurophysiology,* Vol 1. Karger, Basel, 1973.

27. DESMEDT, JE AND BORENSTEIN, S: *Time course of neonatal myasthenia gravis and unsuspectedly long duration of neuromuscular block in distal muscles.* N Engl J Med 296:633, 1977.

28. DONAT, JR AND DONAT, JF: *Tick paralysis with persistent weakness and electromyographic abnormalities.* Arch Neurol 38:59, 1981.

29. EATON, LM AND LAMBERT, EH: *Electromyography and electric stimulation of nerves in diseases of motor units. Observations on myasthenic syndrome associated with malignant tumors.* JAMA 163:1117, 1957.

30. ELMQVIST, D AND LAMBERT, EH: *Detailed analysis of neuromuscular transmission in a patient with the myasthenic syndrome sometimes associated with bronchogenic carcinoma.* Mayo Clin Proc 43:689, 1968.

31. ENGEL, AG AND SANTA, T: *Histometric analysis of the ultrastructure of the neuromuscular junction in myasthenia gravis and in the myasthenic syndrome.* Ann NY Acad Sci 183:46, 1971.

32. ENGEL, AG AND SANTA, T: *Motor endplate fine structure.* In DESMEDT, JE (ED): *New Developments in Electromyography and Clinical Neurophysiology,* Vol 1. Karger, Basel, 1973.

33. ENGEL, AG, LAMBERT, EH, AND GOMEZ, MR: *A new myasthenic syndrome with end-plate acetylcholinesterase deficiency, small nerve terminals and reduced acetylcholine release.* Ann Neurol 1:315, 1977.

34. ENGEL, AG, ET AL: *Ultrastructural localization of the acetylcholine receptor in myasthenia gravis and in its experimental autoimmune model.* Neurology (Minneap) 27:307, 1977.

35. ENGEL, AG, ET AL: *Investigations of 3 cases of a newly recognized familial, congenital myasthenic syndrome.* Ann Neurol 6:146, 1979.

36. ENGEL, WK, ET AL: *Myasthenia gravis.* Ann Intern Med 81:225, 1974.

37. FAMBROUGH, DM, DRACHMAN, DB, AND SATYAMURTI, S: *Neuromuscular junction in myasthenia gravis: Decreased acetylcholine receptors.* Science 182:293, 1973.

38. FENICHEL, GM: *Clinical syndromes of myasthenia in infancy and childhood. A review.* Arch Neurol 35:97, 1978.

39. FUSFELD, RD: *Electromyographic abnormalities in a case of botulism.* Bull LA Neurol Soc 35:164, 1970.

40. GILLIATT, RW: *Applied electrophysiology in nerve and muscle disease.* Proc R Soc Med 59:989, 1966.

41. GREER, M AND SCHOTLAND, M: *Myasthenia gravis in the newborn.* Pediatrics 26:101, 1960.

42. GUTMANN, L: *Heat exacerbation of myasthenia gravis.* Neurology (New York) 28:398, 1978.

43. GUTMANN, L: *Heat-induced myasthenic crisis.* Arch Neurol 37:671, 1980.

44. GUTMANN, L, ET AL: *The Eaton-Lambert syndrome and autoimmune disorders.* Am J Med 53:354, 1972.

45. HALLER, JS AND FABARA, JA: *Tick paralysis. Case report with emphasis on neurological toxicity.* Am J Dis Child 124:915, 1972.

46. HART, ZH, ET AL: *A congenital, familial myasthenic syndrome caused by a presynaptic defect of transmitter resynthesis or mobilization.* Neurology (New York) 29:556, 1979.

47. ITO, Y, ET AL: *Acetylcholine receptors and end-plate electrophysiology in myasthenia gravis.* Brain 101:345, 1978.

48. JOHNSON, RO, CLAY, SA, AND ARNON, SS: *Diagnosis and management of infant botulism.* Am J Dis Child 133:586, 1979.

49. KAO, I, DRACHMAN, DB, AND PRICE, DL: *Botulinum toxin: Mechanism of presynaptic blockade.* Science 193:1256, 1976.

50. KAPLAN, JE, ET AL: *Botulism, type A, and treatment with guanidine.* Ann Neurol 6:69, 1979.

51. KEESEY, J, ET AL: *Anti-acetylcholine receptor antibody in neonatal myasthenia gravis.* N Engl J Med 296:55, 1977.

52. KIMURA, J AND VAN ALLEN, MW: *Post-thymomectomy myasthenia gravis. Report of a case of ocular myasthenia gravis after total removal of a thymoma and review of literature.* Neurology (Minneap) 17:413, 1967.

53. LAMBERT, EH: *Defects of neuromuscular transmission in syndromes other than myasthenia gravis.* Ann NY Acad Sci 135:367, 1966.

54. LAMBERT, EH AND ELMQVIST, D: *Quantal components of end-plate potentials in the myasthenic syndrome.* Ann NY Acad Sci 183:183, 1971.

55. LAMBERT, EH AND ROOKE, ED: *Myasthenic state and lung cancer.* In BRAIN, W AND NORRIS, FH, JR (EDS): *The Remote Effects of Cancer on the Nervous System,* Vol 1. Grune & Stratton, New York, 1965, pp 67–80.

56. LAURITZEN, M, ET AL: *Eaton-Lambert syndrome and malignant thymoma.* Neurology (New York) 30:634, 1980.

57. LEFVERT, AK, ET AL: *Determination of acetylcholine receptor antibody in myasthenia gravis: Clinical usefulness and pathogenetic implications.* J Neurol Neurosurg Psychiatry 41:394, 1978.

58. LEPORE, FE, SANBORN, GE, AND SLEVIN, JT: *Pupillary dysfunction in myasthenia gravis.* Ann Neurol 6:29, 1979.

59. LYON, LW AND VAN ALLEN, MW: *Orbicularis oculi reflex. Studies in internuclear ophthalmoplegia and pseudointernuclear ophthalmoplegia.* Arch Ophthalmol (New York) 87:148, 1972.

60. MATHEW, NT, JACOB, JC, AND CHANDY, J: *Familial ocular myopathy with curare sensitivity.* Arch Neurol 22:68, 1970.

61. MCLENNAN, H AND OIKAWA, I: *Changes in function of the neuromuscular junction occurring in tick paralysis.* Can J Physiol Pharmacol 50:53, 1972.

62. MERSON, MH, ET AL: *Current trends in botulism in the United States.* JAMA 229:1305, 1974.

63. MILLICHAP, JG AND DODGE, PR: *Diagnosis and treatment of myasthenia gravis in infancy, childhood, and adolescence.* Neurology (Minneap) 10:1007, 1960.

64. MORRIS, DH, III: *Tick paralysis: Electrophysiologic measurements.* South Med J 70:121, 1977.

65. MULDER, DW, LAMBERT, EH, AND EATON, LM: *Myasthenic syndrome in patients with amyotrophic lateral sclerosis.* Neurology (Minneap) 9:627, 1959.

66. MURNAGHAN, MF: *Site and mechanism of tick paralysis.* Science 131:418, 1960.

67. MURPHY, A, ET AL: *Critical reexamination of the thymus immunization model of myasthenia gravis.* Muscle and Nerve 3:293, 1980.

68. NAMBA, T, BROWN, SB, AND GROB, D: *Neonatal myasthenia gravis: Report of two cases and review of the literature.* Pediatrics 45:488, 1970.

69. NASTUK, WL AND STRAUSS, AJL: *Further developments in the search for a neuromuscular blocking agent in the blood of patients with myasthenia gravis.* In VIETS, HR (ED): *Myasthenia Gravis.* Charles C Thomas, Springfield, Ill, 1961, pp 229–237.

70. NORRIS, FH, JR: *Neuromuscular transmission in thyroid disease.* Ann Intern Med 64:81, 1966.

71. OOSTERHUIS, HJGH: *Studies in myasthenia gravis. Part I. A clinical study of 180 patients.* J Neurol Sci 1:512, 1964.

72. OOSTERHUIS, H AND BETHLEM, J: *Neurogenic muscle involvement in myasthenia gravis. A clinical and histopathological study.* J Neurol Neurosurg Psychiatry 36:244, 1973.

73. OSSERMAN, KE: *Myasthenia Gravis.* Grune & Stratton, New York, 1958.

74. OSSERMAN, KE AND GENKINS, G: *Studies in myasthenia gravis: Review of a twenty-year experience in over 1200 patients.* Mt Sinai J Med (NY) 38:497, 1971.

75. OSSERMAN, KE, TSAIRIS, P, AND WEINER, LB: *Myasthenia gravis and thyroid disease: Clinical and immunologic correlation.* J Mt Sinai Hosp 34:469, 1967.

76. ÖZDEMIR, C AND YOUNG, RR: *The results to be expected from electrical testing in the diagnosis of myasthenia gravis.* Ann NY Acad Sci 274:203, 1976.

77. PATRICK, J AND LINDSTROM, J: *Autoimmune response to acetylcholine receptor.* Science 180:871, 1973.

78. PATTEN, BM: *Myasthenia gravis: Review of diagnosis and management.* Muscle and Nerve 1:190, 1978.

79. PATTEN, BM, OLIVER, KL, AND ENGEL, WK: *Effect of lactate infusions on patients with myasthenia gravis.* Neurology (Minneap) 24:986, 1974.

80. PEARN, J: *Neuromuscular paralysis caused by tick envenomation.* J Neurol Sci 34:37, 1977.

81. PEREZ, MC, ET AL: *Stable remissions in myasthenia gravis.* Neurology (New York) 31:32, 1981.

82. PERLO, VP, ET AL: *Myasthenia gravis: Evaluation of treatment in 1355 patients.* Neurology (Minneap) 16:431, 1966.

83. PICKETT, J, ET AL: *Syndrome of botulism in infancy: Clinical and electrophysiologic study.* N Engl J Med 295:770, 1976.

84. PITTINGER, C AND ADAMSON, R: *Antibiotic blockade of neuromuscular function.* Ann Rev Pharm 12:169, 1972.

85. PUVANENDRAN, K, ET AL: *Neuromuscular transmission in thyrotoxicosis.* J Neurol Sci 43:47, 1979.

86. RICKER, K AND MERTENS, HG: *Myasthenic reaction in primary muscle fibre disease.* Electro-enceph Clin Neurophysiol 25:413, 1968.

87. RICKER, K, SAMLAND, O, AND PETER, A: *Elektrische und mechanische Muskelreacktion bei Adynamia episodica und Paramyotonia congenita nach Kälteeinwirkung und Kaliumgabe.* J Neurol 208:95, 1974.

88. ROBERTSON, WC, JR, CHUN, RWM, AND KORNGUTH, SE: *Familial infantile myasthenia.* Arch Neurol 37:117, 1980.

89. ROOKE, ED, LAMBERT, EH, AND THOMAS, JE: *Ein myasthenisches Syndrom mit enger Beziehung zu gewissen malignen intrathorakalen Tumoren.* Dtsch Med Wschr 86:1660, 1961.

90. ROSS, RT: *Ocular myopathy sensitive to curare.* Brain 86:67, 1963.

91. ROWLAND, LP, ARANOW, H, JR, AND HOEFER, PFA: *Observations on the curare test in the differential diagnosis of myasthenia gravis.* In VIETS, HR (ED): *Myasthenia Gravis.* Charles C Thomas, Springfield, Ill, 1961, pp 411–434.

92. RUBENSTEIN, AE, HOROWITZ, SH, AND BENDER, AN: *Cholinergic dysautonomia and Eaton-Lambert syndrome.* Neurology (New York) 29:720, 1979.

93. SANDERS, DB, HOWARD, JF, AND JOHNS, TR: *Single-fiber electromyography in myasthenia gravis.* Neurology (New York) 29:68, 1979.

94. SCHILLER, HH AND STÅLBERG, E: *Human botulism studied with a single-fiber electromyography.* Arch Neurol 35:346, 1978.

95. SCHMITT, N, BOWMER, EJ, AND GREGSON, JD: *Tick paralysis in British Columbia.* Can Med Assoc J 100:417, 1969.

96. SCHWARTZ, MS AND STÅLBERG, E: *Myasthenic syndrome studied with single fiber electromyography.* Arch Neurol 32:815, 1975.

97. SEITZ, D, ET AL: *Penicillamine-induced myasthenia in chronic rheumatoid arthritis* (German with English abstract). Dtsch Med Wochenschr 101:1153, 1976.

98. SHAPIRA, Y, ET AL: *A myasthenic syndrome in childhood leukemia.* Dev Med Child Neurol 16:668, 1974.

99. SIMPSON, JA: *Myasthenia gravis: A new hypothesis.* Scott Med J 5:419, 1960.

100. SIMPSON, JA: *Myasthenia gravis: A personal view of pathogenesis and mechanism. Part 1.* Muscle and Nerve 1:45, 1978.

101. SIMPSON, JA: *Myasthenia gravis: A personal view of pathogenesis mechanism. Part 2.* Muscle and Nerve 1:151, 1978.

102. SNEAD, OC, III, ET AL: *Juvenile myasthenia gravis.* Neurology (New York) 30:732, 1980.

103. SPOOR, TC, ET AL: *Dysthyroid and myasthenic myopathy of the medial rectus: A clinical pathologic report.* Neurology (New York) 30:939, 1980.

104. STRICKROOT, FL, SCHAEFFER, RL, AND BERGO, HL: *Myasthenia gravis occurring in an infant born of a myasthenic mother.* JAMA 120:1207, 1942.

105. SWIFT, TR AND IGNACIO, OJ: *Tick paralysis: Electrophysiologic studies.* Neurology (Minneap) 25:1130, 1975.

106. TAKAMORI, M: *Caffeine, calcium, and Eaton-Lambert syndrome.* Arch Neurol 27:285, 1972.

107. TAKAMORI, M, ISHII, N, AND MORI, M: *The role of cyclic 3′, 5′-adenosine monophosphate in neuromuscular transmission.* Arch Neurol 29:420, 1973.

108. TARRAB-HAZDAI, R, ET AL: *Experimental autoimmune myasthenia induced in monkeys by purified acetylcholine receptor.* Nature 256:128, 1975.

109. TOYKA, KV, ET AL: *Myasthenia gravis. Study of humoral immune mechanisms by passive transfer to mice.* N Engl J Med 296:125, 1977.

110. TSUJIHATA, M, ET AL: *Ultrastructural localization of acetylcholine receptor at the motor endplate: Myasthenia gravis and other neuromuscular diseases.* Neurology (New York) 30:1203, 1980.

111. VIETS, HR AND SCHWAB, RS: *Prostigmin in the diagnosis of myasthenia gravis.* N Engl J Med 213:1280, 1935.

112. VINCENT, A AND NEWSOM-DAVIS, J: *Absence of anti-acetylcholine receptor antibodies in congenital myasthenia gravis.* Lancet 1:441, 1979.

113. WALKER, MB: *Myasthenia gravis: A case in which fatigue of the forearm muscles could induce paralysis of the extra-ocular muscles.* Proc R Soc Med 31:722, 1938.

114. WISE, GA AND MCQUILLEN, MP: *Transient neonatal myasthenia. Clinical and electromyographic studies.* Arch Neurol 22:556, 1970.

# MYOPATHIES

Primary diseases of muscle include genetically determined disorders and those of toxic or inflammatory causes. Inherited disorders with progressive clinical courses are traditionally referred to as muscular dystrophies as opposed to congenital myopathies which have less well-defined patterns of inheritance and benign clinical courses.[36] Some metabolic myopathies are also hereditary but are part of a systemic disorder resulting from an inborn error of metabolism. In addition, a wide variety of inflammatory processes may affect muscle, such as dermatomyositis and polymyositis.

Although hypotonia is one of the essential features of the myogenic disorders listed above, not all floppy infants have primary muscle disease. In fact, disorders of the motor unit constitute less than 10 percent of the identifiable causes of muscular hypotonia during infancy.[155] Most common is a disorder of the central nervous system that produces so-called cerebral hypotonia. Other nonmyogenic etiologies of hypotonia include spinal muscular atrophy, poliomyelitis, inflammatory polyneuropathy, myasthenia gravis, and botulism. Differential diagnosis depends, among other things, on the pattern of inheritance, the distribution of muscle weakness, and the time course of progression.

Electromyographic abnormalities are most valuable in differentiating myogenic from neurogenic paresis. However, in some instances the patterns that, on the basis of classic criteria, suggest myopathy may result from neurogenic involvement. This confusing feature, however, rarely occurs in the early stages of a neuropathic process before complex changes of denervation and reinnervation take place. Electromyography is also useful in delineating the distribution of abnormalities and categorizing a number of dystrophies and myopathies. Nerve conduction velocities are generally normal in primary disorders of muscle. However, conduction studies may show decreased amplitude of compound muscle action potentials particularly when recording from a proximal muscle. Sensory nerve potentials and neuromuscular transmission are normal.

## MUSCULAR DYSTROPHY

Muscular dystrophy consists of a group of inherited muscle diseases with a progressive clinical course during early infancy or after a variable period of apparently normal motor function. Most cases of muscular dystrophy probably involve an underlying myogenic lesion in the form of primary muscle fiber degeneration;[172, 173] however, a neurogenic process may play a role in some types.[136] According to currently accepted classification based on genetic criteria and distribution of muscle degeneration, the four main varieties of muscular dystrophy are Duchenne, Becker, facioscapulohumeral, and limb-girdle types. Other categories include oculopharyngeal dystrophy, hereditary distal myopathies, muscular dystrophy of the Emery-Dreifuss type, and myotonic dystrophy. Diagnosis depends on the typical clinical and genetic features and careful electrophysiologic and histologic evaluations.

# Duchenne muscular dystrophy

Duchenne dystrophy,[75] also known as the pseudohypertrophic variety, is a sex-linked recessive disease. A phenotypically normal female transmits the disease, although carriers sometimes are partially symptomatic.[90] Clinical manifestations are less severe in affected girls than in boys as explained by the Lyon hypothesis. Symptomatic young girls may be a carrier of Duchenne dystrophy or may have childhood muscular dystrophy of autosomal recessive inheritance.[97] The pathogenesis is unknown and the neurogenic[7, 135, 136, 137, 157] and vascular[96, 138] theories, once advocated with vigor, are no longer popular.

The membrane theory, which is most prevalent at this time,[141] assumes that an inherited biochemical abnormality alters the composition and function of the muscle membrane.[175] Abnormalities of adenyl cyclase have been demonstrated in homogenates and muscle cells in culture.[132] Various investigators have described abnormalities of erythrocyte membranes,[130, 133, 140] but without subsequent confirmation.[174, 204] Some suggest possible involvement of calcium ($Ca^{++}$) metabolism in the dystrophic process.[17, 131, 142] The main pathologic sequence of events at least in the early stages consists of repeated episodes of muscle fiber necrosis and regeneration.[40] Muscle cells are reduced in number, because regeneration is incomplete. Some fibers are hypertrophic, whereas others are atrophic. Progressive accumulation of collagen finally replaces the muscle cells.

Proximal weakness of the leg begins during early childhood, although histologic evidence indicates that abnormalities already exist at birth. The child normally attains the early developmental milestones such as raising his head or sitting upright. Early difficulty in standing or walking may give an erroneous impression of clumsiness. He tends to walk on his toes and with the feet externally rotated. Weakness becomes apparent by age three or four with inability to run or to climb stairs. The disease is initially only slowly progressive and apparent improvement may even occur as natural growth compensates temporarily for the weakness. However, a steady, downhill course ensues eventually with the development of lumbar lordosis and progressive scoliosis. Frequent falls force the child into a wheelchair, and eventually, contractures of the joints prevent movement of the extremities.

Neurologic findings depend on the stage of illness. Muscles are generally hard and rubbery with reduced or absent stretch reflexes. The quadriceps are particularly vulnerable, but the muscles of the shoulder girdle are also prominently weak. Later, weakness becomes diffuse, sparing only the extraocular muscles. Other features include macroglossia, pseudohypertrophy of the calves, and, in some, mild mental retardation. The serum level of creatine kinase (CK) is very high during the first year, even when the disease is not yet clinically symptomatic.[149] The CK values then fall gradually as the disease advances but never return to normal. Carriers can sometimes be detected by elevated CK levels.[159, 171] Cardiac involvement results in typical electrocardiographic abnormalities that consist of tall, right precordial R waves and deep limb and precordial Q waves.[55, 160]

Electromyographic evaluation reveals characteristic features of myopathy. Insertional activity is initially normal or increased but is lost in the advanced stage when fibrosis has replaced muscle tissues. Fibrillation potentials and positive sharp waves may occur in early stages (see Fig. 13-7 bottom right), but to a much lesser extent compared with myositis or motor neuron disease.[39] The motor unit potentials are polyphasic and low amplitude and of short duration, reflecting random loss of muscle fibers. When present in abundance with early recruitment (see Figs. 13-15 left and 13-18 right), these potentials give rise to a characteristic noise resembling a shower of fibrillation potentials. In mildly affected muscles, however, the abnormalities are so limited in degree and distribution that their detection requires careful exploration. Electromyograpy may show focal abnormalities in certain carriers but generally is of limited value as a test for detection.[24, 87, 143, 198]

## Becker type muscular dystrophy

Becker type of dystrophy, also inherited as a sex-linked recessive trait,[12, 13, 169] bears a close resemblance to the Duchenne dystrophy. However, Becker variety is a distinct entity. Its clinical features include proximal weakness of the upper and lower extremities and pseudohypertrophy. As in Duchenne dystrophy, the patient initially develops difficulty in gait, in climbing stairs, and in rising from the floor. Becker type is a milder disease with later onset than Duchenne dystrophy and considerably longer clinical course with survival into middle adulthood. The patient eventually develops contractures and skeletal deformities, but both features are much less conspicuous than in Duchenne dystrophy. Early myocardial disease and myalgia may develop.[119]

Electromyography shows nearly symmetric abnormalities in the proximal muscles. Fibrillation potentials are common. Complex repetitive discharges may be present, especially in the paraspinal muscles. Motor unit potentials are small and polyphasic and show an early recruitment. In each of eight families recently reviewed,[28] electromyography showed mixed features of myopathy and denervation. Muscle biopsy typically revealed fiber atrophy and hypertrophy with many split and angulated fibers and clumps of pyknotic nuclei. All but one of the patients were able to walk until the age of 16 years and most lived beyond age 20.

## Facioscapulohumeral dystrophy

Facioscapulohumeral dystrophy of Landouzy-Dejerine,[114] inherited as an autosomal dominant trait, affects both sexes equally. The onset is typically towards the end of the first decade, although the symptoms may appear within the first two years.[93] The disease initially involves the muscles of the face, followed by those of the shoulder girdle, including the trapezius, pectoralis, triceps, and biceps. Muscles of the lower extremities become weak later. The disease is very slowly progressive, produces rather minor disability, and is compatible with a normal life expectancy. The patient may have congenital absence of the pectoralis, biceps, or brachioradialis. Occasionally, bilateral foot-drop is the presenting symptom. The last variety is sometimes referred to as scapuloperoneal dystrophy.[195] The level of serum CK is usually normal.

Some authors refer to facioscapulohumeral dystrophy as a syndrome,[200] with divisions into neurogenic, myopathic, and rare myositic subgroups.[74, 150] The patients initially showing myositic features will eventually become clinically indistinguishable from the myopathic type after some months to years. In early stages, electromyography may be normal even in clinically weak muscles. In well-advanced cases, motor unit potentials are short, low amplitude, and polyphasic, with an increased recruitment for the degree of muscle force. The presence of spontaneous discharges suggests the neuropathic form of this syndrome. Weakness in the facioscapulohumeral distribution may occur in other disease entities, notably myasthenia gravis and polymyositis. Complete electrophysiologic testing, including studies of neuromuscular transmission, is helpful in excluding these possibilities.

## Limb-girdle dystrophy

Limb-girdle dystrophy probably includes a group of disorders with progressive weakness of the hip and shoulder muscles. Some are sporadic cases, but an autosomal recessive pattern of inheritance is common, affecting men and women equally. The illness often begins during the second or third decade with weakness in the pelvis that soon spreads to involve the shoulder girdle. Symptoms may be restricted to these areas for many years with only mild progression. Rarely, a limb-girdle syndrome may present with involvement of only one limb without developing other typical features. Facial muscles are usually spared. Pseudohypertrophy may occur in the calves and deltoid. The life span is normal but the patient may eventually be confined to a wheelchair. The serum enzymes may be slightly elevated.

The name limb-girdle syndrome appropriately denotes the heterogeneity of this entity, which can be subdivided into myogenic and neurogenic types based on clinical, histologic, and electrophysiologic findings (see Fig. 12-8 right). In addition, a clinical syndrome of progressive proximal limb-girdle distribution may appear as a secondary manifestation in other well-defined conditions. These include chronic polymyositis,[170] myasthenia gravis, and various metabolic and congenital myopathies, such as late onset acid maltase deficiency and carnitine deficiency. Spinal muscular atrophy also has a similar distribution of weakness,[78, 205] and differentiation between the two may be difficult on clinical grounds. In a recent review of 18 patients with proximal weakness in the limb-girdle distribution, Coërs and Telerman-Toppet[47] were able to firmly diagnose only two patients as having spinal muscular atrophy and two others as having muscular dystrophy even with the help of histologic evaluation. Motor innervation patterns indicated that 4 of the 18 were cases of spinal muscular atrophy and the others were limb-girdle dystrophies. Electromyographic features were suggestive of myopathy in 11 and denervation in 3 and were inconclusive in 4. The terminal innervation ratio more closely correlated with electromyographic results than did histologic changes of the muscle fibers.

## Other dystrophies

Oculopharyngeal dystrophy is a rare form of progressive ophthalmoplegia inherited in an autosomal dominant fashion in French-Canadian families.[203] Progressive ptosis and dysphagia develop late in life. Ptosis may be present without extraocular muscle weakness.[30, 152] Muscle biopsies show variation in fiber size, occasional internal nuclei, small angulated fibers, and a moth-eaten appearance of the intermyofibrillar network with oxidative enzyme reactions.[74] Electromyographic studies reveal no spontaneous activity and abundant brief, low amplitude, and polyphasic motor unit potentials with early recruitment in proximal muscles of the upper extremities.[22] Conduction studies are normal, although the compound muscle action potentials may be of low amplitude in the weak muscles. Differentiation from myasthenia gravis may be a major problem clinically. However, patients with oculopharyngeal dystrophy have absent titers for acetylcholine (ACh) receptor antibody, no response to edrophonium (Tensilon), no decrement of muscle action potentials to repetitive nerve stimulation, and normal single fiber studies for jitter and blocking.

Hereditary distal myopathy, first described by Welander,[206] is a rare autosomal dominant disorder with onset in adulthood.[139] Unlike most other forms of dystrophies, in this entity the distal muscles are predominantly affected. The intrinsic hand muscles are the initial site of involvement in most patients, although the small muscles of the foot may be affected first in some. The dorsiflexors of the wrist and foot are also weak. The disease is slowly progressive, usually with nearly complete sparing of proximal musculature. However, widespread weakness and wasting may occur, especially if the disease appears at an earlier age and progresses rapidly. Serum creatine kinase (CK) levels may be slightly elevated, and muscle biopsies show vacuolar changes.[76, 126] Electromyography demonstrates low amplitude, short duration motor unit potentials, which recruit early.

In a rare type of muscular dystrophy, called Emery-Dreifuss type,[178] weakness develops in the humeroperoneal distribution. Other features include early contractures and cardiac abnormalities. Electromyography and muscle histology show mixed patterns of neurogenic and myopathic changes.

# CONGENITAL MYOPATHY

A number of congenital conditions present with nonprogressive or only slightly progressive muscular weakness. Some of these entities are morphologically distinctive on the basis of muscle biopsy. These include central core disease, nemaline myopathy, myotubular myopathy, congenital fiber type disproportion, and congenital hypotonia with Type I fiber predominance. These rare conditions can be diagnosed only by histologic examination of the muscle. Morphologic changes in the muscle may represent the fundamental pathology or secondary manifestations.

## Central core disease

Central core disease,[187] inherited as an autosomal dominant trait, causes hypotonia shortly after birth and delayed developmental milestones. The patient, who is usually weaker proximally, may have congenital hip dislocations. As an older child, he cannot keep pace with his peers physically but shows no distinct muscular atrophy. The disease may remain unrecognized by the patient or the family unless skeletal deformities develop. These include lordosis, kyphoscoliosis, and abnormalities of the foot.[194] Malignant hyperthermia has occurred in association with central core disease.[59, 79, 85] When these high-risk patients require surgery for musculoskeletal defects, preoperative evaluation should include in vitro tests for malignant hyperthermia described later in this chapter.

Muscle biopsy shows marked Type I fiber predominance. The central region of the muscle fiber contains compact myofibrils but is devoid of oxidative and phosphorylase enzymes because of the virtual absence of mitochondria.[74] These central areas, which are histochemically unreactive with the oxidative enzyme, are referred to as cores. They commonly appear in Type I and to a lesser extent in Type II fibers, but their absence does not preclude the diagnosis.[144] The resemblance of the cores to target fibers (which usually indicate denervation and reinnervation) supports the disputed notion that the disease may be neurogenic in nature.[153] An increased terminal innervation ratio described in this entity is also consistent with a neurogenic process.[48, 108]

Electrophysiologic studies tend to suggest a mixed myopathic-neuropathic process, but findings are variable. Insertional activity is normal, and no spontaneous discharges are seen at rest. Motor unit potentials may be small with early recruitment[146] or large and polyphasic.[108] Fiber density is increased.[51] Nerve conduction studies show reduced amplitude of muscle potentials with either normal[108] or mildly slowed conduction velocity.[101]

## Nemaline myopathy

Nemaline myopathy[188] is so called because of the presence of many rod- or threadlike structures (nemaline in Greek) lying under the sarcolemma. The disease is probably inherited as an autosomal dominant trait.[117] Hypotonia begins at a very early age and is usually nonprogressive. In addition to diffuse weakness, the children are dysmorphic and have reduced muscle bulk or slender musculature. The characteristic clinical features include elongated faces, high-arched palate, high-arched feet, kyphoscoliosis,[120] and an occasional scapuloperoneal distribution of weakness. The serum creatine kinase (CK) level may be slightly elevated.

Patients and carriers both have a predominance of small Type I fibers on muscle biopsy.[14, 54] The characteristic rod-shaped bodies appear optimally with the Gomori trichrome stain and may not be apparent with routine staining. The rods are of unknown origin but contain material identical to the Z-bands of muscle fibers. They may appear predominantly in either Type I or Type II fibers, or in both types.[186] The rods are present in many other conditions and are not specific to this disease. Electromyography may show short, small amplitude motor unit potentials with early recruitment.

## Myotubular or centronuclear myopathy

In myotubular[191] or centronuclear myopathy,[16, 25, 148, 182, 185] fetal myotubes persist into adult life. This is a rare condition with various modes of inheritance.[10, 201] Most patients are hypotonic at birth with ptosis, facial weakness, and extraocular palsy. Proximal or distal muscles of the limbs may be weak. Some patients die in infancy from cardiorespiratory failure, whereas others survive until adulthood with little progression.

Serum CK may be mildly elevated. Muscle biopsies show Type I fiber atrophy and central nuclei (considered characteristic of fetal muscle). The central part of the fiber is devoid of myofibrils and myofibrillar adenosine triphosphate (ATP). Thus, the perinuclear area stains poorly with the ATPase reaction. Oxidative enzymes may be increased or decreased in the central region. Electromyographic abnormalities include an excessive number of polyphasic, low amplitude motor unit potentials, fibrillation potentials, positive sharp waves, and complex repetitive discharges. Myotubular myopathy is the only congenital myopathy consistently associated with spontaneous activity in electromyography. Occasional myotonic discharges may lead to an erroneous diagnosis of myotonic dystrophy, especially in a patient with distal weakness and ptosis.[148, 165] Two sisters with otherwise typical centronuclear myopathy had clinical myotonia.[89]

## Congenital fiber type disproportion

In normal muscles Type II fibers comprise more than 60 percent of the fibers and Type I, 30 to 40 percent. A reversed relationship exists in some children with congenital hypotonia.[34, 53, 106, 125] The disease appears to be genetically determined in some families with an autosomal dominant mode of inheritance. The children are floppy at birth. Contractures are the major source of functional limitation. Additional features include congenital dislocation of the hip joint secondary to intrauterine hypotonia and other skeletal abnormalities such as deformities of the feet and kyphoscoliosis. The disease seems to progress for the first several years and then either stabilizes or improves slightly. The patient is short in stature and fails to attain normal motor skills, although mental development is normal.

The muscle biopsy shows, in addition to fiber type disproportion, small Type I fibers, hypertrophy of Type II fibers, scattered internal nuclei, and occasional nemaline rods. Possible relationships between this condition and nemaline myopathy remain unconfirmed.[116] Electromyography usually demonstrates short, small amplitude motor unit potentials with early recruitment but no spontaneous activity. However, some patients show fibrillation potentials, positive sharp waves, and complex repetitive discharges.

# METABOLIC MYOPATHY

A variety of myopathies result from inborn errors of metabolism.[21] These include certain types of glycogen storage disease and disorders of lipid metabolism. Of the ten glycogen storage diseases identified to date, prominent muscle involvement occurs only in Pompe, Cori-Forbes, McArdle, and Tarui's diseases, which are Types II, III, V, and VII glycogenosis, respectively.[103] Other metabolic myopathies include mitochondrial diseases and malignant hyperpyrexia or hyperthermia.

## Acid maltase deficiency (Type II glycogenosis)

This condition, inherited as an autosomal recessive, results from acid maltase deficiency which leads to accumulation of glycogen in tissue lysosomes.[5, 99] In the infantile type, called Pompe's disease, children develop severe hypotonia shortly after birth and die within the first year from cardiac or respiratory failure.[20] Anterior horn cells contain deposits of glycogen particles. Other organs affected include the heart, tongue, and liver. A large tongue and cardiac abnormalities are important characteristics in differentiating this condition from Werdnig-Hoffmann disease.

In the more benign types, which simulate limb-girdle syndromes or polymyositis, the symptoms are limited to skeletal muscle and appear in childhood or adult life. Patients with the childhood type show proximal weakness of the limb and trunk muscles with variable progression and die of respiratory failure before the end of the second decade.[83, 128] In the adult type the symptoms begin with insidious limb-girdle weakness during the third or fourth decade.[69, 83] Both types show elevated serum enzymes. The muscle biopsy reveals a vacuolar myopathy affecting Type I fibers more than Type II.[45] Glycogen deposits are common in the central nervous system, particularly in the infantile form. The enzymatic defect has been reproduced in tissue culture.[6]

Electromyography shows increased insertional activity, fibrillation potentials, positive sharp waves, and complex repetitive discharges, as expected from anterior horn cell involvement.[80, 83, 100] The insertional activity may be absent in severely affected muscles. As mentioned in Chapter 13, this is one of the few disorders in which true myotonic discharges may occur in the absence of clinical myotonia. The motor unit potentials are polyphasic, low amplitude, and short duration with early recruitment. Widespread abnormalities are common in the infantile type but changes may be restricted to the proximal muscles in the late onset childhood or adult type. The gluteal and paraspinal muscles are common sites of involvement in these cases. Motor and sensory nerve conduction velocities and neuromuscular transmission are normal.

## Debrancher deficiency (Type III glycogenosis)

In the absence of the debrancher enzyme, breakdown of glycogen occurs only in the outer straight glucosyl chains. Consequently, glycogen with short-branched outer chains, called phosphorylase-limit-dextrin, accumulates in the liver and striated and cardiac muscles. The enzymatic defect is generalized,[199] although the skeletal muscles are not necessarily weak on clinical examination.[37, 151] The disease is inherited as an autosomal recessive trait.

Affected children are hypotonic, with proximal weakness and failure to thrive. Accumulation of glycogen in the liver causes hepatomegaly and episodes of hypoglycemia. Clinical features of myopathy may develop after hepatic symptoms have abated and the patient may improve in adolescence, even though the enzymatic defect remains. Distal weakness and wasting sometimes resemble those seen in patients with motor neuron disease.[37, 71] Serum creatine kinase (CK) is markedly elevated. Muscle biopsy shows subsarcolemmal periodic acid-schiff (PAS) positive vacuoles in Type II fibers.[71] Although there are no histochemical signs of denervation, electromyography may show profuse fibrillation potentials, complex repetitive discharges, and small, short duration motor unit potentials.[37, 71]

## Muscle phosphorylase deficiency (Type V glycogenosis)

McArdle[134] first described this rare condition which is usually inherited in an autosomal recessive pattern but sometimes may be inherited in an autosomal dominant pattern.[46] It affects the male more frequently than the female by a ratio of 4 to 1.[68] Myophosphorylase deficiency blocks the conversion of muscle glycogen to glucose during heavy exercise under ischemic conditions. The disease typically becomes symptomatic in childhood or adolescence but, rarely, the patients may be free of muscle weakness or cramps until late adulthood.[118]

The abnormality, confined to skeletal muscles, initially causes only nonspecific complaints of mild weakness and fatigue. Sometime during adolescence the patients begin to notice exercise intolerance.[176, 179] A heavy bout of exercise or repetitive stimulation of the nerve produces painful cramps in the muscle that may last for several hours. Associated breakdown of muscle leads to myoglobinuria causing the urine to become wine-colored. Muscle pain and fatigue may improve during continued exercise if the patient slows down and sustains nonstrenuous activity. This second wind phenomenon is presumably induced by increased mobilization of serum free fatty acids as an alternative source of energy.[161] Exposure to cold during exercise may also delay the development of contracture.

Neurologic examination is not remarkable unless the patient is suffering from muscle cramps at the time. Mild proximal weakness may be present without apparent muscular wasting. The patient may develop permanent limb-girdle weakness later in life. In advanced stages activity is severely limited, because mild exercise may precipitate painful muscle cramps. Atypical clinical presentations in adult patients include progressive muscle weakness without exercise-induced contracture.[129] In infants, generalized hypotonia may lead to respiratory insufficiency and early death.[66]

The ischemic exercise test is of great value in confirming the diagnosis in suspected cases.[147] The test consists of exercising the forearm muscles under ischemic conditions induced by an inflated pneumatic cuff placed around the arm. The inability to convert glycogen to glucose by anaerobic glycolysis promptly precipitates a muscle cramp. The pathogenesis of the cramp has not been clearly elucidated. Depletion of high energy phosphates in the absence of glycogen metabolism may prevent the energy-dependent re-uptake of calcium ($Ca^{++}$) by the sarcoplasmic reticulum,[92] but such an abnormality has not been confirmed.[33] Normally, lactate levels in venous blood should rise with the breakdown of glycogen under ischemic conditions. However, patients with McArdle's disease show no rise in the lactate level when blood is drawn from the exercised arm.

In a contracture, electromyography of a cramped muscle reveals no electrical activity despite muscle shortening (see Fig. 11-3).[121, 177] In contrast, the ordinary muscle cramp or spasm shows abundant discharges of motor unit potentials. In one patient, the post-tetanic mechanical tension of the contracture was only 17 percent of the peak tetanic tension, and twitches superimposed on the contracture were diminished by half, as were their action potentials.[29] Between attacks electromyography may be normal or may reveal fibrillation potentials and polyphasic motor unit potentials.[66] In one study, the mean duration of the motor unit potential in the biceps was 7.1 ms, compared with 9.4 ms in the controls, suggesting myopathic changes.[29] A reduction in the number of motor units has been reported in this syndrome but not confirmed.[197] Motor and sensory nerve conduction velocities are normal, but repetitive nerve stimulation will produce decreased electrical activity associated with the development of muscle contracture.

# Muscle phosphofructokinase deficiency (Type VII glycogenosis)

This disorder, first described by Tarui and associates,[193] results from a defect of muscle phosphofructokinase, which is necessary for the conversion of fructose-6-phosphate to fructose 1-6 diphosphate. The clinical picture, including painful muscle contracture and myoglobinuria, is virtually identical to that of McArdle's disease.[2, 123, 196] However, distinction is possible by means of biochemical or histochemical determination of phosphofructokinase activity in the muscle biopsy. Electromyography is normal between attacks.

# Disorders of lipid metabolism

Whereas glycogen is the major source of energy for rapid strenuous effort, circulating lipid in the form of free fatty acids maintains the energy supply at rest and during prolonged low-intensity exercise. Carnitine palmityl transferase catalyzes the reversible binding of carnitine to plasma fatty acids; once bound, fatty acids can be transported across the mitochondrial membrane for oxidation. Disorders of lipid metabolism include carnitine palmityl transferase deficiency and carnitine deficiency.[67]

Carnitine palmityl transferase deficiency is a rare disorder inherited as an autosomal recessive trait. It presents with painful muscle cramps and recurrent episodes of myoglobinuria induced by prolonged exercise or fasting.[8, 42, 52, 63, 65, 84, 124, 183] In this disorder, impaired oxidation of lipid substrates results, because long chain fatty acids cannot be coupled to carnitine for shuttle across the inner mitochondrial membrane.[122] The first attack of myoglobinuria appears in adolescence, although muscle pain may be present in early childhood. Muscle strength is normal between attacks. Exercise during fasting results in painful muscle cramps. Muscle biopsy may be normal or show a slight excess of intrafiber lipid droplets next to the mitochondria in Type I fibers. Electrophysiologic studies, reported in a few patients, have included normal electromyography and normal motor and sensory nerve conduction velocities.[8, 84]

Carnitine deficiency, probably inherited as an autosomal recessive disorder, was the first biochemical defect identified in muscle lipid metabolism.[4, 81] Two forms of this condition are recognized: In the restricted type, lipid storage occurs predominantly or exclusively in muscle. Reduced muscle carnitine possibly results from a deficit in carnitine uptake in the muscle, since serum carnitine levels are normal in most patients. This entity was called a lipid storage myopathy before recognition of the specific biochemical defect.[27, 82] In the systemic type, reduction in serum liver and muscle carnitine levels presumably results from insufficient synthesis of carnitine.

Carnitine deficiency causes a congenital and slowly progressive myopathy of the limb-girdle type with prominent weakness of the neck muscles and episodic hepatic insufficiency.[23, 113] When the defect is severe it may cause bulbar and respiratory involvement and death at an early age.[23, 50, 95] Some patients show features of both systemic and muscle carnitine deficiency.[43] Since lipid utilization takes place in the mitochondria, there may be some overlap between lipid storage myopathies and the so-called mitochondrial myopathies.[26] The muscle biopsy reveals an excess of lipid droplets mostly in the Type I fibers, which depend on oxidation of long-chain fatty acids to a greater extent than Type II fibers.

Electromyography shows features of myopathy with abundant, small amplitude, short duration, polyphasic motor unit potentials that recruit early. Fibrillation potentials are present in slightly over half of the patients. One may also encounter other forms of spontaneous activity such as complex repetitive discharges. Motor and sensory nerve conduction studies are generally normal, but neuropathy may develop in some.[127] Studies of neuromuscular transmission are normal.

## Mitochondrial disease

Structural abnormalities of the mitochondria apparently cause progressive muscle weakness as a part of complex neurologic and systemic disorders.[73, 115, 145, 189] The most commonly encountered disorder is Kearns-Sayres ophthalmoplegia.[15, 57, 70, 104, 112, 167, 184] The disease occurs sporadically with the initial symptoms of ptosis and extraocular palsy appearing during childhood or adolescence. As indicated by its alternative name, oculocraniosomatic neuromuscular disease with ragged red fibers,[154] characteristic features include progressive weakness of the extraocular muscles, cardiac abnormalities, somatic deficits, and ragged red fibers in the muscle biopsy, indicating a mitchondrial abnormality. Progressive weakness and fatigue may accompany a wide variety of neurologic deficits; for example, pigmentary degeneration of the retina, sensorineuronal deafness, cerebellar degeneration, endocrine abnormalities, sensory motor neuropathy, and demyelinating radiculopathy.[73, 91, 162] Laboratory studies reveal a moderate increase in cerebrospinal fluid protein and a mild elevation of serum CK. Electromyography shows low amplitude, short duration motor unit potentials with early recruitment, but abnormalities are usually mild.

## Malignant hyperpyrexia or hyperthermia

This entity, first described by Denborough and Lovell[58] and Denborough and associates,[60] is a rare condition with an autosomal dominant inheritance. The affected individuals are susceptible to anesthetics in general and the administration of halothane and succinylcholine in particular.[31, 156] After the induction of general anesthesia they develop fasciculations and increased muscle tone. An explosive rise in temperature occurs in conjunction with muscular rigidity and necrosis. The remarkable hyperpyrexia is metabolic in nature and may result from abnormal depolarization of skeletal muscle by halothane,[86] but its exact mechanism is unknown. Patients with malignant hyperthermia characteristically show reduced re-uptake of calcium by the sarcoplasmic reticulum.[107] If untreated, they die of metabolic acidosis and recurrent convulsions.

Without knowledge of a positive family history, malignant hyperthermia is usually not suspected clinically. Susceptible individuals are largely asymptomatic unless subjected to anesthesia. Common physical characteristics include proximal hypertrophy and distal atrophy of the thigh muscles and lumbar lordosis. Some show mild weakness of the proximal muscles, diminution of the muscle stretch reflexes, and elevated serum CK level. The abnormal muscle is hypersensitive to caffeine, which normally causes muscle contracture by increasing the concentration of calcium in the sarcoplasm. In an in vitro screening test for suspected cases, concentrations of halothane and caffeine too low to affect normal muscles produce contracture in specimens obtained from the patients.[32] Malignant hyperthermia may develop in association with central core disease.[59, 85]

# ENDOCRINE MYOPATHY

Endocrine myopathies develop in hyperthyroidism or hypothyroidism, parathyroid disease, and adrenal and pituitary dysfunction. Cushing's syndrome secondary to systemic administration of corticosteroids or adrenocorticotropic hormone (ACTH) is now a common cause of myopathy.

## Thyroid myopathy

Disorders of thyroid function may cause a variety of neuromuscular problems, although muscular symptoms may not be obvious in the face of more fulminating systemic features. Thyrotoxic myopathy is probably the most common.[111] In fact the majority of patients with thyrotoxicosis have some proximal weakness and electromyographic features of low amplitude, short duration motor unit potentials with early recruitment.[166] Myopathy affects men more frequently, even though the incidence of thyrotoxicosis is higher in women. The muscles of the shoulder girdle are weaker than those of the pelvic girdle. Typically, the muscle stretch reflexes are normal or at times even hyperactive. Spontaneous muscle twitching and generalized myokymia may occur but not commonly.[94] Quantitative electromyographic studies have shown short duration motor unit potentials, even if muscle weakness is not evident clinically.[164] Other neuromuscular conditions commonly associated with thyrotoxicosis include exophthalmic ophthalmoplegia, myasthenia gravis, and hypokalemic periodic paralysis.

Hypothyroidism causes proximal muscle weakness, painful muscle spasm, and muscle hypertrophy, especially in children. Hoffmann's sign, or delayed relaxation of contracted muscle, is characteristic of myxedema.[207] The ankle stretch reflex best demonstrates this change in muscle contractibility—a brisk reflex movement of the foot with a slow return to the resting position. Or, a sharp tap to the muscle with a reflex hammer causes a local ridge of muscle to contract. This phenomenon, called myoedema of hypothyroidism, is electrically silent.[180] Electromyography may show increased insertional activity with some repetitive discharges but no evidence of myotonia. Elevations of serum creatine kinase (CK) levels are common.

## Parathyroid disease

The most dramatic neuromuscular complication in hypoparathyroidism is tetany secondary to chronic hypocalcemia. The presence of calcium ($Ca^{++}$) is necessary for the release of acetylcholine (ACh) at the neuromuscular junction. The effect of calcium is apparently opposite at the axonal-cellular junction centrally: a reduction in calcium here results in increased conductance for sodium ($Na^+$) and potassium ($K^+$), thus causing instability and hyperexcitability of the cell membrane. Electromyographic changes in tetany include the presence of motor unit potentials in doublets and triplets.

Varying degrees of proximal muscle weakness develop in patients with hyperparathyroidism.[158, 190] The muscles of the pelvic girdle are weaker than those of the shoulder girdle. The muscle stretch reflexes are characteristically brisk, and some patients show extensor plantar responses. These reflex changes, combined with axial muscle wasting, raise the diagnostic possibility of motor neuron disease. Electromyography may show low amplitude, short duration motor unit potentials with early recruitment in weak muscles. No spontaneous activities are recorded. Nerve conduction studies may reveal reduced amplitude of the compound muscle action potentials, but motor and sensory nerve conduction velocities are normal. Neuromuscular symptoms are most common in hyperparathyroidism but may also occur, less frequently, in hypercalcemia secondary to osteolytic metastases, multiple myeloma, or chronic renal disease.

## Adrenal and pituitary disease

Diseases of the adrenal and pituitary glands may give rise to rather nonspecific muscle weakness, as in Cushing's syndrome, acromegaly, or Addison's disease. Similar weakness also appears after systemic administration of corticosteroids or ACTH. Steroids reduce the intracellular concentration of potassium, but their relationship to myopathy is not clear. Dysfunction of the reticulum or mitochondria may also contribute. Weakness affects the muscles of the pelvic girdle and thigh preferentially. Patients have difficulty rising from a chair or climbing stairs. The neuromuscular symptoms usually improve if the underlying abnormality abates or upon discontinuation of the steroids. Laboratory studies show normal serum enzymes but increased urinary creatine excretion. Muscle biopsy shows Type II fiber atrophy with neither necrosis nor inflammatory changes. These findings are consistent with the degree of muscle wasting observed clinically.[163]

Nerve conduction velocities are normal, but the compound muscle action potentials may be of reduced amplitude especially in proximal muscles. Sensory nerve action potentials are normal. Since electromyography primarily assesses the initially recruited Type I fibers, endocrine or steroid myopathy with Type II fiber atrophy usually reveals no specific abnormality. The insertional activity is normal. Neither fibrillation potentials nor positive sharp waves are present at rest. This finding is important in differentiating steroid myopathy from recurrent inflammatory myopathy in patients with progressive weakness after prolonged steroid therapy. In advanced cases, motor unit potentials may be low amplitude and of short duration and may recruit early, but these abnormalities are generally mild and reversible with withdrawal of steroids.

# MYOSITIS

A variety of inflammatory processes occur in muscle, but the most frequently encountered is polymyositis.[19, 62] The condition is referred to as dermatomyositis if a typical skin rash is present in conjunction with the signs and symptoms of muscle involvement. Both are common diseases but the diagnosis may be difficult in some cases because of the protean clinical presentation. Despite a number of complicated schemes of classifying inflammatory myositis, it is still unclear whether different clinical forms are indeed separate entities or if they represent a spectrum of the same illness. Five subtypes can be identified based on the patient's age and underlying disorder:[18] (1) primary idiopathic polymyositis; (2) primary idiopathic dermatomyositis; (3) dermatomyositis (or polymyositis) associated with neoplasia; (4) childhood dermatomyositis (or polymyositis) associated with vasculitis; and (5) polymyositis or dermatomyositis associated with collagen vascular disease. For the purpose of this discussion it suffices to describe certain clinical features considered characteristic of dermatomyositis and polymyositis as a broad and general category.

## Dermatomyositis

The diagnosis of dermatomyositis depends on the combination of skin rash and muscular weakness. It can occur at any age but is uncommon in adolescence and early adulthood. Thus, the incidence histogram shows a bimodal distribution with peaks in childhood and in the fifth and sixth decades. In dermatomyositis of childhood, the patient rarely suffers from malignancy, but systemic symptoms of collagen vascular disease are very common. In particular, myositis seems to appear in association with Raynaud's phenomenon, lupus erythematosus, polyarteritis nodosa, Sjögren's syndrome, and pneumonitis.

The initial symptoms are often nonspecific and include such systemic manifestations as malaise, fever, anorexia, and loss of weight, and features of respiratory infection. Unfortunately pain and tenderness of affected muscle are overemphasized as diagnostic criteria; they are neither presenting nor primary symptoms in a majority of patients. In some patients, demonstrable tenderness, usually restricted to the muscles of the shoulder, may be present. Vague pain and muscle ache are rather common complaints and are of no specific diagnostic value.

The skin lesions that may precede or follow the onset of weakness consist of a purple-colored rash over the cheeks and eyelids. The discoloration is particularly prominent over the upper eyelids and accompanied by periorbital edema. An erythematous rash may also appear in exposed body parts such as the neck, upper chest, knees, and hands. The affected skin is thick and shows a reddish hue, especially over the interphalangeal joints. Telangiectasia may be present over the chest and the back of the hands in advanced stages. In extreme cases, the skin over the entire body is reddish in color, atrophic, and edematous.

# Polymyositis

No skin lesion is evident in polymyositis, but the signs and symptoms of muscular involvement are very similar to those in dermatomyositis. Initial systemic symptoms are also indistinguishable between the two varieties. Children with myositis usually develop skin rashes. Hence, polymyositis is a disease of adults. Possible underlying conditions include collagen vascular disease and malignancy.[11] The incidence of underlying malignancy is higher in men than in women and can involve bowel, stomach, lung, breast, and ovary.

Weakness is the usual presenting feature, which ordinarily progresses slowly over a matter of weeks. However, the disease may take a fulminating course with the patient crippling during the first week of onset. Pelvic girdle muscles are ordinarily affected first, causing difficulty in climbing stairs or rising from a chair. Weakness of the shoulder girdle follows, rendering the patient incapable of lifting objects or combing the hair. Involvement of neck musculature is common with predilection for the anterior rather than the posterior compartment. Dysphagia can occur, but the bulbar muscles are otherwise spared. Extraocular muscles usually remain entirely normal. Although weakness affects the proximal muscles initially, it soon spreads to involve the distal limb muscles. The muscle stretch reflexes are normal until very late in the course of the disease. Atrophy may be mild and difficult to detect in the deep muscles of the pelvic or shoulder girdle but is sometimes apparent in the orbicularis oculi or other superficial muscles. High dose steroid therapy is effective in a majority of patients,[62] but the outlook is not always optimistic.[168]

The serum level of creatine kinase (CK) is usually helpful in determining the diagnosis and clinical course of the myositis. However, approximately 10 percent of patients with proven diagnoses show normal values even during acute stages. The enzymes may also be normal despite active myositis when muscle atrophy is extensive as in long-standing disease.[18] Nonetheless, elevation of serum CK is one of the most reliable measures of disease activity. The cause of muscle enzyme leakage is not known, but it may be related to defects in the muscle plasma membrane as postulated in Duchenne dystrophy.[149] Alternatively, anastomosis of transverse tubules with terminal cisternae may be a possible source of enzymatic leakage.[44] Other inconsistent laboratory findings include elevated erythrocyte sedimentation rate and gamma globulin.

Muscle biopsy findings include necrosis, phagocytosis, atrophy, degeneration, and regeneration of both Type I and II fibers, internal nuclei, vacuolization, random variation of fiber size, mononuclear inflammatory infiltrates, and endomysial and perimysial fibrosis.[18] Muscle fiber atrophy typically appears in a perifascicular distribution, presumably because the blood supply to the peripheral fibers is interrupted.[1, 9, 18] Single-fiber electromyography (SFEMG) and histochemical investigation have revealed changes of the terminal innervation pattern consistent with reinnervation.[98] Denervation could result either from segmental necrosis of muscle fibers separated from the end-plate region[61] or from involvement of the terminal nerve endings.

A triad of electromyographic abnormalities described by Buchthal and Pinelli[38] nearly always appear in untreated myositis, especially in the clinically weak muscles. They are (1) fibrillation potentials and positive sharp waves (see Fig. 13-7 top right); (2) complex repetitive discharges; and (3) polyphasic motor unit potentials of short duration and low amplitude with early recruitment (see Figs. 13-15 right and 13-18 top). Certain muscles, however, may remain entirely normal, even in patients with moderately advanced disease. For adequate assessment, therefore, one should examine a number of proximal and distal muscles with emphasis on those exhibiting moderate weakness clinically. Electromyographic as well as histologic abnormalities are often greatest in the paraspinal muscles and are occasionally confined to them.[3, 192]

In a retrospective study of 153 patients with polymyositis or dermatomyositis, Bohan and associates[19] found the following electromyographic abnormalities: (1) small amplitude, short duration, polyphasic motor unit potentials (90 percent); (2) fibrillation potentials, positive sharp waves, and insertional irritability (74 percent); (3) complex repetitive discharges (38 percent); (4) a completely normal study with otherwise classic disease (10 percent); and (5) electrical abnormalities restricted to the paraspinal muscle with widespread muscle weakness (1.6 percent). In another large series of 98 patients,[62] electromyographic findings were as follows: (1) fibrillation potentials, positive sharp waves, and polyphasic motor unit potentials of short duration and low amplitude with early recruitment (45 percent); (2) the above changes of motor unit potentials but without spontaneous activity (44 percent); and (3) a normal electromyography (11 percent). No correlation emerged between the grade of impairment at presentation and the electromyographic findings.

Muscle action potentials may show a decrement or, less frequently, increment upon repetitive stimulation of the nerve.[102, 105, 202] These electrophysiologic abnormalities often accompany clinical features of myasthenia. These patients probably have myasthenia gravis with concomitant inflammatory changes of polymyositis and represent an overlap of these two entities. Indeed the electrophysiologic as well as histologic features characteristic of polymyositis commonly occur in patients with severe myasthenia gravis.

Unlike in wallerian degeneration, spontaneous activity in polymyositis diminishes or disappears within a few weeks of successful steroid therapy. Since the time course of this change correlates well with clinical improvement, serial electromyographic evaluation is of value in objectively assessing patient response to various therapies. It is particularly useful in distinguishing a recurrence of myositis from the emergence of steroid myopathy. Clinical recovery is also associated with serial improvement of abnormal motor unit potentials. Progressive increases in amplitude and duration occur initially some weeks or months after therapy, followed by diminution of the number of polyphasic units in a year or two.

## Myositis caused by infectious agents

Although both dermatomyositis and polymyositis are relatively common, bacterial and viral infections of muscle are rare.[49, 64, 110] Parasitic infection is also uncommon in nontropical countries. In trichinosis, *Trichinella spiralis* preferentially invades the extraocular muscles,[56] whereas in cysticercosis *Taenia solium* mostly affects the trunk muscles.[181] Inflammation of muscle may occur in sarcoidosis,[72, 88] sometimes accompanied by a rash typical of dermatomyositis.[109] Myositis may also develop in association with giant cell arteritis.[35] The exact role of infection in these entities is not known. Inclusion body myositis is a distinct but infrequently recognized inflammatory disease of skeletal muscle.[41] In contrast to dermatomyositis, features of collagen vascular disease are absent. The clinical course is benign and only slowly progressive. The disease frequently affects distal muscles in men and does not respond to corticosteroid treatment. Electromyographic abnormalities are similar among different myositic conditions and include fibrillation potentials, positive sharp waves, complex repetitive discharges, and short duration, low amplitude motor unit potentials with early recruitment.

## REFERENCE SOURCES

1. ADAMS, RD: *The pathologic substratum of polymyositis.* In PEARSON, CM AND MOSTOFI, FK (EDS): *The Striated Muscle.* Williams & Wilkins, Baltimore, 1973, pp 292–300.

2. AGAMANOLIS, DP, ET AL: *Muscle phosphofructokinase deficiency: Two cases with unusual polysaccharide accumulation and immunologically active enzyme protein.* Muscle and Nerve 3:456, 1980.

3. ALBERS, JW, ET AL: *Spontaneous electrical activity and muscle biopsy abnormalities in polymyositis and dermatomyositis.* Muscle and Nerve 2:503, 1979.

4. ANGELINI, C, ET AL: *Carnitine deficiency: Acute postpartum crisis.* Ann Neurol 4:558, 1978.

5. ARAOZ, C, ET AL: *Glycogenosis Type II (Pompe's disease): Ultrastructure of peripheral nerves.* Neurology (Minneap) 24:739, 1974.

6. ASKANAS, V, ET AL: *Adult-onset acid maltase deficiency. Morphologic and biochemical abnormalities reproduced in cultured muscle.* N Engl J Med 294:573, 1976.

7. BALLANTYNE, JP AND HANSEN, S: *New method for the estimation of the number of motor units in a muscle. 2. Duchenne, limb-girdle and facioscapulohumeral, and myotonic muscular dystrophies.* J Neurol Neurosurg Psychiatry 37:1195, 1974.

8. BANK, WJ, ET AL: *A disorder of muscle lipid metabolism and myoglobinuria. Absence of carnitine palmityl transferase.* N Engl J Med 292:443, 1975.

9. BANKER, BQ AND VICTOR, M: *Dermatomyositis (systemic angiopathy) of childhood.* Medicine (Baltimore) 45:261, 1966.

10. BARTH, PG, VAN WIJNGAARDEN, GK, AND BETHLEM, J: *X-linked myotubular myopathy with fatal neonatal asphyxia.* Neurology (Minneap) 25:531, 1975.

11. BARWICK, DD AND WALTON, JN: *Polymyositis.* Am J Med 35:646, 1963.

12. BECKER, PE: *Two new families of benign sex-linked recessive muscular dystrophy.* Rev Can Biol 21:551, 1962.

13. BECKER, PE AND KIENER, F: *Eine neue X-chromosomale Muskeldystrophie.* Arch Psychiatr Zeit Neurol 193:427, 1955.

14. BENDER, AN AND WILLNER, JP: *Nemaline (rod) myopathy: The need for histochemical evaluation of affected families.* Ann Neurol 4:37, 1978.

15. BERENBERG, RA, ET AL: *Lumping or splitting? "Ophthalmoplegia-plus" or Kearns-Sayre syndrome?* Ann Neurol 1:37, 1977.

16. BERGEN, BJ, ET AL: *Centronuclear myopathy: Extraocular- and limb-muscle findings in an adult.* Muscle and Nerve 3:165, 1980.

17. BODENSTEINER, JB AND ENGEL, AG: *Intracellular calcium accumulation in Duchenne dystrophy and other myopathies: A study of 567,000 muscle fibers in 114 biopsies.* Neurology (New York) 28:439, 1978.

18. BOHAN, A AND PETER, JB: *Polymyositis and dermatomyositis.* (Second of 2 parts) N Engl J Med 292:403, 1975.

19. BOHAN, A, ET AL: *A computer-assisted analysis of 153 patients with polymyositis and dermatomyositis.* Medicine 56:255, 1977.

20. BORDIUK, JM, ET AL: *Pompe's disease. Electromyographic, electron microscopic, and cardiovascular aspects.* Arch Neurol 23:113, 1970.

21. BOSCH, EP AND MUNSAT, TL: *Metabolic myopathies.* Med Clin of North Am 63:759, 1979.

22. BOSCH, EP, GOWANS, JDC, AND MUNSAT, T: *Inflammatory myopathy in oculopharyngeal dystrophy.* Muscle and Nerve 2:73, 1979.

23. BOUDIN, G, ET AL: *Fatal systemic carnitine deficiency with lipid storage in skeletal muscle, heart, liver, and kidney.* J Neurol Sci 30:313, 1976.

24. BRADLEY, WG AND KELEMEN, J: *Editorial: Genetic counseling in Duchenne muscular dystrophy.* Muscle and Nerve 2:325, 1979.

25. BRADLEY, WG, PRICE, DL, AND WATANABE, CK: *Familial centronuclear myopathy.* J Neurol Neurosurg Psychiatry 33:687, 1970.

26. BRADLEY, WG, TOMLINSON, BE, AND HARDY, M: *Further studies of mitochondrial and lipid storage myopathies.* J Neurol Sci 35:201, 1978.

27. BRADLEY, WG, ET AL: *Myopathy associated with abnormal lipid metabolism in skeletal muscle.* Lancet 1:495, 1969.

28. BRADLEY, WG, ET AL: *Becker-type muscular dystrophy.* Muscle and Nerve 1:111, 1978.

29. BRANDT, NJ, ET AL: *Post-tetanic mechanical tension and evoked action potentials in McArdle's disease.* J Neurol Neurosurg Psychiatry 40:920, 1977.

30. BRAY, GM, KAARSOO, M, AND ROSS, RT: *Ocular myopathy with dysphagia.* Neurology (Minneap) 15:678, 1965.

31. BRITT, BA, KWONG, FHF, AND ENDRENYI, L: *The clinical and laboratory features of malignant hyperthermia management—A review.* In HENSCHEL, EO (ED): *Malignant Hyperthermia: Current Concepts.* Appleton-Century-Crofts, New York, 1977, pp 9–45.

32. BRITT, BA, ET AL: *Malignant hyperthermia: An investigation of five patients.* Can Anaesth Soc J 20:431, 1973.

33. BRODY, IA, GERBER, CJ, AND SIDBURY, JB, JR: *Relaxing factor in McArdle's disease. Calcium uptake by sarcoplasmic reticulum.* Neurology (Minneap) 20:555, 1970.

34. BROOKE, MH: *Congenital fiber type dysproportion.* In KAKULAS, BA (ED): *Clinical Studies in Myology. Part 2.* Excerpta Medica, Amsterdam, 1973, pp 147–159.

35. BROOKE, MH AND KAPLAN, H: *Muscle pathology in rheumatoid arthritis, polymyalgia rheumatica, and polymyositis.* Arch Pathol 94:101, 1972.

36. BROOKE, MH, CARROLL, JE, AND RINGEL, SP: *Congenital hypotonia revisited.* Muscle and Nerve 2:84, 1979.

37. BRUNBERG, JA, MCCORMICK, WF, AND SCHOCHET, SS, JR: *Type III glycogenosis. An adult with diffuse weakness and muscle wasting.* Arch Neurol 25:171, 1971.

38. BUCHTHAL, F AND PINELLI, P: *Muscle action potentials in polymyositis.* Neurology (Minneap) 3:424, 1953.

39. BUCHTHAL, F AND ROSENFALCK, P: *Electrophysiological aspects of myopathy with particular reference to progressive muscular dystrophy.* In BOURNE, GH AND GOLARZ, MN (EDS): *Muscular Dystrophy in Man and Animals.* Hafner, New York, 1963.

40. CARPENTER, S AND KARPATI, G: *Duchenne muscular dystrophy. Plasma membrane loss initiates muscle cell necrosis unless it is repaired.* Brain 102:147, 1979.

41. CARPENTER, S, ET AL: *Inclusion body myositis: A distinct variety of idiopathic inflammatory myopathy.* Neurology (New York) 28:8, 1978.

42. CARROLL, JE, ET AL: *Biochemical and physiologic consequences of carnitine palmityl transferase deficiency.* Muscle and Nerve 1:103, 1978.

43. CARROLL, JE, ET AL: *Carnitine "deficiency": Lack of response to carnitine therapy.* Neurology (New York) 30:618, 1980.

44. CHOU, SM, NONAKA, I, AND VOICE, GF: *Anastomoses of transverse tubules with terminal cisternae in polymyositis.* Arch Neurol 37:257, 1980.

45. CHOU, SM, ET AL: *Adult-type acid maltase deficiency: Pathologic features.* Neurology (Minneap) 24:394, 1974.

46. CHUI, LA AND MUNSAT, TL: *Dominant inheritance of McArdle syndrome.* Arch Neurol 33:636, 1976.

47. COËRS, C AND TELERMAN-TOPPET, N: *Differential diagnosis of limb-girdle muscular dystrophy and spinal muscular atrophy.* Neurology (New York) 29:957, 1979.

48. COËRS, C, ET AL: *Changes in motor innervation and histochemical pattern of muscle fibers in some congenital myopathies.* Neurology (New York) 26:1046, 1976.

49. CONGY, F, ET AL: *Influenzal acute myositis in the elderly.* Neurology (New York) 30:877, 1980.

50. CORNELIO, F, ET AL: *Fatal cases of lipid storage myopathy with carnitine deficiency.* J Neurol Neurosurg Psychiatry 40:170, 1977.

51. CRUZ MARTÍNEZ A, ET AL: *Single fibre electromyography in central core disease.* J Neurol Neurosurg Psychiatry 42:662, 1979.

52. CUMMING, WJK, ET AL: *Carnitine-palmityl-transferase deficiency.* J Neurol Sci 30:247, 1976.

53. CURLESS, RG AND NELSON, MB: *Congenital fiber type disproportion in identical twins.* Ann Neurol 2:455, 1977.

54. DAHL, DS AND KLUTZOW, FW: *Congenital rod disease. Further evidence of innervational abnormalities as the basis for the clinicopathologic features.* J Neurol Sci 23:371, 1974.

55. DANILOWICZ, D, ET AL: *Echocardiography in Duchenne muscular dystrophy.* Muscle and Nerve 3:298, 1980.

56. DAVIS, MJ, ET AL: *Trichinosis: Severe myopathic involvement with recovery.* Neurology (Minneap) 26:37, 1976.

57. DE JESUS, PV: *Neuromuscular physiology in Luft's syndrome.* Electromyogr Clin Neurophysiol 14:17, 1974.

58. DENBOROUGH, MA AND LOVELL, RRH: *Anesthetic deaths in a family.* Lancet 2:45, 1960.

59. DENBOROUGH, MA, DENNETT, X, AND ANDERSON, RMcD: *Central-core disease and malignant hyperpyrexia.* Br Med J 1:272, 1973.

60. DENBOROUGH, MA, ET AL: *Anaesthetic deaths in a family.* Br J Anaesth 34:395, 1962.

61. DESMEDT, JE AND BORENSTEIN, S: *Relationship of spontaneous fibrillation potentials to muscle fibre segmentation in human muscular dystrophy.* Nature 258:531, 1975.

62. DEVERE, R AND BRADLEY, WG: *Polymyositis: Its presentation, morbidity and mortality.* Brain 98:637, 1975.

63. DIDONATO, S, ET AL: *Muscle carnitine palmityltransferase deficiency: A case with enzyme deficiency in cultured fibroblasts.* Ann Neurol 4:465, 1978.

64. DIETZMAN, DE, ET AL: *Acute myositis associated with influenza B infection.* Pediatrics 57:255, 1976.

65. DIMAURO, S AND DIMAURO, PMM: *Muscle carnitine palmityltransferase deficiency and myoglobinuria.* Science 182:929, 1973.

66. DIMAURO, S AND HARTLAGE, PL: *Fatal infantile form of muscle phosphorylase deficiency.* Neurology (New York) 28:1124, 1978.

67. DIMAURO, S, TREVISAN, C, AND HAYS, A: *Disorders of lipid metabolism in muscle.* Muscle and Nerve 3:369, 1980.

68. DIMAURO, S, ET AL: *McArdle disease: The mystery of reappearing phosphorylase activity in muscle culture—A fetal isoenzyme.* Ann Neurol 3:60, 1978.

69. DIMAURO, S, ET AL: *Adult-onset acid maltase deficiency: A postmortem study.* Muscle and Nerve 1:27, 1978.

70. DIMAURO, S, ET AL: *Progressive ophthalmoplegia, glycogen storage, and abnormal mitochondria.* Arch Neurol 29:170, 1973.

71. DIMAURO, S, ET AL: *Debrancher deficiency: Neuromuscular disorder in five adults.* Ann Neurol 5:422, 1979.

72. DOUGLAS, AC, MACLEOD, JG, AND MATTHEWS, JD: *Symptomatic sarcoidosis of skeletal muscle.* J Neurol Neurosurg Psychiatry 36:1034, 1973.

73. DRACHMAN, DA: *Ophthalmoplegia plus. The neurodegenerative disorders associated with progressive external ophthalmoplegia.* Arch Neurol 18:654, 1968.

74. DUBOWITZ, V AND BROOKE, MH: *Muscle Biopsy: A Modern Approach.* WB Saunders, Philadelphia, 1973.

75. DUCHENNE, DE B: *(Recherches sur) la paralysie musculaire pseudohypertrophique ou paralysie myo-sclérosique.* Archives Générales de Médecine, Asselin, Paris, 1868.

76. EDSTRÖM, L: *Histochemical and histopathological changes in skeletal muscle in late-onset hereditary distal myopathy (Welander).* J Neurol Sci 26:147, 1975.

77. EMERY, AEH AND SKINNER, R: *Clinical studies in benign (Becker type) X-linked muscular dystrophy.* Clin Genet 10:189, 1976.

78. EMERY, AEH, ET AL: *International collaborative study of the spinal muscular atrophies. Part I. Analysis of clinical and laboratory data.* J Neurol Sci 29:83, 1976.

79. ENG, GD, ET AL: *Malignant hyperthermia and central core disease in a child with congenital dislocating hips.* Arch Neurol 35:189, 1978.

80. ENGEL, AG: *Acid maltase deficiency in adults: Studies in four cases of syndrome which may mimic muscular dystrophy or other myopathies.* Brain 93:599, 1970.

81. ENGEL, AG AND ANGELINI, C: *Carnitine deficiency of human skeletal muscle with associated lipid storage myopathy: A new syndrome.* Science 179:899, 1973.

82. ENGEL, AG AND SIEKERT, RG: *Lipid storage myopathy responsive to prednisone.* Arch Neurol 27:174, 1972.

83. ENGEL, AG, ET AL: *The spectrum and diagnosis of acid maltase deficiency.* Neurology (Minneap) 23:95, 1973.

84. ENGEL, WK, ET AL: *A skeletal-muscle disorder associated with intermittent symptoms and a possible defect of lipid metabolism.* N Engl J Med 282:697, 1970.

85. FRANK, JP, ET AL: *Central core disease and malignant hyperthermia syndrome.* Ann Neurol 7:11, 1980.

86. GALLANT, EM, GODT, RE, AND GRONERT, GA: *Role of plasma membrane defect of skeletal muscle in malignant hyperthermia.* Muscle and Nerve 2:491, 1979.

87. GARDNER-MEDWIN, D, PENNINGTON, RJ, AND WALTON, JN: *The detection of carriers of X-linked muscular dystrophy genes. A review of some methods studied in Newcastle upon Tyne.* J Neurol Sci 13:459, 1971.

88. GARDNER-THORPE, C: *Muscle weakness due to sarcoid myopathy. Six case reports and an evaluation of steroid therapy.* Neurology (Minneap) 22:917, 1972.

89. GIL-PERALTA, A, ET AL: *Myotonia in centronuclear myopathy.* J Neurol Neurosurg Psychiatry 41:1102, 1978.

90. GOMEZ, MR, ET AL: *Failure of inactivation of Duchenne dystrophy X-chromosome in one of female identical twins.* Neurology (Minneap) 27:537, 1977.

91. GROOTHUIS, DR, ET AL: *Demyelinating radiculopathy in the Kearns-Sayre syndrome: A clinicopathological study.* Ann Neurol 8:373, 1980.

92. GRUENER, R, ET AL: *Contracture of phosphorylase deficient muscle.* J Neurol Neurosurg Psychiatry 31:268, 1968.

93. HANSON, PA AND ROWLAND, LP: *Möbius syndrome and facioscapulohumeral muscular dystrophy.* Arch Neurol 24:31, 1971.

94. HARMAN, JB AND RICHARDSON, AT: *Generalised myokymia in thyrotoxicosis.* Lancet 2:473, 1954.

95. HART, ZH, ET AL: *Muscle carnitine deficiency and fatal cardiomyopathy.* Neurology (New York) 28:147, 1978.

96. HATHAWAY, PW, ENGEL, WK, AND ZELLWEGER, H: *Experimental myopathy after microarterial embolization. Comparison with childhood X-linked pseudohypertrophic muscular dystrophy.* Arch Neurol 22:365, 1970.

97. HAZAMA, R, ET AL: *Muscular dystrophy in six young girls.* Neurology (New York) 29:1486, 1979.

98. HENRIKSSON, KG AND STÅLBERG, E: *The terminal innervation pattern in polymyositis: A histochemical and SFEMG study.* Muscle and Nerve 1:3, 1978.

99. HERS, HG AND DE BARSY, T: *Type II glycogenosis (acid maltase deficiency).* In HERS, HG AND VAN HOOF, F (EDS): *Lysosomes and Storage Diseases.* Academic Press, New York, 1973.

100. HOGAN, GR, ET AL: *Pompe's disease.* Neurology (Minneap) 19:894, 1969.

101. HOOSHMAND, H, MARTINEZ, AJ, AND ROSENBLUM, WI: *Arthrogryposis multiplex congenita. Simultaneous involvement of peripheral nerve and skeletal muscle.* Arch Neurol 24:561, 1971.

102. HOPF, HC AND THORWIRTH, V: *Myasthenie-Myositis-Myopathie.* In HERTEL, G, ET AL (EDS): *Myasthenia Gravis und andere Storumgen der neuromuskularen Synapse.* Thieme, Stuttgart, 1977, pp 142–147.

103. HOWELL, RR: *The glycogen storage diseases.* In STANBURY, JB, WYNGAARDEN, JB, AND FREDRICKSON, DS (EDS): *The Metabolic Basis of Inherited Disease,* ed 3. McGraw-Hill, New York, 1972, pp 149–173.

104. HUDGSON, P, BRADLEY, WG, AND JENKISON, M: *Familial 'mitochondrial' myopathy. A myopathy associated with disordered oxidative metabolism in muscle fibres. Part I. Clinical, electrophysiological and pathological findings.* J Neurol Sci 16:343, 1972.

105. HUFFMANN, G AND LEVEN, B: *Myasthenie und polymyositis.* In HERTEL, G, ET AL (EDS): *Myasthenia Gravis und andere Storumgen der neuromuskularen Synapse.* Thieme, Stuttgart, 1977, pp 147–150.

106. INOKUCHI, T, UMEZAKI, H, AND SANTA, T: *A case of type I muscle fibre hypotrophy and internal nuclei.* J Neurol Neurosurg Psychiatry 38:475, 1975.

107. ISAACS, H AND HEFFRON, JJA: *Morphological and biochemical defects in muscles of human carriers of the malignant hyperthermia syndrome.* Br J Anaesth 47:475, 1975.

108. ISAACS, H, HEFFRON, JJA, AND BADENHORST, M: *Central core disease. A correlated genetic, histochemical, ultramicroscopic, and biochemical study.* J Neurol Neurosurg Psychiatry 38:1177, 1975.

109. ITOH, J, ET AL: *Sarcoid myopathy with typical rash of dermatomyositis.* Neurology (New York) 30:1118, 1980.

110. JEHN, UW AND FINK, MK: *Myositis, myoglobinemia, and myoglobinuria associated with enterovirus echo 9 infection.* Arch Neurol 37:457, 1980.

111. JOHNSTON, DM: *Thyrotoxic myopathy.* Arch Dis Child 49:968, 1974.

112. KARPATI, G, ET AL: *The Kearns-Shy syndrome. A multisystem disease with mitochondrial abnormality demonstrated in skeletal muscle and skin.* J Neurol Sci 19:133, 1973.

113. KARPATI, G, ET AL: *The syndrome of systemic carnitine deficiency. Clinical, morphologic, biochemical and pathophysiologic features.* Neurology (Minneap) 25:16, 1975.

114. KAZAKOV, VM, ET AL: *The facio-scapulo-limb (or the facioscapulohumeral) type of muscular dystrophy. Clinical and genetic study of 200 cases.* Eur Neurol 11:236, 1974.

115. KEARNS, TP: *External ophthalmoplegia, pigmentary degeneration of the retina, and cardiomyopathy: A newly recognized syndrome.* Trans Am Ophthalmol Soc 63:559, 1965.

116. KINOSHITA, M, SATOYOSHI, E, AND KUMAGAI, M: *Familial type I fiber atrophy.* J Neurol Sci 25:11, 1975.

117. KONDO, K AND YUASA, T: *Genetics of congenital nemaline myopathy.* Muscle and Nerve 3:308, 1980.

118. KOST, GJ AND VERITY, MA: *A new variant of late-onset myophosphorylase deficiency.* Muscle and Nerve 3:195, 1980.

119. KUHN, E, ET AL: *Early myocardial disease and cramping myalgia in Becker-type muscular dystrophy: A kindred.* Neurology (New York) 29:1144, 1979.

120. KUITUNEN, P, ET AL: *Nemaline myopathy. Report of four cases and review of the literature.* Acta Paediatr Scand 61:353, 1972.

121. LAYZER, RB AND ROWLAND, LP: *Cramps.* N Engl J Med 285:31, 1971.

122. LAYZER, RB, HAVEL, RJ AND MCILROY, MB: *Partial deficiency of carnitine palmityltransferase: Physiologic and biochemical consequences.* Neurology (New York) 30:627, 1980.

123. LAYZER, RB, ROWLAND, LP, AND RANNEY, HM: *Muscle phosphofructokinase deficiency.* Arch Neurol 17:512, 1967.

124. LAYZER, RB, ET AL: *Muscle carnitine palmitoyl transferase deficiency: A case with diabetes and ketonuria.* Neurology (Minneap) 27:379, 1977.

125. LENARD, HG AND GOEBEL, HH: *Congenital fibre type disproportion.* Neuropädiatrie 6:220, 1975.

126. MARKESBERY, WR, ET AL: *Late onset hereditary distal myopathy.* Neurology (Minneap) 24:127, 1974.

127. MARKESBERY, WR, ET AL: *Muscle carnitine deficiency. Association with lipid myopathy, vacuolar neuropathy and vacuolated leukocytes.* Arch Neurol 31:320, 1974.

128. MARTIN, JJ, DE BARSY, T, AND DEN TANDT, WR: *Acid maltase deficiency in non-identical adult twins. A morphological and biochemical study.* J Neurol 213:105, 1976.

129. MASTAGLIA, FL, ET AL: *Steroid myopathy complicating McArdle's disease.* J Neurol Neurosurg Psychiatry 33:111, 1970.

130. MATHESON, DW AND HOWLAND, JL: *Erythrocyte deformation in human muscular dystrophy.* Science 184:165, 1974.

131. MAUNDER-SEWRY, CA, ET AL: *Element analysis of skeletal muscle in Duchenne muscular dystrophy using x-ray fluorescence spectrometry.* Muscle and Nerve 3:502, 1980.

132. MAWATARI, S, MIRANDA, A, AND ROWLAND, LP: *Adenyl cyclase abnormality in Duchenne muscular dystrophy: Muscle cells in culture.* Neurology (Minneap) 26:1021, 1976.

133. MAWATARI, S, SCHONBERG, M, AND OLARTE, M: *Biochemical abnormalities of erythrocyte membranes in Duchenne dystrophy. Adenosine triphosphatase and adenyl cyclase.* Arch Neurol 33:489, 1976.

134. MCARDLE, B: *Myopathy due to a defect in muscle glycogen breakdown.* Clin Sci 10:13, 1951.

135. MCCOMAS, AJ, SICA, REP, AND CURRIE, S: *An electrophysiological study of Duchenne dystrophy.* J Neurol Neurosurg Psychiatry 34:461, 1971.

136. MCCOMAS, AJ, ET AL: *Sick motoneurons and muscle disease.* Ann NY Acad Sci 228:261, 1974.

137. MCCOMAS, AJ, ET AL: *Multiple muscle analysis of motor units in muscular dystrophy.* Arch Neurol 30:249, 1974.

138. MENDELL, JR, ENGEL, WK, AND DERRER, EC: *Duchenne muscular dystrophy: Functional ischemia reproduces its characteristic lesions.* Science 172:1143, 1971.

139. MILLER, RG, BLANK, NK, AND LAYZER, RB: *Sporadic distal myopathy with early adult onset.* Ann Neurol 5:220, 1979.

140. MILLER, SE, ROSES, AD, AND APPEL, SH: *Erythrocytes in human muscular dystrophy.* Science 188:1131, 1975.

141. MOKRI, B AND ENGEL, AG: *Duchenne dystrophy: Electron microscopic findings pointing to a basic or early abnormality in the plasma membrane of the muscle fiber.* Neurology (Minneap) 25:1111, 1975.

142. MOLLMAN, JE, CARDENAS, JC, AND PLEASURE, DE: *Alteration of calcium transport in Duchenne erythrocytes.* Neurology (New York) 30:1236, 1980.

143. MOOSA, A, BROWN, BH, AND DUBOWITZ, V: *Quantitative electromyography: Carrier detection in Duchenne type muscular dystrophy using a new automatic technique.* J Neurol Neurosurg Psychiatry 35:841, 1972.

144. MORGAN-HUGHES, JA, ET AL: *Central core disease or not? Observations on a family with a non-progressive myopathy.* Brain 96:527, 1973.

145. MORGAN-HUGHES, JA, ET AL: *A mitochondrial myopathy characterized by a deficiency in reducible cytochrome b.* Brain 100:617, 1977.

146. MROZEK, K, STRUGALSKA, M, AND FIDZIAŃSKA, A: *A sporadic case of central core disease.* J Neurol Sci 10:339, 1970.

147. MUNSAT, TL: *A standardized forearm ischemic exercise test.* Neurology (Minneap) 20:1171, 1970.

148. MUNSAT, TL, THOMPSON, LR, AND COLEMAN, RF: *Centronuclear ("myotubular") myopathy.* Arch Neurol 20:120, 1969.

149. MUNSAT, TL, ET AL: *Serum enzyme alterations in neuromuscular disorders.* JAMA 226:1536, 1973.

150. MUNSAT, TL, ET AL: *Inflammatory myopathy with facioscapulohumeral distribution.* Neurology (Minneap) 22:335, 1972.

151. MURASE, T, ET AL: *Myopathy associated with type III glycogenosis.* J Neurol Sci 20:287, 1973.

152. MURPHY, SF AND DRACHMAN, DB: *The oculopharyngeal syndrome.* JAMA 203:1003, 1968.

153. NEVILLE, HE AND BROOKE, MH: *Central core fibers: Structured and unstructured.* In KAKULAS, BA (ED): *Basic Research in Myology.* Excerpta Medica, Amsterdam, 1973.

154. OLSON, W, ET AL: *Oculocraniosomatic neuromuscular disease with "ragged-red" fibers.* Arch Neurol 26:193, 1972.

155. PAINE, RS: *The future of the 'floppy infant': A follow-up study of 133 patients.* Dev Med Child Neurol 5:115, 1963.

156. PALMER, EG, TOPEL, DG, AND CHRISTIAN, LL: *Light and electron microscopy of skeletal muscle from malignant hyperthermia susceptible pigs.* In ALDRETE, JA AND BRITT, BA (EDS): *The Second International Symposium on Malignant Hyperthermia.* Grune & Stratton, New York, 1978.

157. PANAYIOTOPOULOS, CP, SCARPALEZOS, S, AND PAPAPETROPOULOS, T: *Electrophysiological estimation of motor units in Duchenne muscular dystrophy.* J Neurol Sci 23:89, 1974.

158. PATTEN, BM, ET AL: *Neuromuscular disease in primary hyperparathyroidism.* Ann Intern Med 80:182, 1974.

159. PERCY, ME, ET AL: *Serum creatine kinase and pyruvate kinase in Duchenne muscular dystrophy carrier detection.* Muscle and Nerve 2:329, 1979.

160. PERLOFF, JK, ET AL: *The distinctive electrocardiogram of Duchenne's progressive muscular dystrophy.* Am J Med 42:179, 1967.

161. PERNOW, BB, HAVEL, RJ, AND JENNINGS, DB: *The second wind phenomenon in McArdle's syndrome.* Acta Med Scand (suppl 472):294, 1967.

162. PEYRONNARD, JM, ET AL: *Neuropathy and mitochondrial myopathy.* Ann Neurol 7:262, 1980.

163. PLEASURE, DE, WALSH, GO, AND ENGEL, WK: *Atrophy of skeletal muscle in patients with Cushing's syndrome.* Arch Neurol 22:118, 1970.

164. PUVANENDRAN, K, ET AL: *Thyrotoxic myopathy. A clinical and quantitative analytic electromyographic study.* J Neurol Sci 42:441, 1979.

165. RADU, H, ET AL: *Myotubular (centronuclear) (neuro-) myopathy. 1. Clinical, genetical and morphological studies.* Eur Neurol 15:285, 1977.

166. RAMSAY, ID: *Muscle dysfunction in hyperthyroidism.* Lancet 2:931, 1966.

167. RESKE-NIELSEN, E, LOU, HC, AND LOWES, M: *Progressive external ophthalmoplegia. Evidence for a generalised mitochondrial disease with a defect in pyruvate metabolism.* Acta Ophthalmol 54:553, 1976.

168. RIDDOCH, D AND MORGAN-HUGHES, JA: *Prognosis in adult polymyositis.* J Neurol Sci 26:71, 1975.

169. RINGEL, SP, CARROLL, JE AND SCHOLD, SC: *The spectrum of mild X-linked recessive muscular dystrophy.* Arch Neurol 34:408, 1977.

170. ROSE, AL AND WALTON, JN: *Polymyositis: A survey of 89 cases with particular reference to treatment and prognosis.* Brain 89:747, 1966.

171. ROSES, AD, ET AL: *Carrier detection in Duchenne muscular dystrophy.* N Engl J Med 294:193, 1976.

172. ROWLAND, LP: *Are the muscular dystrophies neurogenic?* Ann NY Acad Sci 228:244, 1974.

173. ROWLAND, LP: *Pathogenesis of muscular dystrophies.* Arch Neurol 33:315–321, 1976.

174. ROWLAND, LP (ED): *Pathogenesis of Human Muscular Dystrophies.* Proceedings of the 5th Internat Scientific Conference of the Muscular Dystrophy Association, Excerpta Medica, Amsterdam, 1977.

175. ROWLAND, LP: *Biochemistry of muscle membranes in Duchenne muscular dystrophy.* Muscle and Nerve 3:3, 1980.

176. ROWLAND, LP, FAHN, S, AND SCHOTLAND, DL: *McArdle's disease. Hereditary myopathy due to absence of muscle phosphorylase.* Arch Neurol 9:325, 1963.

177. ROWLAND, LP, ET AL: *The clinical diagnosis of McArdle's disease. Identification of another family with deficiency of muscle phosphorylase.* Neurology (Minneap) 16:93, 1966.

178. ROWLAND, LP, ET AL: *Emery-Dreifuss, muscular dystrophy.* Ann Neurol 5:111, 1979.

179. SAHN, L AND MAGEE, KR: *Phosphorylase deficiency associated with isometric exercise intolerance.* Neurology (Minneap) 26:896, 1976.

180. SALICK, AI AND PEARSON, CM: *Electrical silence of myoedema.* Neurology (Minneap) 17:899, 1967.

181. SAWHNEY, BB, ET AL: *Pseudohypertrophic myopathy in cysticercosis.* Neurology (Minneap) 26:270, 1976.

182. SCHOCHET, SS, JR, ET AL: *Centronuclear myopathy: Disease entity or a syndrome? Light- and electron-microscopic study of two cases and review of the literature.* J Neurol Sci 16:215, 1972.

183. SCHOLTE, HR, JENNEKENS, FGI, AND BOUVY, JJBJ: *Carnitine palmitoyltransferase II deficiency with normal carnitine palmitoyltransferase I in skeletal muscle and leucocytes.* J Neurol Sci 40:39, 1979.

184. SCHOTLAND, DL, ET AL: *Neuromuscular disorder associated with a defect in mitochondrial energy supply.* Arch Neurol 33:475, 1976.

185. SERRATRICE, G, ET AL: *Centronuclear myopathy: Possible central nervous system origin.* Muscle and Nerve 1:62, 1978.

186. SHAFIQ, SA, ET AL: *Nemaline myopathy: Report of a fatal case, with histochemical and electron microscopic studies.* Brain 90:817, 1967.

187. SHY, GM AND MAGEE, KR: *A new congenital non-progressive myopathy.* Brain 79:610, 1956.

188. SHY, GM, ET AL: *Nemaline myopathy. A new congenital myopathy.* Brain 86:793, 1963.

189. SHY, GM, ET AL: *A generalized disorder of nervous system, skeletal muscle and heart resembling Refsum's disease and Hurler's syndrome. Part I. Clinical, pathologic and biochemical characteristics.* Am J Med 42:163, 1967.

190. SMITH, R AND STERN, G: *Myopathy, osteomalacia and hyperparathyroidism.* Brain 90:593, 1967.

191. SPIRO, AJ, SHY, GM, AND GONATAS, NK: *Myotubular myopathy.* Arch Neurol 14:1, 1966.

192. STREIB, EW, WILBOURN, AJ, AND MITSUMOTO, H: *Spontaneous electrical muscle fiber activity in polymyositis and dermatomyositis.* Muscle and Nerve 2:14, 1979.

193. TARUI, S, ET AL: *Phosphofructokinase deficiency in skeletal muscle. A new type of glycogenosis.* Biochem Biophys Res Commun 19:517, 1965.

194. TELERMAN-TOPPET, N, GERARD, JM, AND COËRS, C: *Central core disease. A study of clinically unaffected muscle.* J Neurol Sci 19:207, 1973.

195. THOMAS, PK, SCHOTT, GD, AND MORGAN-HUGHES, JA: *Adult onset scapuloperoneal myopathy.* J Neurol Neurosurg Psychiatry 38:1008, 1975.

196. TOBIN, WE, ET AL: *Muscle phosphofructokinase deficiency.* Arch Neurol 28:128, 1973.

197. UPTON, ARM, MCCOMAS, AJ, AND BIANCHI, FA: *Neuropathy in McArdle's syndrome.* N Engl J Med 289:750, 1973.

198. VALLI, G, SCARLATO, G, AND CONTARTESE, M: *Quantitative electromyography in the detection of the carriers in Duchenne type muscular dystrophy.* J Neurol 212:139, 1976.

199. VAN HOOF, F AND HERS, HG: *The subgroups of type III glycogenosis.* Eur J Biochem 2:265, 1967.

200. VAN WIJNGAARDEN, GK AND BETHLEM, J: *The facioscapulohumeral syndrome.* In KAKULAS, BA (ED): *Clinical Studies in Myology,* Part 2. Excerpta Medica, Amsterdam, 1973.

201. VAN WIJNGAARDEN, GK, ET AL: *Familial "myotubular" myopathy.* Neurology (Minneap) 19:901, 1969.

202. VASILESCU, C, ET AL: *Myasthenia in patients with dermatomyositis. Clinical, electrophysiological and ultrastructural studies.* J Neurol Sci 38:129, 1978.

203. VICTOR, M, HAYES, R, AND ADAMS, RD: *Oculopharyngeal muscular dystrophy. A familial disease of late life characterized by dysphagia and progressive ptosis of the eyelids.* N Engl J Med 267:1267, 1962.

204. WAKAYAMA, Y, ET AL: *Alteration in erythrocyte membrane structure in Duchenne muscular dystrophy.* Ann Neurol 4:253, 1978.

205. WALTON, JN: *Some changing concepts in neuromuscular disease.* In KAKULAS, BA (ED): *Clinical Studies in Myology,* Part 2. Excerpta Medica, Amsterdam, 1973.

206. WELANDER, L: *Myopathia distalis tarda hereditaria.* Acta Med Scand (suppl 265)141:1, 1951.

207. WILSON J AND WALTON, JN: *Some muscular manifestations of hypothyroidism.* J Neurol Neurosurg Psychiatry 22:320, 1959.

# 26

# NEUROMUSCULAR DISEASES CHARACTERIZED BY ABNORMAL MUSCLE ACTIVITY

Pathologic muscle stiffness may result from abnormalities of the central nervous system, peripheral nerve trunk, axon terminal, or muscle membrane. Myotonia is the clinical phenomenon of delayed relaxation of voluntarily or reflexively contracted muscle. It is accompanied by a characteristic electrical discharge if the affected muscles are tested electromyographically. Both clinical myotonia and associated electrical phenomena occur in a number of syndromes. These include myotonic dystrophy, myotonia congenita, paramyotonia congenita, and a form of periodic paralysis. Involuntary contraction of skeletal muscle is an essential part of neuromyotonia or continuous muscle fiber discharge, the Schwartz-Jampel syndrome, and myokymia. In the stiff-man syndrome, sustained muscle contractions also occur, but the spontaneous discharges probably originate centrally rather than in the peripheral neuromuscular system. Other conditions with abnormal muscle activity include the common cramp, contracture, tetanus, tetany, and hemifacial spasm.

Several techniques are available for determining the site of abnormal discharges. Nerve blocks will eliminate abnormal muscular activity originating in the central nervous system or the proximal part of the peripheral nerve. In this instance, repetitive nerve stimulation distal to the block fails to induce the abnormal muscle activity. Discharges originating in the distal or terminal nerve segment cease after neuromuscular transmission block by curare. Curarization does not affect abnormal discharges originating from intrinsic muscle fibers, however. Some cramp syndromes display a distinctive pattern of abnormalities on electromyography. Others produce a normal interference pattern, although the number and frequency of discharging motor units are not under voluntary control. Contracture is distinguished from true cramps, because the contracted muscle is electrically silent.

## MYOTONIA

In myotonia, the muscle membrane, once activated, tends to discharge repetitively. This has its clinical counterpart in delayed muscle relaxation. Myotonia is painless, unlike cramp or spontaneous spasm. Postactivation myotonia typically occurs at the beginning of voluntary movement after a period of rest. Percussion myotonia follows a brisk tap over the thenar eminence. During volitional activity, the myotonia may worsen initially but improve following a warm-up period. Cold aggravates both postactivation and percussion myotonia. Characteristic electrophysiologic findings[160] include myotonic discharges that wax and wane at varying frequencies up to 150 impulses per second, as discussed in Chapter 13, and declining muscle action potentials with repetitive nerve stimulation, as described in Chapter 9. Voluntary contraction, muscle percussion, and needle insertion provoke myotonic discharges.

Myotonia and myositis may be parts of the symptom complex seen in multicentric reticulohistiocytosis.[5] Myotonic discharge with or without clinical myotonia may be seen in a number of metabolic muscle diseases such as hyperkalemic periodic paralysis, acid maltase deficiency,[49] hyperthyroidism,[119] or malignant hyperpyrexia as discussed in Chapter 25. Administration of the hypocholesterolemic agent diazocholesterol can induce a myopathy in which myotonia is sometimes seen.[161] In these entities, however, myotonia is neither predominant nor essential as it is in myotonic dystrophy, myotonia congenita, and paramyotonia.

Although the underlying defect in myotonia remains unknown, recent studies implicate the sarcolemmal membrane.[97, 141] After-depolarization occurs following activation of the muscle membrane, presumably because potassium ions ($K^+$) accumulate in the transverse tubular system. This negative after-potential is normally not large enough to generate an action potential but may initiate repetitive discharges in the electrically unstable membrane with low conductance.[2] Instability of the muscle membrane may result from abnormally low chloride permeability in the myotonia seen in goats or induced experimentally with drugs.[10, 27, 58, 97] In humans, however, low chloride permeability occurs only in myotonia congenita and not in myotonic dystrophy. As part of a diffuse involvement of different organ systems, erythrocytes may demonstrate biochemical and biophysical abnormalities.[32, 116, 138, 139, 140, 173] This has not, however, been universally confirmed.[59]

## Myotonic dystrophy

Myotonic dystrophy is transmitted as an autosomal dominant trait but may show incomplete penetrance or anticipation with earlier and more severe symptomatology in successive generations. Some claim that the latter may simply reflect earlier recognition or inaccurate histories. Typically, the illness begins in adolescence or early adult life. Neuromuscular symptoms consist of weakness and myotonia. Patients may have muscle stiffness and cramps, but usually distal muscle weakness prompts them to seek medical advice. On questioning, they usually admit to difficulty with grip release, which seems to be more of an inconvenience than a disability to them. Weakness may begin in the hands and feet but eventually spreads to involve all the muscles, including the flexors of the neck.

In adults the diagnosis can be suspected from a hatchet-faced appearance, which results from relatively selective atrophy of the temporalis and masseter. Prominent wasting of the neck muscles, particularly of the sternocleidomastoids, gives rise to a swan-neck. The head supported by a slender neck appears unstable. In recumbency, the patient is unable to lift the head from a pillow against gravity. Facial weakness produces a blank expression and ptosis. In the absence of this characteristic appearance, milder cases of myotonic dystrophy may escape detection. Usually, however, grip or percussion myotonia can be demonstrated. Myotonic phenomena become less prominent as the muscle wasting and weakness advance. Myotonia tends to diminish with continued exercise, and indeed the muscle may become almost normal clinically or electrically after repetitive testing. Muscle biopsy usually reveals Type I fiber atrophy and long chains of internal nuclei.

Additional features include early frontal baldness, cataracts, gynecomastia, and testicular or ovarian atrophy. The disease affects numerous other systems as evidenced by cardiac abnormalities, bowel symptoms, respiratory infections, mental disturbances, and low intelligence. Unusual susceptibility to certain medications such as barbiturates increases the risks of general anesthesia.[131]

In congenital myotonic dystrophy, neuromuscular and systemic manifestations are evident in the neonatal period.[70, 71, 166] But these hypotonic infants show no evidence of clinical or electrical myotonia until the age of five years or later. Weakness produces a triangular mouth in which the upper lip points upward in the middle. Clubfeet are common. Many children are mentally retarded. Diaphragmatic elevation is also characteristic.[22, 38] Infants frequently die of respiratory infections. Curiously, congenital myotonia nearly always appears in children born to myotonic mothers; paternal inheritance is rare. Some biopsied specimens have shown severe deficiency in Type IIB fibers.[6]

Electromyography shows myotonic discharges (see Fig. 13-6) in all affected adults and approximately one half of the relatives at risk for myotonic dystrophy.[127] Thus, in adults, the test helps to establish the diagnosis, even if the clinical features are limited to mild distal weakness and atrophy. Unfortunately, during infancy and early childhood, patients tend to show neither the characteristic electrical discharges nor clinical myotonic phenomenon.[44] Genetic counselling may therefore have to await adolescence or adulthood. Low amplitude, short duration, polyphasic motor unit potentials indicate a myopathic process.[28] Additional neurogenic features occur as part of the generalized membrane abnormality. These include: (1) mildly slowed motor nerve conduction velocities;[9, 33, 122] (2) striking reduction in the number of functioning motor units;[8, 108, 109] and (3) occasional hypertrophy of peripheral nerves.[21] However, the severity of the neuropathic changes does not correlate with the degree of muscular atrophy and weakness.[122] Peripheral nerve morphometry has shown no significant abnormality in the cutaneous branches of the common peroneal nerve.[128]

## Myotonia congenita

Two different varieties of myotonia congenita show different genetic and clinical characteristics. The type originally described by Thomsen[169] in four generations of his own family is transmitted as an autosomal dominant and involves both sexes equally. Myotonia appears in infancy or early childhood but remains mild throughout life. Occasional asymptomatic patients with electromyographic evidence of myotonic discharge may represent sporadic cases of Thomsen's disease. The second more common type described by Becker[12, 15, 16, 17] appears in an autosomal recessive fashion but affects men more frequently. Myotonia is more severe in the recessive type, although the two varieties otherwise share similar clinical features.[87, 184] In a third, rare type of myotonia congenita, the patient may have, in addition to myotonia, painful muscle cramps induced by exercise.[14] A contracted muscle is electrically silent, that is, a contracture, probably resulting from some defect of muscle metabolism.[148, 163]

Myotonia often predominates in the lower extremities causing difficulty in ambulation. Movements are initiated slowly and with difficulty, especially after prolonged rest. With continued exercise, movement may become almost normal. This warm-up phenomenon is not a systemic effect, since repetitive movements of one set of muscles do not limber up another set of adjacent muscles. Although the patient may appear weak, normal muscle power becomes evident once myotonia disappears. Retarded motor development is common in children. In some patients muscular hypertrophy develops as a result of continuous involuntary exercise and may produce a Herculean appearance, which contrasts strikingly with the muscular wasting in myotonic dystrophy. This degree of hypertrophy, however, does not appear as commonly as previously publicized. No other systems seem to be affected, and the patient has a normal life expectancy.

Diagnosis depends on family history and clinical features. Percussion myotonia is readily demonstrated. In equivocal cases, exposure to cold serves as a useful provocative test. Muscle biopsy reveals internal nuclei—but to a lesser extent than in myotonic dystrophy—and the absence of Type IIB fibers.[40] A spin-labelled study has shown increased fluidity of the erythrocyte membrane in myotonia congenita as compared with myotonic dystrophy.[32]

Electromyography plays an important role in establishing the nonspecific diagnosis of myotonia. As discussed in Chapter 24, repetitive nerve stimulation may cause significant decline in successive evoked muscle action potentials as a result of increased muscle fiber refractoriness. Unlike in myasthenia gravis, the decrementing tendency does not diminish towards the end of a train, and a faster rate of stimulation produces greater change. The decremental motor response, though known to occur in any type of myotonic disorder, is particularly impressive in Becker variety.[4]

## Paramyotonia congenita

Paramyotonia congenita of Eulenberg,[51] transmitted by a single autosomal dominant gene, affects both sexes equally.[13, 16, 17, 133, 170] The symptoms begin at birth or in early childhood and do not improve with age. The myotonia paradoxically intensifies rather than improves with exercise. When exposed to cold, the patient may develop stiffness of the tongue, eyelids, face, and extremity muscles. The pathophysiology of the cold-induced rigidity remains unclear. It may not represent true myotonia, since the electric discharges disappear with cooling, despite increasing muscular stiffness.[179]

The disorder closely resembles hyperkalemic periodic paralysis. Attacks of flaccid weakness accompanied by myotonia are not unlike the spells of periodic paralysis. In various members of the same family, intermittent paralysis may occur without myotonia, or vice versa. Laboratory findings include elevated or high normal levels of serum potassium. Electromyography shows evidence of myotonia and a decrementing response of the compound muscle action potential to repetitive nerve stimulation.[30, 31] During episodes of paralysis, stimulation of the nerve fails to elicit muscle action potentials. Nerve conduction studies are normal between attacks.

# PERIODIC PARALYSIS

Periodic paralysis results from reversible inexcitability of muscle membrane. Traditional classification distinguishes three types according to the serum level of potassium ($K^+$) during a paralytic attack: hypokalemic, hyperkalemic, and normokalemic. However, all three categories share a number of clinical features, and changes in serum potassium show no direct cause and effect relationship to paralytic events. Indeed, episodes of weakness associated with either hypokalemia or hyperkalmia can occur in a given individual.[37] More recent classification divides the periodic paralyses into primary hereditary and secondary acquired types.[142] Primary hereditary types consist of hypokalemic periodic paralysis and potassium-sensitive hyperkalemic or normokalemic periodic paralysis. The last two are usually accompanied by myotonia and possibly represent the same entity as paramyotonia congenita. The second group includes thyrotoxic hypokalemic periodic paralysis, acute or chronic potassium depletion and retention, hypokalemia secondary to renal tubular acidosis,[18] and chronic hypernatremia.[101]

During an attack of periodic paralysis the muscle membrane is inexcitable to direct or indirect stimulation.[25, 66, 73, 158] An end-plate potential persists during the paralytic episodes, but no action potentials are propagated along the muscle fibers.[69] In the hypokalemic types, inexcitability results from membrane dysfunction, since contraction occurs normally when calcium ($Ca^{++}$) is applied to fibers stripped of their outer membranes.[48] An important finding common to hypokalemic[73, 135] and hyperkalemic periodic paralyses[25] is substantial depolarization of the resting potential, presumably because of increased sodium ($Na^+$) conductance.[73, 121] These observations suggest that depolarization block leads to muscle fiber inexcitability at least in hypokalemic periodic paralysis.

# Hypokalemic periodic paralysis

This familial disease, inherited as an autosomal dominant, occurs with higher incidence in men.[50, 60, 61] Although variable in onset, episodes of paralysis typically begin in the second decade. During an attack, weakness starts in the legs and gradually spreads to involve all the muscles of the body, with the exception of the ocular muscles, diaphragm, and other respiratory muscles. At the height of paralysis the patient may be immobilized. The episodes characteristically occur after rest, especially on waking in the morning. A heavy carbohydrate meal may precipitate the attack. Each paralytic episode lasts several hours to a day, but a few days may elapse before complete recovery. Serum potassium is low during an attack. Administration of potassium chloride usually relieves the paralysis. These attacks vary in frequency and severity but tend to remit after 35 years of age. Eyelid myotonia, originally described in the hyperkalemic type of periodic paralysis, may also appear in the hypokalemic variety.[132] The light microscope reveals few structural abnormalities, but electron microscopic studies show vacuoles arising from local dilation of the transverse tubules and sarcoplasmic reticulum.[47]

Between attacks, clinical and electrophysiologic abnormalities may be absent, although some patients have progressive myopathy.[46, 50, 125] Hypokalemic myopathy may also develop in other conditions associated with potassium loss.[137, 143, 144] During severe paralytic episodes, electrophysiologic studies show a reduction in the number of voluntarily recruited motor unit potentials and decreased muscle excitability to electrical stimulation. Stimulation of the nerve supplying the muscle elicits no muscle action potentials. In less severe cases the amplitude of the compound muscle action potentials diminishes in proportion to the degree of weakness.[66] Repetitive nerve stimulation at a rate of 10 to 25 per second may produce an incremental response in mildly weakened muscles[69] but no change in very weak muscles.[35] Corresponding to electrical recovery with repetitive stimulation, temporary improvement of strength occurs after gentle exercise. However, severe rebound weakness usually follows.

# Hyperkalemic periodic paralysis
# (Adynamia episodica hereditaria)

In this autosomal dominant disorder, which affects the two sexes equally, episodes of flaccid weakness accompany elevated serum potassium.[23, 60, 61, 93, 107] The disease begins in infancy or early childhood with spells of generalized hypotonia. Sudden weakness develops after a short period of rest following exercise, upon exposure to cold, or after the administration of potassium. Further exercise or administration of carbohydrates temporarily delays what actually becomes a more severe paralytic episode. Paralysis usually lasts less than one hour but may be more prolonged. Weakness probably results from muscle release of potassium rather than from the high serum level of potassium. Myotonia commonly involves the muscles of the face, eyes, and tongue. This finding suggests that hyperkalemic periodic paralysis and paramyotonia congenita may be equivalent syndromes.[42, 57, 93] Both entities may appear in a single family.

Between attacks, electromyography may show increased insertional activity with myotonic and complex repetitive discharges. During an attack, muscle irritability and myotonic discharges increase but electrical or mechanical stimulation fails to excite the muscle. Abundant low amplitude, short duration motor unit potentials with early recruitment suggests progressive myopathy. In the presence of prominent myotonia, repetitive nerve stimulation may cause a decrement of the evoked muscle action potentials,[99] a tendency accentuated by cooling.[134] The physiologic mechanism underlying episodic paralysis remains unknown. Pertinent findings include a reduced resting muscle membrane potential,[39] reversible depolarization during the attacks,[23, 25, 29] and possible neural hyperexcitability.[155]

## Normokalemic periodic paralysis

This very rare condition also seems to have some enigmatic relationship to potassium. Only a few reports have appeared since Poskanzer and Kerr[129] described attacks of flaccid quadriplegia in infancy with normal serum levels of potassium. The clinical features closely resemble those of hyperkalemic periodic paralysis,[113] of which the normokalemic type may be a variant.

# NEUROMYOTONIA

In myotonia abnormal muscle activity occurs only after voluntary or induced muscle contraction. In contrast, neuromyotonia is characterized by sustained or repetitive spontaneous activity of the muscle fibers. In a severe form, continuous and excessive muscle contraction may give rise to abnormal posture. In a milder form, asynchronous contraction of single or multiple motor units produces generalized myokymia. Isaacs[77] originally described two patients with progressive painless stiffness and rigidity of the trunk and extremities. This syndrome has since been referred to as continuous muscle fiber activity,[78, 79, 98, 100] neuromyotonia,[112] neurotonia,[175] or pseudomyotonia.[76, 159] The term pseudomyotonia used here distinguishes persistent muscle activity originating from peripheral nerve from true myotonia, which represents disorders of the muscle membrane.

The disease appears sporadically. Symptoms begin at any age, although rarely in the neonatal period.[19] The patient initially notices muscle twitching, especially in the legs. The affected muscles are stiff and fail to relax completely following voluntary contraction. The patient moves slowly and deliberately, as if imitating a slow motion picture. Stiffness seems to vary from one movement to the next. Excessive sweating occurs, probably because of continuous muscle activity. The patient has reduced or absent muscle stretch reflexes. Laryngeal spasm may develop.[80, 96] In advanced stages the patient holds the arms rigidly with the wrist flexed and the fingers extended. In milder forms of the syndrome the abnormal activity appears restricted in degree and distribution.[11, 149]

Electromyography reveals characteristic spontaneous discharges in all involved muscle groups. Waveforms of varying configuration appear at high frequencies up to 300 impulses per second, representing either motor unit potentials or fibrillations. A marked decrement in successive motor unit potential amplitude suggests that the motor units are unable to follow rapidly recurring nerve impulses. This high-frequency, decrementing discharge produces a unique musical sound, pings, that differs from other spontaneous potentials including myotonic discharge.[89] During voluntary contraction, many motor units fire successively with overlap. Artificially induced ischemia or electrical stimulation of the nerve may abruptly initiate the spontaneous discharge.

The motor activity persists during sleep, general or spinal anesthesia, or after procaine block of the peripheral nerve.[19, 77, 79] Local administration of curare abolishes the activity. Other therapeutic agents include diphenylhydantoin and carbamazepine for some[76, 77, 79, 174] but not all patients.[11] Microelectrode studies of end-plate potentials (EPP) in an intercostal muscle biopsy have demonstrated normal miniature end-plate potentials (MEPP) and no evidence of quantal squander.[89] The peripheral nerve may show associated abnormalities.[19, 180] These findings suggest that the high-frequency discharge originates at the distal motor axon. Two members of a family demonstrated hyperexcitability of motor and sensory neurons.[91]

# SCHWARTZ-JAMPEL SYNDROME

Continuous muscle fiber activity occurs in osteochondromuscular dystrophy originally described by Schwartz and Jampel.[154] This is a rare disease of autosomal recessive inheritance. The characteristic clinical features include short stature, muscular hypertrophy, diffuse bone disease, ocular and facial anomalies, and severe voluntary and percussion myotonia.[1, 55, 85, 124, 145] The muscle biopsy may reveal myopathic and neurogenic features.[53] Electromyographic findings resemble the neuromyotonia of Isaacs and Merten or complex repetitive discharges. Unlike myotonia, the repetitive high frequency discharges do not wax or wane. They persist following nerve block or even nerve degeneration. However, most but not all of the spontaneous activity disappears after administration of curare[167] or succinylcholine.[34] Some authors have reported increased insertional activity and absence of the silent period (SP) following muscle contraction. The defect responsible for the continuous muscle contraction presumably lies in the muscle component of the neuromuscular junction, but the exact mechanism remains unknown.[154, 167]

# MYOKYMIA

Myokymia has a distinctive clinical appearance and association with certain neurologic disorders. In this entity, spontaneous repetitive contraction of narrow muscle strips occurs for several seconds. Each strip of muscle, 1 to 2 cm in width, slowly contracts along the longitudinal axis. Different strips show independent irregular undulations that have been likened to a cutaneous race of worms. Schultze[153] first introduced the term myokymia in describing a patient with leg cramps associated with spontaneous muscle contractions of the calves, thighs, chest, and arms. He considered myokymia to be a manifestation of benign neuromuscular irritability.[65] Gamstorp and Wohlfart[62] also described a number of patients with delayed relaxation clinically and with continuous spontaneous motor unit discharges electromyographically.

The name has since been applied to muscle twitches in a variety of conditions, including lead poisoning, thyrotoxicosis, scleroderma, systemic infections, intoxications, and spinal cord lesions.[149, 174] Myokymia of the superior oblique muscle may cause oscillopsia.[165] Generalized myokymia with impaired muscle relaxation may develop in association with the syndromes of continuous muscle fiber activity,[80, 149] restless leg syndrome,[75] and with peripheral neuropathy.[180] Thus, myokymia occurs in a heterogenous group of disorders and probably represents a nonspecific neuronal response to injury. In most limb myokymia, discharges arise focally at the site of a chronic peripheral nerve lesion.[3] In one study, carbamazepine (Tegretol) led to nearly total symptomatic relief.[123]

Whereas electromyographic abnormalities vary slightly from one patient to another, the prolonged undulating movements of myokymia all seem to result from brief tetanic contractions of repetitively discharging single or multiple motor units; that is, grouped fasciculation.[117] Interestingly, however, myokymia is usually accompanied by neither fibrillation potentials nor positive sharp waves. Myokymia does not wax or wane but may be associated with myotonia.[62, 68, 172] Sleep or volitional movement does not affect clinical myokymia or the electrical discharges. They also remain unchanged with rest, percussion, electrical stimulation, or needle movement.[76, 123] However, xylocaine infusion of a peripheral nerve trunk blocks myokymic discharges.

The term myokymia is most commonly used to describe undulating, wormlike movement of the facial muscles.[90] Facial myokymia is typically seen with the pontine lesions of multiple sclerosis[72] (see Fig. 13-9 top) or glioma,[36, 168] but also appears after Bell's palsy or polyradiculoneuropathy[41, 177] (see Fig. 13-9 bottom). Metastatic tumor that interrupts the supranuclear pathways descending upon the facial nucleus may also give rise to myokymia.[156, 178] Two electromyographic patterns characterize facial myokymic discharges.[130] In the continuous type, rhythmic single or paired discharges of one or a few motor units recur with striking regularity at intervals of 100 to 200 ms. In the discontinuous type, bursts of motor unit activity at 30 to 40 impulses per second last for 100 to 900 ms, and repeat in regular intervals of 100 ms to 10 seconds (see Fig. 13-9 top).

Although the continuous versus discontinuous types tend to appear with multiple sclerosis and brain stem glioma, respectively, clinical specificity has not emerged.

# HEMIFACIAL SPASM

Hemifacial spasm may develop spontaneously or as a late complication of Bell's palsy or other disorders of the facial nerve. Unlike focal convulsive twitches of the face, the spasmodic contractions often follow blinking and consist of simultaneous rapid twitching in several facial muscles. Less commonly, one side of the face may show prolonged contraction with irregular, fluctuating movements. Spontaneous movement of this type nearly exclusively occurs in the facial muscles, but masticatory spasm may rarely accompany facial hemiatrophy.[83] Various hypotheses for the spontaneous occurrence of unilateral synkinetic facial movement include aberrant regeneration,[176] fiber excitation by ephaptic transmission (cross-talk) at the site of injury,[146, 183] and hyperexcitability of the facial nucleus following axonal injury.[54] The idiopathic type may result from vascular compression of the facial nerve.[52, 64, 81, 104, 126]

Characteristic electromyographic findings include isolated bursts of high frequency repetitive motor unit discharges at rates ranging from 200 to 400 impulses per second. But slow irregular discharge around 20 to 40 impulses per second may also occur.[72] The diagnosis of hemifacial spasm usually depends on simple visual inspection or electromyographic recording of synkinesis.[182] In clinically equivocal cases the electrically elicited blink reflex[7, 84] may document synkinesis by demonstrating the presence of R1 and R2 components not only in the orbicularis oculi but also in the orbicularis oris, platysma, or other facial muscles as discussed in Chapter 16 (see Fig. 16-9).

# TETANUS

The toxin of *Clostridium tetani* travels from wound to central nervous system via blood or retrograde axonal transport. After an incubation period of one to two weeks the patient develops either generalized or localized manifestations of neuromuscular irritability. These include spasm of the masticatory muscles (trismus) and facial grimacing (risus sardonicus). These symptoms become maximal within a few days and may improve in several weeks, though chronic manifestations of tetanic contraction may occur. The continuous motor unit discharges seen in electromyography resolves during sleep, with administration of general or spinal anesthesia, and after peripheral nerve block.

Tetanus toxin presumably blocks postsynaptic inhibition in the spinal cord and brain stem, thereby increasing the excitability of alpha motor neurons.[26] The shortened or absent silent period (SP) probably results from failure of Renshaw inhibition. This characteristic electrodiagnostic feature of tetanus seldom occurs in other disorders with motor unit hyperactivity.[136, 164] Although the exact pathophysiology is not known, the muscle spasms and rigidity almost certainly result from the effect of tetanus toxin on the central nervous system. Some clinical and electrophysiologic findings suggest peripheral nerve involvement in severe tetanus.[157] Facial nerve conduction studies may[63] or may not[171] show abnormalities.

# STIFF-MAN SYNDROME

Moersch and Woltman[115] and many others have described the typical clinical and electrophysiologic features of the stiff-man syndrome.[56, 67, 102, 110, 152] It usually occurs sporadically in adult men and women, but a congenital form has also been reported.[86, 147] Muscle stiffness develops insidiously, progressing from tightness to painful, sustained contraction. The disease has some predilection for the pelvic and shoulder girdle muscles. The tightness of the chest muscles may interfere with breathing and swallowing.

The extremities may be immobilized in unnatural positions with simultaneous contraction of agonistic and antagonistic muscles. Inversion and plantarflexion of the feet reflect the overpowering force of the posterior versus anterior calf muscles. Movement, either active or passive, aggravates the pain.

The excessive muscle contraction resembles physiologic cramps but it is continuous and involves many muscle groups simultaneously. Patients with the stiff-man syndrome may be mistaken for hysterics because of their facial grimacing, unusual posture, and complaints of muscle cramps that superficially mimick voluntary contraction. Conspicuous absence of other neurologic abnormalities may strengthen this erroneous impression. Close observation, however, reveals that the powerful spasms are unlike any voluntary contraction. Indeed, fractures of the long bones have resulted. Various conditions described in association with stiff-man–like pictures include nocturnal myoclonus and epilepsy,[105] focal cortical atrophy with increased spinal fluid gammaglobulin,[102] and ingestion of alcohol.[20]

Electromyography shows a sustained interference pattern consisting of normal motor unit potentials in agonistic as well as antagonistic muscles.[103, 162] The persistent electrical activity associated with painful muscle cramps probably originates in the central nervous system. The spasm and spontaneous discharges disappear during sleep, with administration of general or spinal anesthesia, following procaine block of the peripheral nerve, and following infusion of curare.[67, 111] The exact neurophysiologic mechanism underlying the abnormal discharge remains unknown. Clinical similarities with chronic tetanus suggest a possible relationship between these two entities.[67, 74, 115] Tetanus toxin causes hyperexcitability of motor units by blocking spinal inhibitory postsynaptic potentials. Similarly, the motor neuron pool may become excessively excitable in the absence of the inhibitory spinal mechanisms in the stiff-man syndrome.[74, 120] However, the silent period (SP), which is ordinarily absent in patients with tetanus, has been reported to remain normal in the stiff-man syndrome.[103, 162] Rigidity and the electrical discharges markedly improve with the administration of diazepam (Valium), which suppresses interneurons at spinal and supraspinal levels,[74] or baclofen.[114, 181]

# CRAMPS

Skeletal muscle cramps, either spontaneous or induced by ischemia or exercise, occur in a broad spectrum of illnesses. Cramps represent briefly sustained, painful or painless involuntary contractions lasting seconds to minutes.[92] This definition excludes such involuntary movements as tremor, chorea, hemiballisms, or myoclonus, and isolated muscle twitches associated with fasciculations or complex repetitive discharges.

Electrically, muscle cramps result from high frequency motor unit discharge at rates ranging from 200 to 300 impulses per second.[43, 118] It usually involves a large part of the muscle synchronously, as opposed to the asynchronous activation of motor units during voluntary muscle contraction. Despite effective inhibition by nerve block or spinal anesthesia, repetitive nerve stimulation distal to the block still induces cramping. These findings suggest a peripheral origin.

Painful cramps commonly occur in the calf muscles and other flexors of the lower limb. It may start after maintaining a certain posture for a prolonged period of time, and may improve by rubbing or lengthening the muscle. Numerous predisposing factors include salt depletion, other causes of hyponatremia, hypocalcemia, and vitamin deficiency. Most cases of cramps in healthy subjects have no detectable underlying cause.

Muscle cramp constitutes an early feature of motor neuron disease. It may also occur in association with sciatica or peripheral neuropathies. Patients with certain inborn errors of metabolism may complain of exertional cramps, but not as an essential feature. Satoyoshi[150, 151] has described a syndrome of progressive muscle spasm, alopecia, and diarrhea. In this syndrome, which affects women more frequently than men, painful intermittent cramps involve the limb muscles initially, then the neck, trunk, and mastication muscles several years later. These painful muscle spasms originate centrally and, except for normal serum calcium ($Ca^{++}$) levels, resemble tetani. The symptoms begin at about age 10 and slowly progress, leading to malnutrition and possible death.

Cramps also occur in familial[82, 94] and sporadic cases[75] of the muscular pain-fasciculation syndrome. The familial variety with an autosomal dominant inheritance affects both sexes. The symptoms appear during the first or second decade. Exercise-induced painful cramps, although generalized, predominantly affect the hands and feet. Motor and sensory conduction velocities are either normal or mildly decreased. Electromyography reveals normal motor unit potentials with no fibrillation potentials or positive sharp waves. Sporadic cases occur in both sexes with onset of symptoms during the third to seventh decades. Although painful cramps primarily involve the calves, fasciculations develop in the lower extremities diffusely. Nerve conduction studies show decreased conduction and increased distal latencies. Needle studies may reveal fibrillation potentials and positive sharp waves. The possible relationship between the tubular aggregates reported in biopsy specimens and muscle cramps remains to be elucidated.[95]

The physiologic term tetanus is used to describe tetany caused by hypocalcemia and alkalosis.[92] Decreased extracellular calcium increases sodium ($Na^+$) conductance, which leads to membrane depolarization and repetitive nerve firing. Hypomagnesemia and hyperkalemia also induce carpopedal spasm. Electromyography reveals grouped motor unit potentials firing asynchronously at a rate of 4 to 15 impulses per second, with periods of relative silence in between. Tetanic contraction abates with infusion of curare but not with peripheral nerve block. Thus, the spontaneous discharge seems to occur at some point along the length of the peripheral nerve. Various maneuvers precipitate clinical or electrical neuromuscular irritability. They include a gentle tap over the facial nerve (Chvostek's sign) or the lateral surface of the fibula (peroneal sign), and artificially induced ischemia of the forearm (Trousseau's sign).

## CONTRACTURE

Contracture refers to intense mechanical muscle shortening in the absence of muscle action potentials. Thus, electromyography reveals no electrical activity in the contracted muscle.[45] Contracture most commonly develops with ischemia in muscle phosphorylase (see Fig. 11-3) and muscle phosphofructokinase deficiencies.[106] In these entities, failure to produce adenosine triphosphate (ATP) prohibits reaccumulation of calcium ($Ca^{++}$) by the sarcoplasmic reticulum, the essential initial step for muscle relaxation, as described in Chapter 11.

Painless exertional contracture may occur in some patients without enzymatic deficiency.[24] Here, electromyography during voluntary muscle contraction is normal. After strong contraction, however, the muscle relaxes only slowly over a period of 10 seconds. During this period the stiff muscle is electrically silent.[88] Normal motor unit potentials reappear if the patient voluntarily contracts the stiff muscle. Needle insertion or voluntary contraction initiates no myotonic discharge. Isolated sarcoplasmic reticulum has a decreased capacity to accumulate calcium. Painful contracture has also been described in a hereditary myopathy associated with electromyographic signs of generalized myotonia.[148, 163]

## REFERENCE SOURCES

1. ABERFELD, DC, HINTERBUCHNER, LP, AND SCHNEIDER, M: *Myotonia, dwarfism, diffuse bone disease and unusual ocular and facial abnormalities. (A new syndrome.)* Brain 88:313, 1965.

2.  ADRIAN, RH AND BRYANT, SH: *On the repetitive discharge in myotonic muscle fibres.* J Physiol (Lond) 240:505, 1974.

3.  ALBERS, JW, ET AL: *Limb myokymia.* Muscle and Nerve 4:494, 1981.

4.  AMINOFF, MJ, ET AL: *The declining electrical response of muscle to repetitive nerve stimulation in myotonia.* Neurology (Minneap) 27:812, 1977.

5.  ANDERSON, TE, ET AL: *Myositis and myotonia in a case of multicentric reticulohistiocytosis.* Br J Derm 80:39, 1968.

6.  ARGOV, Z, ET AL: *Congenital myotonic dystrophy. Fiber type abnormalities in two cases.* Arch Neurol 37:693, 1980.

7.  AUGER, RG: *Hemifacial spasm: Clinical and electrophysiologic observations.* Neurology (New York) 29:1261, 1979.

8.  BALLANTYNE, JP AND HANSEN, S: *New method for the estimation of the number of motor units in a muscle. 2. Duchenne, limb-girdle and facioscapulohumeral, and myotonic muscular dystrophies.* J Neurol Neurosurg Psychiatry 37:1195, 1974.

9.  BALLANTYNE, JP AND HANSEN, S: *Neurogenic influence in muscular dystrophies.* In ROWLAND, LP (ED): *Pathogenesis of Human Muscular Dystrophies.* Proceedings of the Fifth International Scientific Conference of the Muscular Dystrophy Association, Excerpta Medica, Amsterdam, 1977, pp 187–199.

10. BARCHI, RL: *Myotonia. An evaluation of the chloride hypothesis.* Arch Neurol 32:175, 1975.

11. BARRON, SA AND HEFFNER, RR, JR: *Continuous muscle fiber activity. A case with unusual clinical features.* Arch Neurol 36:520, 1979.

12. BECKER, PE: *Zur Genetik der Myotonien.* In KUHN, E (ED): *Progressive Muskeldystrophie Myotonie, Myasthenie.* Springer-Verlag, Berlin, 1966, pp 247–255.

13. BECKER, PE: *Fortschritte der allgemeinen und klinischen Humangenetik. Paramyotonia congenita (Eulenburg),* Vol III. Georg Thieme, Stuttgart, 1970.

14. BECKER, PE: *Genetic approaches to the nosology of muscle disease: Myotonias and similar diseases.* In BERGSMA, D (ED): *The Second Conference on the Clinical Delineation of Birth Defects: Part VII. Muscle.* Williams & Wilkins, Baltimore, 1971, pp 52–62.

15. BECKER, PE: *Generalized non-dystrophic myotonia. The dominant (Thomsen) type and the recently identified recessive type.* In DESMEDT, JE (ED): *New Developments in Electromyography and Clinical Neurophysiology,* Karger, Basel, 1973, pp 407–412.

16. BECKER, PE: *Myotonia congenita and syndromes associated with myotonia. Clinical-genetic studies of the nondystrophic myotonias.* In BECKER, PE, ET AL: (EDS): *Topics in Human Genetics,* Vol 3. Georg Thieme, Stuttgart, 1977.

17. BECKER, PE: *Syndromes associated with myotonia: Clinical-genetic classification.* In ROWLAND, LP (ED): *Pathogenesis of Human Muscular Dystrophies.* Proceedings of the Fifth International Scientific Conference of the Muscular Dystrophy Association, Excerpta Medica, Amsterdam, 1977, pp 699–703.

18. BENNETT, RH AND FORMAN, HR: *Hypokalemic periodic paralysis in chronic toluene exposure.* Arch Neurol 37:673, 1980.

19. BLACK, JT, ET AL: *Muscle rigidity in a newborn due to continuous peripheral nerve hyperactivity.* Arch Neurol 27:413, 1972.

20. BLANK, NK, MEERSCHAERT, JR, AND RIEDER, MJ: *Persistent motor neuron discharges of central origin present in the resting state. A case report of alcohol-induced muscle spasms.* Neurology (Minneap) 24:277, 1974.

21. BORENSTEIN, S, ET AL: *Myotonic dystrophy with nerve hypertrophy. Report of a case with electrophysiological and ultrastructural study of the sural nerve.* J Neurol Sci 34:87, 1977.

22. BOSSEN, EH, SHELBURNE, JD, AND VERKAUF, BS: *Respiratory muscle involvement in infantile myotonic dystrophy.* Arch Pathol 97:250, 1974.

23. BRADLEY, WG: *Adynamia episodica hereditaria. Clinical, pathological and electrophysiological studies in an affected family.* Brain 92:345, 1969.

24. BRODY, IA: *Muscle contracture induced by exercise. A syndrome attributable to decreased relaxing factor.* N Engl J Med 281:187, 1969.

25. BROOKS, JE: *Hyperkalemic periodic paralysis. Intracellular electromyographic studies.* Arch Neurol 20:13, 1969.

26. BROOKS, VB, CURTIS, DR, AND ECCLES, JC: *The action of tetanus toxin on the inhibition of motoneurones*. J Physiol (Lond) 135:655, 1957.

27. BRYANT, SH: *The physiological basis of myotonia*. In ROWLAND, LP (ED): *Pathogenesis of Human Muscular Dystrophies*. Proceedings of the Fifth International Scientific Conference of the Muscular Dystrophy Association, Excerpta Medica, Amsterdam, 1977.

28. BUCHTHAL, F: *Diagnostic significance of the myopathic EMG*. In ROWLAND, LP (ED): *Pathogenesis of Human Muscular Dystrophies*. Proceedings of the Fifth International Conference of the Muscular Dystrophy Association, Excerpta Medica, Amsterdam, 1977.

29. BUCHTHAL, F, ENGBAEK, L, AND GAMSTORP, I: *Paresis and hyperexcitability in adynamia episodica hereditaria*. Neurology (Minneap) 8:347, 1958.

30. BURKE, D, SKUSE, NF, AND LETHLEAN, AK: *Contractile properties of the abductor digiti minimi muscle in paramyotonia congenita*. J Neurol Neurosurg Psychiatry 37:894, 1974.

31. BURKE, D, SKUSE, NF, AND LETHLEAN, AK: *An analysis of myotonia in paramyotonia congenita*. J Neurol Neurosurg Psychiatry 37:900, 1974.

32. BUTTERFIELD, DA, ET AL: *Spin label study of erythrocyte membrane fluidity in myotonic and Duchenne muscular dystrophy and congenital myotonia*. Nature 263:159, 1976.

33. CACCIA, MR, NEGRI, S, AND PARVIS, VP: *Myotonic dystrophy with neural involvement*. J Neurol Sci 16:253, 1972.

34. CADILHAC, J, ET AL: *EMG studies of two family cases of the Schwartz and Jampel syndrome (osteo-chondro-muscular dystrophy with myotonia)*. Electromyogr Clin Neurophysiol 15:5, 1975.

35. CAMPA, JF AND SANDERS, DB: *Familial hypokalemic periodic paralysis. Local recovery after nerve stimulation*. Arch Neurol 31:110, 1974.

36. CHERINGTON, M, SADLER, KM, AND RYAN, DW: *Facial myokymia*. Surg Neurol 11:478, 1979.

37. CHESSON, AL, JR, SCHOCHET, SS, JR, AND PETERS, BH: *Biphasic periodic paralysis*. Arch Neurol 36:700, 1979.

38. CHUDLEY, AE AND BARMADA, MA: *Diaphragmatic elevation in neonatal myotonic dystrophy*. Am J Dis Child 133:1182, 1979.

39. CREUTZFELDT, OD, ET AL: *Muscle membrane potentials in episodic adynamia*. Electroenceph Clin Neurophysiol 15:508, 1963.

40. CREWS, J, KAISER, KK, AND BROOKE, MH: *Muscle pathology of myotonia congenita*. J Neurol Sci 28:449, 1976.

41. DAUBE, JR, KELLY, JJ, JR, AND MARTIN, RA: *Facial myokymia with polyradiculoneuropathy*. Neurology (New York) 29:662, 1979.

42. DELWAIDE, PJ AND PENDERS, CA: *Paramyotonie familiale et crises parétiques avec hypokaliémie*. Rev Neurol (Paris) 125:287, 1971.

43. DENNY-BROWN, D AND FOLEY, JM: *Myokymia and the benign fasciculation of muscular cramps*. Trans Assoc Am Phys 61:88, 1948.

44. DODGE, PR, ET AL: *Myotonic dystrophy in infancy and childhood*. Pediatrics 35:3, 1965.

45. DYKEN, ML, SMITH, DM, AND PEAKE, RL: *An electromyographic diagnostic screening test in McArdle's disease and a case report*. Neurology (Minneap) 17:45, 1967.

46. DYKEN, M, ZEMAN, W, AND RUSCHE, T: *Hypokalemic periodic paralysis. Children with permanent myopathic weakness*. Neurology (Minneap) 19:691, 1969.

47. ENGEL, AG: *Evolution and content of vacuoles in primary hypokalemic periodic paralysis*. Mayo Clin Proc 45:774, 1970.

48. ENGEL, AG AND LAMBERT, EH: *Calcium activation of electrically inexcitable muscle fibers in primary hypokalemic periodic paralysis*. Neurology (Minneap) 19:851, 1969.

49. ENGEL, AG, ET AL: *The spectrum and diagnosis of acid maltase deficiency*. Neurology (Minneap) 23:95, 1973.

50. ENGEL, AG, ET AL: *Clinical and electromyographic studies in a patient with primary hypokalemic periodic paralysis*. Am J Med 38:626, 1965.

51. EULENBURG, A: *Ueber eine familiäre, durch 6 Generationen verfolgbare Form congenitaler Paramyotonie*. Neurologisches Centralblatt 5:265, 1886.

52. FABINYI, GCA AND ADAMS, CBT: *Hemifacial spasm: Treatment by posterior fossa surgery.* J Neurol Neurosurg Psychiatry 41:829, 1978.

53. FARIELLO, R, ET AL: *A case of Schwartz-Jampel syndrome with unusual muscle biopsy findings.* Ann Neurol 3:93, 1978.

54. FERGUSON, JH: *Hemifacial spasm and the facial nucleus.* Ann Neurol 4:97, 1978.

55. FOWLER, WM, JR, ET AL: *The Schwartz-Jampel syndrome. Its clinical, physiological and histological expressions.* J Neurol Sci 22:127, 1974.

56. FRANCK, G, ET AL: *Le syndrome de l'homme raide. Etude clinique, polygraphique et histoenzymologique.* Acta Neurol Belg 74:221, 1974.

57. FRENCH, EB AND KILPATRICK, R: *A variety of paramyotonia congenita.* J Neurol Neurosurg Psychiatry 20:40, 1957.

58. FURMAN, RE AND BARCHI, RL: *The pathophysiology of myotonia produced by aromatic carboxylic acids.* Ann Neurol 4:357, 1978.

59. GAFFNEY, BJ, ET AL: *Spin-label studies of erythrocytes in myotonic dystrophy: No increase in membrane fluidity.* Neurology (New York) 30:272, 1980.

60. GAMSTORP, I: *Adynamia episodica hereditaria.* Acta Paediatrica (suppl 108)45:43, 1956.

61. GAMSTORP, I: *A study of transient muscular weakness.* Acta Neurol Scand 38:3, 1962.

62. GAMSTORP, I AND WOHLFART, G: *A syndrome characterized by myokymia, myotonia, muscular wasting and increased perspiration.* Acta Psych Neurol Scand 34:181, 1959.

63. GARCIA-MULLIN, R AND DAROFF, RB: *Electrophysiological investigations of cephalic tetanus.* J Neurol Neurosurg Psychiatry 36:296, 1973.

64. GARDNER, WJ AND SAVA, GA: *Hemifacial spasm—A reversible pathophysiologic state.* J Neurosurg 19:240, 1962.

65. GARDNER-MEDWIN, D AND WALTON, JN: *Myokymia with impaired muscular relaxation.* Lancet 1:127, 1969.

66. GORDON, AM, GREEN, JR, AND LAGUNOFF, D: *Studies on a patient with hypokalemic familial periodic paralysis.* Am J Med 48:185, 1970.

67. GORDON, EE, JANUSZKO, DM, AND KAUFMAN, L: *A critical survey of stiff-man syndrome.* Am J Med 42:582, 1967.

68. GREENHOUSE, AH, ET AL: *Myotonia, myokymia, hyperhidrosis, and wasting of muscle.* Neurology (Minneap) 17:263, 1967.

69. GROB, D, JOHNS, RJ, AND LILJESTRAND, Ä: *Potassium movement in patients with familial periodic paralysis. Relationship to the defect in muscle function.* Am J Med 23:356, 1957.

70. HARPER, PS: *Congenital myotonic dystrophy in Britain. I. Clinical aspects.* Arch Dis Child 50:505, 1975.

71. HARPER, PS: *Congenital myotonic dystrophy in Britain. II. Genetic basis.* Arch Dis Child 50:514, 1975.

72. HJORTH, RJ AND WILLISON, RG: *The electromyogram in facial myokymia and hemifacial spasm.* J Neurol Sci 20:117, 1973.

73. HOFMANN, WW AND SMITH, RA: *Hypokalaemic periodic paralysis studied in vitro.* Brain 93:445, 1970.

74. HOWARD, FM, JR: *A new and effective drug in the treatment of the stiff-man syndrome. Preliminary report.* Mayo Clin Proc 38:203, 1963.

75. HUDSON, AJ, BROWN, WF, AND GILBERT, JJ: *The muscular pain-fasciculation syndrome.* Neurology (New York) 28:1105, 1978.

76. HUGHES, RC AND MATTHEWS, WB: *Pseudo-myotonia and myokymia.* J Neurol Neurosurg Psychiatry 32:11, 1969.

77. ISAACS, H: *A syndrome of continuous muscle-fibre activity.* J Neurol Neurosurg Psychiatry 24:319, 1961.

78. ISAACS, H: *Continuous muscle fibre activity in an Indian male with additional evidence of terminal motor fibre abnormality.* J Neurol Neurosurg Psychiatry 30:126, 1967.

79. ISAACS, H AND HEFFRON, JJA: *The syndrome of 'continuous muscle-fibre activity' cured: Further studies.* J Neurol Neurosurg Psychiatry 37:1231, 1974.

80. JACKSON, DL, ET AL: *Isaacs syndrome with laryngeal involvement: An unusual presentation of myokymia.* Neurology (New York) 29:1612, 1979.

81. JANNETTA, PJ, ET AL: *Etiology and definitive microsurgical treatment of hemifacial spasm. Operative techniques and results in 47 patients.* J Neurosurg 47:321, 1977.

82. JUSIC, A, DOGAN, S, AND STOJANOVIC, V: *Hereditary persistent distal cramps.* J Neurol Neurosurg Psychiatry 35:379, 1972.

83. KAUFMAN, MD: *Masticatory spasm in facial hemiatrophy.* Ann Neurol 7:585, 1980.

84. KIMURA, J, RODNITZKY, RL, AND OKAWARA, SH: *Electrophysiologic analysis of aberrant regeneration after facial nerve paralysis.* Neurology (Minneap) 25:989, 1975.

85. KIRSCHNER, BS AND PACHMAN, LM: *IgA deficiency and recurrent pneumonia in the Schwartz-Jampel syndrome.* J Pediatrics 88:1060, 1976.

86. KLEIN, R, HADDOW, JE, AND DELUCA, C: *Familial congenital disorder resembling stiff-man syndrome.* Am J Dis Child 124:730, 1972.

87. KUHN, E, ET AL: *The autosomal recessive (Becker) form of myotonia congenita.* Muscle and Nerve 2:109, 1979.

88. LAMBERT, EH: *Neurophysiological techniques useful in the study of neuromuscular disorders.* In ADAMS, RD, EATON, LM, AND SHY, GM (EDS): *Neuromuscular Disorders,* Vol 38. Williams & Wilkins, Baltimore, 1960, pp 247–273.

89. LAMBERT, EH: *Muscle spasms, cramps, and stiffness.* Am Acad Neurol Spec Course #17, 1978.

90. LAMBERT, EH, LOVE, JG, AND MULDER, DW: *Facial myokymia and brain tumor: Electromyographic studies* Am Assoc Electromyograph Electrodiag Newsletter 8:8, 1961.

91. LANCE, JW, BURKE, D, AND POLLARD, J: *Hyperexcitability of motor and sensory neurons in neuromyotonia.* Ann Neurol 5:523, 1979.

92. LAYZER, RB AND ROWLAND, LP: *Cramps.* N Engl J Med 285:31, 1971.

93. LAYZER, RB, LOVELACE, RE, AND ROWLAND, LP: *Hyperkalemic periodic paralysis.* Arch Neurol 16:455, 1967.

94. LAZARO, RP, ROLLINSON, RD, AND FENICHEL, GM: *Familial cramps and muscle pain.* Arch Neurol 38:22, 1981.

95. LAZARO, RP, ET AL: *Cramps, muscle pain, and tubular aggregates.* Arch Neurol 37:715, 1980.

96. LEVINSON, S, CANALIS, RF, AND KAPLAN, HJ: *Laryngeal spasm complicating pseudomyotonia.* Arch Otolaryngol 102:185, 1976.

97. LIPICKY, RJ: *Studies in human myotonic dystrophy.* In ROWLAND, LP (ED): *Pathogenesis of Human Muscular Dystrophies.* Proceedings of the Fifth International Scientific Conference of the Muscular Dystrophy Association, Excerpta Medica, Amsterdam, 1977.

98. LUBLIN, FD, ET AL: *Myokymia and impaired muscular relaxation with continuous motor unit activity.* J Neurol Neurosurg Psychiatry 42:557, 1979.

99. LUNDBERG, PO, STÅLBERG, E, AND THIELE, B: *Paralysis periodica paramyotonica. A clinical and neurophysiological study.* J Neurol Sci 21:309, 1974.

100. LÜTSCHG, J, ET AL: *The syndrome of 'continuous muscle fiber activity.'* Arch Neurol 35:198, 1978.

101. MADDY, JA AND WINTERNITZ, WW: *Hypothalamic syndrome with hypernatremia and muscular paralysis.* Am J Med 51:394, 1971.

102. MAIDA, E, ET AL: *Stiff-man syndrome with abnormalities in CSF and computerized tomography findings. Report of a case.* Arch Neurol 37:182, 1980.

103. MAMOLI, B, ET AL: *Electrophysiological studies on the "stiff-man" syndrome.* J Neurol 217:111, 1977.

104. MAROON, JC: *Hemifacial spasm. A vascular cause.* Arch Neurol 35:481, 1978.

105. MARTINELLI, P, ET AL: *Stiff-man syndrome associated with nocturnal myoclonus and epilepsy.* J Neurol Neurosurg Psychiatry 41:458, 1978.

106. MCARDLE, B: *Myopathy due to a defect in muscle glycogen breakdown.* Clin Sci 10:13, 1951.

107. MCARDLE, B: *Adynamia episodica hereditaria and its treatment.* Brain 85:121, 1962.

108. MCCOMAS, AJ, CAMPBELL, MJ, AND SICA, REP: *Electrophysiological study of dystrophia myotonica.* J Neurol Neurosurg Psychiatry 34:132, 1971.

109. McComas, AJ, Sica, REP, and Toyonaga, K: *Incidence, severity, and time-course of moto-neurone dysfunction in myotonic dystrophy: Their significance for an understanding of anticipation.* J Neurol Neurosurg Psychiatry 41:882, 1978.

110. Mertens, HG and Ricker, K: *Übererregbarkeit der γ-Motoneurone beim "Stiff-man" Syndrom.* Klin Wschr 46:33, 1968.

111. Mertens, HG and Ricker, K: *The differential diagnosis of the 'stiff-man' syndrome.* In Walton, JN, Canal, N, and Scarlato, G (eds): *Muscle Diseases.* Excerpta Medica, Amsterdam, 1970, pp 635–638.

112. Mertens, HG and Zschocke, S: *Neuromyotonie.* Klin Wschr 43:917, 1965.

113. Meyers, KR, et al: *Periodic muscle weakness, normokalemia, and tubular aggregates.* Neurology (Minneap) 22:269, 1972.

114. Miller, F and Korsvik, H: *Baclofen in the treatment of stiff-man syndrome.* Ann Neurol 9:511, 1981.

115. Moersch, FP and Woltman, HW: *Progressive fluctuating muscular rigidity and spasm ("stiff-man" syndrome): Report of a case and some observations in 13 other cases.* Proc Staff Meet Mayo Clin 31:421, 1956.

116. Nagano, Y and Roses, AD: *Abnormalities of erythrocyte membranes in myotonic muscular dystrophy manifested in lipid vesicles.* Neurology (New York) 30:989, 1980.

117. Norris, FH, Jr: *Myokymia.* Letter to the editor. Arch Neurol 34:133, 1977.

118. Norris, FH, Jr, Gasteiger, EL, and Chatfield, PO: *An electromyographic study of induced and spontaneous muscle cramps.* Electroenceph Clin Neurophysiol 9:139, 1957.

119. Okuno, T, et al: *Myotonic dystrophy and hyperthyroidism.* Neurology (New York) 31:91, 1981.

120. Olafson, RA, Mulder, DW, and Howard, FM: *"Stiff-man" syndrome: A review of the literature, report of three additional cases and discussion of pathophysiology and therapy.* Proc Staff Meet Mayo Clin 39:131, 1964.

121. Otsuka, M and Ohtsuki, I: *Mechanism of muscular paralysis by insulin with special reference to periodic paralysis.* Am J Physiol 219:1178, 1970.

122. Panayiotopoulos, CP and Scarpalezos, S: *Dystrophia myotonica. Peripheral nerve involvement and pathogenic implications.* J Neurol Sci 27:1, 1976.

123. Parry-Jones, NO, et al: *Myokymia, not myotonia.* Br Med J 2:300, 1977.

124. Pavone, L, et al: *Schwartz-Jampel syndrome in two daughters of first cousins.* J Neurol Neurosurg Psychiatry 41:161, 1978.

125. Pearson, CM: *The periodic paralyses: Differential features and pathological observations in permanent myopathic weakness.* Brain 87:341, 1963.

126. Pierry, A and Cameron, M: *Clonic hemifacial spasm from posterior fossa arteriovenous malformation.* J Neurol Neurosurg Psychiatry 42:670, 1979.

127. Polgar, JG, et al: *The early detection of dystrophia myotonica.* Brain 95:761, 1972.

128. Pollock, M and Dyck, PJ: *Peripheral nerve morphometry in myotonic dystrophy.* Arch Neurol 33:33, 1976.

129. Poskanzer, DC and Kerr, DNS: *A third type of periodic paralysis, with normokalemia and a favourable response to sodium chloride.* Am J Med 31:328, 1961.

130. Radü, EW, Skorpil, V, and Kaeser, HE: *Facial myokymia.* Eur Neurol 13:499, 1975.

131. Ravin, M, Newmark, Z, and Saviello, G: *Myotonia dystrophica—An anesthetic hazard: Two case reports.* Anesth Analg 54:216, 1975.

132. Resnick, JS and Engel, WK: *Myotonic lid lag in hypokalaemic periodic paralysis.* J Neurol Neurosurg Psychiatry 30:47, 1967.

133. Ricker, K and Meinck, HM: *Paramyotonia congenita (Eulenburg). Neurophysiologic studies of a case.* Z Neurol 203:13, 1972.

134. Ricker, K, Samland, O, and Peter, A: *Elektrische und mechanische Muskelreaktion bei Adynamia episodica und Paramyotonia congenita nach Kälteeinwirkung und Kaliumgabe.* J Neurol 208:95, 1974.

135. Riecker, G and Bolte, HD: *Membranpotentiale einzelner Skeletmuskelzellen bei hypokaliämischer periodischer Muskelparalyse.* Klin Wschr 44:804, 1966.

136. RISK, WS, ET AL: *Chronic tetanus: Clinical report and histochemistry of muscle.* Muscle and Nerve 4:363, 1981.

137. RIVERA, VM: *Interpretation of serum creatine phosphokinase.* JAMA 225:993, 1973.

138. ROSES, AD AND APPEL, SH: *Protein kinase activity in erythrocyte ghosts of patients with myotonic muscular dystrophy (inborn error of metabolism membrane).* Proc Nat Acad Sci USA 70:1855, 1973.

139. ROSES, AD AND APPEL, SH: *Muscle membrane protein kinase in myotonic muscular dystrophy.* Nature 250:245, 1974.

140. ROSES, AD AND APPEL, SH: *Phosphorylation of component a of the human erythrocyte membrane in myotonic muscular dystrophy.* J Membr Biol 20:51, 1975.

141. ROWLAND, LP: *Pathogenesis of muscular dystrophies.* Arch Neurol 33:315, 1976.

142. ROWLAND, LP AND LAYZER, RB: *Muscular dystrophies, atrophies, and related diseases.* In BAKER, AB AND BAKER, LH (EDS): *Clinical Neurology,* Vol 3. Harper & Row, Hagerstown, Md, 1973, pp 1–100.

143. RUBENSTEIN, AE AND WAINAPEL, SF: *Acute hypokalemic myopathy in alcoholism. A clinical entity.* Arch Neurol 34:553, 1977.

144. RUFF, RL: *Insulin-induced weakness in hypokalemic myopathy.* Ann Neurol 6:139, 1979.

145. SAADAT, M, ET AL: *Schwartz syndrome: Myotonia with blepharophimosis and limitation of joints.* J Pediatrics 81:348, 1972.

146. SADJADPOUR, K: *Postfacial palsy phenomena: Faulty nerve regeneration or ephaptic transmission?* Brain Res 95:403, 1975.

147. SANDER, JE, LAYZER, RB, AND GOLDSOBEL, AB: *Congenital stiff-man syndrome.* Ann Neurol 8:195, 1980.

148. SANDERS, DB: *Myotonia congenita with painful muscle contractions.* Arch Neurol 33:580, 1976.

149. SAROVA-PINCHAS, I, GOLDHAMMER, Y, AND BRAHAM, J: *Multifocal myokymia.* Muscle and Nerve 1:253, 1978.

150. SATOYOSHI, E: *Recurrent muscle spasms of central origin.* Trans Am Neurol Assoc 92:153, 1967.

151. SATOYOSHI, E: *A syndrome of progressive muscle spasm, alopecia, and diarrhea.* Neurology (New York) 28:458, 1978.

152. SCHMIDT, RT, STAHL, SM, AND SPEHLMANN, R: *A pharmacologic study of the stiff-man syndrome. Correlation of clinical symptoms with urinary 3-methoxy-4-hydroxy-phenyl glycol excretion.* Neurology (Minneap) 25:622, 1975.

153. SCHULTZE, FR: *Beiträge zur Muskelpathologie.* Dtsch Z Nervenheilk 6:65, 1895.

154. SCHWARTZ, O AND JAMPEL, RS: *Congenital blepharophimosis associated with a unique generalized myopathy.* Arch Ophthalmol 68:52, 1962.

155. SEGURA, RP AND PETAJAN, JH: *Neural hyperexcitability in hyperkalemic periodic paralysis.* Muscle and Nerve 2:245, 1979.

156. SETHI, PK, SMITH, BH, AND KALYANARAMAN, K: *Facial myokymia: A clinicopathological study.* J Neurol Neurosurg Psychiatry 37:745, 1974.

157. SHAHANI, M, ET AL: *Neuropathy in tetanus.* J Neurol Sci 43:173, 1979.

158. SHY, GM, ET AL: *Studies in familial periodic paralysis.* Exp Neurol 3:53, 1961.

159. SIGWALD, J, ET AL: *Pseudo-myotonie. Forme particulière d'hypertonie musculaire à prédominance distale.* Rev Neurol (Paris) 115:1003, 1966.

160. SIMPSON, JA: *Neuromuscular diseases.* In RÉMOND, A (ED): *Handbook of Electroencephalography and Clinical Neurophysiology,* Vol 16B. Elsevier, Amsterdam, 1973.

161. SOMERS, JE AND WINER, N: *Reversible myopathy and myotonia following administration of a hypocholesterolemic agent.* Neurology (Minneap) 16:761, 1966.

162. STÖHR, M AND HECKL, R: *Das stiff-man syndrom. Klinische, elektromyographische und pharmakologische Befunde bei einem eigenen Fall.* Arch Psychiat Nervenkr 223:171, 1977.

163. STÖHR, M, ET AL: *Myopathia myotonica. Fallbericht über eine neuartige hereditäre metabolische myopathie.* J Neurol 210:41, 1975.

164. STRUPPLER, A, STRUPPLER, E, AND ADAMS, RD: *Local tetanus in man.* Arch Neurol 8:162, 1963.

165. SUSAC, JO, SMITH, JL, AND SCHATZ, NJ: *Superior oblique myokymia.* Arch Neurol 29:432, 1973.

166. SWIFT, TR, IGNACIO, OJ, AND DYKEN, PR: *Neonatal dystrophia myotonica.* Am J Dis Child 129:734, 1975.

167. TAYLOR, RG, ET AL: *Continuous muscle fiber activity in the Schwartz-Jampel syndrome.* Electroenceph Clin Neurophysiol 33:497, 1972.

168. TENSER, RB AND CORBETT, JJ: *Myokymia and facial contraction in brain stem glioma. An electromyographic study.* Arch Neurol 30:425, 1974.

169. THOMSEN, J: *Tonische Krämpfe in willkürlich beweglichen Muskeln in Folge von ererbter psychischer Disposition (Ataxia muscularis?).* Arch Psychiatr Nervenkr 6:702, 1876.

170. THRUSH, DC, MORRIS, CJ, AND SALMON, MV: *Paramyotonia congenita: A clinical, histochemical and pathological study.* Brain 95:537, 1972.

171. VAKIL, BJ, ET AL: *Cephalic tetanus.* Neurology (Minneap) 23:1091, 1973.

172. VALENSTEIN, E, WATSON, RT, AND PARKER, JL: *Myokymia, muscle hypertrophy and percussion "myotonia" in chronic recurrent polyneuropathy.* Neurology (New York) 28:1130, 1978.

173. VICKERS, JD, McCOMAS, AJ AND RATHBONE, MP: *Myotonia muscular dystrophy: Abnormal temperature response of membrane phosphorylation in erythrocyte membranes.* Neurology (New York) 29:791, 1979.

174. WALLIS, WE, VAN POZNAK, A, AND PLUM, F: *Generalized muscular stiffness, fasciculations, and myokymia of peripheral nerve origin.* Arch Neurol 22:430, 1970.

175. WARMOLTS, JR AND MENDELL, JR: *Neurotonia: Impulse-induced repetitive discharges in motor nerves in peripheral neuropathy.* Ann Neurol 7:245, 1980.

176. WARTENBERG, R: *Hemifacial Spasm: A Clinical and Pathophysiological Study.* Oxford University Press, New York, 1952.

177. WASSERSTROM, WR AND STARR, A: *Facial myokymia in Guillain-Barré syndrome.* Arch Neurol 34:576, 1977.

178. WAYBRIGHT, EA, GUTMANN, L, AND CHOU, SM: *Facial myokymia. Pathological features.* Arch Neurol 36:244, 1979.

179. WEGMÜLLER, E, LUDIN, HP, AND MUMENTHALER, M: *Paramyotonia congenita. A clinical, electrophysiological and histological study of 12 patients.* J Neurol 220:251, 1979.

180. WELCH, LK, APPENZELLER, O, AND BICKNELL, JM: *Peripheral neuropathy with myokymia, sustained muscular contraction and continuous motor unit activity.* Neurology (Minneap) 22:161, 1972.

181. WHELAN, JL: *Baclofen in treatment of the 'stiff-man' syndrome.* Arch Neurol 37:600, 1980.

182. WILLIAMS, HL, LAMBERT, EH, AND WOLTMAN, HW: *The problem of synkinesis and contracture in cases of hemifacial spasm and Bell's palsy.* Ann Oto Rhino Laryngol 61:850, 1952.

183. WOLTMAN, HW, WILLIAMS, HL, AND LAMBERT, EH: *An attempt to relieve hemifacial spasm by neurolysis of the facial nerves: A report of two cases of hemifacial spasm with reflections on the nature of the spasm, the contracture and mass movement.* Proc Staff Meet Mayo Clin 26:236, 1951.

184. ZELLWEGER, H, ET AL: *Autosomal recessive generalized myotonia.* Muscle and Nerve 3:176, 1980.

# APPENDICES

# 1

# HISTORICAL REVIEW

Clinical electrophysiology began towards the end of the eighteenth century with Galvani's discovery of animal electricity and has since progressed steadily during the past two centuries. Electrophysiologic assessments of muscle and nerve are now considered indispensable in the practice of neurology, physiatry, and other related clinical disciplines. The historical growth of this medical field may be divided arbitrarily into four relatively distinct but overlapping eras. They represent (1) early development; (2) classical electrodiagnosis; (3) electromyography and nerve stimulation techniques; and (4) recent developments.

During the first period, ending at about the mid-nineteenth century, the existence of bioelectricity was firmly established by Galvani and others. The basic concepts of electricity were also founded during this period by a series of scientific achievements of Volta and his pupils. The progress in these two branches of science was complementary despite the initial controversy that arose over the existence of animal electricity. A number of studies in the last half of the nineteenth century established the relationship between the duration of stimulation and current strength in eliciting muscle contractions. This led to the development of classic electrodiagnosis, the study of muscle response to electrical stimulation as a diagnostic test. The method gained popularity during the first half of this century as the recording apparatus was improved from the capillary electrometer to the string galvanometer.

Modern techniques began with the invention of the cathode ray oscilloscope in 1922 and the concentric needle electrode a few years later. Aided by these technical advances, electromyography became a clinically useful tool. The nerve stimulation technique was then introduced, first for studies of neuromuscular transmission, and later for assessments of conduction velocity. Since then, there has been wide application of these techniques, which are now considered conventional. More recently, an increasing number of newer electrophysiologic tests have been designed to evaluate anatomic regions not accessible by the conventional methods. These include studies of human reflexes and other late potentials, recordings of somatosensory evoked potentials, and single fiber electromyography.

# EARLY DEVELOPMENT

Ancient physicians used electrical discharges from the black torpedo fish for the treatment of headaches and arthritis. However, it was not until the turn of the seventeenth century when the word electric was first used by William Gilbert[51] in his book *De Magnete*. Static discharges were also well known after the invention of the Leyden jar by Musshenbroek in 1745. In the same year Kratzenstein first induced muscle contraction by static electricity. The next year he wrote the first report on the use of electricity in medical therapy.[77] Many similar studies followed towards the end of the eighteenth century, each describing muscle contraction induced by electrical stimulation.

It was Galvani who laid the foundation for clinical electrophysiology: He introduced the idea that electricity was generated by nervous tissue, after a series of experiments on muscle contraction in frog legs. This observation was first published in 1791 in his now famous article *De viribus electricitatis in motu musculari commentarius* which appeared in the Proceedings of the Bologna Academy.[45] His concept of animal electricity was received with considerable skepticism in his time. Controversy arose chiefly from Volta's belief that the two plates of different metals were responsible for the electricity observed in Galvani's experiments.[121] Fowler[43] agreed with Volta that dissimilar metals and the muscle had to be connected to generate frog current.

Later, Galvani was able to produce muscle contraction by draping the free end of the nerve across the muscle without the use of metals. This finding was reproduced by Humboldt[70] and Matteucci.[97] In the meantime, Volta's conviction that animal electricity was in reality the effect of a very weak artificial current induced by application of two different metals lead to the development of the Voltanic pile in 1799. He also noted that muscle contraction occurred only at the closing and opening of the circuit. Although Galvani's view on intrinsic electrical current in frog legs was correct, Volta's new invention was so dramatic and convincing that his view of electricity of metallic origin was widely upheld. This is understandable, since the Voltanic pile produced all the phenomena attributed to animal electricity by Galvani.[122] Indeed Galvani's experiment was all but forgotten until much later when Nobili[104] and Matteucci[96] reported electrical activity from muscle in 1830 and 1842, respectively.

In 1822, Magendie,[92] who is credited for distinguishing between motor and sensory nerves, tried to insert a needle into the nerve for electrical stimulation, a practice soon abandoned because of the patient's discomfort! Sarlandiere[113] was the first to introduce electropuncture for direct electrical activation of muscle. One of Volta's pupils, Marianini,[94] found in 1829 that ascending (negative) current was more effective than descending current in eliciting muscle contraction. Nobili[104] recognized different stages of excitability based on the degree of muscle contraction after turning on and off the electrical current supplied by a battery. This concept was later used clinically by Erb[39] in the assessment of abnormal excitabilities of disordered muscles.

According to Licht,[88] the concept of current flow was introduced by Ampère who witnessed Oersted's 1819 demonstration that metallic wire extended from the two poles of a battery acted on a magnetic needle at a distance. In 1831, Henry found the augmenting action of a long coil of wire on direct current, and in the same year Faraday introduced alternating current induced in a coil of wire by another coil that was periodically charged. In 1833, Duchenne de Boulogne found that a muscle could be stimulated electrically from the skin surface using cloth-covered electrodes. This was the first surface stimulation employed for activation of muscle. He was also the first to use Faradic current for stimulation.[30]

Carlo Matteucci[96,97] of Pisa demonstrated that stimulation of the nerve proximal to the application of a ligature or section failed to elicit muscle contraction. Electrical activity originating from contracting muscles was also first detected by him in 1838. In his experiment published a few years later, sciatic nerve still connected to the leg muscles was placed on the thigh muscles dissected from the other leg.[96] He observed that contraction of the thigh muscles was followed by movements of the other leg provided that its sciatic nerve was not insulated from bared muscle. In his experiment, electrical activity of contracting muscle was detected using a neuromuscular preparation, the only means available in those days. Inspired by the work of Matteucci, Du-Bois-Reymond[28] registered action potentials generated in the muscle.[100] In 1851, he identified the action potential of voluntarily contracting arm muscles, using jars of liquid as electrodes.[29] This was perhaps the beginning of electromyography.[101]

In 1850, Helmholtz[59] succeeded in measuring the conduction velocity of the nerve impulse in the frog by mechanically recording the muscle twitch. Using the same procedure, a conduction velocity of 61.0 $\pm$ 5.1 m/s was found in the human median nerve.[60] Helmholtz also determined the conduction rate in sensory nerve of man to be 60 m/s by measuring the difference in reaction time. Hermann[61, 62] stimulated the brachial plexus in the axilla and recorded the muscle action potential from the surface of the forearm. The term action current was first introduced by Hermann in 1878. Burdon Sanderson[14] was the first to show in 1895 that this wave of excitation preceded the mechanical response.

## CLASSIC ELECTRODIAGNOSIS

Although Duchenne[31] was aware that certain localized areas of muscle were more easily stimulated, it was Remak[108] who discovered that these points represented entry zones of the muscular nerves. In 1857, Ziemssen[129] carefully mapped out the whole skin surface of the body in agonal patients and proved by dissection immediately after the death that the motor points were indeed entrances of the nerve into the muscle. Krause,[78] who is remembered for his description of the skin corpuscle, suggested that motor impulses were transmitted through the end-plates, the name coined by Kühne[81] to describe the nerve endings of striated muscle in 1862.

Electrical stimulation of the muscle as a diagnostic test was discussed comprehensively by Meyer and translated into English by Hammond[99] in 1869. Using galvanic current, he found that less current was required to activate paralytic limbs caused by cerebral disease than to activate the normal limb. In contrast, more current was necessary for activation when paralysis was caused by lesions of the spinal (peripheral) nerve. There had been a few reports[3] indicating that diseased muscle might respond better to continuous current (Galvanic) than interrupted current (Faradic). It was Neumann,[103] however, who found in 1864 that the critical parameter that determined the effectiveness of a current was its duration.

In agreement with Neumann, Erb noted that the paralyzed muscle no longer contracted in response to stimuli if the current was interrupted too frequently. This phenomenon was called the reaction of degeneration.[39] Studying the quantitative relationship between muscle contraction and current strength, Erb found that excitability was different among various disorders and described marked irritability in tetany. He also introduced in 1882 a formula of polar contraction in normals and its reversal in some disease states, and is generally credited as a founder of classic electrodiagnosis.

DuBois-Reymond believed that a muscle response was determined by change in current rather than by the absolute value of current strength. This view prevailed until the end of the nineteenth century. However, in 1870 Engelman showed a relationship between current intensity and duration in eliciting muscle contraction and determined the strength-duration curve in laboratory animals.[86] The concept of DuBois-Reymond was further challenged by Hoorweg,[68] who stated that nerve excitation was a function of stimulus time and intensity, a view also supported by Lapicque. Waller and Watteville[124] suggested a duration-intensity relationship for optimal stimulation in 1883.

Towards the end of the nineteenth century, abnormal localization of motor points was noted in degenerated muscle by some investigators.[27, 50] Lewis Jones[75] pointed out that the phenomenon of "displacement of the motor point" was a result of abnormal sensitivity of muscle, even in regions distinct from the motor point. In 1907 Bordet reported that, during passage of a sustained current, the critical excitatory level changed less rapidly in the denervated muscle compared with normally innervated muscle.[109] This observation led to accommodation measurements and the galvanic-tetanic ratio—electrodiagnostic tests used widely until recent years.

The galvanometer built by Sturgeon in 1836 was further improved by d'Arsonval,[17] who constructed the reflecting coil galvanometer. Lippmann[91] introduced the capillary-electrometer in 1872. Weiss[128] first attempted to produce a rectangular stimulus pulse, using a ballistic rheotome. Lapicque[86,87] developed a more accurate apparatus with a circuit breaker operated by gravity in 1907. Using this instrument, he defined rheobase as the minimal continuous current intensity required for muscle excitation and chronaxie as the minimal current duration required at an intensity twice the rheobase.[87] A battery of condensors was first used for diagnostic purposes by Lewis Jones[75] in 1913. Using this apparatus, Bourguignon[7] was the first to study chronaxie in man. Strength duration curves in man were first reported by Adrian[1] in 1916. He noted that healthy muscles showed fairly constant curves. There was a predictable shift of the curve when the muscle degenerated and during different phases of recovery. A constant current stimulator designed by Bauwens[4] improved the accuracy in determining strength-duration curves.

# ELECTROMYOGRAPHY
# AND NERVE STIMULATION TECHNIQUES

Oscillation (fasciculation) of denervated muscle was first observed by Schiff[115] after section of the hypoglossal nerve in 1851. This spontaneous movement ceased if the muscle became atrophic or nerve regeneration occurred. The term action potential was introduced by Bernstein[5] in 1866. Fibrillation was described as a tremor of denervated muscle in experimental animals by Rogowicz[111] and Ricker.[110] The first electromyography after DuBois-Reymond was performed by Piper,[106] who recorded voluntary activity of muscles using the string galvanometer at the turn of the century. He claimed a constant frequency of discharge independent of the muscle force. He thought this reflected the rhythm of neural impulses, whereas others considered the rate of discharge to be inherent in the muscle.[46, 47] Buchanan,[11] using the capillary electrometer, found the frequency of the electromyogram far from constant during different degrees of contraction. She concluded in 1908 that the mechanism of neural innervation could not be studied from the interference pattern. Langley and Kato[85] and Langley[84] studied fibrillation in muscular dystrophy.

Much progress in the study of muscle action potentials followed the development of sensitive recording apparatus. The cathode ray tube was invented by Braun[8] in 1897. Einthoven[37] designed the string galvanometer with a fiber of quartz. In 1920, Forbes and Thacher[42] were the first to use the electron tube to amplify the action potential and a string galvanometer to record it. The cathode ray oscilloscope, introduced by Gasser and Erlanger[48] in 1922, was one of the most important advances in technology, as it eliminated the mechanical limitation of galvanometers.[49] Their book *Electrical Signs of Nervous Activity* laid the foundation of modern clinical electrophysiology.[40]

Liddell and Sherrington[89] introduced the concept of the motor unit in 1925. Clinical electromyography in patients was first performed by Proebster[107] in 1928. Studying neurogenic weakness, he found spontaneous potentials in the denervated muscles after brachial plexus injury at birth, as well as in cases of long-standing poliomyelitis. Another major advancement in clinical electromyography came when Lord Adrian and Detlov Bronk[2] introduced the concentric needle electrode in 1929. They found no spontaneous activity in normal resting muscles. The use of this electrode made it possible for the first time to record from single motor units. Adrian also introduced the use of a loudspeaker so that electromyographers could use not only visual but acoustic cues as well. Motor unit potentials were studied by Denny-Brown in the same year[22] and later by Eccles and Sherrington,[35] Clark,[15] and Hoefer and Putnam.[65]

Introduction of the differential amplifier by Matthews[98] in 1934 made the recording of small muscle potentials possible, as it minimized electrical interference from other sources. Lindsley[90] noted unusual fluctuation of motor units in a patient with myasthenia gravis. Further work on denervation potentials came from Brown,[10] who tested the effect of acetylcholine on the denervated muscles. Using a bipolar electrode, Denny-Brown and Pennybacker[24] differentiated fibrillation from fasciculation in 1938, a finding later substantiated by Eccles[34] using a refined method. In 1941, Denny-Brown and Nevin[23] recorded myotonic discharges. Buchthal and Clemmesen[13] confirmed the electromyographic findings of atrophic muscles in the same year.

The demand for electrical testing increased markedly during the two World Wars because of the large number of battlefield peripheral nerve injuries. This tendency was particularly prominent during the Second World War when there was an accelerated growth of electronic devices such as radar and oscilloscopes. War casualties demanded development of procedures to determine quickly the presence and extent of nerve injury and the status of regeneration. Polio epidemics also increased the need for electrical studies of muscle. Many fundamental contributions to electromyography and nerve conduction studies came from this combination of circumstances.

The first attempt to standardize clinical testing of electromyography was reported in 1943 by Weddell, Feinstein, and Pattle.[126, 127] They noted that spontaneous discharges occurred 18 to 20 days after denervation in man. In the same year, Watkins, Brazier, and Schwab[125] recorded spontaneous activities in poliomyelitis, using surface electrodes placed at various recording sites. In 1944, Hoefer and Guttman[64] recorded spontaneous activity in patients with spinal cord lesions, using surface electrodes placed longitudinally. They reported that spontaneous electrical activity was sometimes helpful in localizing the lesions. The monopolar electrode was introduced in the same year by Jasper and Notman.[72] Jasper, Johnston, and Geddes[71] built a portable apparatus for electromyography. Further clinical applications of the needle electrode were reported by Huddleston and Golseth[69] in poliomyelitis, Golseth and Huddleston[54] in lower motor neuron disease, and Shea, Woods, and Werden[116] in nerve root compression. The first book of electromyography since Piper was published by Marinacci[95] in 1955. Buchthal[12] contributed a monograph two years later.

Jolly[74] described abnormal fatigability of the orbicularis oculi muscle to intermittent, direct-current stimulation in myasthenic patients in 1895. However, Harvey and Masland[58] were the first to quantitate this clinical observation by stimulating the nerve repetitively and recording the muscle action potentials. This technique, reported in 1941, was later applied to the study of myasthenic syndromes[33] and other disorders of the neuromuscular junction. It became an important part of our electrodiagnostic armamentarium in the early 1960s,[83] and was recently standardized by Desmedt.[26]

In measuring motor nerve conduction, Piper[105] in 1909 and Münnich[102] in 1916 recorded the muscle action potential instead of the muscle twitch. Around the same time, inspired by Sherrington's work[117] on the stretch reflex, Hoffmann[66, 67] demonstrated the monosynaptic reflex in man by stimulating the tibial nerve and recording the muscle action potential from the soleus. While recording latencies of the H-reflex, Schäffer[114] noted a velocity of 60 to 65 m/s for the human sensory nerve. Interest in nerve injury and repair during the war prompted basic scientists to study conduction velocity of regenerating nerve in experimental animals.[6, 41, 112] In 1944, Harvey and Kuffler[56] and Harvey, Kuffler, and Tredway[57] studied peripheral neuritis in man, stimulating the nerve and recording muscle action potentials. It was Hodes, Larrabee, and German,[63] however, who in 1948 first calculated the conduction velocity, stimulating the nerve at different levels in neurologic patients. Around the same time, nerve stimulation was used by Kugelberg[79] to study the effect of ischemia on nerve excitability.

This work was extended by Cobb and Marshall,[16] who showed that the rate of impulse propagation was slowed in the ischemic nerve.

Eichler[36] was the first to report percutaneous recording of nerve action potential in response to electrical stimulation of the median and ulnar nerves in 1937. The modern technique of sensory nerve conduction studies, however, was developed 10 years later as a by-product when Dawson[18] was attempting to record cortical potentials by stimulating peripheral nerves in patients with myoclonus. He used photographic superimposition[44] of a number of faint traces to improve resolution of the recorded response. The same technique was applied by Dawson and Scott[21] when they needed to assess the growth of the sensory action potential of the peripheral nerve with increasing stimulus strength to prove the origin of their cortical potential.[52] Dawson[20] subsequently developed the technique of digital nerve stimulation to differentiate sensory potentials from antidromic impulses in motor fibers. Although some felt that for routine electrodiagnostic investigation the measurement of latency was all that was required, study of nerve conduction velocity became an integral part of electrodiagnostic assessment in the 1960s.

These studies, initiated independently in the U.S. and Europe, started the whole field of electromyography and nerve conduction measurements, which developed very rapidly. Important contributions came from Magladery and McDougal,[93] Wagman and Lesse,[123] Gilliatt and Wilson,[53] Lambert,[82] Simpson,[118] Buchthal,[12] Thomas, Sears, and Gilliatt,[120] Johnson and Olsen,[73] Kato,[76] Thomas and Lambert,[119] and Desmedt[25,26] to name only a few. The First International Congress of Electromyography, held at Pavia, Italy, in 1961, was an indication of the rapidly growing worldwide interest in this relatively new branch of medicine.

# RECENT DEVELOPMENT

Conventional methods of nerve conduction study were mainly concerned with diseases affecting the distal portion of the peripheral nerve in the four extremities and seldom contributed to the investigation of the remainder of the nervous system. Several neurophysiologic methods have recently emerged as diagnostic tests in evaluating the function of these less accessible anatomic regions. These include studies of human reflexes and other late responses. Of these, the most extensively investigated have been the H-reflex of Hoffmann,[66, 67] F-wave of Magladery and McDougal,[93] and blink reflex of Kugelberg.[80]

Somatosensory evoked potentials provide another electrophysiologic means for study of the central nervous system. Although the technique of signal averaging introduced by Dawson[19] was extensively used for peripheral conduction studies, its clinical application for cerebral signals was limited. With the wide availability of minicomputers and averagers, however, there has been an increasing trend to evaluate neural conduction in the central nervous system by determining latencies of the somatosensory responses recorded over the scalp or cervical or lumbar spine.[25] This development is historically interesting, since photographic superimposition, forerunner of electrical averaging, was originally used by Dawson[18] in the study of somatosensory cerebral potentials. Visual and auditory cerebral evoked potentials have also been introduced as clinical tests. They are less likely to be performed in an electromyography laboratory, however, because of the nature of stimulus modalities required to elicit these responses.

The technique of single fiber electromyography was introduced by Ekstedt and Stålberg[38] to study electrophysiologic characteristics of individual muscle fibers. This is in contrast to the conventional use of coaxial or monopolar recording needles for assessment of the motor unit, the smallest functional unit of muscle contraction. The technique has since been refined and simplified for research application and clinical use as a supplement to conventional electromyography. Some other newer techniques, although directly related to electromyography and nerve conduction studies, have not yet found their way into the clinical laboratory. These include the in vitro technique of sural nerve conduction studies developed by Dyck and Lambert[32] and electroneurography, introduced by Hagbarth and Vallbo.[55]

Most of the major events that have taken place in the history of clinical electrophysiology of muscle and nerve have been outlined above. Inclusion of further details, although tempting because of a number of intriguing anecdotes, is outside the scope of this book. Interested readers are referred to previous publications on this matter by Mottelay,[101] Marinacci,[95] Licht,[88] Gilliatt,[52] and Brazier.[9]

# REFERENCE SOURCES

1. ADRIAN, ED: *The electrical reactions of muscles before and after nerve injury.* Brain 39:1, 1916.

2. ADRIAN, ED AND BRONK, DW: *The discharge of impulses in motor nerve fibres. Part II. The frequency of discharge in reflex and voluntary contractions.* J Physiol (Lond) 67:119, 1929.

3. BAIERLACHER, E: *Beiträge zur therapeutischen Verwerthung des galvanischen Stromes.* Aerztliches Intelligenz-Blatt 4:37, 1859.

4. BAUWENS, P: *The thermionic control of electric currents in electro-medical work.* Proc R Soc Med 34:715, part 2, 1941.

5. BERNSTEIN, J: *Untersuchungen über die Natur des elektrotonischen Zustandes und der negativen Schwankung des Nervenstroms.* Arch Anat Physiol 596, 1866.

6. BERRY, CM, GRUNDFEST, H, AND HINSEY, JC: *The electrical activity of regenerating nerves in the cat.* J Neurophysiol 7:103, 1944.

7. BOURGUIGNON, G: *La Chronaxie Chez l'homme.* Masson, Paris, 1923.

8. BRAUN, F: *Ueber ein Verfahren zur Demonstration und zum Studium des zeitlichen Verlaufes variabler Ströme.* Annalen der Physik und Chemie 60:552, 1897.

9. BRAZIER, MAB: *The emergence of electrophysiology as an aid to neurology.* In AMINOFF, MJ (ED): *Electrodiagnosis in Clinical Neurology.* Churchill Livingstone, New York, 1980.

10. BROWN, GL: *The actions of acetylcholine on denervated mammalian and frog's muscle.* J Physiol (Lond) 89:438, 1937.

11. BUCHANAN, F: *The electrical response of muscle to voluntary, reflex, and artificial stimulation.* Quart J Exper Physiol 1:211, 1908.

12. BUCHTHAL, F: *An Introduction to Electromyography.* Scandinavian University Books, Copenhagen, 1957.

13. BUCHTHAL, F AND CLEMMESEN, S: *On the differentiation of muscle atrophy by electromyography.* Acta Psych Neurol 16:143, 1941.

14. BURDON SANDERSON, J: *The electrical response to stimulation of muscle, and its relation to the mechanical response.* J Physiol (Lond) 18:117, 1895.

15. CLARK, DA: *Muscle counts of motor units: A study in innervation ratios.* Am J Physiol 96:296, 1931.

16. COBB, W AND MARSHALL, J: *Repetitive discharges from human motor nerves after ischaemia and their absence after cooling.* J Neurol Neurosurg Psychiatry 17:183, 1954.

17. D'ARSONVAL, D: *Électricité. Galvanomètre apériodique.* Acad Sci Compt Rend 94:1347, 1882.

18. DAWSON, GD: *Cerebral responses to electrical stimulation of peripheral nerve in man.* J Neurol Neurosurg Psychiatry 10:137, 1947.

19. DAWSON, GD: *A summation technique for the detection of small evoked potentials.* Electroenceph Clin Neurophysiol 6:65, 1954.

20. DAWSON, GD: *The relative excitability and conduction velocity of sensory and motor nerve fibres in man.* J Physiol (Lond) 131:436, 1956.

21. DAWSON, GD AND SCOTT, JW: *The recording of nerve action potentials through skin in man.* J Neurol Neurosurg Psychiatry 12:259, 1949.

22. DENNY-BROWN, D: *On the nature of postural reflexes.* Proc R Soc Lond 104b:252, 1929.

23. DENNY-BROWN, D AND NEVIN, S: *The phenomenon of myotonia.* Brain 64:1, Part 1, 1941.

24. DENNY-BROWN, D AND PENNYBACKER, JB: *Fibrillation and fasciculation in voluntary muscle.* Brain 61:311, 1938.

25. DESMEDT, JE: *Somatosensory cerebral evoked potentials in man.* In RÉMOND, A (ED): *Handbook of Electroencephalography and Clinical Neurophysiology,* Vol 9. Elsevier, Amsterdam, 1971.

26. DESMEDT, JE: *The neuromuscular disorder in myasthenia gravis. 1. Electrical and mechanical response to nerve stimulation in hand muscles.* In DESMEDT, JE (ED): *New Developments in Electromyography and Clinical Neurophysiology,* Vol 1. Karger, Basel, 1973.

27. DOUMER, E: *Note sur un nouveau signe électrique musculaire.* Compt Rend de la Societe Biol 9:656, 1891.

28. DUBOIS-REYMOND, E: *Vorläufiger Abrifs einer Untersuchung über den sogenannten Froschstrom und über die elektromotorischen Fische.* Annalen der Physik Und Chemie 58:1, Series 2, 1843.

29. DUBOIS-REYMOND, E: *On the time required for the transmission of volition and sensation through the nerves.* Roy Inst Great Britain Proc, Vol 4, p 575, 1866.

30. DUCHENNE, G: *De L'électrisation Localisée et de son application a la Physiologie, a la Pathologie et a la Therapeutique.* JB Baillière, Paris, 1855. Translated into English by TIBBITS, LINDSAY, AND BLAKISTON, Philadelphia, 1871.

31. DUCHENNE, G: *Physiologie des mouvements demonstrée d'laide de l'experimentation électrique et de l'observations cliniques et applicable a l'étude de paralysies et des déformations,* 1867. Translated into English by KAPLAN, EB, WB Saunders, Philadelphia, 1959.

32. DYCK, PJ AND LAMBERT, EH: *Numbers and diameters of nerve fibers and compound action potential of sural nerve: Controls and hereditary neuromuscular disorders.* Trans Am Neurol Assoc 91:214, 1966.

33. EATON, LM AND LAMBERT, EH: *Electromyography and electric stimulation of nerves in diseases of motor unit. Observations on myasthenic syndrome associated with malignant tumors.* JAMA 163:1117, 1957.

34. ECCLES, JC: *Changes in muscle produced by nerve degeneration.* J Med Australia 1:573, 1941.

35. ECCLES, JC AND SHERRINGTON, CS: *Numbers and contraction-values of individual motor-units examined in some muscles of the limb.* Proc R Soc London 106b:326, 1930.

36. EICHLER, W: *Über die Ableitung der Aktionspotentiale vom menschlichen Nerven in situ.* Zeit Biol 98:182, 1937.

37. EINTHOVEN, W: *Ein neues Galvanometer.* Drude's Annalen Physik 12:1059, 1903.

38. EKSTEDT, J AND STÅLBERG, E: *A method of recording extracellular action potentials of single muscle fibres and measuring their propagation velocity in voluntarily activated human muscle.* Bull Am Assoc Electromyogr Electrodiagn 10:16, 1963.

39. ERB, W: *Handbuch der Electrotherapie.* FCW Vogel, Leipzig, 1882. Translated into English by PUTZEL, L, William Wood and Company, New York, 1883.

40. ERLANGER, J AND GASSER, HS: *Electrical Signs of Nervous Activity.* University of Pennsylvania Press, Philadelphia, 1937.

41. ERLANGER, J AND SCHOEPFLE, GM: *A study of nerve degeneration and regeneration.* Am J Physiol 147:550, 1946.

42. FORBES, A AND THACHER, C: *Amplification of action currents with the electron tube in recording with the string galvanometer.* Am J Physiol 52:409, 1920.

43. FOWLER, R: *Experiments and observations relative to the influence lately discovered by M. Galvani, and commonly called animal electricity.* Printed for T Duncan, P Hill, Robertson and Berry, and G Mudie; and J Johnson, St. Paul's Churchyard, London, 1793.

44. GALAMBOS, R AND DAVIS, H: *The response of single auditory-nerve fibers to acoustic stimulation.* J Neurophysiol 6:39, 1943.

45. GALVANI, L: *De Viribus Electrocitatis In Motu Musculari Commentarius.* Proc Bologna Academy and Institute of Sciences and Arts 7:363, 1791. Translated into English by GREEN, RM, Elizabeth Licht, Cambridge, 1953.

46. GARTEN, S: *Beiträge zur Kenntnis des Erregungsvorganges im Nerven und Muskel des Warmblüters.* Z Biol 52:534, 1908.

47. GARTEN, S: *Über die zeitliche Folge der Aktionsströme im menschlichen Muskel bei willkürlicher Innervation und bei Erregung des Nerven durch den konstanten Strom.* Z Biol 55:29, 1910.

48. GASSER, HS AND ERLANGER, J: *A study of the action currents of nerve with the cathode ray oscillograph.* Am J Physiol 62:496, 1922.

49. GASSER, HS AND ERLANGER, J: *The nature of conduction of an impulse in the relatively refractory period.* Am J Physiol 73:613, 1925.

50. GHILARDUCCI, F: *Sur une nouvelle forme de la réaction de dégénérescence. (Réaction de Dégénérescence à distance.)* Arch D Electricite Medicale et de Physiotherapie du Cancer 4:17, 1896.

51. GILBERT, W: *De Magnete, Magneti-Cisqve Corporibvs, et Demagno magnete tellure; Phyfiologia noua, plurimis et argumentis, et experimentis demonftrata.* London, 1600. Translated into English by MOTTELAY, PF, John Wiley & Sons, New York, 1893.

52. GILLIATT, RW: *History of nerve conduction studies.* In LICHT, S (ED): *Electrodiagnosis and Electromyography,* ed 3. Waverly Press, Baltimore, 1971, pp 412–418.

53. GILLIATT, RW AND WILSON, TG: *Ischaemic sensory loss in patients with peripheral nerve lesions.* J Neurol Neurosurg Psychiatry 17:104, 1954.

54. GOLSETH, JG AND HUDDLESTON, OL: *Electromyographic diagnosis of lower motor neuron disease.* Arch Phys Med 30:495, 1949.

55. HAGBARTH, KE AND VALLBO, AB: *Single unit recordings from muscle nerves in human subjects.* Acta Physiol Scand 76:321, 1969.

56. HARVEY, AM AND KUFFLER, SW: *Motor nerve function with lesions of the peripheral nerves. A quantitative study.* Arch Neurol Psychiatry 52:317, 1944.

57. HARVEY, AM, KUFFLER, SW, AND TREDWAY, JB: *Peripheral neuritis. Clinical and physiological observations on a series of twenty cases of unknown etiology.* Bull Johns Hopk Hosp 77:83, 1945.

58. HARVEY, AM AND MASLAND, RL: *The electromyogram in myasthenia gravis.* Bull Johns Hopk Hosp 69:1, 1941.

59. HELMHOLTZ, H: *Vorläufiger Bericht über die Fortpflanzungsgeschwindigkeit der Nervenreizung.* Arch Anat Physiol Wiss Med 71, 1850.

60. HELMHOLTZ, H AND BAXT, N: *Neue Versuche über die Fortpflanzungsgeschwindigkeit der Reizung in den motorischen Nerven der Menschen.* Monatsberichte Der Königlich Preussischen, Akademie der Wissenschaften Zu Berlin, pp 184–191, 1870.

61. HERMANN, L: *Ueber den Actionsstrom der Muskeln im lebenden Menschen.* Pflugers Arch Ges Physiol 16:410, 1878.

62. HERMANN, L: *Untersuchungen über die Actionsströme des Muskels.* Pflugers Arch Ges Physiol 16:191, 1878.

63. HODES, R, LARRABEE, MG, AND GERMAN, W: *The human electromyogram in response to nerve stimulation and the conduction velocity of motor axons. Studies on normal and on injured peripheral nerves.* Arch Neurol Psychiatry 60:340, 1948.

64. HOEFER, PFA AND GUTTMAN, SA: *Electromyography as a method for determination of level of lesions in the spinal cord.* Arch Neurol Psychiatry 51:415, 1944.

65. HOEFER, PFA AND PUTNAM, TJ: *Action potentials of muscles in "spastic" conditions.* Arch Neurol Psychiatry 43:1, 1940.

66. HOFFMANN, P: *Über die Beziehungen der Sehnenreflexe zur willkürlichen Bewegung und zum Tonus.* Z Biol 68:351, 1918.

67. HOFFMANN, P: *Untersuchungen Über die Eigenreflexe (Sehnenreflexe) Menschlicher Muskeln.* Julius Springer, Berlin, 1922.

68. HOORWEG, JL: *Ueber die elektrische Nervenerregung.* Arch Ges Physiol 52:87, 1892.

69. HUDDLESTON, OL AND GOLSETH, JG: *Electromyographic studies of paralyzed and paretic muscles in anterior poliomyelitis.* Arch Phys Med 29:92, 1948.

70. HUMBOLDT, FA: *Versuche über die gereizte Muskel-und Nervenfaser nebst Vermutunge über den chemischen Process des Lebens in der Thier-und Pflanzenwelt,* Vol 2. Decker, Posen, und Rottmann, Berlin, 1797.

HISTORICAL REVIEW

71. JASPER, HH, JOHNSTON, RH, AND GEDDES, LA: *The R.C.A.M.C. Electromyograph, Portable Mark II.* National Research Council of Canada, Montreal, 1945.

72. JASPER, H AND NOTMAN, R: *Electromyography in Peripheral Nerve Injuries.* National Research Council of Canada, Montreal, Report #3, 1944.

73. JOHNSON, EW AND OLSEN, KJ: *Clinical value of motor nerve conduction velocity determination.* JAMA 172:2030, 1960.

74. JOLLY, F: *Myasthenia gravis pseudoparalytica.* Berliner Klinische Wochenschrift 32:33, 1895.

75. JONES, HL: *The use of condenser discharges in electrical testing.* Proc R Soc Med 6:49, Part 1, 1913.

76. KATO, M: *The conduction velocity of the ulnar nerve and the spinal reflex time measured by means of the H wave in average adults and athletes.* Tohoku J of Exper Med 73:74, 1960.

77. KRATZENSTEIN, C: *Physicalische Briefe I. Nutzen der Electricitat in der Arzeneiwissenschaft.* Halle, 1746.

78. KRAUSE, W: *Die terminalen Körperchen der einfach sensiblen Nerven.* Hahn'sche Hofbuchhandlung, Hannover, 1860.

79. KUGELBERG, E: *Accommodation in human nerves and its significance for the symptoms in circulatory disturbances and tetany.* Acta Physiol Scand (suppl 24)8:7, 1944.

80. KUGELBERG, E: *Facial reflexes.* Brain 75:385, 1952.

81. KÜHNE, W: *Über die Peripherischen Endorgane der Motorischen Nerven.* W Engelmann, Leipzig, 1862.

82. LAMBERT, EH: *Electromyography and electric stimulation of peripheral nerves and muscles.* In Mayo Clinic: *Clinical Examinations in Neurology.* WB Saunders, Philadelphia, 1956, pp 287–317.

83. LAMBERT, EH: *Neurophysiological techniques useful in the study of neuromuscular disorders.* In ADAMS, RD, EATON, LM, AND SHY, GM (EDS): *Neuromuscular Disorders.* Williams & Wilkins, Baltimore, 1960, pp 247–273.

84. LANGLEY, JN: *Observations on denervated muscle.* J Physiol (Lond) 50:335, 1916.

85. LANGLEY, JN AND KATO, T: *The physiological action of physostigmine and its action on denervated skeletal muscle.* J Physiol (Lond) 49:410, 1915.

86. LAPICQUE, L: *Première approximation d'une loi nouvelle de l'excitation électrique basée sur une conception physique du phénomène.* Compt Rend Societe Biol 62:615, 1907.

87. LAPICQUE, L: *Actualitiés Scientifiques et Industrielles #624. Physiologie Générale Due Système Nerveux. Vol 5, La Chronaxie et ses applications physiologiques.* Hermann and Company, Paris, 1938.

88. LICHT, S: *History of electrodiagnosis.* In LICHT, S (ED): *Electrodiagnosis and Electromyography,* ed 3. Waverly Press, Baltimore, 1971, pp 1–23.

89. LIDDELL, EGT AND SHERRINGTON, CS: *Recruitment and some other features of reflex inhibition.* Proc R Soc B 97:488, 1925.

90. LINDSLEY, DB: *Myographic and electromyographic studies of myasthenia gravis.* Brain 58:470, 1935.

91. LIPPMANN, MG: *Unités Électriques Absolues.* Georges Carré et C Naud, Paris, 1899.

92. MAGENDIE, F: *Expériences sur les fonctions des racines des nerfs rachidiens.* J Physiol Exp Pathol 2:276, 1822.

93. MAGLADERY, JW AND McDOUGAL, DB, JR: *Electrophysiological studies of nerve and reflex activity in normal man. I. Identification of certain reflexes in the electromyogram and the conduction velocity of peripheral nerve fibres.* Bull Johns Hopk Hosp 86:265, 1950.

94. MARIANINI, S: *Memoire sur la secousse qu'éprouvent les animaux au moment où ils cessent de servir d'arc de communication entre les pôles d'un électromoteur, et sur quelques autres phénomènes physiologiques produits par l'électricité.* Ann Chimie Physique 40:225, Series 2, 1829.

95. MARINACCI, AA: *Clinical Electromyography.* San Lucas Press, Los Angeles, 1955.

96. MATTEUCCI, C: *Sur un phénomène physiologique produit par les muscles en contraction.* Ann Chimie Physique 6:339, 1842.

97. MATTEUCCI, C: *Traité des Phénomènes Électro-physiologiques des Animaux*. Fortin, Masson, Paris, 1844.

98. MATTHEWS, BHC: *A special purpose amplifier*. J Physiol (Lond) 81:28, 1934.

99. MEYER, M: *Electricity in its relation to practical medicine*. Translated into English from 3rd German Edition by HAMMOND, WA. D Appleton and Company, New York, 1869.

100. MORGAN, CE: *Electro-physiology and Therapeutics*. William Wood and Company. New York, 1868.

101. MOTTELAY, PF: *Bibliographical History of Electricity and Magnetism*. Charles Griffin and Company, London, 1922.

102. MÜNNICH, F: *Über die Leitungsgeschwindigkeit im motorischen Nerven bei Warmblütern*. Z Biol 66:1, 1916.

103. NEUMANN, E: *Ueber das verschiedene Verhalten gelähmter Muskeln gegen den constanten und inducirten Strom und die Erklärung desselben*. Deutsche Klinik 7:65, 1864.

104. NOBILI, L: *Analyse expérimentale et théorique des phénomènes physiologiques produits par l'électricité sur la grenouille; avec un appendice sur la nature du tétanos et de la paralysie, et sur les moyens de traiter ces deux maladies par l'électricité*. Ann Chimie Physique 44:60, Series 2, 1830.

105. PIPER, H: *Weitere Mitteilungen über die Geschwindigkeit der Erregungsleitung im markhaltigen menschlichen Nerven*. Pflugers Arch Ges Physiol 127:474, 1909.

106. PIPER, H: *Elektrophysiologie menschlicher Muskeln*. Julius Springer, Berlin, 1912.

107. PROEBSTER, R: *Über Muskelaktionsströme am Gesunden und Kranken Menschen*. Zeit fur Orthopadische Chirurgie (suppl 2)50:1, 1928.

108. REMAK, R: *Galvanotherapie Der Nerven-und Muskelkrankheiten*. August Hirschwald, Berlin, 1858.

109. RICHARDSON, AT AND WYNN PARRY, CB: *The theory and practice of electrodiagnosis*. Ann Phys Med 4:3, 1957.

110. RICKER, G: *Beiträge zur Lehre von der Atrophie und Hyperplasie*. Arch Path Anat Physiol 165:263, 1901.

111. ROGOWICZ, N: *Ueber pseudomotorische Einwirkung der Ansa Vieussenii auf die Gesichtsmuskeln*. Arch Ges Physiol 36:1, 1885.

112. SANDERS, FK AND WHITTERIDGE, D: *Conduction velocity and myelin thickness in regenerating nerve fibres*. J Physiol (Lond) 105:152, 1946.

113. SARLANDIERE, C: *Mémoires sur l'electro-puncture*. L'Auteur and M. Delaunay, Paris, 1825.

114. SCHÄFFER, H: *Eine neue Methode zur Bestimmung der Leitungsgeschwindigkeit im sensiblen Nerven beim Menschen*. Dtsch Zeit Nervenheilk 73:234, 1922.

115. SCHIFF, M: *Ueber motorische Lähmung der Zunge*. Arch Physiol Heilkunde 10:579, 1851.

116. SHEA, PA, WOODS, WW, AND WERDEN, DH: *Electromyography in diagnosis of nerve root compression syndrome*. Arch Neurol Psychiatry 64:93, 1950.

117. SHERRINGTON, CS: *On the proprio-ceptive system, especially in its reflex aspect*. Brain 29:467, 1906.

118. SIMPSON, JA: *Electrical signs in the diagnosis of carpal tunnel and related syndromes*. J Neurol Neurosurg Psychiatry 19:275, 1956.

119. THOMAS, JE AND LAMBERT, EH: *Ulnar nerve conduction velocity and H-reflex in infants and children*. J Applied Physiol 15:1, 1960.

120. THOMAS, PK, SEARS, TA, AND GILLIATT, RW: *The range of conduction velocity in normal motor nerve fibres to the small muscles of the hand and foot*. J Neurol Neurosurg Psychiatry 22:175, 1959.

121. VOLTA, A: *Account of some discoveries made by Mr. Galvani, of Bologna; with experiments and observations on them*. Phil Trans R Soc Lond 83:10, 1793.

122. VOLTA, A: *Collezione dell' opere del cavliere conte alessandro Volta*. Florence, 1816.

123. WAGMAN, IH AND LESSE, H: *Maximum conduction velocities of motor fibers of ulnar nerve in human subjects of various ages and sizes*. J Neurophysiol 15:235, 1952.

124. WALLER, A AND WATTEVILLE, A: *On the influence of the galvanic current on the excitability of the motor nerves of man*. Phil Trans R Soc Lond, Part 3, 173:961, 1883.

125. WATKINS, AL, BRAZIER, MAB, AND SCHWAB, RS: *Concepts of muscle dysfunction in polio-myelitis based on electromyographic studies.* JAMA 123:188, 1943.

126. WEDDELL, G, FEINSTEIN, B, AND PATTLE, RE: *The clinical application of electromyography.* Lancet 1:236, 1943.

127. WEDDELL, G, FEINSTEIN, B, AND PATTLE, RE: *The electrical activity of voluntary muscle in man under normal and pathological conditions.* Brain 67:178, 1944.

128. WEISS, G: *Technique d'Électrophysiologie.* Gauthier-Villars, Paris, 1892.

129. ZIEMSSEN, H: *Die Electricität in der Medicin.* August Hirschwald, Berlin, 1866.

# FUNDAMENTALS OF ELECTRONICS AND INSTRUMENTATION

Peter J. Seaba, M.S.E.E.
D. David Walker, M.S.E.E.

## A. BASIC ELECTRONICS

Knowledge of basic electronics is most important in the discussion of instrumentation. However, it is also essential in explaining the origin of physiologic signals, field distribution, electrical safety, and other areas related to electromyography and nerve conduction studies. A solid background in electronics and instrumentation will aid the electromyographer in improving recording techniques, selecting and operating new instruments, recognizing and correcting instrument faults, and understanding new techniques.

The purpose of this section is to provide a general outline of the material with which the electromyographer should be familiar. Any good text on basic electronics should be adequate for the reader interested in a more comprehensive review.[2, 6] An excellent self-study course is the Heath Continuing Education Series in Electronics.[3]

## ELECTRICITY

### Charge

A primary electrical concept is that of *charge*. A neutral atom or molecule has an equal number of positively charged particles (protons) and negatively charged particles (electrons). If electrons are removed, the substance becomes positively charged. This is easily accomplished by friction, and is readily noticed in the dry winter months when, for example, a large amount of charge may accumulate on combs or shoe soles. The first electrical generators operated on the basis of friction. Using various means of generating charged materials, it was noted that the like charges repel, whereas opposite charges attract each other.

### Voltage, current, and resistance

Positively charged protons and neutral neutrons are bound tightly in the nucleus of the atom, whereas electrons are found in shells or levels around the nucleus. In some atoms, classed as metals, the outermost shell contains a single electron that can be easily removed by chemical action. Loss of the electron is called ionization. This process generates a certain force, or voltage, that tends to restore the electron. For example, the ionization potential of silver is 0.799 V or 799,000 $\mu$V. Two metals placed in an acid provide a source of voltage, a battery cell. If a material that easily relinquishes its outer electrons is placed between the two poles of a battery, a *current* of electrons will flow. Materials that readily allow the flow of electrons are called *conductors*.

Current is measured in *amperes* or amps (A). If one coulomb of charge (that is, $6.24 \times 10^{18}$ electrons) flows past a point in one second, the current is 1 A. Current is a mathematical concept, and flow is represented from $+$ to $-$. Actual *electron flow* occurs from $-$ to $+$. Electron flow, or flow of charge from $-$ to $+$, will be used in this text. Often engineering texts will use current flowing from $+$ to $-$.

Resistance is the opposition to flow exhibited by the conductor. Materials that exhibit extremely high resistance are called insulators. The unit of resistance is the *ohm*.

# OHM'S LAW AND OTHER FORMULAS

## Ohm's Law

Ohm's law relates voltage, current, and resistance. The voltage (E) across a resistor is equal to the product of the current (I) through the resistor times the resistance (R). Ohm's law has an analogy in the hydraulics of blood flow. The pressure is equal to the product of the rate of flow times the resistance of the vessel to flow.

$$E = I \times R$$
$$I = E/R$$
$$R = E/I$$

## Power

A simple circuit consists of a voltage supply such as a battery and a resistance such as a lamp. Power (energy) is expended by the flow of electrons through resistance and is expressed in *watts* as follows:

$$Power = Voltage \times Current$$
$$P = E \times I$$

For example, a 60 W bulb connected to 120 V will have $\frac{1}{2}$ A flowing through it. The formula for power can be rearranged by replacing E by I $\times$ R or replacing I by E/R:

$$P = E \times I$$
$$P = (I \times R) \times I = I^2 R$$
$$P = E \times (E/R) = E^2/R$$

## Resistors in series

Ohm's law is used for a single resistor. A string of resistors are said to be connected in *series* (App. Fig. 2-1). Voltage, V, applied to a string of resistors is equal to the sum of the individual voltages across each resistor.

$$V = V_1 + V_2 + V_3 + \ldots + V_n$$

Ohm's law then can be used to describe the voltage across the *individual* resistors:

$$V_1 = I_1 \times R_1 \qquad V_2 = I_2 \times R_2 \ldots$$

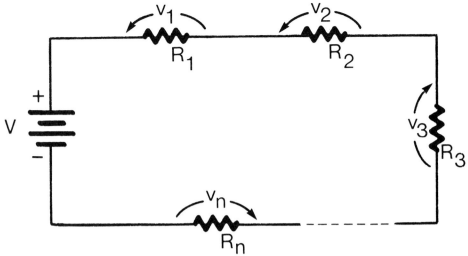
Appendix Figure 2-1
Deriving the equivalent series resistance.

The rate of electron flow (that is, current) would not change from one resistor to the next, so the original equation becomes:

$$V = (I \times R_1) + (I \times R_2) + (I \times R_3) + \ldots + (I \times R_n)$$

and collecting terms:

$$V = I \times (R_1 + R_2 + R_3 + \ldots + R_n)$$

Thus the total resistance, R, equivalent to several resistors in series is:

$$R = R_1 + R_2 + R_3 \ldots + R_n.$$

## The voltage divider

If a voltage is applied to a number of resistors connected in series, a portion of this total voltage appears across each resistor and can be determined from Ohm's law. For example, 1 V is applied to three resistors in series: 90K, 9K, and 1K ohms (App. Fig. 2-2). Since the voltage and equivalent series resistance is known:

$$
\begin{aligned}
I &= E/R \\
&= 1 \text{ V}/(90K + 9K + 1K) \text{ ohms} \\
&= 1V/100K \text{ ohms} \\
&= 10^{-5} \text{ A} \\
&= 10 \ \mu A
\end{aligned}
$$

Because the current flowing through all resistors, including the 1K resistor, is 10 $\mu A$, the voltage across the 1K resistor is:

$$
\begin{aligned}
E &= I \times R \\
&= 10^{-5}A \times 1K \text{ ohm} \\
&= 10^{-2} \text{ V} \\
&= 10 \text{ mV}
\end{aligned}
$$

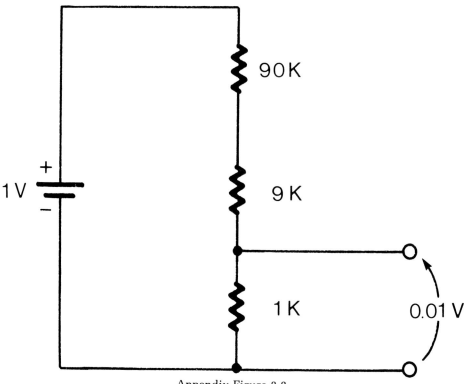

Appendix Figure 2-2

A 100:1 voltage divider. The output voltage is equal to the input voltage divided by 100. If the output is taken across the 9K + 1K resistors, the divider ratio would be 10:1.

The ratio of 1 V to 10 mV is 100:1. The above circuit will divide the applied voltage across the resistors, so that 1/100 of the input voltage will appear across the 1K resistor.

The ratio of input voltage to output voltage is equal to the ratio of total resistance to output resistance. Thus, in the last case, it was 100K:1K or 100:1. The voltage divider is widely used. For example, the above circuit might be used to provide precision millivolt calibration signals. Also, the electrode resistance and the input resistance of the amplifier form a voltage divider; the voltage seen at the input of the amplifier is a portion of the actual voltage of the original signal.

## Resistors in parallel

Resistors may also be arranged in *parallel* (App. Fig. 2-3). Here, the total current, I, is the sum of the individual currents:

$$I = I_1 + I_2 + I_3 + \ldots + I_n$$

The voltages across each resistor are the same, E. The individual currents are then equal to E divided by the respective resistances.

$$I = E/R_1 + E/R_2 + E/R_3 + \ldots E/R_n$$

Collecting terms:

$$I = E (1/R_1 + 1/R_2 + 1/R_3 + \ldots + 1/R_n)$$

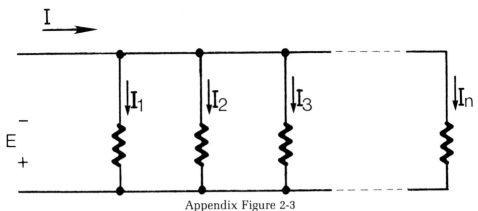

Appendix Figure 2-3
Deriving the equivalent parallel resistance.

Algebraic manipulation into the form of Ohm's law (E = IR) yields:

$$E = I \left( \frac{1}{1/R_1 + 1/R_2 + 1/R_3 \ldots 1/R_n} \right)$$

Thus, the total resistance, R, is:

$$R = \frac{1}{1/R_1 + 1/R_2 + 1/R_3 \ldots 1/R_2}$$

For two resistors in parallel the formula is reduced to:

$$R = \frac{R_1 \times R_2}{R_1 + R_2}$$

# CAPACITANCE, FILTERS, AND INDUCTANCE

## Factors influencing capacitance

If voltage is applied to two closely spaced neutral conductors electrons will flow from one conductor to the positive pole and from the negative pole to the other conductor (App. Fig. 2-4). This will continue until the voltage between the two conductors equals the applied voltage. If the original voltage source is then removed, a voltage difference will remain between the two conductors. The two conductors are usually called *plates*, and the resulting charge storage is called capacitance. Capacitance is measured in *farads* as the ratio of the number of electrons in coulombs (q) stored on one plate to the voltage applied. Since a farad is very large, capacitance units of micro- ($10^{-6}$), nano- ($10^{-9}$), and pico- ($10^{-12}$) farads are often encountered. Capacitance depends on parameters such as plate size and the material between the plates (termed the dielectric). It is inversely proportional to the distance between the two plates.

## The high frequency (low-pass) RC filter

A simple high frequency filter consists of a capacitor and a resistor (App. Fig. 2-5). Voltage applied to the input terminals of this circuit does not immediately appear at the output. Because the voltage across a capacitor (the output voltage) cannot change immediately, the input voltage initially appears across the resistor. As electrons flow from

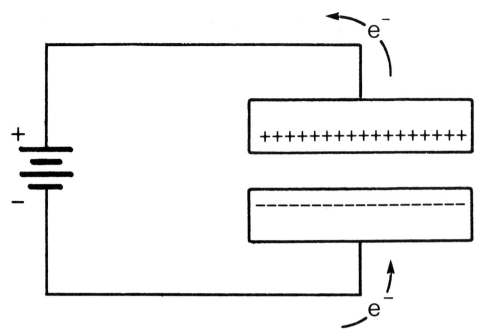

Appendix Figure 2-4

Applying a voltage to two closely spaced conductors causes the electrons to flow from one conductor to another.

one plate and accumulate on the other, the capacitor voltage rises and eventually equals that of the input voltage. The reason for the characteristic rise is easily understood. Initially the voltage across the capacitor is zero. Therefore, the voltage across the input (for example 100 V) appears entirely across the resistor. The current charging the capacitor will then be 100/R. As electrons flow, the voltage across the capacitor rises. When the voltage across the capacitor reaches 10 V, the voltage across the resistor will be 90 V, since the total must equal the 100 V input. The current will then be 90/R, and it will take longer for the voltage across the capacitor to rise another 10 V. When the voltage across the capacitor reaches 20 V, the voltage across the resistor will have dropped to 80 V, and the charging current will be only 80/R at this point. It will take even longer for the voltage to rise another 10 V. Thus, as the voltage across the capacitor rises, the current decreases slowing the rate of charge. Mathematically, the curve of the output voltage is described by:

$$1 - e^{-t/RC}$$

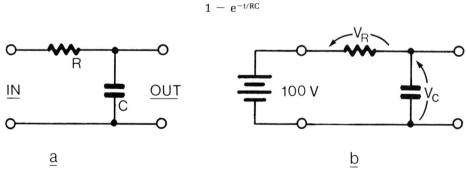

a

b

Appendix Figure 2-5

A simple RC filter; the schematic diagram (a) and deriving the step response (b), when a 100-V step is applied to the input.

where t is the time in seconds (after the input voltage is applied), R is the resistance in ohms, C the capacitance in farads, and e is a constant (base of the Naperian Logarithmic System). If, for example, the resistance was 1 megohm ($10^6$ ohms) and the capacitance 1 microfarad ($10^{-6}$ farads), then R $\times$ C would equal 1. The equation would then be: $1 - e^{-t}$

At time 0, $e^{-0}$ $= 1$ output $= 1 - 1$ or 0 percent
At time 1 second, $e^{-1} = 1/2.718$ output $= 1 - 0.37$ or 63 percent
At time 2 second, $e^{-2} = 1/2.718^2$ output $= 1 - 0.135$ or 86.5 percent
At time 3 second, $e^{-3} = 1/2.718^3$ output $= 1 - 0.05$ or 95 percent

Each second the ouput will have increased 63 percent of the remaining difference. The time taken for the output to rise to 63 percent is called the *Rise Time Constant.* In this case, it is 1 second. The value will be equal to the product of the resistance and capacitance (R $\times$ C). For example, if the capacitor was changed to 2 μfarads, the product R $\times$ C would be 2 seconds. With this change it would take 2 seconds for the output $(1 - e^{-t/2})$ to rise to 63 percent of its final value.

If a slowly varying sine wave is applied to the input, the capacitor has time to charge. The output voltage, which is proportional to charge, will be about the same as the input (Gain $= 1$) (App. Fig. 2-6). If a very fast signal is applied to the input, the capacitor will not have time to charge. The output is then near zero at high frequencies. The cutoff frequency of the filter is commonly defined as that frequency at which the output amplitude is 70 percent (actually $1/\sqrt{2}$) of the input. There is no abrupt drop-off of the output at a given frequency. The cutoff frequency can be calculated from the value of the resistor and capacitor:

$$\text{FREQ}_{70\%} = \frac{1}{2 \pi R C} \text{ Hz}$$

Thus, the rise time constant (R $\times$ C) indicates the frequency response of the filter. For electromyography the high frequency filter is usually changed by selecting various capacitors. A high frequency filter also affects output phase. The peak of the output is

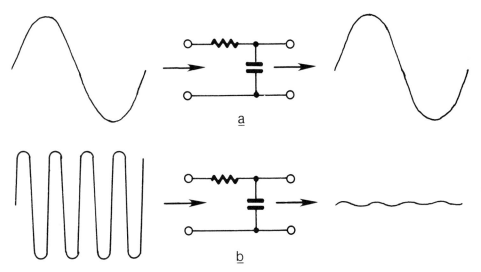

Appendix Figure 2-6
The frequency response of the high-frequency (low-pass) filter. The filter passes low frequencies (a) but filters out high frequencies (b).

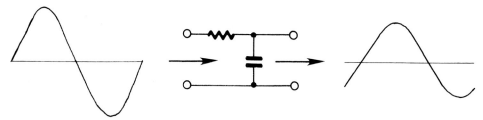

Appendix Figure 2-7

When the input frequency equals $1/(2\pi RC)$, the output waveform is attenuated *and* delayed by 45 degrees.

shifted to the right or delayed in phase compared with the input, since it takes time for the capacitor to charge and discharge. At the cutoff frequency, the output wave is delayed 45 degrees of a complete 360-degree cycle (App. Fig. 2-7). At much lower frequencies there is little phase shift, whereas at high frequencies the shift approaches 90 degrees.

## The low frequency (high-pass) RC filter

A simple low frequency (high-pass) filter is formed by reversing the positions of the resistor and capacitor from the low-pass. The response of this filter to square wave input (or calibration) can be deduced by observing that the voltage across the resistor plus the voltage across the capacitor must equal the input voltage. Subtracting the voltage across the capacitor (which was just described for the high frequency filter)

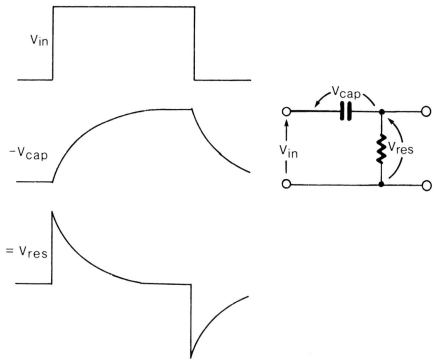

Appendix Figure 2-8

The step response of the low-frequency (high-pass) filter can be derived by subtracting the high frequency filter response from the input step.

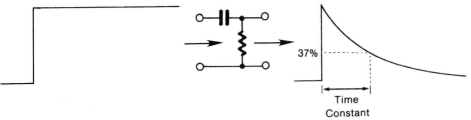

Appendix Figure 2-9

The decay time constant of the low-frequency filter.

from the input voltage provides the voltage across the resistor (App. Fig. 2-8). Thus, the characteristic response of a low-frequency filter to a step or square wave input is an abrupt rise, followed by an exponential decay back to baseline. The formula for this curve is $e^{-t/RC}$. At time zero (when the voltage step is applied) the output is $e^0$ or 100 percent. At time $t = RC$, output is $e^{-1}$ or approximately 37 percent. The product, RC, is the time taken for the output to drop to 37 percent of its initial value (or approach 63 percent of its final value) and is called the *Decay Time Constant* (App. Fig. 2-9). The frequency response of low-frequency filters may be summarized as follows (App. Fig. 2-10). At low frequencies (slow changes) the capacitor has time to charge and discharge, so that the voltage appears across it and not across the resistor, so the output is nearly zero. High frequency signals do not have time to charge or discharge the capacitor and appear as the output across the resistor.

The frequency at which the output voltage is 70 percent of the input voltage is used to indicate the cutoff frequency of the filter. This frequency can be calculated from the value of the resistor and capacitor:

$$\text{FREQ}_{70\%} = \frac{1}{2\pi R C} \text{ Hz}$$

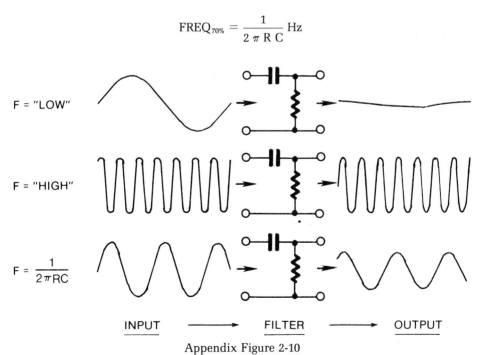

Appendix Figure 2-10

The frequency response of the low frequency filter. Low frequencies are filtered out; high frequencies are passed. When the input frequency equals $1/(2\pi RC)$, the output is attenuated *and* shifted ahead in time by 45 degrees.

**FUNDAMENTALS OF ELECTRONICS AND INSTRUMENTATION**

Thus, the decay time constant indicates the value of the filter. If a calibration trace decayed to 37 percent of its initial value in 10 ms (0.01 sec) the cutoff frequency would be F = 1/(2π × 0.01) Hz or about 16 Hz. The low frequency filter is usually changed by selecting various capacitors.

In addition to affecting the amplitude, the low frequency filter also affects the phase of the output. The peak of the output is shifted to the left or ahead in time, since it starts to decay before the input has reached its peak. The phase shift caused by low and high frequency filters alters latency measurements in nerve conduction studies. Care must be taken in the selection of filter settings, so that amplitude and latency are minimally affected. Normal control and patient data must be recorded with identical filter settings.

## Inductance

The capacitor stores energy in an electrical field between two plates. The inductor stores energy in a magnetic field. When a wire moves through a magnetic field or a magnetic field changes around the wire, voltage is induced in the wire. This electromagnetic effect is used in generators or alternators. This effect is also responsible for the generation of small voltages when a magnetic tape is drawn past the wire coil of a tape recorder head.

When current flows through a wire, a magnetic field is generated around the wire. If the power supplying the current is suddenly removed, the magnetic field collapses around the wire. This in turn induces current, which acts to maintain the flow of current in the wire. If power is suddenly applied to a wire, the expanding magnetic field will induce an opposing current. Thus, inductance opposes any change in current, as its mechanical analog, inertia, opposes any change in the velocity of a mass. The unit of inductance is the *henry*. The symbol L is used to designate the value of inductance and the schematic symbol is a coil (App. Fig. 2-11).

Inductance can be increased by forming a coil of wire. Adding a core of magnetic material to the center of the coil concentrates the magnetic field, increasing the inductance of the coil. Previously the inductor was widely used in power supplies to filter out 60 Hz ripple, since inductors oppose any change in current. However, the physical size of inductors used at power frequencies made them impractical and other means of 60 Hz filtering were developed. A small inductor is effective at high frequencies since inductive reactance (opposition to changes in current) is proportional to frequency. They may be found in the input circuitry of the electromyographic amplifier to filter out high frequency radio transmissions, such as paging systems. They are still found in modern power supplies but are used to remove radio, not line, frequencies.

Stray or unintentional inductance and capacitance occur in all circuits. Stray inductance and capacitance in the input circuit of an amplifier, coupled with high electrode impedance, can severely affect the high frequency response.

# TRANSFORMERS

## Turns ratio

If an alternating voltage is applied to a coil of wire, surrounding a metal core, the varying current will cause the magnetic field to vary. A second coil can be placed on the metal core, and the varying magnetic field will induce a voltage in this second coil of wire (App. Fig. 2-11). The voltage appearing across this second coil (called the secondary) depends on the voltage applied to the first coil (primary) and the turns ratio of the secondary to the primary coils. The output voltage is the input voltage multiplied by the ratio of secondary turns to primary turns. In the figure there are 10 turns of the primary coil for every turn in the secondary. If 120 V is applied to the primary, the secondary voltage will be 120 × 1/10 V or 12 V.

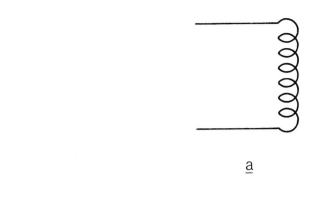

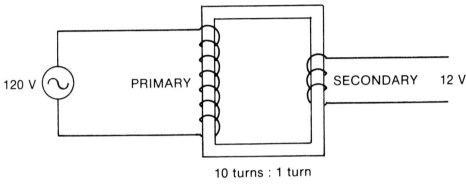

10 turns : 1 turn

b

Appendix Figure 2-11

The flow of current generates a magnetic field that in the inductor (a) is used to store energy and in the transformer (b) generates voltage in a second coil.

Transformers are found in instrument power supplies, transforming the normal 120 V supply to the low voltage levels required by solid state devices. The transformer is also often found at the output of a stimulator, where it isolates the stimulating voltage and increases it to the desired level.

## The ground loop

The transformer effect may also be observed while recording electromyography. Lamp ballasts, motors, and power lines all serve as primaries—generating magnetic fields. The secondary may be any conductor in the area, such as input cables to the amplifier. Conductors that form a loop act as a shorted secondary of a transformer.[5] High current can be generated in such a loop. A ground loop is often formed by connections through the power or outlet ground and shielded cables between the instruments. If the currents generated are near the inputs of the amplifier, 60 Hz interference will occur. Current may also be induced in the input leads or electrodes directly by the transformer effect.

# DC VERSUS AC

## Reactance and impedance

As noted earlier, resistance is the opposition to current flow, specifically to direct current (DC) flow. Constant voltage is applied to measure resistance. However, capacitors and inductors exhibit time-varying currents when a constant voltage is applied. Capacitive and inductive reactance is measured by applying a sinusoidal alternating current (AC) voltage and measuring the current flow. Reactance is the resistance to alternating current. Impedance is the combination of resistance, capacitive reactance, and inductive reactance (App. Fig. 2-12). In electromyography the signal of interest is a mixture of AC signals, commonly in the range of 10 Hz to 10 KHz. The input impedance of the amplifier combined with the electrode impedance determines the effect of the amplifier on these signals.

Electrode impedance consists mainly of resistive and capacitive components. These components are affected by such variables as electrode material, electrolyte, skin condition, and time.[1,4] Not only do fine needle electrodes and large surface electrodes record from different areas, but their impedance is so different that the frequency response of the recordings is affected.

Amplifier input impedance also consists mainly of resistive and capacitive components. The input signal is often conducted by shielded wire, which is composed of two closely spaced conductors. This forms a capacitive path to ground for the electromyographic signal. The longer the input cable is, the larger the plate area is, and the greater is the capacitive path to ground. Input capacitive effects may be reduced by placing the first stage of the amplifier close to the patient or using electronically driven shields.

The symbol for impedance is the letter Z, and the units are ohms. The magnitude of capacitive reactance is $1/(2\pi CF)$, where C is the capacitor in farads and F is frequency. At high frequencies the capacitor has very little reactance and approaches a short circuit. When the frequency is very low, the capacitive reactance becomes very large, approaching an open circuit.

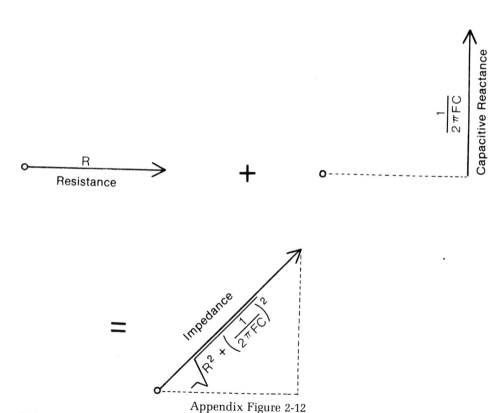

Appendix Figure 2-12

Resistance and capacitive reactance must be added as a vector sum, thus the complicated looking formula for this sum.

The magnitude of inductive reactance is $2\pi LF$, where L is the inductance and F is the frequency. At low frequencies the inductive reactance is small and approaches a short circuit. At high frequencies the reactance is large, approaching an open circuit. Resistance, capacitive reactance, and inductive reactance cannot be added directly, they must be added as a vector summation (App. Fig. 2-12).

## Root mean square

The measurement of a DC voltage waveform is unambiguous—it is constant for all time. On the other hand, a continually varying waveform, for example, the sine wave, can be characterized by its peak-to-peak voltage, zero-to-peak voltage, or average voltage. A commonly used measure is the root mean square (RMS) voltage.

The RMS voltage is derived as the square root of the mean square voltage over the period of interest (such as the full cycle for a sine wave). For a sine wave this value corresponds to 0.707 of the zero-to-peak value. Since power is proportional to the square of the voltage, the RMS voltage indicates the effective power that the voltage will deliver to a resistance load. Thus, a 1 V DC and 1 V RMS AC signal will deliver the same power to a given resistor. The 120 V RMS outlet voltage actually varies from plus to minus 170 V during a cycle, but delivers the same power to a resistor as 120 V direct current. The 0.707 value holds true only for sine waves and not for other waveforms. For random noise (nonrepetitive signals) the RMS may be computed by digital methods or measured by applying the signal to a resistor and measuring the temperature rise, which is proportional to power expended in the resistor.

## Changing AC to DC

Amplifiers require various levels of DC voltage, but our normal outlet supplies a rather fixed AC voltage. Although transformers can supply voltages at various levels using different turns ratios, the voltage continues to alternate. Devices that change alternating into direct current are called rectifiers or diodes. They conduct current in one direction, but not the other.

The vacuum tube rectifier was popular for many years but has been replaced by its solid-state equivalent. Specially treated semiconductor materials, such as silicon, have either extra electrons (N-type) or missing electrons (P-type) in their crystal structure. The two types join at a P-N junction. If a positive voltage is applied to the P-type material and a negative voltage applied to the N-type material, holes and electrons, respectively, are repelled to the P-N junction, where they combine, and current flows. If the voltages are reversed, holes are drawn to the negative voltage, electrons are drawn to the positive voltage, and no current flows. The P-N junction accomplishes in a solid crystalline state that which was accomplished by the vacuum tube in a gaseous state.

The schematic symbol for the diode is an arrow, which points in the direction of conventional current flow (opposite to electron flow). Appendix Figure 2A-13a is a diagram of a transformer and diode supplying current to a resistor load. The voltage supplied to the load is not just DC, but is DC plus AC ripple. This can be smoothed by adding a capacitor (App. Fig. 2-13b), which stores energy and supplies it to the load during the half cycles when the transformer output is of the wrong polarity. Between peaks there will be the characteristic exponential decay through the load resistor. If the time constant (R × C) is very long compared with the 16.7 ms between 60 Hz peaks, the ripple will be small. The DC voltage obtained will vary with changes in the line voltage and changes in current drawn by the load. Voltage regulator circuits may be added to this basic arrangement to provide voltages that are independent of line and load changes and have very little ripple.

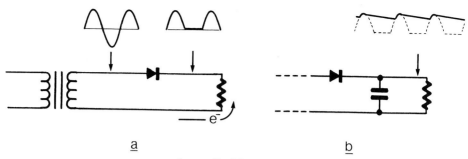

a                  b

Appendix Figure 2-13

A simple power supply. The diode allows current to flow in one direction only, thus only the positive portions (a) are seen across the load (resistor). The voltage supplied to the load is not a smooth, constant level. To smooth out the voltage, a capacitor is added (b). Between peaks energy stored in the capacitor is released, tending to keep the voltage constant.

# AMPLIFIERS

## The transistor and electron tube

In amplifying devices, the input signal is used to control elements that are driven by the power supply. Amplified reproduction of the input signal is illustrated by the following voltage divider circuit. A power supply provides 10 V DC to two resistors; one is a 5 K ohm resistor, while the other is a variable resistor (App. Fig. 2-14a). The output is the voltage across the variable resistor. If the variable resistor was 0 ohms, the output voltage would be 0 V. If the variable resistor was 5 K, the output would be ½ of 10 or 5 V. If the resistance was very high (infinite), the output voltage would be the full 10 V. This circuit will function as an amplifier if the resistance of the variable resistor changes in response to a small input voltage. The transistor is such a device. Here, a small input current greatly alters the apparent resistance (App. Fig. 2-14b). A vacuum tube triode circuit is very similar, but the supply voltage must be higher (App. Fig. 2-14c). A grid of wire in the vacuum tube is placed between the cathode and plate. A small voltage on this grid will greatly affect the flow of electrons/current through the tube. The British term for the electron tube is valve, which refers to its hydraulic analog.

The NPN transistor consists of two pieces of N-type semiconductor with a slice of P-type material in between (thus N-P-N). A small amount of current flowing in the P-type material (the base) controls the current flowing from one piece of N-type material (the emitter) to the other piece of N-type material (the collector). The PNP transistor has a complementary arrangement of N and P type materials, with currents flowing in the opposite direction. In the N-channel field effect transistor, the center of a bar of N-type material (which normally is a fair conductor) is circumscribed by material of the opposite type, P-type. When this P-type gate is made negative, a flow of current through the N-type bar is restricted. A major advantage of this transistor is that the gate draws very little current and thus has very high input impedance.

## The integrated circuit amplifier

In the transistor, the area performing the amplification is quite small. The remaining volume consists of support and connections for the NPN materials. In the 1960s several transistors were integrated; that is, an entire circuit was made of semiconductor material. This construction allowed the entire circuit to be built with only one case and set of leads. At present, most electromyographs are compact, because they are constructed using various types of these integrated circuits.

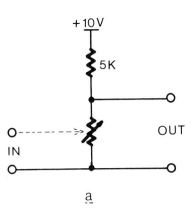

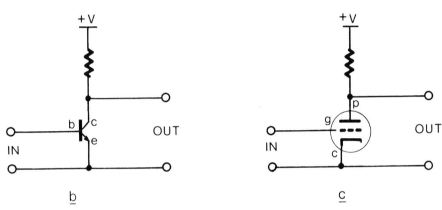

Appendix Figure 2-14

A simple amplifier. If a device that varies its resistance in response to an input voltage is placed in series with a fixed resistor across a power supply (a) the output voltage will vary. Such a device is the NPN transistor (b). A small amount of current flowing from the base allows many times that current to flow from emitter to collector. The electron tube (c) controls the flow of electrons from cathode to plate by negative voltage placed on the grid.

# DIGITAL ELECTRONICS

The electronics discussed so far have dealt with the analog signal, which continually varies in time. In addition, digital circuits are used in the electromyograph. Timing circuits present stimuli, control rate, and measure latencies, whereas logic circuits simplify and improve the operation of the instrument. Recent advances in technology have also made it possible to add digital processing at a reasonable cost. This enables one to convert an amplified analog signal to a string of numbers (digits) that can then be used for complex computations.

## Combinational and sequential logic

One class of digital circuits is combinational logic. Three basic operations are represented by the AND Gate, OR Gate, and the inverter. Two states, usually represented as 0 and 1, are used as inputs and outputs for these circuits. The AND gate requires that both inputs be high (1) before the output will be high. With two inputs, each with two possible states, four possible combinations of inputs exist. These, with their associated output states are shown in Appendix Figure 2-15a. The OR gate is shown in Appendix

Figure 2-15b. The inverter merely converts a 1 input to an 0 output and vice versa. Other complex functions can be expressed as a combination of these three functions. The application may be as simple as ORing two inputs, such as a foot switch and a hand switch to control stimulation. Or it may be a complex system to protect the patient.

The other class of logic is sequential logic—output depending on the previous inputs. One common sequential circuit is the counter, whose output depends on all of the past inputs.

Complex combinations of these circuits can be interconnected (hard-wired) to perform routine functions. The microprocessor is such a combination, but with the advantage that it may be programmed to follow a sequence of steps. Thus, the function is controlled not by fixed wire connections (hardware) but by a program. The program, called firmware, is stored in a Read Only Memory (ROM), which can be changed by changing an integrated circuit. More complex clinical and research instruments are programmable. The program is readily changed by the operator and is referred to as software.

## Binary arithmetic

There are two binary digits (bits) 0 and 1. Given only one bit there are two combinations, 0 and 1. With two bits, there are 4 combinations possible: 00, 01, 10, and 11 (corresponding to the decimal numbers 0, 1, 2, 3). With 8 bits, $2^8$ or 256 combinations are possible. Thus with enough bits, any decimal integer can be represented. Most microcomputers use 8 bits (256 combinations), and memory is blocked into groups of 8 bits. Some newer microprocessors and many minimicrocomputers use a 16-bit word length, thus, 65,536 possible combinations. In microcomputers the keyboard may be in HEXADECIMAL, a shorthand notation for 4 bits. Since 4 bits can represent 16 combinations, the characters 0, 1, 2, . . . 9, A, B, C, D, E, F are used as shorthand. One character takes the place of each 4 bit combination (for example, C = 1100).

## Analog-to-digital converters

The analog-to-digital converter (A/D or ADC) converts voltage to a binary number that then can be used by a digital computer. There is a limited range of voltage, such as −5

| INPUT A | INPUT B | OUTPUT |
|---------|---------|--------|
| 0 | 0 | 0 |
| 0 | 1 | 0 |
| 1 | 0 | 0 |
| 1 | 1 | 1 |

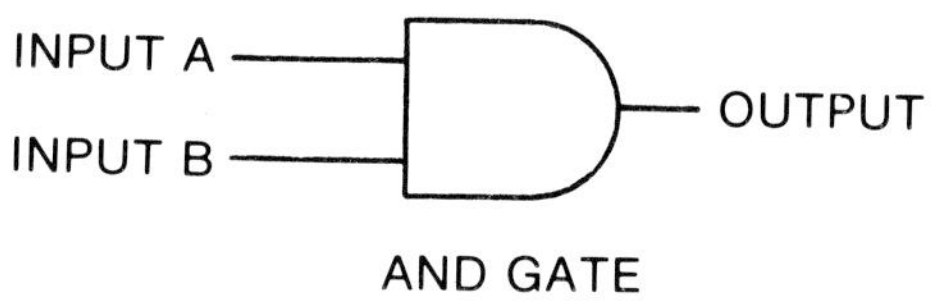

INPUT A ———

INPUT B ———

OUTPUT

AND GATE

a

| INPUT A | INPUT B | OUTPUT |
|---------|---------|--------|
| 0 | 0 | 0 |
| 0 | 1 | 1 |
| 1 | 0 | 1 |
| 1 | 1 | 1 |

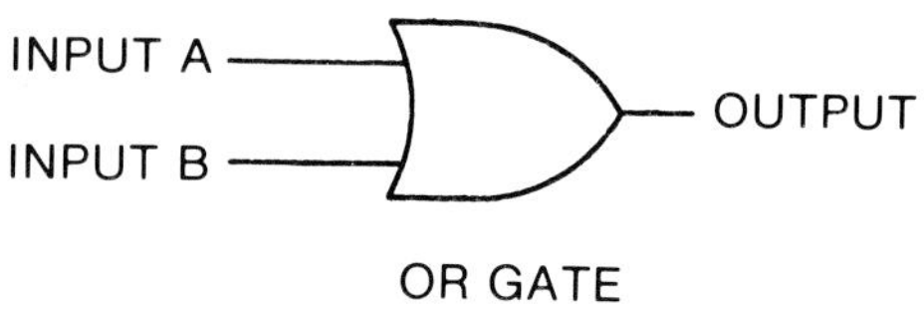

INPUT A ———

INPUT B ———

OUTPUT

OR GATE

b

Appendix Figure 2-15
Digital Logic. If both inputs (A and B) are high or 1, the output of the AND gate (a) is high. The output of the OR gate (b) is high, if either input (A or B) is high.

to $+5$ V, that can be accurately converted to a number. If the converter had 1-bit resolution, it could resolve voltages into positive and negative. With two bits it could resolve the polarity and indicate whether the magnitude was greater or less than 2.5 V (for a range of $-5$ to $+5$). Converters with 8 or 10 bits of resolution are common in systems that process physiologic signals. These divide the range into 256 and 1024 levels, respectively.

The A/D converter converts the voltage to a number, stores it, and samples another voltage in like fashion. The conversion and storage must be done rapidly in order to retain the information of the original analog waveform. In general, the samples must be acquired at a rate greater than twice the highest frequency of interest in the analog signal. For frequencies up to 10 KHz, the sampling rate must be greater than 20 KHz (the time between samples must be less than 50 $\mu$s). Once the numbers are obtained, the microprocessor can be used to add one response to another and thus average; digitally filter the response; measure various parameters; and store data along with clinical information.

# REFERENCE SOURCES

1.  GEDDES, LA: *Electrodes and the Measurement of Bioelectric Events.* John Wiley & Sons, New York, 1972.

2.  GROB, B: *Basic Electronics.* McGraw-Hill, New York, 1977.

3.  HEATH COMPANY: *Heath Continuing Education Series in Electronics.* Heath Company, Benton Harbor, Michigan.

4.  STOLOV, W: *Instrumentation and Measurement in Electrodiagnosis.* Minimonograph #16, American Association of Electromyography and Electrodiagnosis, Rochester, Minnesota, 1981.

5.  STRONG, P: *Grounding-safety.* In: *Biophysical Measurements.* (Tektronix part no. 062-1247-00) Tektronix, Inc., Beaverton, Oregon, 1973.

6.  YANOF, HM: *Biomedical Electronics,* ed 2. FA Davis, Philadelphia, 1972.

# B. INSTRUMENTATION

The electromyograph consists of an amplifier, a stimulator, an oscilloscope with time base for signal display, and a device for data storage such as magnetic tape recorder or paper write out. This section will outline the basic structure and function of these components pertinent to the understanding of their operation. Electronic amplifiers are found in all phases of life: stereos, radios, televisions, and other recording equipment. The amplifiers used in electromyography and in these familiar devices are similar in many ways, but some critical differences exist.[5]

We will also describe some of the recording problems encountered during electromyography in general and with stimulus artifact in particular. In this regard, electrodes can no longer be considered simple connections between the patient and the instrument. Rather, they represent complex series-parallel connections of capacitance, resistance, and voltage sources. Finally, the last few pages briefly discuss the rapidly expanding use of microcomputers in electromyography.

# THE AMPLIFIERS

## The basic amplifier

A single-ended input amplifier diagram is shown in Appendix Figure 2-16. The main characteristic of the amplifier is gain or amplification, the ratio of the output to input voltage. With a gain of $+100$ (often the $+$ is understood), a $-5$ mV signal applied between the input and ground will result in an output of $-500$ mV ($-5$ mV $\times$ $+100$).

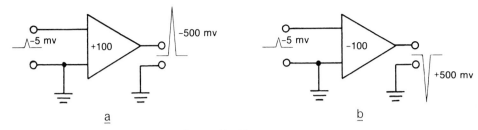

a

b

Appendix Figure 2-16

The single-ended input amplifier may have positive gain (a) where the output is of the same polarity as the input, or negative gain (b) where the output is inverted. The output is equal to the input multiplied by the gain.

If, in the process of amplification, the signal is inverted the gain is considered to be negative. If the gain were $-100$, the input signal above ($-5$ mV) would result in an output voltage of $+500$ mV ($-5$ mV $\times -100$).

Amplifiers have some important limitations. The input impedance may be high, but not infinite, as assumed in ideal amplifiers. The actual voltage seen by the amplifier is determined by the ratio of the input impedance of the amplifier to the combined impedance of the amplifier and the recording electrode (App. Fig. 2-17). Connecting a measuring instrument (electromyograph) to the system (patient) alters the original signal. Noise or unwanted signal is introduced by the amplifier components. One component of this noise is proportional to the electrode impedance; the lower the electrode impedance is, the lower the noise is.

The excursion of the output voltage is restricted by the voltages provided to the amplifier by the power supply. Most modern amplifiers are powered by low voltages, usually less than $+20$ and $-20$ V. If the supplies were $+12$ and $-12$ V, the output of the amplifier might be within the range of $+10$ and $-10$ V. With a gain of 100, this would limit any input voltage to a range of $-100$ to $+100$ mV (100 mV $\times$ 100 = 10 V limit).

The frequency response of the amplifier imposes limits at both ends of the spectrum. Filters are thus added to predictably control the frequency response of the amplifier. Rarely is DC amplification needed, but there are trade-offs between gain and the desired high-frequency response.

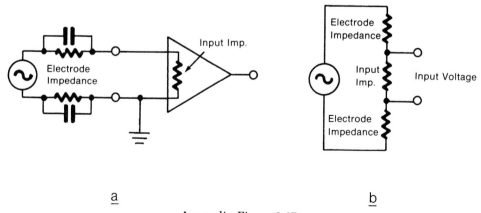

a

b

Appendix Figure 2-17

The voltage at the input of the amplifier is not the physiologic voltage (a). The electrode impedances and the input impedance of the amplifier form a voltage divider (b).

# The differential amplifier

The single-ended amplifier uses the ground as one input lead. Hence, noise induced on the ground lead is amplified. The differential amplifier was developed to circumvent this problem in recording low-level signals such as those encountered in electromyography. It consists of two separate, single-ended input amplifiers. One amplifier has positive gain and the input may be labeled + or noninverting. The other amplifier has an identical negative gain and is often labeled − or inverting. The outputs of these two amplifiers are added; the result is then filtered, amplified by single-ended input amplifiers, and further conditioned for display. The sum of the inverting and noninverting amplifiers is the amplified difference of the two input signals. For example, if a −5 mV spike was applied commonly to both inputs (between ground and both inputs), one amplifier would amplify this to −500 mV, whereas the other would amplify this to +500 mV (App. Fig. 2-18). The sum would be zero, since there is no difference between the signal applied to the inputs. The differential amplifier is represented by a triangle with + and − inputs (App. Fig. 2-19).

With the differential amplifier, external radiated interference, which affects both leads equally, will cancel. For example, noise appearing on the ground lead will be applied simultaneously to both inputs and not amplified, leaving an output consisting only of the amplified differential signal. Physiologic signals that affect both leads, such as the electrocardiogram, would also be cancelled, provided that the signal is of the same amplitude at the two input leads.

The range of input signal amplitudes over which a differential amplifier functions properly is determined by two major factors. One is the common-mode range: the range of voltage that may be applied to both + and − inputs simultaneously and still allows true differential amplification at the output. Beyond this range, differential amplification deteriorates rapidly. The difference between the leads of an ungrounded patient and the ground may easily reach a few volts and exceed the common-mode range. Even if the patient is well grounded, external interference may generate more common-mode signals than the amplifier is capable of cancelling.

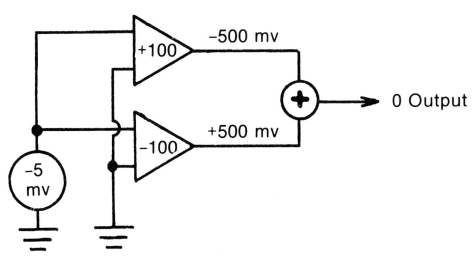

Appendix Figure 2-18

The differential amplifier is formed by two single-ended input amplifiers that theoretically have identical gain but opposite signs. The outputs of the two amplifiers are then summed to form a single output. If a signal is applied *commonly* to both inputs, the outputs of the amplifiers are of the same magnitude but opposite polarity. The outputs then sum to zero.

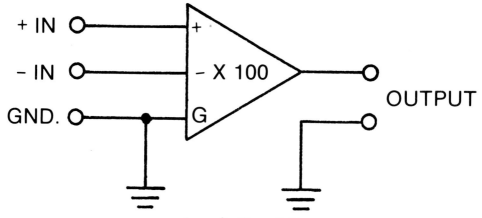

The symbol for the differential amplifier is similar to the symbol for the single-ended input amplifier, but with an extra input terminal. Often the + input is called the noninverting input, and the − input is called the inverting input. The ground terminals on both the input and output may be deleted in some diagrams.

The second input limitation is the differential-mode range. Although the voltage on each input might be within the common-mode range, the difference between the two (the desired signal) may overload succeeding stages of amplification. The output swing of an amplifier refers to the maximum output voltage that can be achieved in either the + or − direction. Dividing the maximum output swing (either peak-to-peak or in one direction) by the voltage gain of the amplifier yields the maximum input voltage difference that can be amplified correctly. With a larger voltage difference, the amplifier output remains at its maximum value and is said to be saturated. Both common-mode range and output swing are affected by signal frequency.

## Factors that influence differential amplification

The foregoing describes the theoretical function of the differential amplifier. However, several factors qualify actual operation.[1,6] In the example, the gains of the input amplitude were said to be +100 and −100. In actuality, these will not be perfectly matched. For example, if 1 percent precision resistors were used, the gains might be +100 and −99 (App. Fig. 2-20). The outputs, when −5 mV is applied commonly, would then be −500 mV and +495 mV. The sum then would be −5 mV, not zero.

The Common-Mode Rejection Ratio (CMRR) indicates how well the input amplifiers are matched. CMRR is the ratio of the differential gain to the common mode gain. In the above example, −5 mV applied commonly to both inputs resulted in −5 mV output, or a common mode gain of 1. If the −5 mV is applied differentially, perhaps −2½ mV to one input and +2½ mV to the other input, the output would be −500 mV or a differential gain of 100 (App. Fig. 2-20b). The CMRR in this case is then 100:1 (where input gains are matched 1 part in 100).

Often CMRR is expressed in decibels (dB), which is 20 $\log_{10}$ ratio. It is common for modern amplifiers to have CMRR greater than 10,000 (80 dB). It is far more difficult to match the response of the two inputs over a wide frequency range than at only one frequency. Some amplifiers may have the CMRR specified for 60 Hz only. CMRR is meaningful only if the applied input voltage and the test frequency are indicated. It should be specified over the entire bandwidth, as the ability to reject all common mode signals is desired.

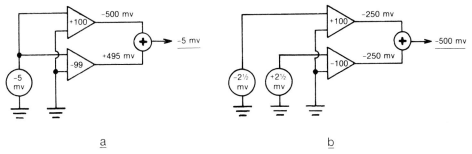

a                            b

Appendix Figure 2-20

The ability of the differential amplifier to reject signals common to both inputs is called the common-mode rejection ratio (CMRR). This is dependent on the matching of the two input amplifiers. If the difference between the two is 1 part in 100, some of the common-mode signal appears at the output (a). Here, the common-mode gain is 1. The differential gain is 100 (b). The CMRR is then 100:1.

Little can be done to optimize the CMRR, other than careful initial amplifier selection and periodic maintenance. However, there are factors over which we have control. Unbalanced electrode impedances severely degrade the overall CMRR even though the amplifier has very high CMRR. The physiologic signal of interest is connected to an amplifier through electrode and tissue impedance. This impedance and the input impedance of the amplifier form a voltage divider (see App. Fig. 2-17b). The CMRR of this input circuit is equal to the ratio of the input impedance of the amplifier to the difference between the two electrode impedances. Thus, if the input impedance of the amplifier is 10 megohms (10,000K) and the electrode impedances are 10K and 7K ohms, the overall CMRR is then limited to $10,000K/(10K - 7K) = 3333:1$ even if the amplifier CMRR were infinitely high.

For effective cancellation, external interference must affect both input leads equally. When the two input leads are widely separated and the interference source is relatively close, a considerable difference in the interference signal at the two inputs will be amplified. Thus, the two input leads should be kept in close proximity so that they are affected equally by external interference. For the same reason, stimulus artifact is minimized when the two recording electrodes are approximately equidistant from the stimulating electrodes.

# Filters

One method of optimizing electromyographic information is filtering. If the frequency spectra of the noise and the signal of interest differ, filtering can be useful. However, if applied indiscriminately, filtering will also distort the signal of interest. The three basic types of filters encountered in electromyography are the high-frequency/low-pass filter; the low-frequency/high-pass filter; and the 60 Hz/notch filter.[1]

In instruments intended for routine clinical use, high- and low-frequency filters may not be independently accessible. For example, the high-frequency filter may be controlled by the gain/sensitivity control. At the high sensitivities used for sensory recordings, a lower high-frequency filter setting would be automatically selected, filtering out high-frequency noise. At lower sensitivities used for motor recordings, in which high frequency noise is not as problematic, a higher high frequency filter setting would be used.

As discussed in part A, filter characteristics are determined by selecting different fixed capacitors (App. Fig. 2-21a). The ultimate high-frequency response is limited by such factors as the type of electrode, capacitance in the input cables, and stray capaci-

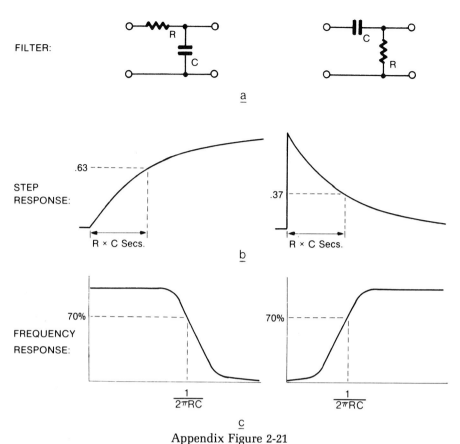

FILTER:

STEP RESPONSE:

.63

R × C Secs.

.37

R × C Secs.

a

b

FREQUENCY RESPONSE:

70%

$$\frac{1}{2\pi RC}$$

70%

$$\frac{1}{2\pi RC}$$

c

Appendix Figure 2-21

The schematic diagram of the high-frequency (low-pass) and low-frequency (high-pass) filters. Filters are diagrammed in (a). The response of the filter to a step input is diagrammed in (b), and the frequency response in (c).

tance within the amplifier. The step (or calibration) response indicates the type and value of the filters being used (App. Fig. 2-21b). The high-frequency filter controls the rise of the output signal. The low-frequency filter results in the output returning to baseline with a characteristic negative-exponential curve. The rise time constant is the time taken for the voltage to rise to 63 percent $(1-1/e)$ of its final value. The decay time constant is the time taken for the voltage to decay to 37 percent $(1/e)$ of its peak value (or 63 percent of the transition from initial to final value).

The frequency responses of the two types of filters show gradual changes (App. Fig. 2-21c). Since there is no abrupt drop off, the filter is arbitrarily labeled for the frequency at which output has dropped to 70 percent of the passband value. For either the basic RC high- or low-frequency filter discussed previously, this value is equal to $1/(2\pi RC)$ Hz.

Filters not only attenuate signals but also shift the phase. This may alter latency measurements. The low-frequency filter produces an apparent shift ahead in time, shortening recorded latencies, while the high-frequency filter delays the signals, increasing the recorded latency. Signals that are well within the passband of the amplifier (that is, at least 2 to 4 times the low-frequency filter setting and less than ¼ to ½ of the high-frequency filter setting) are minimally affected by this phase shift.

As previously mentioned, overall frequency response is affected by the input leads. Often the input leads are shielded to reduce external interference. The shield, wrapped about the inner conductor, forms a capacitor between the inputs and ground, which filters out higher frequencies. If each input signal (amplified by a gain-of-one driver amplifier) is fed back to the shield, the difference between the voltage of the incoming signal and that of the shield is eliminated. This in turn abolishes the capacitance and filtering effects of the input cables. In practice the amplifiers that drive the shields have gains slightly less than one; nonetheless, the resulting capacitance and filtering effect are greatly diminished. Another variation is to drive both input shields with the common-mode signal which reduces the degradation of CMRR even with unequal electrode impedances.[6]

# THE ELECTRICAL STIMULATOR

## Electrical requirements

For nerve conduction studies electrical stimulation of the nerve provides a clearly defined reproducible response of minimum latency. A current of short duration is induced in the fluid surrounding a nerve bundle by applying a potential to electrodes usually on the skin surface, but sometimes inserted subcutaneously. The current is directed primarily along the direction of the nerve so that one point is depolarized and another point is hyperpolarized. The current is increased until every nerve fiber in the bundle is reliably activated as evidenced by a maximum and constant response. Surface electrode stimulation requires 100 to 600 V, which induces currents of 20 to 75 mA for 50 to 1000 $\mu$s. The higher values are necessary when the stimulating electrodes are distant from the nerve or when neuropathy decreases nerve excitability. There is an inverse relationship between the stimulus intensity and duration necessary for effective depolarization: a stimulus of less intensity may be equally effective if applied for a longer duration. Stimulus durations in excess of 1 ms are not generally tolerated well. Stimuli of less than 50 $\mu$s duration are ineffective, since they are limited by rise time considerations and other capacitive effects. The circuit formed by the tissue impedance is similar to a high frequency filter (see App. Fig. 2-21) and the voltage at the stimulating site will not have reached full potential in 50 $\mu$s.

The stimulator must also provide control and timing of the stimuli for different types of measurements. This may require pairs of shocks at the same or different electrodes, with adjustable delays between the shocks and independent intensity control. Some collision techniques require three precisely timed but adjustable stimuli, while train stimulus techniques require many shocks to be delivered at adjustable repetitive rates. In one type of paired shock technique the first shock is adjusted in intensity to give only a subliminal excitation of the motor neuron pool. It requires the application of two shocks with independent intensity control at the same electrode site within a short latency. For this purpose, independent stimulus generators must be designed such that their outputs can be connected together to the same stimulating electrodes without affecting the separate stimuli or harming the circuits.

## Stimulus isolation

A line operated electrical stimulator is easier to design and less expensive if one of the outputs is grounded. However, using the ground as one of the outputs presents many problems (App. Fig. 2-22). Stimulating current will flow not only from the stimulating electrode to the stimulator ground but also to the amplifier ground and inputs. This will overload the amplifier, exceeding the common-mode and/or differential input voltage limits. The uncontrolled current may also produce stimulation at sites other than the one intended.

An isolated stimulus is one which is not referenced (connected) to ground. For safety and reduction of stimulus artifact, stimulus isolation should be high. Merely not

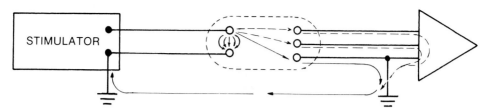

Appendix Figure 2-22

The nonisolated stimulator (having one output terminal grounded) causes two problems. The stimulating current is divided between the stimulator ground and amplifier ground. Some of the current will also find its way to the inputs of the amplifier and overload the amplifier.

grounding one side of the output is not sufficient, because within the stimulator there are many alternate resistive and capacitive pathways to ground. Usually a nonisolated stimulator is used to produce the desired pulse, and an isolation circuit is interposed between the stimulator and the patient. There are a number of devices that may isolate output (App. Fig. 2-23).

These include: 1. Transformer: Coupling the energy magnetically to the patient, 2. RF Unit: Using the stimulus pulse to drive a radio frequency (RF) oscillator, and "transmitting" the energy to the patient side of the circuit, and 3. Battery: Using a battery to supply the stimulating current, and controlling it via an optically coupled isolator/switch.

## Constant voltage versus constant current

Stimulators are divided into two types: constant-voltage and constant-current. The constant-voltage type provides an adjustable voltage across the stimulating electrodes, which is more or less independent of the stimulating current. The voltage is adjusted until it provides the desired stimulation. This voltage level depends on the impedance of the electrodes and body tissues. The constant-current stimulator provides an adjustable current through the stimulating electrode essentially independent of the output voltage required to achieve this (up to a maximum voltage limit). Current is adjusted until it provides the desired stimulation. One advantage is that changes in electrode

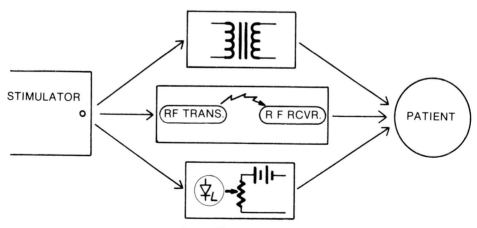

Appendix Figure 2-23

The output of the stimulator may be *isolated* from ground in a number of ways. The energy may be transferred magnetically (through a transformer) to the patient; transmitted via radio frequencies; or the output of the stimulator may be used to control the output of an isolated battery via a light emitting diode.

impedance, based on factors such as repositioning or electrode or electrolyte change, do not alter the stimulating current in the body circuit.

In our laboratory, measurement of actual stimulating voltage and current reveals that the stimulating electrode-electrolyte circuit has a considerable capacitive component. With constant-voltage stimulators current initially peaks while this capacitance is being charged, the magnitude depending for one thing on the rise time of the applied voltage. If the constant-voltage stimulator has a very fast rise time (5 $\mu$s) and is very stiff (that is, is capable of providing large currents with little reduction in output voltage), the initial peak capacitive current may be many times the average current value and stimulation may be accompanied by sharp pain.

With constant-current stimulators, stimulus voltage rises slowly to its maximum value as the capacitance is charged. When metal pin electrodes of a constant-current stimulation are touched very lightly to the skin surface, the stimulating voltage abruptly rises because of the high electrode impedance and a sharp pain is felt. If the pressure of the pins against the skin is increased the pain is reduced. We speculate that the capacitive component of the stimulator load engenders greater current flow near the skin surface where it will also stimulate superficial pain fibers.

# STIMULUS ARTIFACT

When an electrical stimulus is applied, some amplifier output deviation invariably occurs simultaneously with stimulus onset. This stimulus artifact results from many factors and is generally of no consequence as long as it terminates before the onset of the response. In fact, the artifact conveniently marks the stimulus event on the response trace. However, the duration of the stimulus artifact limits the minimum latency that can be accurately measured.

## Origin of stimulus artifact

There are several pathways by which the stimulus voltage arrives at the inputs of the recording amplifiers.[4] One route is by volume conduction. Because of the large difference between the stimulus (hundreds of volts) and the recorded signal (mV or $\mu$V) spread of potential from the stimulating to the recording electrode is significant. Within a few millimeters of the stimulating electrodes a field in the tens of volts can be recorded. A few more millimeters distant, the signal falls to the 1 to 10 volt range, and so on. Thus at the recording site stimulus artifact can be quite sizable relative to the recorded signal.

The orientation of the stimulus and recording electrodes can affect stimulus artifact amplitude. If both pick-up electrodes lie along an isopotential line with regard to the stimulus, they register similar voltages that will be suppressed by the differential amplifier (as long as the common-mode range is not exceeded). This is most likely to occur if the orientation of the stimulating electrodes is nearly perpendicular to that of the recording electrodes. Since the intervening volume is neither geometrically regular nor homogeneous, some artifact will always exist. Nonetheless, when there is some freedom in electrode placement, it is worth trying various orientations (usually changing the stimulating electrodes) to minimize the artifact.

Conduction of stimulus current to the recording electrode is enhanced by perspiration and electrode cream. Thus, cleaning and drying the skin between the stimulating and recording electrodes with alcohol may reduce the artifact. Placing the ground strap between the stimulus and recording electrodes also reduces stimulus artifact. This shields the recording electrodes by creating an isopotential surface in the volume conductor which distorts but does not entirely eliminate the stimulus potential spread. However, the ground electrode should not be located too far from the recording electrode, as common-mode interference signals increase with distance. For best shielding effect and patient safety, this should be the only ground to the patient.

Stimulus leakage to ground provides pathways for stimulus current to flow to amplifier inputs and represents a second source of stimulus artifact. In spite of the precautions taken to isolate the stimulator, some stimulus current will always flow to ground. The wires to stimulating electrodes should be kept as far as possible from any ground. If one of these wires is close to a ground, there is capacitive connection to ground reducing the isolation of the stimulus. Unshielded recording electrode wires allow coupling of the stimulus potential into the recording amplifier. It is best to keep the stimulating and recording cables as far from each other as possible and to minimize electrode impedances.

Another pathway occurs when using a high- or radio-frequency transformer isolater. High frequencies tend to flow over the grounds, over the body surface, and through the air to the amplifier inputs. This is then detected by the electrodes or input circuitry and appears on the output.

## Reducing stimulus artifact

As just discussed, technique can have a profound effect on stimulus artifact. Factors to consider are the position of the stimulus and input cables, stimulating electrode size and material, skin preparation, recording electrode impedance, electrode orientation, and placement of the ground electrode. The low- and high-frequency filters of the recording amplifier also affect stimulus artifact. The higher the value of the low-frequency filter is: the smaller the capacitor, the less energy stored, and thus the faster a stimulus artifact will recover to baseline. The high-frequency filter has an integrating effect on short, fast impulses. It tends to reduce their amplitude but increase their duration at the output. A very low high-frequency filter may satisfactorily reduce artifact amplitude, or a very high value may allow the artifact to peak and recover quickly without extending its duration. In general, however, filters are not adequate to deal with stimulus artifact problems, because the values required excessively distort the signal of interest or are incompatible with other considerations such as noise. As previously discussed, an amplifier common-mode rejection ratio (CMRR) is usually specified at 60 Hz for the line interference rejection. Since the stimulus is a fast-rising signal, it has relatively high-frequency components. Thus, for stimulus artifact rejection, the CMRR at higher frequencies (several KHz) is also important in assessing amplifier performance.

Obviously, stimulus magnitude and duration affect the amount of artifact. Additionally, the stimulus wave shape can have an effect. Both the rise time and fall time of the stimulus are of particular interest. If the rise of the stimulus current is too fast, various problems can occur. The coupling of signals from the stimulating wires to the electrode leads is enhanced with faster rising stimulus voltages, as is artifact via ground loop current and stray capacitive effects. Also the common-mode rejection of these high frequency components is probably less. If the stimulus current is slow to return to zero at the end of stimulus, the effect is a longer duration artifact. Thus decay of stimulus current must be prompt. Because of the magnitudes of difference between stimulus and response voltage, the duration of the stimulus artifact may be many times greater than the actual stimulus duration. The stimulus fall time may be prolonged by capacitance in the stimulator or in the electrode.

Stimulus artifact poses a problem only when it becomes superimposed upon responses of interest. High voltage stimuli of long duration combined with stray capacitance and a high frequency filter result in a distorted and prolonged stimulus artifact. Modification of filter settings and electrode position will reduce some of the stimulus artifact. If the voltages are large enough to overload the amplifier the problem becomes more complex. In this situation the amplifier circuitry will enter a nonlinear mode. A capacitor may be rapidly charged through a low resistance path and then left to discharge slowly through a large resistance. The output is then disturbed for an exceptionally long time.

## Artifact suppression circuits

Using the shortest possible stimulating wires, having a remote shielded preamp near the electrode site, and placing the ground between stimulating and recording electrodes are all common ways of reducing stimulus artifact. Isolation of the stimulator output eliminates the connection between stimulus current and ground except via stray capacitance. However, in situations in which excessive stimulus artifact remains a problem, more elaborate techniques have been devised.

In measuring latencies shorter than 10 ms the above conventional means of reducing stimulus artifact may prove inadequate, so various electronic manipulations are used. One method is cancellation. In the amplifier a signal (derived from the stimulator) with the proper amplitude, shape, and polarity is added to exactly cancel the stimulus artifact. This is generally done at or near the input stage where the artifact has not saturated the amplifier. Cancellation has some drawbacks: it requires special adjustment of the compensating signal for each stimulus arrangement, and even successive stimuli are not the same. Also, the shape of the stimulus at the electrodes and later in the amplifier is not the same as in the stimulator.

Electronic circuits have also been directed at reducing the duration of amplifier overload. One electronic technique to enhance amplifier recovery is called limiting or clamping. At the input or at later stages, signal response is limited. The magnitude of an overload is diminished and recovery is faster. With the so-called blocking technique the amplifier is switched off during stimulation. Electronic and mechanical switches have been used to disconnect the electrode inputs, or to open or short some other signal path during stimulus time, so that overload will not occur. This technique also has drawbacks. Mechanical switches are, of course, slow. Electrical switching can induce additional artifacts. Switching some circuits may affect their operating state and produce a transient refractory period when the circuit is restored.

A stimulus suppression circuit for faster recovery has been recently developed in our laboratory.[7] It might be called a DC blocking amplifier. Most amplifiers used in electrophysiology consist of several stages to achieve the required gain. Conventionally, these stages are AC (capacitor) coupled to block DC operating levels. To allow selection of the low-frequency cutoff, one or more of the coupling capacitors are varied. In the quiescent state, charge exists on each of the coupling capacitors according to the DC voltage difference between the stages. If an overloading input saturates the stage 1, the charge on the coupling capacitor to the stage 2 will be altered and will require a longer time to recover (App. Fig. 2-24).

To reduce the recovery time of such an amplifier the coupling time constants may be shortened or the voltage gains reduced and judiciously appropriated. However, this results in a loss of low-frequency response or loss in sensitivity. A point is reached at which the amplifier cannot meet all the specifications required for electrophysiologic recording. To solve this problem the input and interstage coupling capacitors are eliminated in our design (App. Fig. 2-25) so that the feed-forward path from electrodes to output is strictly DC. This amplifier recovers almost immediately, because it contains no significant capacitors to store charge. To establish a low-frequency cutoff and to eliminate DC electrode offset, an integrator feedback loop subtracts an offset signal from the stage 1 input (shown as a subtraction in the negative electrode lead). This sets a single low-frequency break point at $f = K/(2\pi RC)$ Hz where K is the (fixed) gain from the stage 1 offset input to the stage 1 output.

Thus, C can be varied to change the low-frequency cutoff. This capacitor is the only place in the amplifier where significant charge could be stored during overload. To

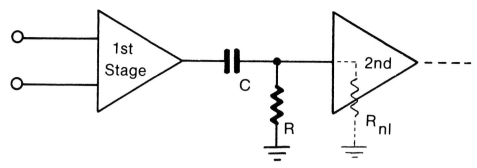

Appendix Figure 2-24

Energy of the stimulus artifact is stored in capacitor C of the low frequency filter. If the 2nd stage is overloaded, the capacitor may be charged through a nonlinear resistance in addition to the normal input resistance. It is then left to discharge slowly through R only, creating an artifact of long duration.

achieve fast recovery, a circuit monitors the stage 1 output and, by various schemes, responds to stage 1 overdrive and opens the feedback loop. The charge on C, representing the average offset value needed to keep the amplifier at baseline, holds until the overload is gone and then, when the loop is reclosed, it restores the amplifier to baseline. The control circuit may be designed to hold the loop open for a fixed time on each overload; or it may hold the loop open until the overload recovers, with or without a fixed maximum time. In contrast to a conventional amplifier such as the one depicted in Appendix Figure 2-24, the lower the low-frequency cutoff (large C) is, the better is the recovery from the overload in this fast-recovery amplifier.

# THE DISPLAY

Once the recorded potential is properly amplified and filtered, the electrical signal is displayed for evaluation. The muscle action potentials recorded by a needle electrode are within the audio frequency range. Thus, one early method of analysis was to reproduce the signal acoustically through an audio amplifier and speaker. The speaker and its enclosure drastically affect the tonal quality of the sound and will vary widely from one manufacturer to another. Indeed, the most faithful reproduction may not be the

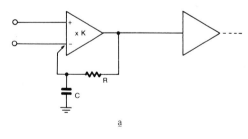

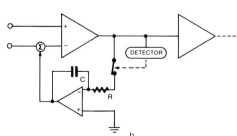

Appendix Figure 2-25
An amplifier with similar characteristics can be constructed by using direct-coupled stages and feeding back the DC offset (a). The fast recovery amplifier (b) detects large signals and disconnects them from the feedback circuit. This avoids storing stimulus artifact on the low-frequency filter capacitor.

most pleasant or useful. Auditory reproduction is widely used, but is not as objective as the visual display.

The common ink-writer used for displaying the electrocardiogram and electroencephalogram is not suitable for the high-frequency signals encountered in electromyography. With regard to the pen-writer analogies may be drawn between electrical and mechanical concepts: inductance/inertia, resistance/drag, or capacitance/spring-restoring force. The mechanical circuit forms a sharp low–pass filter that limits it frequency response to 100 Hz or less. Many methods have been introduced to minimize the moving mass of the writing element, which is the primary limiting factor.

## The cathode ray tube

The cathode ray tube (CRT) offers a means to display high-frequency signals. The electron, which has very little mass, is used as the moving element. A fine beam of electrons moves through a vacuum and strikes light-emitting phosphor. By applying voltages to plates above and below the beam (vertical deflection plates), the electrons are deflected vertically. Similar plates on either side deflect the beam horizontally (horizontal deflection plates). With the proper plate voltages, the phosphorescent dot can be positioned anywhere on the screen. By using CRT phosphors that continue to phosphoresce for a brief time (up to 300 ms), visualization of the signal trace is facilitated.

Usually a sawtooth generator is used to supply the signal to horizontal deflection plates. At first the left plate is made more positive than the right, which starts the beam at the left edge of the screen. The voltage difference between the plates decreases linearly, which moves the beam towards the center of the screen. Then the right plate becomes more positive, drawing the beam to the right side of the screen. As the beam ends the sweep at the right edge of the screen, it returns instantaneously to the left plate, which now is positive. This portion is called the retrace. The sequence then repeats. The rate at which the beam moves across the screen is controlled by the sawtooth generator. This can be varied in steps so that the screen is horizontally calibrated in milliseconds (or microseconds) per centimeter. Duration or latency are calculated along the X axis, multiplying the distance by the horizontal scale.

The vertical or Y axis deflection is controlled by the output of the amplifier. The vertical deflection factor is called sensitivity and is related to the voltage of the signal at the input of the amplifier. These units are in millivolts (or microvolts) per centimeter. A sensitivity of 5 mV per cm means that the beam will move vertically (either up or down, depending on the polarity of the input voltage) 1 cm for every 5 mV difference in voltage at the amplifier input. The voltage of a waveform is determined by multiplying the corresponding vertical deflection by the sensitivity. The result is an amplitude versus time display (oscilloscope) of the recorded activity.

A third axis of the display is intensity, and is referred to as the Z axis. This axis is used when the sweep is retraced. As the beam retraces, the Z axis is modulated so that the intensity is very low and the retracing beam is not visible. Another term for this is blanking.

The sawtooth generator, which gives rise to the time or X axis sweep, may be left in a free-run or continuous mode while viewing ongoing electromyography. Alternatively, a triggered mode can be used. The sweep is initiated by the amplified signal, retraces, then holds (no beam is visible with the Z axis off) until the next signal triggers the sweep again. The operator manually selects the trigger level. The sweep may also be triggered externally, by devices such as an electrical stimulator. If the stimulus initiates the sweep, the latency of the response can be measured. When the response to stimulation contains early and late components, the sweep time must be set to accommodate the later response. This results in poor horizontal resolution. One solution is to use a rapid sweep, display the initial response on the first half of the screen, hold the sweep at that point while no response is generated, and then resume the rapid sweep in time for the later response. Thus only the segments of interest are displayed.

Some applications may require that two channels be observed simultaneously. This is accomplished by chopping the signal, alternately connecting the output of two amplifiers to the vertical deflection plates. This is done thousands of times per second. In addition, a DC offset signal is added to one of the signals, so that it is displaced vertically from the other signal. During the transition from displaying one amplifier output to the other, the intensity is blanked so that the display appears as two solid traces, without any transitions between.

## Storing the signal

The standard oscilloscope (with a long-persistence phosphor) and an audio amplifier/ speaker are adequate for most applications. A permanent copy may be desirable to provide an objective patient record. The standard storage oscilloscope, used with a Polaroid camera, provides a relatively inexpensive method. The storage oscilloscope in the store mode retains and displays the waveform. With a storage oscilloscope, one may repeat a trial, with the beginning of each response erasing the previous response, until a clean response is obtained. Then the stored trace is photographed. Alternatively, several responses may be stored on the screen if each trace is vertically or Y-shifted from the preceding trace.

After a waveform is stored, a cursor is helpful in accurately measuring latencies. In early instruments the marker was added at the time of recording, but each change in marker position required a new stimulus. A technique of displaying a nonstoring marker on a stored display was developed, so that various measurements could then be made without repeating the shock.

Another method of storage is digital. The signal is conditioned by an amplifier; converted to a series of numbers by an analog-digital converter; then stored in memory. Recently digital memory has become more popular and is offered by major manufacturers at a reasonable cost.

Several other methods, in addition to the instant camera, have been used for producing permanent records. Film can be used to record ongoing data from the face of the CRT. To do this the horizontal sweep of the oscilloscope is disabled, causing the trace to move only in the vertical direction. The film is then moved to provide the time axis. With sufficient film speed, the fastest activity can be recorded. Delay caused by film processing has been circumvented by ultraviolet-sensitive instant image papers or rapid processors. However, these are expensive and the images are not truly permanent. Another process for permanently recording high-frequency signals involves a technique similar to that used in copy machines. As paper is drawn over a grid of wire, a static electrical charge is placed on the surface in the appropriate spot. A suspension of graphite is used to develop the image. The particles settle on the charged area of the paper.

## Magnetic tape recording

Signals may be recorded in entirety on tape for future analysis, or the tape can be played back and only the sections of interest written out. The tape medium is relatively inexpensive and reuseable. However, the common home entertainment tape recorder is inadequate because of its variability in amplitude and speed. Amplitude variation is not as critical as speed variation, which would affect latency measurements. Specially designed tape transports and the use of special purpose tape reduce the amplitude variations from 30 percent or more to less than 10 percent. With amplitude modulation (AM), the signal is recorded directly (direct mode) on tape. Disadvantages of this type of recording include amplitude variability and a limited low-frequency response of approximately 100 Hz. With frequency modulation (FM), the incoming potentials determine the frequency of a signal generator whose output is then recorded on tape; that is, the potential is carried by the signal from the generator. Thus, amplitude is converted to frequency and recorded. Frequency is then converted to amplitude on playback. FM recording has no low frequency limit and amplitude variation in the carrier signal has little effect on the output. However, the high-frequency response, which is proportional to tape speed, is only one tenth or less than that of the direct mode recording. Higher tape speeds must be used to cover the bandwidth of electromyographic signals.

# SIGNAL PROCESSING

New technology in microcomputers has been widely applied to the processing of conditioned electrical signals.[2,3] This includes signal display, memory, frequency analysis, and averaging. An excellent review of signal analysis is available.[1]

The microprocessor is becoming common in electromyographic instrumentation. In the past, signal processing was performed by large, central computing facilities or by specialized instruments that were expensive but limited in capability. Now the popularity of small home and office computers has provided a wide range of microcomputers and peripheral equipment at relatively low prices. Special computations, which previously required recording the data on tapes in a laboratory and processing them at a computer center for later analysis, are now performed in the laboratory by a portable microcomputer. In the near future, circuit boards within the electromyography instruments will provide complex signal processing.

One contribution of microcomputers has been to provide storage and hard copy of the signal. The biologic signal is amplified and filtered and then input to an analog-to-digital converter (A/D). At discrete points in time input voltages are converted to numbers and stored at different points (addresses in memory). The points can then be transferred at high speed from memory onto an oscilloscope on which (if there are enough points) the display appears as a solid line. Alternatively, they can be read back slowly to be displayed by a standard, inexpensive plotter.

Another logical application is signal averaging. This is particularly useful for low amplitude sensory responses. Any portion of the signal that is time-locked to the stimulus will be preserved as the signal is averaged. Ongoing activity or noise that is not temporally related to the stimulus will be positive one time, negative another, and will tend to average to zero. Single responses that are barely detectable can thus be greatly enhanced. This also permits use of stimuli much lower in intensity. A unique corollary of signal averaging is reverse averaging. Signals can be processed and stored successively until a motor response is seen. The processor can then store a portion of data that has occurred before the motor response. This process can be repeated until several preresponse waveforms are averaged.

Microcomputers can be programmed to find peaks, display latencies, calculate nerve conduction velocities, and list normal values. Clinical history, data, and results can also be stored on flexible disks for mass storage. In addition to assisting with standard electromyographic recording, the processor can perform analyses that have been too complex or unavailable until recently. One popular use is digital filtering of the stored signal. The biologic signal may be recalled from memory, smoothed and measured, while the signal remains stored in its original form for comparison. The raw signal can be rectified and digitally summed (integrated) to provide a measure of relative activity, or it may be digitally differentiated to enhance rate of change. Another promising application of the microprocessor is the extraction of an objective measure from waveforms. The Fourier transform, which breaks down a given signal into its various frequency components, represents one example. These techniques will allow different laboratories to compare data and greatly expand the data base.

The microprocessor-based system is very attractive, because only programs need be changed as new techniques are developed. Fixed programs may be contained in integrated circuits. However, the electromyographer must recognize that these instruments will not make electromyography simpler. They will, if properly used, provide a useful adjunct, speed up diagnosis, and make diagnosis more reliable. They will not operate at the touch of a button. Indeed, the operator will have to be more sophisticated to run the instrument properly and to understand its advantages and disadvantages.

# REFERENCE SOURCES

1. COOPER, R, OSSELTON, JW, AND SHAW, JC: *EEG Technology,* ed 3. Butterworth & Co, Boston, 1980.

2. GANS, BM: *Signal extraction and analysis. A primer for clinical electromyographers.* Minimonograph #12, American Association of Electromyography and Electrodiagnosis, 1979.

3. REINER, S AND BOGOFT, JB: *Instrumentation.* In JOHNSON, EW (ED): *Practical Electromyography.* Williams & Wilkins, Baltimore, 1980.

4. McGILL, KC, ET AL: *On the nature and elimination of stimulus artifact in nerve signals evoked and recorded using surface electrodes.* I EEE Trans Biomed Eng BME-29:129, 1982.

5. STOLOV, W: *Instrumentation and Measurement in Electrodiagnosis.* Minimonograph #16, American Association of Electromyography and Electrodiagnosis, Rochester, Minnesota, 1981.

6. STRONG, P: *Amplifiers.* In: *Biophysical Measurements.* (Tektronix part no. 062-1247-00) Tektronix, Inc., Beaverton, Oregon, 1973.

7. WALKER, DD AND KIMURA, J: *A fast-recovery electrode amplifier for electrophysiology.* Electroenceph Clin Neurophysiol 45:789, 1978.

# C. ELECTRICAL SAFETY

All devices leak some current to their cases and patient leads. If this becomes excessive, and the ground fails, current can flow through the patient to ground. Most electrical safety recommendations are concerned with detecting or preventing loss of ground and excessive leakage current. All personnel involved in recording bioelectrical potentials should be briefed on electrical safety. Furthermore, measures intended to insure safety, such as effective grounding, minimizing leakage current, and removing ground loops, also greatly reduce recording interference.

Increasing concern for patient safety over the last 10[9] years is reflected in documents that regulate the manufacture and maintenance of instruments and the wiring in both hospitals and private offices.[6, 8, 11, 12] Official recommendations pertaining to such factors as leakage current and ground integrity are changing. The importance of these recommendations will be discussed and typical limits given as guidelines.[1] The electromyographer should understand the rationale for safe technique to cope with unfamiliar situations and revisions of the safety standards.[2]

# GENERAL ELECTRICAL SAFETY

## Electrical power distribution

Electrical power is transmitted to communities at high voltages to minimize power loss. Transformers reduce the high voltage to 120 volts alternating current (VAC) used in the home and hospital (App. Fig. 2-26). As the power enters the building, one side (called neutral) is grounded. The other line (termed hot) is 120 VAC with respect to neutral, or ground. Thus, one need only touch the hot side and any ground to receive a shock. Normally one would not come in direct contact with a hot line, but there are many opportunities for indirect contact.

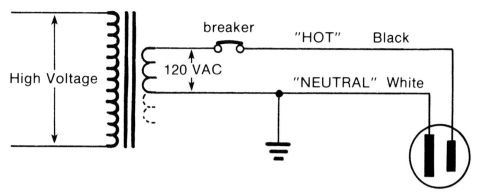

Appendix Figure 2-26

Simplified diagram of power distribution to outlets in the hospital and home. The longer slot of the outlet is (if wired correctly) connected to the grounded neutral line. The shorter slot is connected to the "HOT" side of the line.

Theoretically, current enters an instrument or appliance, flows through the electronics, and exits. In practice, some of the current leaks to the case or chassis of the instrument (App. Fig. 2-27). Therefore electrical hazards abound wherever contacts with ground are plentiful, as in bathrooms, kitchens, basements, outdoors, and other wet areas.

A third wire (ground) added to the outlet circumvents this problem (App. Fig. 2-28). The chassis of the instrument is connected to this ground so that current leaking to the chassis will flow harmlessly to ground[5] (App. Fig. 2-29).

The grounded three-wire system is a necessity in the hospital where: 1. Grounds are abundant, 2. Many instruments may be attached to the patient, resulting in multiple sources of leakage current, 3. Attachment of electrodes bypasses the insulating, outer layer of skin, 4. Instruments and outlets receive constant, rough handling, and 5. The patient may be weak, unable to withdraw from a shock, and susceptible to lower levels of current than normal.

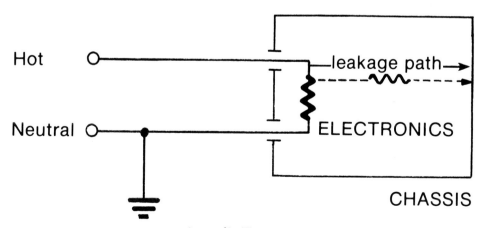

Appendix Figure 2-27

Ideally current should enter an instrument, flow through the electronics and exit. In practice, some current flows to the chassis of the instrument. If a grounded person were to touch the instrument, this *leakage current* would flow through him to ground.

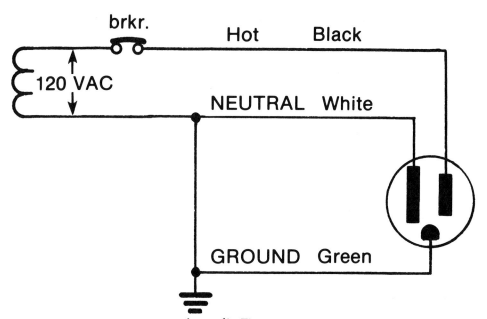

Appendix Figure 2-28

An extra terminal is added to the three wire/grounded outlet. A separate green wire is connected to the building ground.

## Leakage current and loss of ground

Although it would seem that the third wire (ground) eliminates need for concern about leakage current, a break in the ground path would allow the leakage current to flow to the patient or operator. In electromyography the patient is grounded (via amplifier ground lead) to avoid excessive interference. If, for example, the ground pin of the power plug were to break off, the leakage current normally flowing to the outlet ground could now flow to the patient through the amplifier ground lead. The patient need only be in contact with an operational ground (such as another instrument or a grounded bed) to complete the circuit. Thus a hazard exists when there is *excessive leakage current* and *loss of chassis ground*. Electrical safety standards and inspections are aimed at the detection and prevention of these two conditions.

## Documents concerned with patient safety

The National Electrical Code of the National Fire Protection Association (NFPA) includes a section entitled "Electricity in Health Care Facilities."[8] This document, which specifies the wiring of the laboratory (as opposed to the wiring of the instrument), is often called the Code and applies to the private office as well as the hospital. This section requires, among other things, that all outlets in the patient area have a separate third wire for grounding.[7] In the past the U-shaped outlet ground was often connected to the metal conduit that contained the hot and neutral wires. Paint, corrosion, and poor installation of the conduit often made this ground connection ineffective.

One of the documents concerned with the electrical safety of instruments is Underwriters Laboratories' "Standard for Medical and Dental Equipment, UL544." This standard specifies the construction, performance (including leakage current and grounding), and labelling of medical instruments. Instruments must be submitted to rigorous tests in order to be listed under UL544. Requirements for initial and periodic

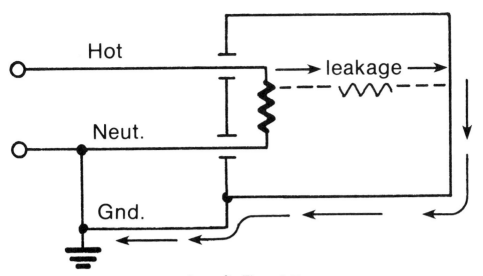

Appendix Figure 2-29

The third connection, ground, returns the leakage current harmlessly to the power distribution system.

inspection of wiring and medical instruments are included in the Joint Commission on Accreditation of Hospitals' "Functional Safety and Sanitation"[6] as well as the Veterans Administration Circular 10-77-111.[12] A summary of standards affecting hospitals may be found in the "Hospital Electrical Standards Symposium."[3]

# PROTOCOL FOR MAINTAINING SAFE OPERATION

## Ongoing electrical safety tests

It is the responsibility of the director of the laboratory to verify that laboratory wiring and medical instruments are periodically inspected. Small or private laboratories may find it necessary to perform the tests themselves. A multi-function electrical safety test instrument will cost from $500 to $1000 and requires training in its use.

Outlets in the laboratory should be checked at regular intervals, at least once a year. The tests include polarity (that is, the longer slot of the outlet, neutral, should be at 0 V; the shorter slot, hot, at 120 V; and the U-shaped terminal, ground, at 0 V). Contact tension, the ability of the receptacle to hold each pin of the plug, is especially important for the ground pin. The quality of each outlet ground is measured with an ohmmeter which can resolve a few milliohms. The resistance between each outlet ground and a common ground point should be no more than 0.20 ohms (0.10 ohms for new installations). An equipotential ground bus may be used to ground larger metal objects in the room or provide a redundant ground for electrically operated instruments. The voltage on outlet grounds, measured in reference to the common ground point, should be less than 20 mV. Although the National Electrical Code allows 500 mV, this would indicate a problem developing in the grounding circuitry.

The instrument must also be tested for ground integrity. The path from the instrument chassis to the ground pin on the power plug should not exceed 0.15 ohms. The instrument cord should be moved vigorously during this test to detect any intermittent problems.

The chassis leakage current is measured by disconnecting the ground, placing a load between the chassis and ground, and measuring the current flowing through the load (App. Fig. 2-30). Since threshold of perception and the physiologic effect of current varies with frequency,[10] a load is used that simulates the physiologic response to various frequencies. Instrument leakage is also tested with the polarity of the outlet connection reversed. This is done because some outlets may be incorrectly wired and the leakage current in this instance could be appreciably higher. The leakage current measured with the instrument both on and off, normal and reverse polarity, should be less than 100 μA.

Patient-lead leakage current is measured by placing the load between a patient lead and ground. Again the measurement is made with the instrument ungrounded, with polarity both normal and reversed, and with power on and off. The limit for lead leakage current is 50 μA. Since the patient is connected to a ground lead, this lead must also be tested. If the instrument uses a patient ground lead that is directly connected to the chassis or power ground, the patient lead leakage (ground) will equal the chassis leakage. In this case the chassis leakage current (above) will also be limited to 50, not 100 μA.

The JCAH Accreditation Manual for Hospitals requires that policies and procedures be established for the above tests and that corrective measures be taken when the limits are exceeded.

## Routine laboratory protocol

Laboratory personnel should remove any two-wire (ungrounded) devices (TV, clock, radio, lamp, and other electrical instruments) from the patient area. Liquids must be kept off, out of, and away from the instrument. Spilled liquids can increase leakage current and corrode the ground connection. Daily instrument inspections should include looking for instrument spills, frayed cords, broken plugs, and plugs not fully inserted in outlets. Employees should be initially briefed on electrical safety protocol and given annual reviews.

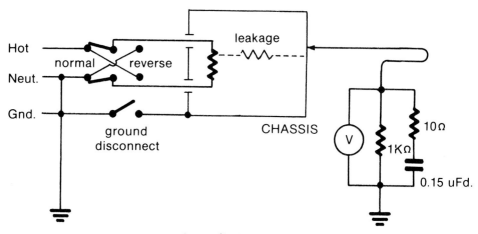

Appendix Figure 2-30

Chassis leakage becomes important when the ground fails. If a grounded person were to touch the case (or be attached to the ground electrode of the instrument), the current would flow through the person. This current is measured by intentionally disconnecting the ground and measuring the voltage across a grounded network in contact with the chassis. This network simulates the physiologic sensitivity to various frequencies. The hot and neutral lines are also reversed to simulate the effect of an improperly wired outlet.

## Special precautions during portable recordings

Special precautions should be taken during recordings performed outside the laboratory. Written policies and procedures must also be established for precautions to be observed during portable recordings. Instruments used portably are subject to rough treatment and age much faster. The electrical environment at a remote site is usually unknown. A major problem may arise if the instrument plugs and receptacles are not Hospital Grade, and are unable to maintain high contact tension. Standard outlets may be initially satisfactory, but their contact tension drops to less than an ounce after a few uses.

The measures mentioned above for the fixed laboratory instrument must also be followed when recording portably. After arriving at the recording site one should again check the physical condition of the instrument, looking for spills and damaged cords or plugs. Extension cords add another source of leakage current as well as another set of contacts where the ground connection might be interrupted. The patient should not be connected when an instrument is turned on or off, since surges of current may occur at this time.

The patient ground lead should ideally incorporate some current-limiting device. A ground lead connected directly to the circuit ground provides a low impedance path to ground for leakage current from the electromyograph (and other instruments), should its ground fail. The other pathways for leakage—through the amplifier inputs—have impedance on the order of a few thousands ohms. For maximum safety when recording portably it may be desirable to use isolated inputs on all leads. Isolated inputs can be connected directly to 120 VAC and the resulting current will be less than 20 μA. If the instrument were to fail, very little current could flow to the patient.

Devices connected to the patient should all be plugged into the same group of outlets because different grounds may not be the same potential. Current could flow from one grounded instrument, through the patient, to an instrument connected to another ground. The difference in voltage between two widely spaced grounds may be caused by leakage currents or fault currents flowing through the room from other instruments. If a ground path is broken and the patient is connected through instruments to grounds on either side of the break, all of the current could flow through the patient. Magnetic fields from motors, transformers, and other electrical devices induce current in the gound lead. If the patient is connected to two widely spaced outlets a ground loop is formed.[10] This loop acts like the secondary of a transformer, producing little voltage but considerable current. If only current-limited grounds are connected to the patient and all instruments are connected to the same area, these problems will be alleviated.

# THE ELECTRICALLY SENSITIVE PATIENT

## Inherent body protection from electrocution

The human body is protected from electrical shock by the high resistance of dry skin. In the hospital this is often violated by electrodes, transducers, and other devices. The risk is offset by providing good grounding systems and instruments with low leakage current. The large amount of tissue that surrounds the heart provides another form of protection to the organ most sensitive to electrical shock. Current flowing from arm to arm will spread as it enters the trunk, with only a small portion (perhaps 1/1000) of the total current flowing through the sensitive part of the heart. However, this second form of protection is bypassed when conductors, such as pacemaker leads or dye injection catheters, are inserted directly into the heart. For example, if a grounded catheter is within the heart and an instrument is leaking current to the patient, all the current would be directed to the heart. Or if the catheter is connected to some device that is leaking current, it would flow through the heart to any ground. Thus, whether the catheter is the sink for or the source of external current, the effect is the same. The term microshock has been used to describe this situation in which very small currents can be lethal.

Electrically sensitive patients can be affected by small voltages and currents such as those between two outlet grounds. Thus, extra care must be taken in grounding instruments in the room of an electrically sensitive patient. A limit of 20 $\mu$A has been set as the maximum acceptable leakage current for the electrically sensitive patient.[1] It would take a voltage difference of only 20 mV to produce 20 $\mu$A in the standard test 1 K ohm load.

## Isolated inputs

Two common fallacies should be pointed out. First, battery operated devices are not inherently safe. Battery voltages are well above the 20 mV calculated to induce 20 $\mu$A in the standard 1 K ohm load. Battery operated devices should also be UL544 listed. Second, a patient is not necessarily safe when his ground lead is removed. Leakage current flows not only to the ground lead but also into the amplifier inputs. These inputs present very high input impedance only as long as the input voltage is kept low. When input voltage becomes very high (that is, a few volts), the input impedance drops significantly and allows a large current to flow, unless isolated inputs are used. At present most hospitals require that any instrument connected to an electrically sensitive patient or neonate have isolated inputs. These inputs, as previously described, can withstand 120 VAC and pass less than 20 $\mu$A current. Catheters are now being made that are also electrically isolated.

# SPECIAL CIRCUITS AND DEVICES ENCOUNTERED IN THE HOSPITAL

## Isolated power systems

The term isolated power is unrelated to isolated inputs. One problem, stated earlier, is that one side of the standard power system is grounded. If neither side is grounded, a person has to make contact with both sides of the power line to receive a shock. This is the concept of the isolated power supply. Isolated power is usually supplied by a 1:1 transformer, with the secondary floating, so that neither side is connected to ground.[4] A healthy person can come into direct contact with either side of the line and only a limited amount of current will flow. However, this current can be 100 times the safe limit for the electrically sensitive patient. Thus isolated power systems do not protect this class of patient. Isolated power was required in surgery suites where everyone is grounded to prevent a static discharge in an explosive atmosphere. Fixed location isolated power supplies have two disadvantages. First of all they are expensive. Second the lines must be continually checked for isolation, to ensure that neither side is grounded. One type of device used for this purpose generates interference on the power line, and this interference often finds its way into the inputs of physiologic amplifiers. Small isolation transformers, which do not have these disadvantages, are now found in portable medical instrumentation systems. In portable systems there may be several line-operated devices with the total leakage current well in excess of limits. If they are all operated from an isolated transformer, the leakage current is essentially only that of the transformer.

## Redundant ground bus and ground fault interrupter

Another safety feature is the redundant ground bus. Portable instruments often have an extra cable for grounding. This cable plugs into a ground bus, which is tied into the outlet grounds. If the ground path in the power cord were to break, the instrument would still be grounded through this redundant ground.

The ground fault interrupter (GFI) is found in wet areas of the home as well as the hospital. The GFI senses the current flowing through the hot and neutral conductors supplying an outlet. Normally this will sum to zero (the current leaving on the hot line will return on the neutral). If a small difference develops (usually 5 mA) the GFI will disconnect the power. Thus if a person touches the hot line, returning some of the current through ground (ground fault) instead of through neutral, power is interrupted. These GFIs are found, for example, in hydrotherapy where patients and staff are well grounded and are in contact with electrically operated equipment. The GFI can only be used in areas where the power can be interrupted: Areas with life sustaining instruments must be excluded. As with isolated power the trip-level of 5 mA makes it useless in cases that involve the electrically sensitive patient.

# REFERENCE SOURCES

1.  AAMI: *Safe Current Limits for Electromedical Apparatus.* Association for the Advancement of Medical Instrumentation (AAMI), Arlington, Virginia, 1978.

2.  AAMI: *Interim Rationale Statement for the American National Standard: Safe Current Limits for Electromedical Apparatus.* Association for the Advancement of Medical Instrumentation (AAMI), Arlington, Virginia, 1980.

3.  American Society for Hospital Engineering: *Hospital Electrical Standards Compendium.* American Society for Hospital Engineering, Chicago, Illinois, 1981.

4.  DALZIEL, CF: *Electric shock hazards.* IEEE Spectrum 9 (2):41, 1972.

5.  HATCH, DJ AND RABER, MB: *Grounding and safety.* IEEE Trans Biomed Eng BME-22:62, 1975.

6.  Joint Commission on Accreditation of Hospitals: *Functional Safety and Sanitation.* In: *Accrediation Manual for Hospitals.* Joint Commission on Accreditation of Hospitals, Chicago, Illinois, 1982 Edition.

7.  MCPARTLAND, JF, MCPARTLAND, JM, AND MCPARTLAND, GI: *McGraw-Hill's National Electrical Code Handbook,* ed 17. McGraw-Hill, New York, 1981.

8.  National Fire Protection Association: Article 517. *Health Care Facilities.* In: *National Electrical Code,* NFPA 70-1981. National Fire Protection Association, Boston, Massachusetts, 1981.

9.  SEABA, P: *Electrical safety.* Am J EEG Technol 20:1, 1980.

10. STRONG, P: *Grounding-safety.* In: *Biophysical Measurements,* (Tektronix part no. 062-1247-00) Tektronix, Inc., Beaverton, Oregon, 1973.

11. Underwriters Laboratories, Inc.: *Standard for Medical and Dental Equipment,* UL544, ed 2. Underwriters Laboratories, Inc., Northbrook, Illinois, 1980.

12. Veterans Administration: *Veterans Administration Documents on Electrical Safety and Service Manuals.* J Clin Eng 3:64, 1978.

# GLOSSARY*

**Absolute Refractory Period —** See *Refractory Period.*

**Accommodation —** The reduced efficacy of a prolonged constant current or a gradually increasing current in generating action potentials from nervous tissue.

**Accommodation Curve —** A curve obtained by plotting the strength of current (in multiples of *Rheobase*) required to produce a response from an excitable tissue against the time required by a slowly rising current pulse to reach that value.

**Action Current —** The electrical current associated with an *Action Potential.*

**Action Potential —** (Abbr. *AP*). Strictly defined, the all-or-none, self-propagating, non-decrementing voltage change recorded from an excitable cell. The source of the action potential should be specified, e.g. nerve (fiber) action potential or muscle (fiber) action potential. Commonly, the term refers to the nearly synchronous summated action potentials of a group of cells, e.g., *Motor Unit Potential.* To avoid ambiguity in reference to the recording of nearly synchronous summated action potentials of nerve and muscle as done in nerve conduction studies, it is recommended that the terms *Compound Nerve Action Potential* and *Compound Muscle Action Potential* be used, respectively, or the specific named responses, e.g., *M Wave, F Wave, H wave, R1 and R2 Waves.*

**Active Electrode —** Synonymous with *Exploring Electrode.* See *Recording Electrode.*

**Adaptation —** A transient state at the initiation of an abrupt depolarization in which the impulse frequency first increases and then diminishes before the cell reaches a steady firing frequency.

**After Discharge —** Repetitive electrical firing that persists after initiation by some other process, usually muscle contraction. It may have variable form and be regular or irregular at long or short intervals.

---

* Reprinted with permission from *A Glossary of Terms Used in Clinical Electromyography*, 1980. Compiled by the Nomenclature Committee: the American Association of Electromyography and Electrodiagnosis: George H. Kraft, Chairman; Jasper R. Daube; Joel A. DeLisa; Joseph Goodgold; Charles K. Jablecki; Edward H. Lambert; J. A. Simpson; Albrecht Struppler; and David O. Wiechers.

**Afterpotential** — Membrane potential following the spike component of an *Action Potential* and not yet returned to a steady resting value. It first has a positive phase (positive afterpotential), which is followed by a negative phase (negative afterpotential).

**Amplitude** — With reference to an *Action Potential,* the maximum voltage difference between two points, usually baseline to peak or peak to peak. By convention, the amplitude of the *Compound Muscle Action Potential* is measured from the baseline to the most negative peak. In contrast, the amplitude of a *Compound Sensory Nerve Action Potential, Motor Unit Potential, Fibrillation Potential, Positive Sharp Wave, Fasciculation Potential,* and most other *Action Potentials* is measured from the most positive to the most negative peak.

**Anodal Block** — A local block of nerve conduction caused by hyperpolarization of the nerve cell membrane by an electrical stimulus. See *Stimulating Electrode.*

**Anode** — The positive terminal of a source of electrical current.

**Antidromic** — Said of an action potential or of the stimulation causing the action potential that propagates in the direction opposite to the normal (dromic or *Orthodromic*) one for that fiber—i.e., conduction along motor fibers toward the spinal cord and conduction along sensory fibers away from the spinal cord. Contrast with *Orthodromic.*

**Artifact** — A voltage change generated by a biological or nonbiological source other than the ones of interest. The *Stimulus Artifact* is the potential recorded at the time the stimulus is applied and includes the *Electrical* or *Shock Artifact,* which is a potential due to the volume conducted electrical stimulus. The stimulus and shock artifacts usually precede the activity of interest. A *Movement Artifact* refers to a change in the recorded activity due to movement of the recording electrodes.

**Auditory Evoked Potential** — Electrical waveform of biological origin elicited by a sound stimulus. See *Evoked Potential.*

**Backfiring** — Recurrent discharge of an antidromically activated motor neuron.

**BAER** — Abbreviation for brain stem auditory evoked response. Synonym: *Brain Stem Auditory Evoked Potential.*

**Baseline** — The potential difference recorded from the biological system of interest while the system is at rest.

**Benign Fasciculation** — Use of term discouraged. See *Fasciculation Potential.*

**BER** — Abbreviation for brain stem evoked response. See *Brain Stem Auditory Evoked Potential.*

**Bifilar Needle Electrode** — See *Bipolar Needle Electrode.*

**Biphasic Action Potential** — An action potential with two phases.

**Biphasic Spike Potential** — See *End-Plate Activity, Biphasic.*

**Bipolar Needle Electrode** — A recording electrode with two insulated wires side by side in a metal cannula whose bare tips act as the active and reference electrodes. The metal cannula may be grounded.

**Bizarre High-Frequency Discharge** — See *Complex Repetitive Discharge.*

**Bizarre Repetitive Potential** — See *Complex Repetitive Discharge.*

**Blink Reflex** — See *Blink Responses.*

**Blink Response** — Strictly defined, one of the *Blink Responses.* See *Blink Responses.*

**Blink Responses** — *Compound Muscle Action Potentials* evoked from obicularis oculi muscles as a result of brief electrical or mechanical stimuli to the cutaneous area innervated by the supraorbital (or less commonly the infraorbital) branch of the trigeminal nerve. Typically, there is an early compound muscle action potential (*R1 Wave*) ipsilateral to the stimulation site with a latency of about 10 msec and a bilateral late compound muscle action potential (*R2 Wave*) with a latency of approximately 30 msec. Generally, only the *R2 Wave* is associated with a visible twitch of the orbicularis oculi. The configuration, amplitude, duration, and latency of the two components, along with the sites of recording and the sites of stimulation, should be specified. Both *R1* and *R2 Waves* are probably due to a polysynaptic brain stem reflex, the *Blink Reflex*, with the afferent arc provided by the sensory branches of the trigeminal nerve and the efferent arc provided by the facial nerve motor fibers.

**Brain Stem Auditory Evoked Potential** — (Abbr. *BAEP*). Early (latency less than 10 msec) electrical waveforms of biological origin elicited in response to sound stimuli. See *Evoked Potential*.

**Brain Stem Auditory Evoked Response** — (Abbr. *BAER, BER*). Synonymous with *Brain Stem Auditory Evoked Potential*.

**Breakthrough Voluntary Activity** — A burst of voluntary activity occurring within the *S-X Interval*.

**BSAP** — Abbreviation for brief, small, abundant potentials. Use of term is discouraged. It is used to describe a recruitment pattern of brief-duration, small-amplitude, overly abundant motor unit action potentials. Quantitative measurements of motor unit potential duration, amplitude, numbers of phases, and recruitment frequency are to be preferred to qualitative descriptions such as this. See *Motor Unit Potential*.

**BSAPP** — Abbreviation for brief, small, abundant, polyphasic potentials. Use of term is discouraged. It is used to describe a recruitment pattern of brief-duration, small-amplitude, overly abundant, polyphasic motor unit action potentials. Quantitative measurements of motor unit potential duration, amplitude, numbers of phases, and recruitment frequency are to be preferred to qualitative descriptions such as this. See *Motor Unit Potential*.

**Cathode** — The negative terminal of a source of electrical current.

**Cerebral Evoked Potential** — Electrical waveforms of biological origin recorded over the head and elicited by sensory stimuli. See specific evoked potentials, e.g., *Somatosensory Evoked Potential, Visual Evoked Potential, Auditory Evoked Potential*.

**Chronaxie** — The time required for an electrical current stimulus at a voltage twice the *Rheobase* to elicit the first visible muscle twitch. See *Strength-Duration Curve*.

**Clinical Electromyography** — Loosely used to refer to all electrodiagnostic studies of peripheral nerves and muscle. See *Electrodiagnosis*.

**Coaxial Needle Electrode** — See synonym, *Concentric Needle Electrode*.

**Collision** — When used with reference to nerve conduction studies, the interaction of two action potentials propagated toward each other from opposite directions on the same nerve fiber so that the refractory periods of the two potentials prevent propagation past each other.

**Complex Action Potential** — See preferred term, *Serrated Action Potential*.

**Complex Motor Unit Potential** — See preferred term, *Serrated Action Potential*.

**Complex Repetitive Discharge** — Polyphasic or serrated action potentials that may begin spontaneously or after a needle movement. They have a uniform frequency, shape, and amplitude, with abrupt onset, cessation, or change in configuration. Amplitude ranges from 100 $\mu$V to 1 mV and frequency of discharge from 5 to 100 Hz.

**Compound Action Potential** — See *Compound Mixed Nerve Action Potential, Compound Motor Nerve Action Potential, Compound Nerve Action Potential, Compound Sensory Nerve Action Potential,* and *Compound Muscle Action Potential.*

**Compound Mixed Nerve Action Potential** — A compound nerve action potential is considered to have been evoked from afferent and efferent fibers if the recording electrodes detect activity on a mixed nerve with the electrical stimulus applied to a segment of the nerve which contains both afferent and efferent fibers.

**Compound Motor Nerve Action Potential** — A compound nerve action potential is considered to have been evoked from efferent fibers to a muscle if the recording electrodes detect activity only in a motor nerve or a motor branch of a mixed nerve, or if the electrical stimulus is applied only to such a nerve or a ventral root. The amplitude, latency, duration, and phases should be noted. See *Compound Nerve Action Potential.*

**Compound Muscle Action Potential** — The summation of nearly synchronous muscle fiber action potentials recorded from a muscle commonly produced by stimulation of the nerve supplying the muscle either directly or indirectly. Baseline-to-peak amplitude, duration, and latency of the negative phase should be noted, along with details of the method of stimulation and recording. Use of specific named potentials is recommended, e.g., *M Wave, F Wave, H Wave,* and *R1 Wave* or *R2 Wave (Blink Responses).*

**Compound Nerve Action Potential** — The summation of nearly synchronous nerve fiber action potentials recorded from a nerve trunk, commonly produced by stimulation of the nerve directly or indirectly. Details of the method of stimulation and recording should be specified, together with the fiber type (sensory, motor, or mixed).

**Compound Sensory Nerve Action Potential** — A compound nerve action potential is considered to have been evoked from afferent fibers if the recording electrodes detect activity only in a sensory nerve or in a sensory branch of a mixed nerve, or if the electrical stimulus is applied to such a nerve or a dorsal nerve root, or an adequate stimulus is applied synchronously to sensory receptors. The amplitude, latency, duration, and configuration should be noted. Generally, the amplitude is measured as the maximum peak-to-peak voltage, the latency as either the *Latency* to the initial deflection or the *Peak Latency* to the negative peak, and the duration as the interval from the first deflection of the waveform from the baseline to its final return to the baseline. The compound sensory nerve action potential has been referred to as the *Sensory Response* or *Sensory Potential.*

**Concentric Needle Electrode** — Recording electrode that measures the potential difference between the bare tip of a central insulated wire in the bare shaft of a metal cannula. The bare tip of the central wire (active electrode) is flush with the bevel of the cannula (reference electrode).

**Conditioning Stimulus** — A stimulus, preceding a *Test Stimulus,* used to modify the response elicited by the test stimulus alone. See *Stimulus.*

**Conduction Block** — Failure of an action potential to be conducted past a particular point in the nervous system. In practice, a conduction block is documented by demonstration of a reduction in amplitude of an evoked potential greater than that normally seen with electrical stimulation at two different points on a nerve trunk; anatomical nerve variations and technical factors related to nerve stimulation must be excluded as the source of the reduction in amplitude.

**Conduction Distance** — See *Conduction Velocity.*

**Conduction Time** — See *Conduction Velocity.*

**Conduction Velocity** — Speed of propagation of an *Action Potential* along a nerve or muscle fiber. The nerve fiber studied (motor, sensory, autonomic, or mixed) should be specified. For a nerve trunk, the maximum conduction velocity is calculated from the *Latency* of the evoked potential (muscle or nerve) at maximal or supramaximal intensity of stimulation at two different points. The distance between the two points (*Conduction Distance*) is divided by the difference between the corresponding latencies (*Conduction Time*). The calculated velocity represents the conduction velocity of the fastest fibers and is expressed as meters per second (m/sec). As commonly used, the term *Conduction Velocity* refers to the *Maximum Conduction Velocity*. By specialized techniques, the conduction velocity of other fibers can be determined as well and should be specified, e.g., minimum conduction velocity.

**Contraction** — A voluntary or involuntary reversible muscle shortening that may or may not be accompanied by *Action Potentials* from muscle. This term is to be contrasted with the term *Contracture,* which refers to a condition of fixed muscle shortening.

**Contracture** — An electrically silent, involuntary state of maintained muscle contraction, as seen in phosphorylase deficiency. The term is also used to refer to immobility of a joint due to other local processes.

**Cortical Evoked Potential** — See *Cerebral Evoked Potential.*

**Coupled Discharge** — See preferred term, *Late Component.*

**Cramp Discharge** — Repetitive firing of action potentials with the configuration of *Motor Unit Potentials* at a high frequency in a large area of muscle, associated with an involuntary, painful muscle contraction (cramp).

**Cycles Per Second** — Unit of frequency. (Abbr. *C/sec* or *CPS*). Preferred equivalent is *Hertz* (Abbr. *Hz*).


**Decrementing Response** — A progressive decline in the amplitude associated with a decrease in the area of the negative phase of the *M Wave* of successive responses to a series of supramaximal stimuli. The rate of stimulation and the number of stimuli should be specified. Contrast with *Incrementing Response.*

**Delay** — Interval between onset of oscilloscope sweep and onset of a stimulus. Had been used in the past to designate the interval from the stimulus to the response. Compare with *Latency.*

**Denervation Potential** — Use of term discouraged. See *Fibrillation Potential.*

**Depolarization** — A decrease in the electrical potential difference across a membrane from any cause, to any degree, relative to the normal resting potential. See *Polarization.*

**Depolarization Block** — Failure of an excitable cell to respond to a stimulus because of *Depolarization* of the cell membrane.

**Discharge** — Synonymous with *Action Potential.*

**Discharge Frequency** — The rate of repetition of an *Action Potential.* When potentials occur in groups, the rate of recurrence of the group and the rate of repetition of the individual components in the groups should be specified. See *Firing Rate.*

**Discrete Activity** — The pattern of electrical activity at full voluntary contraction of the muscle is reduced to the extent that each individual *Motor Unit Potential* can be identified. The firing frequency of each of these potentials should be specified together with the force of contraction.

**Distal Latency** — See *Motor Latency* and *Sensory Latency.*

**"Dive Bomber" Potential** — Use of term discouraged. See preferred term, *Myotonic Discharge.*

**Double Discharge** — Two action potentials of the same form and nearly the same amplitude, occurring consistently in the same relationship to one another at intervals of 2 to 20 msec. Contrast with *Paired Discharge.*

**Doublet** — Synonymous with *Double Discharge.*

**Duration** — The time during which something exists or acts. (1) The duration of individual potential *Waveforms* is defined as the interval from the first deflection from the baseline to its final return to the baseline, unless otherwise specified. One common exception is the duration of the *M Wave*, which usually refers to the interval from the deflection of the first negative phase from the baseline to its return to the baseline. (2) The duration of a single electrical stimulus refers to the interval of the applied current or voltage. (3) The duration of recurring stimuli or action potentials refers to the interval from the beginning to the end of the series.

**Earthing Electrode** — Synonymous with *Ground Electrode.*

**Electrical Artifact** — See *Artifact.*

**Electrical Silence** — The absence of measureable electrical activity due to biological or nonbiological sources. The sensitivity, or signal-to-noise level, of the recording system should be specified.

**Electrode** — A device capable of conducting electricity. The material (metal, fabric), size, configuration (disc, ring, needle), and location (surface, intramuscular, intracranial) should be specified. Electrodes may be used to record an electrical potential difference (*Recording Electrodes*) or to apply an electrical current (*Stimulating Electrodes*). In both cases, two electrodes are always required. Depending on the relative size and location of the electrodes, however, the stimulating or recording condition may be referred to as "Monopolar." See *Ground Electrode, Recording Electrode,* and *Stimulating Electrode.* Also see specific needle electrode configurations: *Monopolar, Concentric, Bipolar,* and *Multilead Needle Electrodes.*

**Electrodiagnosis** — (Abbr. *EDX*). General term used to refer to the recording of responses of nerves and muscle to electrical stimulation and the recording of insertional, spontaneous, and voluntary action potentials from muscle. It was originally used to refer to *Strength-Duration Curve* determinations and other early techniques.

**Electromyelography** — The recording and study of electrical activity from the spinal cord. The term is also used to refer to studies of electrical activity from the cauda equina.

**Electromyogram** — The record obtained by *Electromyography.*

**Electromyograph** — An instrument for detecting and displaying *Action Potentials* from muscle and nerve.

**Electromyography** — (Abbr. *EMG*). Strictly defined, the recording and study of insertional, spontaneous, and voluntary electrical activity of muscle. It is commonly used to refer to nerve conduction studies as well. Compare with *Clinical Electromyography* and the more general term, *Electrodiagnosis.*

**Electroneurography** — The recording and study of the action potentials of peripheral nerves. See preferred term, *Nerve Conduction Studies,* and the more general term, *Electrodiagnosis.*

**Electroneuromyography** — A newly fabricated word used to refer to the combined studies of *Electromyography* and *Electroneurography.* See preferred terms, *Clinical Electromyography* and *Electrodiagnosis.*

**Electrospinogram** — The record obtained by *Electromyelography.*

**End-Plate Activity** — Spontaneous electrical activity recorded with a needle electrode close to muscle end-plates. May be either of two forms:
    1. **Monophasic.** Low-amplitude (10–20) $\mu V$, short-duration (0.5–1 msec), monophasic (negative) potentials that occur in a dense, steady pattern and are restricted to a localized area of the muscle. Because of

the multitude of different potentials occcurring, the exact frequency, although appearing to be high, cannot be defined. These potentials are miniature end-plate potentials recorded extracellularly. This form of end-plate activity has been referred to as *End-Plate Noise* and is associated with a sound not unlike that of a seashell, which has been called a *Sea Shell Noise* or *Roar*.

2. **Biphasic.** Moderate-amplitude (100–300 $\mu$V), short-duration (2–4 msec), biphasic (negative-positive) spike potentials that occur irregularly in short bursts with a high frequency (50–100 Hz), restricted to a localized area within the muscle. These potentials are generated by muscle fibers excited by activity in nerve terminals. These potentials have been referred to as *Biphasic Spike Potentials*, *End-Plate Spikes*, and, incorrectly, "*Nerve*" *Potentials*.

**End-Plate Noise** — See *End-Plate Activity, Monophasic*.

**End-Plate Potential** — Graded, nonpropagated potential recorded by microelectrodes from muscle fibers in the region of the neuromuscular junction.

**End-Plate Spike** — See *End-Plate Activity, Biphasic*.

**End-Plate Zone** — The site of the neuromuscular junction, a localized area of the muscle fiber in which activity identified as end-plate activity may be recorded.

**Evoked Action Potential** — Action potential elicited by a stimulus.

**Evoked Compound Muscle Action Potential** — The electrical activity of a muscle produced by stimulation of the nerves supplying the muscle. Baseline-to-peak amplitude of the negative phase, duration of the negative phase, and *Latency* should be measured, and details of the method of stimulation should be recorded. See specific named potentials: *M Wave, F Wave, H Wave, R1 and R2 Waves*, and *Blink Responses*.

**Evoked Potential** — Electrical waveform elicited by and temporally related to a stimulus, most commonly an electrical stimulus delivered to a sensory receptor or nerve, or applied directly to a discrete area of the brain, spinal cord, or muscle. See *Auditory Evoked Potential, Brain Stem Auditory Evoked Potential, Spinal Evoked Potential, Somatosensory Evoked Potential, Visual Evoked Potential, Cerebral Evoked Potential, Compound Muscle Action Potential*, and *Compound Sensory Nerve Action Potential*.

**Evoked Response** — Tautology. Use of term discouraged. Suggested term is *Evoked Potential*.

**Excitability** — Capacity to be activated by or react to a stimulus.

**Excitatory Postsynaptic Potential** — (Abbr. *EPSP*). A local, graded depolarization of a neuron in response to activation by a nerve terminal at a synapse. Contrast with *Inhibitory Postsynaptic Potential*.

**Exploring Electrode** — Synonymous with *Active Electrode*. See *Recording Electrode*.

**Facilitation of Neuromuscular Transmission** — An increase in the amplitude of an end-plate potential of a muscle fiber with stimulation of the axon in a variety of physiological and pharmacological settings. Use of the term is not recommended for description of the phenomenon recorded in repetitive stimulation studies.

**Fasciculation** — The random, spontaneous twitching of a group of muscle fibers which may be visible through the skin. The electrical activity associated with the spontaneous contraction is called the *Fasciculation Potential*. Compare with *Myokymia*.

**Fasciculation Potential** — The electrical potential associated with *Fasciculation* which has dimensions of a motor unit potential that occurs spontaneously as a single discharge. Most commonly these potentials occur sporadically and are termed "single fasciculation potentials." Occasionally, the potentials occur as a grouped discharge and are termed "grouped fasciculation potentials." The occurrence of large numbers of either simple or grouped fasciculations may produce a writhing, vermicular movement of the skin called *Myokymia*. Use of the terms *Benign Fasciculation* and *Malignant Fasciculation* is discouraged. Instead, the configuration of the potentials, peak-to-peak amplitude, duration, number of phases, and stability of configuration, in addition to frequency of occurrence, should be specified.

**Fatigue** — Reduction in the force of contraction of muscle fibers as a result of repeated use or electrical stimulation. More generally, it is a state of depressed responsiveness resulting from protracted activity and requiring appreciable recovery time.

**Fiber Density** — (1) Anatomically, fiber density is a measure of the number of muscle or nerve fibers per unit area. (2) In single-fiber EMG, the fiber density is the mean number of muscle fiber potentials under voluntary control encountered during a systematic search. See *Single Fiber Electromyography*.

**Fibrillation** — The spontaneous contractions of individual muscle fibers which are ordinarily not visible through the skin. This term has been used loosely in electromyography for the preferred term, *Fibrillation Potential*.

**Fibrillation Potential** — The electrical activity associated with fibrillating muscle fibers, reflecting the action potential of a single muscle fiber. The action potentials may occur spontaneously or after movement of the needle electrode. The potentials usually occur repetitively and regularly. Classically, the potentials are biphasic spikes of short duration (usually less than 5 msec) with an initial positive phase and a peak-to-peak amplitude of less than 1 mV. The firing rate has a wide range (1–50 Hz) and often decreases just before cessation of an individual discharge. A high-pitched regular sound is associated with the discharge of fibrillation potentials and has been described in the old literature as "rain on a tin roof." In addition to this classic form of fibrillation potentials, *Positive Sharp Waves* may also be recorded from fibrillating muscle fibers; the difference in the configuration of the potentials is due to the position of the recording electrode.

**Firing Pattern** — Qualitative and quantitative description of the sequence of discharge of potential waveforms recorded from muscle or nerve.

**Firing Rate** — Frequency of repetition of a potential. The relationship of the frequency to the occurrence of other potentials and the force of muscle contraction may be described. See *Discharge Frequency*.

**Fractionation of Motor Unit Potentials** — Use of term discouraged. This term has been used to describe polyphasic, short-duration, low-amplitude motor unit potentials, a configuration thought to imply failure to activate all of the muscle fibers in a motor unit.

**F Reflex** — Use of term discouraged, as it is incorrect. No reflex is considered to be involved. See *F Wave*.

**Frequency** — Number of complete cycles of a repetitive waveform in 1 second. Measured in *Hertz* (Hz), a unit preferred to its equivalent, *Cycles Per Second* (C/sec).

**Frequency Analysis** — Determination of the range of frequencies composing a potential waveform, with a measurement of the absolute or relative amplitude of each component frequency. It is similar to the mathematical technique of Fourier analysis.

**F Response** — Synonymous with *F Wave*. See *F Wave*.

**Full Interference Pattern** — See *Interference Pattern*.

**F Wave** — A late compound action potential evoked intermittently from a muscle by a supramaximal electrical stimulus to the nerve. Compared with the maximal amplitude M wave of the same muscle, the F wave has a reduced amplitude and variable configuration and a longer and more variable latency. It can be found in many muscles of the upper and lower extremities, and the latency is longer with more distal sites of stimulation. The F wave is due to antidromic activation of motor neurons. It was named by Magladery and McDougal in 1950. Contrast with *H Wave*.

**G1, G2** — Synonymous with Grid 1, Grid 2. See *Recording Electrodes*.

**"Giant" Motor Unit Action Potential** — Use of term discouraged. It refers to a motor unit potential with a peak-to-peak amplitude and duration much greater than the range recorded in corresponding muscles in normal subjects of similar age. Quantitative measurements of amplitude and duration are preferable.

**Ground Electrode** — An electrode connected to a large conducting body (such as the earth) used as a common return for an electrical circuit and as an arbitrary zero potential reference point.

**Grouped Discharge** — Intermittent repetition of a group of *Action Potentials* with the same or nearly the same waveform and a relatively short interpotential interval within the group in comparison with the time interval between each group. It may occur spontaneously or with voluntary activity and may be regular or irregular in its firing pattern.

**Habituation** — Decrease in amplitude and/or duration of a response with repeated stimuli. Response may be eliminated.

**Hertz** — (Abbr. Hz). Unit of frequency representing cycles per second.

**Hoffman Reflex** — See *H Wave*.

**H Reflex** — Abbreviation for Hoffman reflex. See *H Wave*.

**H Response** — Synonymous with *H Wave*.

**H Wave** — A late compound muscle action potential having a consistent latency evoked regularly, when present, from a muscle by an electrical stimulus to the nerve. It is regularly found only in a limited group of physiologic extensors, particularly the calf muscles. The reflex is most easily obtained with the cathode positioned proximal to the anode. Compared with the maximal amplitude *M Wave* of the same muscle, the H wave has a reduced amplitude, a longer latency, and a lower optimal stimulus intensity; its configuration is constant. The latency is longer with more distal sites of stimulation. A stimulus intensity sufficient to elicit a maximal-amplitude M wave reduces or abolishes the H wave. The H wave is thought to be due to a spinal reflex, the Hoffman reflex, with electrical stimulation of afferent fibers in the mixed nerve to the muscle and activation of motor neurons to the muscle through a monosynaptic connection in the spinal cord. The reflex and wave are named in honor of Hoffman's description (1918). Compare with *F Wave*.

**Hyperpolarization** — See *Polarization*.

**Increased Insertional Activity** — See *Insertional Activity*.

**Incremental Response** — See synonym, *Incrementing Response*.

**Incrementing Response** — A progressive increase in amplitude associated with an increase in the area of the negative phase of the *M Wave* of successive responses to a series of supramaximal stimuli. The rate of stimulation and the number of stimuli should be specified. Contrast with *Decrementing Response*.

**Indifferent Electrode** — Synonymous with *Reference Electrode*. See *Recording Electrode*.

**Inhibitory Postsynaptic Potential** — (Abbr. *IPSP*). A local graded hyperpolarization of a neuron in response to activation at a synapse by a nerve terminal. Contrast with *Excitatory Postsynaptic Potential.*

**Injury Potential** — The potential difference between a normal region of the surface of a nerve or muscle and a region that has been injured; also called a demarcation potential. This potential was studied before intracellular recording was introduced. The injury potential approximates the potential across the membrane because the injured surface is almost at the potential of the inside of the cell. This term has been loosely used to describe *Insertional Activity* encountered in *Clinical Electromyography.*

**Insertional Activity** — Electrical activity caused by insertion or movement of a needle electrode. The amount of the activity may be described qualitatively as *Normal, Reduced, Increased,* or *Prolonged.*

**Interdischarge Interval** — Time between consecutive discharges of the same potential. Measurements should be made between the corresponding points on each waveform.

**Interference** — Unwanted electrical activity arising outside the system being studied.

**Interference Pattern** — Electrical activity recorded from a muscle with a needle electrode during maximal voluntary effort, in which identification of each of the contributing action potentials is not possible, because of the overlap or interference of one potential with another. When no individual potentials can be identified, this is known as a *Full Interference Pattern.* A *Reduced Interference Pattern* is one in which some of the individual potentials may be identified while other individual potentials cannot be identified because of overlapping. The term *Discrete Activity* is used to describe the electrical activity recorded when each of the motor unit potentials can be identified. It is important that the force of contraction associated with the interference pattern be specified.

**Interpotential Interval** — Time between two different potentials. Measurement should be made between the corresponding parts on each waveform.

**Intramuscular Electrode** — An electrode usually used for recording and usually shaped like a needle to facilitate placement within a muscle belly.

**Involuntary Activity** — Action potentials that are not under voluntary control. The condition under which they occur should be described, e.g., spontaneous, or, if elicited by a stimulus, the nature of the stimulus. Compare with *Spontaneous Activity.*

**Isoelectric Discharge** — Recording obtained from a pair of equipotential electrodes.

**Iterative Discharge** — See preferred term, *Repetitive Discharge.*


**Jitter** — Synonymous with "single fiber electromyographic jitter." Jitter is the variability of the *Interpotential Interval* between two muscle fiber action potentials belonging to the same motor unit. It is usually expressed quantitatively as the mean value of the difference between the interpotential intervals of consecutive discharges (the mean consecutive difference, abbr. MCD). Under certain conditions, jitter is expressed as the mean value of the difference between the interpotential intervals arranged in the order of decreasing interpotential intervals (the mean sorted difference, abbr. MSD).

**Jolly Test** — A technique, described in 1895 by Jolly, of application of a Faradic current to a motor nerve while recording the muscle contraction. This test has been refined and replaced by the technique of *Repetitive Stimulation* of motor nerves and the recording of successive M waves to detect a defect of neuromuscular transmission; use of the term is discouraged for modern testing techniques.

**Late Component of a Motor Unit Potential** — A potential separated from a *Motor Unit Potential* by a segment of baseline recording, but firing in a time-locked relationship to the motor unit potential.

**Late Response** — A general term used to describe an evoked potential having a longer latency than the *M Wave*. See *H Wave, F Wave*.

**Latency** — Interval between the onset of a stimulus and the onset of a response unless otherwise specified. Latency always refers to the onset unless specified, as in *Peak Latency*.

**Latency of Activation** — The time required for an electrical stimulus to depolarize a nerve. In the past this had been estimated to be 0.1 msec.

**Latent Period** — See synonym, *Latency*.

**Malignant Fasciculation** — Use of term discouraged. See *Fasciculation Potential*.

**Maximal Stimulus** — See *Stimulus*.

**Maximum Nerve Conduction Velocity** — See *Conduction Velocity*.

**Membrane Instability** — Tendency of a cell membrane to depolarize spontaneously or after mechanical irritation or voluntary activation.

**Microneurography** — The technique of recording peripheral nerve action potentials in man by means of intraneural microelectrodes.

**Miniature End-Plate Potential** — When recorded with microelectrodes, monophasic negative discharges with amplitudes less than 100 $\mu$V and duration of 4 msec or less, occurring irregularly and recorded in an area of muscle corresponding to the myoneural junction. They are thought to be due to small quantities (quanta) of acetylcholine released spontaneously. Compare with *End-Plate Activity*.

**Mixed Nerve Action Potential** — See *Compound Nerve Action Potential*.

**Monophasic Action Potential** — An action potential with one phase.

**Monphasic End-Plate Activity** — See *End-Plate Activity*.

**Monopolar Needle Electrode** — A solid wire, usually of stainless steel, coated, except at its tip, with an insulating material. Variations in voltage between the tip of the needle (active or exploring electrode) positioned in a muscle and a conductive plate on the skin surface or a bare needle in subcutaneous tissue (reference electrode) are measured. By convention, this recording condition is referred to as a monopolar needle electrode recording; it should be emphasized, however, that potential differences are always recorded between two electrodes.

**Motor Latency** — Interval between the onset of a stimulus and the onset of the resultant *Compound Muscle Action Potential*. The term may be qualified as *Proximal Motor Latency* or *Distal Motor Latency*, depending on the relative position of the stimulus.

**Motor Nerve Action Potential** — See *Compound Motor Nerve Action Potential*.

**Motor Nerve Conduction Velocity** — (Abbr. MNCV). See *Conduction Velocity*.

**Motor Point** — The point over a muscle where a contraction of a muscle may be elicited by a minimal-intensity, short-duration electrical stimulus.

**Motor Response** — Either (1) the compound muscle action potential recorded over a muscle with stimulation of the nerve to the muscle or (2) the muscle twitch or contraction elicited by stimulation of the nerve to a muscle. As commonly used, the motor response refers only to the evoked potential, the *M Wave*.

**Motor Unit** — The anatomical unit of an anterior horn cell, its axon, the neuromuscular junctions, and all of the muscle fibers innervated by the axon.

**Motor Unit Action Potential** — (Abbr. MUAP). See synonym, *Motor Unit Potential*.

**Motor Unit Potential** — (Abbr. MUP). Action potential reflecting the electrical activity of that part of a single anatomical motor unit that is within the recording range of an electrode. The action potential is characterized by its consistent appearance with and relationship to the force of a voluntary contraction of a muscle. The following parameters should be specified, quantitatively if possible, after the recording electrode is placed so as the minimize the *Rise Time* (which by convention should be less than 0.5 msec), which generally also maximizes the amplitude:

    I.  Configuration
- A. *Amplitude*, peak-to-peak ($\mu$V or mV)
- B. *Duration*, total (msec)
- C. Number of *Phases (Monophasic, Biphasic, Triphasic, Tetraphasic, Polyphasic)*
- D. Direction of each *Phase* (negative, positive)
- E. Number of *Turns of Serrated Potential*
- F. Variation of shape with consecutive discharges
- G. Presence of *Late Components*

    II.  *Recruitment* characteristics
- A. Threshold of activation (first recruited, low threshold, high threshold)
- B. *Onset Frequency* (Hz)
- C. *Recruitment Frequency* (Hz) or *Recruitment Interval* (msec) of individual potentials

Descriptive terms implying diagnostic significance are not recommended, e.g., *Myopathic, Neuropathic, Regeneration, Nascent, Giant, BSAP,* and *BSAPP.*

**Motor Unit Subunit** — Abandoned concept of muscle physiology. Fibers of a motor unit were considered to be arranged in groups of subunits containing an average of 10 fibers that fired synchronously. This is no longer accepted.

**Motor Unit Territory** — (1) The area in which *Motor Unit Potentials* from a single motor unit may be recorded with a *Rise Time* of less than 0.5 msec. (2) The area in a muscle over which the muscle fibers of an individual motor unit are distributed anatomically.

**Movement Artifact** — See *Artifact.*

**M Response** — See synonym, *M Wave.*

**MUAP** — Abbreviation for motor unit action potential. See synonym, *Motor Unit Potential.*

**Multielectrode** — See *Multilead Electrode.*

**Multilead Electrode** — Three or more insulated wires inserted through a common metal cannula with their bared tips at an aperture in the cannula and flush with the outer circumference of the cannula. The arrangement of the bare tips relative to the axis of the cannula and the distance between each tip should be specified.

**Multiple Discharge** — Four or more motor unit action potentials of the same form and nearly the same amplitude occurring consistently in the same relationship to one another. See *Double* and *Triple Discharge.*

**Multiplet** — See *Multiple Discharge.*

**MUP** — Abbreviation for *Motor Unit Potential.*

**Muscle Action Potential** — Strictly defined, the term refers to the action potential recorded from a single muscle fiber. However, the term is commonly used to refer to a compound muscle action potential. See *Compound Muscle Action Potential.*

**Muscle Fiber Conduction Velocity** — The speed of propagation of a single muscle fiber action potential, usually expressed as meters per second. The muscle fiber conduction velocity is usually less than most nerve conduction velocities, varies with the rate of discharge of the muscle fiber, and requires special techniques for measurement.

**Muscle Unit** — An anatomical term referring to the group of muscle fibers innervated by a single motor neuron. See *Motor Unit.*

**M Wave** — *A Compound Action Potential* evoked from a muscle by a single electrical stimulus to its motor nerve. By convention, the M wave elicited by supramaximal stimulation is used for motor nerve conduction studies. The recording electrodes should be placed so that the initial deflection of the evoked potential is negative. The *Latency*, commonly called *Motor Latency*, is the latency (milliseconds) to the onset of the first negative phase. The amplitude (millivolts) is the baseline-to-peak amplitude of the first negative phase, unless otherwise specified. The *Duration* (milliseconds) refers to the duration of the first negative phase, unless otherwise specified. Normally, the configuration of the M wave (usually biphasic) is quite stable with repeated stimuli at slow rates (1–5 Hz). See *Repetitive Stimulation.*

**Myokymia** — Involuntary, continuous quivering of muscle fibers which may be visible through the skin as a vermiform movement. It is associated with spontaneous, rhythmic discharge of *Motor Unit Potentials*. See *Myokymic Discharges, Fasciculation,* and *Fasciculation Potential.*

**Myokymic Discharges** — Action potentials with the configuration of *Motor Unit Potentials* that occur spontaneously, recur regularly, and may be associated with clinical myokymia. Two distinct firing patterns are recognized. Commonly, the discharges are grouped with a short period (up to a few seconds) of firing at a uniform rate (2–20 Hz) followed by a short period (up to a few seconds) of silence, with repetition of the same sequence for a particular potential. Less commonly, the potential recurs continuously at a fairly uniform firing rate (1–5 Hz). Myokymic discharges are a subclass of *Grouped Discharges* and *Repetitive Discharges.*

**Myopathic Motor Unit Potential** — Use of term discouraged. It is used to refer to low-amplitude, short-duration, polyphasic motor unit action potentials. The term incorrectly implies specific diagnostic significance of a motor unit potential configuration. See *Motor Unit Potential.*

**Myopathic Recruitment** — Use of term discouraged. It is used to describe an increase in the number of and firing rate of motor unit potentials compared with normal for the strength of muscle contraction.

**Myotonic Discharge** — Repetitive discharge of 20–80 Hz of biphasic (positive-negative) spike potentials less than 5 msec in duration or monophasic positive waves of 5–20 msec recorded after needle insertion, or less commonly after voluntary muscle contraction or muscle percussion. The amplitude and frequency of the potentials must both wax and wane to be identified as myotonic discharges. This change produces a characteristic musical sound in the audio display of the electromyograph due to the corresponding charge in pitch, which has been likened to the sound of a "dive bomber." Contrast with *Waning Discharge.*

**Myotonic Potential** — See preferred term, *Myotonic Discharge.*

**Myotonic Response** — Delayed relaxation of muscle after voluntary contraction or percussion and associated with a myotonic discharge. See *Myotonic Discharge.*

**Nascent Motor Unit Potential** — From the Latin *nascens,* to be born. Use of term is discouraged as it incorrectly implies diagnostic significance of a motor unit potential configuration. Term has been used to refer to very low-amplitude, long-duration, highly polyphasic motor unit potentials observed during early stages of reinnervation of muscle. See *Motor Unit Potential.*

**Nascent Unit** — Use of term discouraged. See *Nascent Motor Unit Potential.*

**Needle Electrode** — An electrode for recording or stimulating, shaped like a needle. See specific electrodes: *Bipolar Needle Electrode, Concentric Needle Electrode, Monopolar Needle Electrode, Multilead Electrode.*

**Nerve Action Potential** — Strictly defined, refers to an action potential recorded from a single nerve fiber. The term is commonly used to refer to the compound nerve action potential. See *Compound Nerve Action Potential.*

**Nerve Conduction Studies** — Refers to all aspects of electrodiagnostic studies of peripheral nerves. However, the term is generally used to refer to the recording and measurement of *Compound Nerve* and *Compound Muscle Action Potentials* elicited in response to a single supramaximal electrical *Stimulus* under standardized conditions that permit establishment of normal ranges of amplitude, duration, and latency of *Evoked Potentials* and the calculation of the *Maximum Conduction Velocity* of individual nerves. See *Compound Nerve Action Potential, Compound Muscle Action Potential, Conduction Velocity,* and *Repetitive Stimulation.*

**Nerve Conduction Velocity** — (Abbr. NCV). Loosely used to refer to the maximum nerve conduction velocity. See *Conduction Velocity.*

**Nerve Potential** — Equivalent to *Nerve Action Potential.* Also commonly, but inaccurately, used to refer to the biphasic form of *End-Plate Activity.* The latter use is incorrect because muscle fibers, not nerve fibers, are the source of these potentials.

**Nerve Trunk Action Potential** — See preferred term, *Compound Nerve Action Potential.*

**Neuromyotonia** — Clinical syndrome of continuous muscle fiber activity manifested as continuous muscle rippling and stiffness. It may be associated with a variety of electrical discharges.

**Neuromyotonic Discharges** — Bursts of *Motor Unit Potentials* firing at more than 150 Hz for ½ to 2 sec. The amplitude of the response typically wanes. Discharges may occur spontaneously or be initiated by needle movement.

**Neuropathic Motor Unit Potential** — Use of term discouraged. It is used to refer to abnormally high-amplitude, long-duration, polyphasic *Motor Unit Potentials.* The term incorrectly implies a specific diagnostic significance of a motor unit potential configuration. See *Motor Unit Potential.*

**Neuropathic Recruitment** — Use of term discouraged. It has been used to describe a recruitment pattern with a decreased number of *Motor Unit Potentials* firing at a rapid rate. See preferred terms, *Discrete Activity, Reduced Interference Pattern.*

**Noise** — Strictly defined, an *Artifact* consisting of low-amplitude, random potentials produced by an amplifier and unrelated to the input signal. It is most apparent when high gains are used. It is loosely used to refer to end-plate noise. Compare with *End-Plate Activity.*

**Onset Frequency** — The lowest stable frequency of firing for a single *Motor Unit Potential* that can be voluntarily maintained by a subject.

**Onset Latency** — Tautology. See *Latency.*

**Order of Activation** — The sequence of appearance of different *Motor Unit Potentials* with increasing strength of voluntary contraction. See *Recruitment.*

**Orthodromic** — Said of *Action Potentials* or stimuli eliciting action potentials propagated in the same direction as physiological conduction, e.g., motor nerve conduction away from the spinal cord and sensory nerve conduction toward the spinal cord. Contrast with *Antidromic.*

**Paired Discharge** — Two action potentials of the same form and nearly the same amplitude occurring consistently in the same relationship to each other at intervals of 20–80 msec. Contrast with *Double Discharge.*

**Paired Response** — Loosely used to refer to either the preferred term *Paired Discharge* or the preferred term *Late Component*.

**Paired Stimuli** — Two temporally linked stimuli. The time interval between the two stimuli and the intensity of each stimulus should be specified. The first is called the *Conditioning Stimulus* and the second the *Test Stimulus*.

**Parasite Potential** — See preferred term, *Late Component of a Motor Unit Potential*.

**Peak Latency** — Interval between the onset of a stimulus and a specified peak of the evoked potential (usually the negative peak).

**Phase** — That portion of a *Wave* between the departure from and the return to the *Baseline*.

**Polarization** — As used in neurophysiology, the presence of an electrical *Potential* difference across an excitable cell membrane. The potential across the membrane of a cell when it is not excited by input or spontaneously active is termed the *Resting Potential*; it is at a steady state with regard to the electrical potential difference across the membrane. *Depolarization* describes a decrease in polarization to any degree, relative to the normal resting potential. *Hyperpolarization* describes an increase in polarization relative to the resting potential. *Repolarization* describes an increase in polarization from the depolarized state toward, but not above, the normal or resting potential.

**Polyphasic Action Potential** — An *Action Potential* having five or more phases. See *Phase*. Contrast with *Serrated Action Potential*.

**Positive Sharp Wave** — Strictly defined, one form of electrical activity associated with fibrillating muscle fibers. It is recorded as a biphasic, positive-negative *Action Potential* initiated by needle movement and recurring in a uniform, regular pattern at a rate of 2–50 Hz, which may decrease just before cessation of discharge. The amplitude and duration vary considerably but the initial positive deflection is usually less than 5 msec in duration and up to 1 mV in amplitude. The negative phase is of low amplitude, with a duration of 10–100 msec. A sequence of positive sharp waves is commonly referred to as a *Train of Positive Sharp Waves*. Positive sharp waves are recorded from the damaged area of fibrillating muscle fibers. Loosely defined, positive sharp waves refer to any action potential recorded with the wave-form of a positive wave, without reference to the firing pattern or method of generation.

**Positive Wave** — Strictly defined, the positive phase of a waveform. Loosely defined, the term refers to a positive sharp wave. See *Positive Sharp Wave*.

**Postactivation Depression** — The reduction in the amplitude of an *Evoked Potential* in response to a single *Stimulus* which occurs after *Repetitive Stimulation* or after voluntary contraction.

**Postactivation Exhaustion** — The reduction of the amplitude associated with a decrease in the area of the negative phase of the initial *M Wave* and/or the exaggeration of the *Decrementing Response* seen 2–4 min after either a brief (10–30 sec), strong voluntary contraction or a period of nerve stimulation causing tetanic muscle contraction. Compare with *Postactivation Facilitation*.

**Postactivation Facilitation** — The increase in amplitude associated with an increase in the area of the negative phase of the initial *M Wave* and/or the diminution of the *Decrementing Response* seen a few seconds after either a brief (10–30 sec), strong voluntary contraction or a period of nerve stimulation causing tetanic muscle contraction. Compare with *Postactivation Exhaustion*.

**Postactivation Potentiation** — Synonymous with preferred term, *Postactivation Facilitation*.

**Posttetanic Potentiation** — Enhancement of excitability following a long period of high-frequency stimulation. This phenomenon is known mainly in the mammalian spinal cord, where it lasts minutes or even hours. Use of the term is not recommended to describe the phenomenon of *Postactivation Facilitation.*

**Potential** — Strictly, *Voltage;* loosely, synonymous with *Action Potential.* See *Polarization.*

**Prolonged Insertional Activity** — See *Insertional Activity.*

**Propagation Velocity of a Muscle Fiber** — The speed of transmission of a muscle fiber action potential.

**Proximal Latency** — See *Motor Latency* and *Sensory Latency.*

**Pseudofacilitation (of Neuromuscular Transmission)** — Use of term discouraged. It refers to an increase in amplitude with a corresponding reduction in duration of the negative phase of the *M Wave,* resulting in no change in the area of the negative phase of the M wave. This probably reflects a reduction in the temporal dispersion of a constant number of summated muscle fiber action potentials, and must be differentiated from *Postactivation Facilitation.* See *Postactivation Facilitation.*

**Pseudomyotonic Discharge** — Use of term discouraged. It has been used to refer to different phenomena, including (1) *Myotonic Discharges* occurring in the presence of a neurogenic disease, (2) *Complex Repetitive Discharges,* and (3) *Repetitive Discharges* that wax or wane in either frequency or amplitude but not in both. See *Waning Discharge.*

**Pseudopolyphasic Action Potential** — Use of term discouraged. See preferred term, *Serrated Action Potential.*


**R1, R2 Waves** — See *Blink Responses.*

**Recording Electrode** — Device used to monitor electrical current or potential. All electrical recordings require two *Electrodes.* The electrode close to the source of the activity to be recorded is called the *Active* or *Exploring Electrode,* and the other electrode is called the *Reference Electrode.* Active electrode is synonymous with the older terminology G1 or Grid 1, and the reference electrode with G2 or Grid 2. By current convention, a potential difference that is negative at the active electrode relative to the reference electrode causes an upward deflection on the oscilloscope screen. The term "monopolar recording" is not recommended, because all recording requires two electrodes; however, it is commonly used to describe the use of an intramuscular needle exploring electrode in combination with a surface disc or subcutaneous needle reference electrode.

**Recruitment** — The orderly activation of the same and new motor units with increasing strength of voluntary muscle contraction. See *Motor Unit Potential.*

**Recruitment Frequency** — Firing rate of a *Motor Unit Potential* when an additional motor unit potential first appears during gradually increasing strength of voluntary muscle contraction.

**Recruitment Interval** — The *Interdischarge Interval* between two consecutive discharges of a *Motor Unit Potential* when an additional motor unit potential first appears during gradually increasing strength of voluntary muscle contraction. The reciprocal of the recruitment interval is the *Recruitment Frequency.*

**Recruitment Pattern** — A qualitative and/or quantitative description of the sequence of appearance of *Motor Unit Potentials* with increasing strength of voluntary muscle contraction. The *Recruitment Frequency* and *Recruitment Interval* are two quantitative measures commonly used. See *Interference Pattern* for qualitative terms commonly used.

**Reduced Insertional Activity** — See *Insertional Activity.*

**Reduced Interference Pattern** — See *Interference Pattern.*

**Reference Electrode** — See *Recording Electrode.*

**Reflex** — A stereotyped *Motor Response* elicited by a *Stimulus.*

**Refractory Period** — Time after an *Action Potential* during which the response to an additional stimulus is altered. The *Absolute Refractory Period* is that segment of the refractory period during which no stimulus, however strong, evokes an additional action potential. The *Relative Refractory Period* is that segment of the refractory period during which a stimulus must be greater than a normal threshold stimulus to evoke a second action potential.

**Relative Refractory Period** — See *Refractory Period.*

**Repetitive Discharges** — General term for the recurrence of an *Action Potential* with the same or nearly the same form. The term may refer to recurring potentials recorded in muscle at rest, during voluntary contraction, or in response to single nerve stimulus. The discharge may be named for the number of times a potential recurs in a group (e.g., *Double Discharge, Triple Discharge, Multiple Discharge, Coupled Discharge*) or other characteristics (e.g., *Complex Repetitive Discharge, Myokymic Discharge*).

**Repetitive Stimulation** — The technique of utilizing repeated supramaximal stimulation of a nerve while quantitatively recording M *Waves* from muscles innervated by the nerve. It should be described in terms of the frequency of stimuli and number of stimuli (or duration of the total group). For descriptions of specific patterns of responses, see the terms *Incrementing Response, Decrementing Response, Postactivation Facilitation,* and *Postactivation Exhaustion.*

**Repolarization** — See *Polarization.*

**Residual Latency** — Refers to the calculated time difference between the measured distal latency of a motor nerve and the expected distal latency, calculated by dividing the distance between the stimulus cathode and the active recording electrode by the maximum conduction velocity measured in a more proximal segment of a nerve.

**Response** — Used to describe an activity elicited by a *Stimulus.*

**Resting Membrane Potential** — Voltage across the membrane of an excitable cell at rest. See *Polarization.*

**Rheobase** — The intensity of an electrical current of infinitely long duration necessary to produce a minimal visible twitch of a muscle when the cathode is applied to the motor point of the muscle. In practice a duration of at least 300 msec is used to determine the rheobase.

**Rise Time** — By convention, the shortest interval from the nadir of a positive phase to the peak of a negative phase of a *Wave.*

**Satellite Potential** — Synonymous with preferred term, *Late Component.*

**Sea Shell Noise (Sea Shell Roar)** — Use of term discouraged. See *End-Plate Activity, Monophasic.*

**Sensory Delay** — See preferred terms, *Sensory Latency* and *Sensory Peak Latency.*

**Sensory Latency** — Interval between the onset of a stimulus and the onset of the *Compound Sensory Nerve Action Potential.* This term has been loosely used to refer to the *Sensory Peak Latency.* The term may be qualified as *Proximal Sensory Latency* or *Distal Sensory Latency,* depending on the relative position of the stimulus.

**Sensory Nerve Action Potential** — See *Compound Sensory Nerve Action Potential.*

**Sensory Nerve Conduction Velocity** — See *Conduction Velocity.*

**Sensory Peak Latency** — Interval between the onset of a *Stimulus* and the peak of the negative phase of the *Compound Sensory Nerve Action Potential.* Note that the term "*Latency*" refers to the interval between the onset of a stimulus and the onset of a response.

**Sensory Potential** — Used to refer to the compound sensory nerve action potential. See *Compound Sensory Nerve Action Potential.*

**Sensory Response** — Used to refer to a sensory evoked potential, e.g., *Compound Sensory Nerve Action Potential.*

**Serrated Action Potential** — An action potential waveform with several changes in direction (turns) which do not cross the baseline. This term is preferred to the terms *Complex Action Potential* and *Pseudopolyphasic Action Potential.* See *Turns.*

**Shock Artifact** — See *Artifact.*

**Silent Period** — Time during which there is no electrical activity in muscle following rapid unloading of a muscle.

**Single Fiber Electromyography** — (Abbr. SFEMG). General term referring to the technique and conditions that permit recording of a single muscle fiber *Action Potential.* See *Single Fiber Needle Electrode.*

**Single Fiber Needle Electrode** — A needle *Electrode* with a small recording surface (usually 25 μm in diameter) permitting the recording of single muscle fiber action potentials. See *Single Fiber Electromyography.*

**Somatosensory Evoked Potential** — (Abbr. SSEP). Electrical *Waves* recorded from the head or trunk in response to electrical or physiological stimulation of peripheral sensory fibers. Recordings over the spine may be referred to as *Spinal Evoked Potentials.*

**Spike** — Transient *Wave* with a pointed peak and a short duration (a few milliseconds or less). See *End-Plate Spike* and *Fibrillation Potentials.*

**Spinal Evoked Potential** — Electrical *Wave* recorded over the spine in response to electrical stimulation of peripheral sensory fibers. See *Somatosensory Evoked Potential.*

**Spontaneous Activity** — Action potentials recorded from muscle or nerve at rest after insertional activity has subsided and when there is no voluntary contraction or external stimulus. Compare with *Involuntary Activity.*

**Staircase Phenomenon** — The progressive increase in the force of a muscle contraction observed with repeated nerve stimulation at low rates.

**Stigmatic Electrode** — Synonymous with active or exploring electrode. See *Recording Electrodes.*

**Stimulating Electrode** — Device used to apply electrical current. All electrical stimulation requires two electrodes; the negative terminal is termed the *Cathode* and the positive terminal, the *Anode.* By convention, the stimulating electrodes are called "*Bipolar*" if they are roughly equal in size and separated by less than 5 cm. The stimulating electrodes are called "*Monopolar*" if the cathode is smaller in size than the anode and is separated from the anode by more than 5 cm. Electrical stimulation for *Nerve Conduction Studies* generally requires application of the cathode to produce depolarization of the nerve trunk fibers. If the anode is inadvertently placed between the cathode and the recording electrodes, a focal block of nerve conduction (*Anodal Block*) may occur and cause a technically unsatisfactory study.

**Stimulus** — Any external agent, state, or change that is capable of influencing the activity of a cell, tissue, or organism. In clinical *Nerve Conduction Studies*, an electrical stimulus is generally applied to a nerve or a muscle. The electrical stimulus may be described in absolute terms or with respect to the evoked potential of the nerve or muscle. In absolute terms, the electrical stimulus has a strength or intensity measured in voltage (volts) or current (milliamperes) and a duration (milliseconds). With respect to the evoked potential, the stimulus may be graded as subthreshold, threshold, submaximal, maximal, or supramaximal. A *Threshold Stimulus* is that electrical stimulus just sufficient to produce a detectable response. Stimuli less than the threshold stimulus are termed *Subthreshold*. The *Maximal Stimulus* is the stimulus intensity after which a further increase in the stimulus intensity causes no increase in the amplitude of the evoked potential. Stimuli of intensity below this and above threshold are *Submaximal*. Stimuli of intensity greater than the maximal stimulus are termed *Supramaximal*. Ordinarily, supramaximal stimuli are used for nerve conduction studies. By convention, an electrical stimulus of approximately 20% greater voltage than required for the maximal stimulus may be used for supramaximal stimulation. The frequency, number, and duration of a series of stimuli should be specified.

**Stimulus Artifact** — See *Artifact*.

**Strength-Duration Curve** — Graphic presentation of the relationship between the intensity (Y axis) and various durations (X axis) of the threshold electrical stimulus for a muscle with the stimulating cathode positioned over the motor point.

**Submaximal Stimulus** — See *Stimulus*.

**Subthreshold Stimulus** — See *Stimulus*.

**Supramaximal Stimulus** — See *Stimulus*.

**Surface Electrode** — Conducting device for stimulating or recording placed on a skin surface. The material (metal, fabric), configuration (disc, ring), size, and separation should be specified. See *Electrode (Ground, Recording, Stimulating)*.

**S-X Interval** — The total duration of the *Silent Period* produced by electrical stimulation of the mixed nerve to a voluntarily contracting muscle, measured from the stimulus artifact to resumption of uninterrupted voluntary activity.

**Temporal Dispersion** — A waveform of longer duration than normal. Commonly used to refer to an increase in the duration of an evoked potential with more proximal sites of stimulation of a greater degree than that normally seen.

**Terminal Latency** — Synonymous with preferred term, *Distal Latency*. See *Motor Latency* and *Sensory Latency*.

**Test Stimulus** — The stimulus producing the event being measured. Contrast with *Conditioning Stimulus*.

**Tetanic Contraction** — State of a muscle in sustained contraction resulting from stimulation at a frequency high enough for individual twitches to summate to a smooth tension and with associated electrical activity of muscle action potentials. It may be attained in normal muscle voluntarily or in response to repetitive nerve stimulation. Contrast with *Cramp Discharge*.

**Tetanus** — Loosely used to refer to *Tetanic Contraction*. The term is also used to refer to the acute infectious disease. See *Tetanic Contraction* and *Tetany*.

**Tetany** — A clinical syndrome manifested by muscle twitching, cramps, and sustained muscle contraction (*Tetanus*). These clinical signs are manifestations of peripheral and central nervous system nerve irritability from several causes. In these conditions, *Repetitive Discharges* (double discharge, triple discharge, multiple discharge) occur frequently with voluntary activation of motor unit potentials or may appear as spontaneous activity with systemic alkalosis or local ischemia.

**Tetraphasic Action Potential** — *Action Potential* with four phases.

**Threshold** — The level at which a clear and abrupt transition occurs from one state to another. The term is generally used to refer to the voltage level at which an *Action Potential* is initiated in a single axon or a group of axons. It is also operationally defined as the intensity that produced a response in about 50% of equivalent trials.

**Threshold Stimulus** — See *Stimulus*.

**Time Constant of Accommodation** — (lambda, λ). The time constant of the rate at which, after accommodation, the threshold of an excitable tissue reverts to its initial level. It is the reciprocal of the slope of the *Accommodation Curve*.

**Train of Positive Sharp Waves** — See *Positive Sharp Waves*.

**Train of Stimuli** — A group of stimuli. The duration of the group and the frequency of the individual components should be specified.

**Triphasic Action Potential** — *Action Potential* with three phases.

**Triple Discharge** — Three action potentials of the same form and nearly the same amplitude, occurring consistently in the same relationship to one another. The interval between the second and the third action potential often exceeds that between the first two, and both are usually in the range of 2–20 msec.

**Triplet** — See *Triple Discharge*.

**Turns** — Changes in direction of a waveform which do not necessarily pass through the baseline. The minimal excursion required to constitute a turn should be specified.

**Unipolar Needle Electrode** — See synonym, *Monopolar Needle Electrode*.

**Visual Evoked Potential** — Electrical waveforms of biological origin recorded over the cerebrum and elicited by light stimuli.

**Visual Evoked Response** — (Abbr. VER). See *Visual Evoked Potential*.

**Voltage** — Potential difference between two points.

**Volume Conduction** — Spread of current from a potential source through a conducting medium, such as the body tissues.

**Voluntary Activity** — In electromyography, the electrical activity recorded from a muscle with consciously controlled muscle contraction. The effort made to contract the muscle, e.g., minimal, moderate, or maximal, and the strength of contraction in absolute terms or relative to a maximal voluntary contraction of a normal corresponding muscle should be specified.

**Waning Discharge** — General term referring to a repetitive discharge that decreases in frequency or in amplitude. Compare with *Myotonic Discharge*.

**Wave** — An undulating line constituting a graphic representation of a change, e.g., a changing potential difference.

**Waveform** — The shape of a *Wave*. The term is often used synonymously with wave.

**Wedensky-Like Neuromuscular Failure** — Use of term discouraged. The term has been used to describe a decrease in the strength of the sustained muscle contraction during repeated nerve stimulation at frequencies within the physiological range (less than 50 Hz). See preferred term, *Decrementing Response*.

**Wedensky Phenomenon** — A decrease in strength of a sustained muscle contraction during sustained nerve stimulation at frequencies above the physiological range, e.g., greater than 50 Hz. This phenomenon is seen in normal muscle.

# INDEX

A *t* following a page number indicates a table; an italic page number indicates an illustration.

Action potential(s)—(*continued*)
   depolarization and, 175
   generation of, 175
   recording of
     sources of error in, 89–91
   negative spike and, *34*
   nerve. *See* Nerve action potential(s).
   of human muscle fiber, *311*
   propagation of, 63–64
   recording of, *36*
   repolarization and, 36
   sensory, 86. *See also* Sensory potential(s).
     antidromic, 86
     orthodromic, 93
   serrated, 244
   subthreshold activation and, 31
   triphasic wave and, 36
   turns of, 244
Action potential complex
   duration of
     fiber density and, 310
Acute intermittent porphyria, 475–476
   dying back phenomenon and, 74
Addison's disease, 537
Adductor brevis muscle. *See under* Muscle(s).
Adductor hallucis muscle. *See under* Muscle(s).
Adductor longus muscle. *See under* Muscle(s).
Adductor magnus muscle. *See under* Muscle(s).
Adductor pollicis muscle. *See under* Muscle(s).
Adrenal disease, 537–538
Adrenoleukodystrophy
   F-waves in, *367*
Adynamia episodica hereditaria, 553
Afferent fibers, 66
After-potential
   negative, 33
     in B fibers, 66
   positive, 33
Age
   effects of
     in nerve conduction measurement, 99, *99*
Alcoholic neuropathy, 465–466. *See also under* Neuropathy, alcoholic.
   axonal degeneration in, 74–75
   electromyographic abnormalities in, 74
Alkalosis
   tetany and, 558
All median hand, 17, 153
All ulnar hand, 17, 153
All-or-none phenomenon
   action potentials and, 31–33, 175
   depolarization and, 31
   repolarization and, 32
Alpha-bungarotoxin
   myasthenia gravis and, 178

Amplifier(s), 594
   basic, 597–603
   common mode voltage and, 45
   differential, 45, 599–600, *599, 600, 601*
     factors influencing, 600–601
   electrode, 45
   fast-recovery, 85
   frequency band of, 46
   integrated circuit, 594, *595*
   settings of
     in single fiber electromyography, 307
   single-ended input, 597, *597*
Amplifier noise, 50–51
Amplitude
   vs. latency, 160, 162–163
   of miniature end-plate potential (MEPP), 174
   of motor unit potential, 44, 242, *243*
   of sensory nerve potentials, 95
   reduction in, *92*
Amplitude modulation (AM), 48, 87
Amyloid neuropathy, 467
Amyloidosis, 467
   carpal tunnel syndrome and, 494
Amyotrophic lateral sclerosis
   axon reflex and, 356
   bulbar signs in, 432
   clinical signs of, 433
   conduction velocities in, 434
   cooling and, 191
   cramps in, 432
   diagnosis of, 433
   electromyographic abnormalities in, 434
   electrophysiologic findings in, 435
   fasciculations in, 433
   fasciculation potentials and, 272
   F-wave abnormalities in, 363
   H-reflex in, 434
   motor unit potentials in, *249, 278*
   muscle biopsies in, 433
   neuromuscular transmission in, 434
   pathology of, 432–433
   sphincter muscle in, 301
   spontaneous activity in, *268*
   vs. cervical spondylosis, 433
   vs. chronic mercurialism, 433
   vs. lead intoxication, 433
Anal sphincter. *See* Sphincter(s), anal.
Analog-to-digital converters, 596–597
Anastomosis(es)
   Martin-Gruber, 17, 150–153
   median-to-ulnar, 150
Anconeus muscle. *See under* Muscle(s).
AND gate, 595, *596*
Anemia
   pernicious, 471
Annulospiral endings
   muscle spindles and, 223
Anodal block, 158

Anode(s), 83–84
Anomaly(ies)
  all median hand, 153
  as sources of error, 150–154
  Martin-Gruber, 150–153
  of innervation, 16–17
Anterior horn cell disease(s). See also Motor
      neuron disease.
  fibrillation potentials and, 267, 270
Anterior interosseous nerve. See under
      Nerve(s).
Anterior interosseous syndrome, 494
Anterior rami. See under Ramus(i).
Anterior root, 7
Anterior thoracic nerve. See under Nerve(s).
Anterior tibial muscle. See under Muscle(s).
Anterior tibial nerve. See Nerve(s), peroneal,
      deep.
Anti-acetylcholine receptor antibody
  in myasthenia gravis, 178
Antibiotic toxicity
  depressed neuromuscular transmission in,
     179–180, 200
Anticholinesterase drugs
  administration of
    neuromuscular transmission and, 191
  overdose of
    fasciculation potentials and, 272
Antidromic impulse
  blocking of, 355
Apparatus
  defective, 53
  diathermy
    interference from, 53
Aran-Duchenne syndrome, 435
Arcade of Frohse, 493
Arm-diaphragm synkinesis, 452
Arnold-Chiari malformation, syringomyelia
    and, 442
Arsenic poisoning, 473
Arthrogryposis multiplex congenita,
    440
Artifact(s), 48–49
  friction, 53
  from cardiac pacemaker, 49
  from transcutaneous stimulator, 50
  movement-induced, 53, 190
    and temperature, 191–192
    detection of, 190
  shock, 85–86
  60 Hz, 48, 51, 53
  stimulus, 85–86, 605–608, 608
    control of, 85
    ground electrode and, 86
  surface electrodes and, 43
Artifact suppression circuits, 607–608
Asthma
  poliomyelitislike syndrome and, 442
Autonomic nerve(s). See under Nerve(s).

Averaging technique
  in signal recording, 86, 87
Axilla(ae)
  stimulation at
    median nerve and, 145–146
    ulnar nerve and, 145–146
Axillary nerve. See under Nerve(s).
Axon(s)
  conduction velocity of
    activation threshold and, 228
  degeneration of, 61, 74–75
  diameter of
    activation threshold and, 228
    conduction velocity and, 65
  vs. myelin
    in nerve disease, 74–76
  conduction of, 156
  degeneration of, 72
  refractory period and, 157–165. See also
    Refractory period.
  transport of, 61
Axon reflex(es)
  clinical significance of, 356
  of tibial nerve, 358, 359
  physiologic characteristics of, 356
  repetitive discharges vs., 360
Axonotmesis, 71–73
Axoplasmic resistance
  conduction velocity and, 64

B FIBERS, 65–66
Backfiring
  of motor neurons, 355
Bacillus botulinus
  types of, 518
Bacteremia
  needle examination and, 237
Baker's cyst
  sural nerve compression and, 502
Baldness
  myotonic dystrophy and, 550–551
Becker type muscular dystrophy, 529
Bell's palsy, 335, 336, 490
  blink reflex and, 333–334, 490
  direct response in, 490
  facial myokymia and, 555
  hemifacial spasm and, 556
  latency of R1 in, 344
  nerve excitability in, 490
  site of lesion in, 5
Belly-tendon recording, 88, 190
  anticholinesterase drugs and
    administration of, 191
  temperature and, 191–192
  movement-induced artifacts and, 190
Beriberi, 471
Beta-lipoprotein
  absence of, 477
Biceps brachii muscle. See under Muscle(s).

Biceps femoris muscle. *See under* Muscle(s).
Binary arithmetic, 596
Biopsy
  nerve, 66
Bipolar concentric needle, *43, 44*
Bleeding tendency
  patients with
    electromyography in, 237
Blink reflex, 6, 323–351
  abnormalities of, *324*
    neurological disorders with, 333–343
  Charcot-Marie-Tooth disease and, *341, 474*
  direct response and, *334t*
  hemifacial spasm and, 556
  in Bell's palsy, 490
  in Guillain-Barré syndrome, 470
  in syringomyelia, 443
  normal values of *334t*, 343
  recording of
    technique for, *328*
  stimulation for, *324*
  with cavernous sinus lesion, *330*
Blocking
  jitter and, 311
  myasthenia gravis and, 211
Botulinum
  presynaptic abnormalities and, 179–180
Botulism, 518–519
  clinical symptoms of, 518–519
  cooling and, 191
  electrophysiologic tests for, 519
  fibrillation potentials and, 270
  infant, 518
  motor unit potentials and, 280
    fatigue of, 278
  muscle action potentials in, *199*
    amplitude of, 199–200
  repetitive stimulation and
    amplitude decrement with, 196
Brachial neuralgia. *See* Idiopathic brachial
    neuritis.
Brachial plexus. *See* Plexus(es), brachial.
Brachial plexus lesions
  axon reflex and, 356
Brachialis muscle. *See under* Muscle(s).
Brachioradialis muscle. *See under* Muscle(s).
Bulbar palsy
  progressive, 435
    juvenile, 439
Bulbar signs
  in amyotrophic lateral sclerosis, 432
  in infantile spinal muscular atrophy, 437

C Fibers, 65–66
Calcium
  in sarcoplasm, 176
Calcium ions
  in muscle action potential, 176
Calcium-dependent facilitation
  neuromuscular transmission and, 183

Calcium-receptive protein
  muscle contraction and, 219
Calibration signals, 47
Calibration waveform, *257*
Cannula-recorded end-plate spikes, 241
Capacitance, 585–590
  factors influencing, 585, *586*
Carbamazepine
  in neuromyotonia, 554
Carbon disulfide
  toxic neuropathy and, 472
Carcinoma
  bronchogenic
    neuropathy and, 466, 467
Cardiac catheter(s)
  nerve stimulation and 84–85
Carnitine palmityl transferase deficiency, 535
Carpal ligament. *See* Ligament(s), carpal.
Carpal tunnel syndrome, 71, 494–496
  conduction velocity and, 99
  electrophysiologic studies of, 495
  F-wave in, *372*
  incidence of, 495
  median-to-ulnar communication in, *153*
  nerve conduction in, *146*
  pathologic studies of, 495
  sensory nerve potentials in, *113*
  symptoms of, 495
Carpopedal spasm, 558
Cataract(s)
  myotonic dystrophy and, 550–551
Cathodal block, 158
Cathode, 63, 83–84
Cathode ray tube, 47, 609–610
Cauda equina, 17
  lesions of, 456
    vs. peripheral lesions, 130
Cauda equina syndrome
  H-reflex in, *385*
Cell(s)
  ionic concentration of
    transmembrane potential and, 28
  Renshaw, 355
Cell membrane
  local current in, 33
Central core disease, 531
  malignant hyperthermia and, 536
  Type I fiber predominance in, 531
Centronuclear myopathy
  fibrillation potentials and, 270
Ceramide trihexose, 477
Cerebellopontine angle, 5
Cerebral lipidosis, 476
Cerebral stroke
  blink reflex in, *346*
Cerebroside sulfate, 476
Cervical disc
  herniated, 450
Cervical plexus. *See* Plexus(es), cervical.
Cervical rib syndrome, 454–455

Cramp(s), 285, 557–558
  in amyotrophic lateral sclerosis, 432
Cranial nerve(s). *See under* Nerve(s).
Creatine kinase (CK)
  electromyography and, 237
  in Duchenne muscular dystrophy, 528
  in infantile spinal muscular atrophy, 437
  in juvenile spinal muscular atrophy, 439
  in polymyositis, 539
Cross-bridges
  myosin-actin
    muscle contraction and, 219
Cross-talk. *See* Ephaptic transmission.
Cubital tunnel
  ulnar nerve and, 111
Cubital tunnel syndrome, 496–497
  electrophysiologic assessment of, 497
Curare
  neuromuscular transmission and, 209–210
Curarization, 549
Current, 581–582
  constant
    vs. constant voltage, 604–605
  Faradic, 571
  Galvanic, 571
  local
    in action potential, 63
    in cell membrane, 33
  stimulating
    spread of, 144
Current density
  in volume conduction, 35
Current flow
  in volume conduction, 34
Current leaks, 613, *613*
Cushing's syndrome, 537
Cutaneous nerve(s). *See under* Nerve(s).
Cutoff frequency, 587, 589
Cyst(s)
  dermoid, 456
Cysticercosis
  myositis and, 540

Dapsone
  toxic neuropathy and, 472
Debrancher deficiency, 533–534
Decay time constant, 589, *589*
Deep peroneal nerve. *See* Nerve(s), peroneal, deep.
Degeneration
  wallerian, *72*
    nerve conduction during, 72
Dejerine-Sottas disease, 473, 474–475
Delay line, 47
Delta aminolevulinic acid, 475
Deltoid muscle. *See under* Muscle(s).
Demyelination
  conduction velocity and, 65

experimental, 75
  diphtheria toxin in, 75
  in neurapraxia, 70
  segmental, 75–76
    conduction abnormalities and, 92
    nerve conduction in, 75
    Schwann cells in
      disturbance of, 75
Denervation
  complex repetitive discharges and, 274
  fibrillation potentials in, 270
  insertional positive waves and, 261
  spontaneous activity in, 266–276
Denervation hypersensitivity, 266
Depolarization
  action potential and, 31, 36
  cathodal, 63
  critical level of, 175
*Dermacentor andersoni*, 519
*Dermacentor paridulis*, 519
Dermatomyositis, 538–539
  early recruitment in, *284*
  fibrillation potentials and, 270
  spontaneous activity in, *269*
Dermoid cyst
  of conus medullaris, 456
Desynchronization
  of nerve volley, 76
Diabetes
  ischemia and, 100
Diabetic amyotrophy, 464
Diabetic neuropathy. *See* Neuropathy, diabetic
Diaphragm. *See under* Muscle(s).
Diathermy apparatus
  interference from, 53
Diazepam
  blink reflex and, 345
  stiff-man syndrome and, 557
Differential amplifier. *See under* Amplifier.
Digital circuitry, 47
Digital electronics, 595–597
Digital nerve entrapment, 496, 498
Diode(s), 593, *594*
Diphenylhydantoin
  in neuromyotonia, 554
  toxic neuropathy and, 472
Diphtheria toxin
  in experimental demyelination, 75
Diphtheric neuropathy, 470
Diplegia
  facial
    direct response in, *327*
    traumatic
      stimulation in, *145*
Dipole(s)
  of transmembrane potential, 36
  volume conduction and, 34
Direct response
  blink reflex and, 334*t*

Impulse(s)
   antidromic, *159*
   orthodromic, *159*
Inclusion body myositis, 540
Incontinence
   anal sphincter and
      recording of, *300*
Inductance, 585–590, *591*
Infantile spinal muscular atrophy, 437–438
   bulbar signs in, 437
   clinical features of, 437
   electromyography in, 437
   fasciculations in, 437
   nerve conduction velocities in, 438
Inferior gemelli muscle. *See under* Muscle(s).
Inferior gluteal nerve. *See under* Nerve(s).
Inferior oblique muscle. *See under* Muscle(s).
Inferior rectus muscle. *See under* Muscle(s).
Infraorbital nerve. *See under* Nerve(s).
Infraspinatus muscle. *See under* Muscle(s).
Innervation
   anomalies of, 16–17
   muscle contraction and, 222
   rules for, 16–17
Innervation ratio
   motor units and, 226, 226*t*
   motor unit potentials and, 241–242
   of extraocular muscles, 293
Input impedance, 46, 598, *598*
   in preamplifier, 45
   use of electrodes and, 42
Insertional activity, 238, *238*
   absence of, 259–260
   clinical significance of, 238–239
   decreased, 259–262
   increase in, 260
Insertional positive waves, 260–262
   of denervation, 261
Instrumentation, 581–619
   in electromyography, 41
Insulation
   of needle electrodes, 42
Integrated circuit, 594, *595*
Integration, 253
Intercostal muscles. *See under* Muscle(s).
Interdigital nerve syndrome, 501
Interference
   electromagnetic, 53
   electrostatic, 53
   from diathermy apparatus, 53
   radio, 53–54
   radio frequency and, 53
   reduction of, 46
   60 Hz, 48, *51*, 53
Interference pattern, 228–229, 282–285. *See also* Recruitment pattern.
Internal auditory meatus, 5
Interneuron(s)
   excitability of, 346–348

Internodal capacitance
   conduction velocity and, 65
Internodal distance
   conduction velocity and, 64
   in myelinated fibers, 61
Internodal length spectrum(a)
   in sural nerve fibers, 67, 69
Internuclear ophthalmoplegia, 296
Interossei muscles. *See under* Muscle(s).
Intrafusal muscle fibers, 223, *223*
Intraocular pressure
   measurement of
      tonography and, 212
Inverter, 595
Involuntary movement, 285
Ion(s). *See under individual names.*
Ischemia
   effect of
      conduction velocity and, 99
      diabetes and, 100
      neurapraxia and, 70
      somatosensory evoked potentials and, 415, 418–419
   uremia and, 99
Ischemic exercise test
   in McArdle's disease, 534
Ischemic test, 208
   for neuromuscular transmission
Isolated inputs, 617, 618
Isolated power system, 618
Isoniazid
   toxic neuropathy and, 472
*Ixodes holocyclus,* 519

Jakob-Creutzfeldt disease, 440–441
   use of needle electrodes in, 42, 441
Jaw reflex, 385–386, 386*t*
   clinical applications of, 386
   following chin tap, *387*
   masseteric silent period and, 386
   normal values of, 385–386
Jitter, 310–313
   determination of, 312–313, *313*
   in normal subjects, 315*t*
   manual calculation of, *314*
   muscle temperature and, 313
   myasthenia gravis and, 211
Junctional folds, 173
Juvenile progressive bulbar palsy, 439
Juvenile spinal muscular atrophy
   creatine kinase in, 439
   electromyography in, 439
   fasciculations in, 438
   nerve conduction studies in, 439

Kanamycin
   myasthenia gravis and, 520
   presynaptic abnormalities and, 179–180
Kearns-Sayres ophthalmoplegia, 536

Lumbar disc(s)
  herniated, 456
    complex repetitive discharges and, *275,
      276*
    electromyography in, 457
Lumbar plexus. *See* Plexus(es), lumbar.
Lumbosacral roots, 455–457
Lumbrical muscles. *See under* Muscle(s).
Lupus erythematosus
  carpal tunnel syndrome and, 494
  dermatomyositis and, 538
Lymphoma(s)
  neuropathy in, 466
Lyon hypothesis, 528

MAGNESIUM
  presynaptic abnormalities and, 179–180
Magnetic tape recorder, 48
Magnetic tape recording, 610–611
Main sensory nucleus, 6
Malignancy(ies)
  neuropathies and, 466–467
Malignant hyperpyrexia, 536
Malignant hyperthermia, 536
Manganese
  presynaptic abnormalities and, 179–180
Mapping technique
  motor unit overlap and, 226
Martin-Gruber anastomosis, 17, 150–153
Masseter muscle. *See* Muscle(s), masseter.
Masseter reflex, 6
Mastication
  muscles of, 5
    cell bodies of, 6
McArdle's disease, 534
  contracture in, *220*
  decremental response in, 520
  repetitive stimulation in, 203
Mean interspike interval (MISI), 310
Mean value of consecutive difference (MCD),
  313
Medial cord
  of brachial plexus
    formation of, 12
    lesions of
      symptoms in, 452
      ulnar nerve sensory potential in, 112
    stimulation of, 116
Medial dorsal cutaneous nerve. *See under*
  Nerve(s).
Medial plantar nerve. *See under* Nerve(s).
Medial rectus muscle. *See under* Muscle(s).
Median nerve. *See under* Nerve(s).
Medullary syndrome
  left lateral, *342*
Membrane(s)
  muscle
    conduction velocity and, 175
  postsynaptic, 173

  presynaptic, 173
Membrane capacitance
  action potential and, 63
Membrane conductance
  action potential and, 63
Membrane physiology, 27–28
Mental nerve. *See under* Nerve(s).
Meralgia paresthetica, 498
Mercurialism
  vs. amyotrophic lateral sclerosis, 433
Mesencephalic nucleus, 6
Metabolic neuropathies, 471, 473
Metabolism
  lipid
    disorders of, 535
Metachromatic leukodystrophy, 476
Metastasis
  neuropathy and, 466
Methyl n-butyl ketone
  toxic neuropathy and, 472
Metronidazol
  toxic neuropathy and, 472
Microelectrode(s)
  glass, 45
Microelectrode recording, 211
Microprocessor, 596
Middle trunk
  of brachial plexus
    formation of, 9, 12
    lesions of
      radial sensory potential in, 115
      symptoms in, 452
    stimulation of, 106–107
Miniature end-plate potentials (MEPP), 174
  amplitude of, 174
  end-plate noise and, 241
  in myasthenia gravis, 177
  quantum size and, 174
Mitochondrial disease, 536
Mobilization store
  acetylcholine quanta and, 174
Möbius syndrome, 296
  extraocular muscle in, *298*
Mononeuropathy(ies), 489–508
  fibrillation potentials and, 267, 270
Monopolar needles, *43,* 44
Monosynaptic reflex
  H-reflex and, 379
Morphometric assessment
  in sural nerve fibers, 66
Morton's neuroma, 501
Motor end-plate(s). *See* End-plate(s), motor.
Motor latency, 96–97
Motor nerve conduction. *See* Nerve conduction, motor.
Motor neuron(s)
  recurrent activation and, 355
  reflexive activation of
    recurrent activation vs., 353, 355

Muscle(s)—(*continued*)
abductor hallucis, 17t–18t, 125
F-wave from, *354, 365, 373*
tibial nerve conduction and, *354, 365, 373*
abductor pollicis brevis, 10t–11t, 15
median nerve conduction and, 106
abductor pollicis longus, 10t–11t, 13–14
adductor hallucis, 17t–18t
anconeus, 10t–11t, 13
biceps brachii, 10t–11t, 13
biceps femoris, 17t–18t
brachial plexus conduction and, 122–123
brachialis, 10t–11t, 13
brachioradialis, 10t–11t, 13
contraction of
mechanism of, 219
cooling of
fibrillation potentials and, 267
coracobrachialis, 10t–11t, 13
deltoid, 10t–11t, 13
brachial plexus conduction and, 193
denervated
needle insertion and, 239
diaphragm
innervation of, 4t
digastric
innervation of, 4t
diseases of, 520–521
electrical properties of, 27–39
extensor carpi radialis brevis, 10t–11t, 13–14
extensor carpi radialis longus, 10t–11t, 13–14
extensor carpi ulnaris, 10t–11t, 13–14
extensor digiti minimi, 10t–11t, 13–14
extensor digitorum, 10t–11t, 13–14
extensor digitorum brevis, 17t–18t
peroneal nerve conduction and, 128
extensor digitorum longus, 17t–18t
extensor indicis, 10t–11t
radial nerve conduction and, 113
extensor pollicis brevis, 10t–11t, 13–14
extensor pollicis longus
innervation of, 13–14
external oblique
examination of, 296
extraocular
electromyography of, 291–296
examination of, 291–296
fast twitch fibers in, 293
innervation ratio of, 293
slow twitch fibers in, 293
unique properties of, 293–294
facial, 193
examination of, 289–291
fast, 221–222
flexor carpi ulnaris, 10t–11t, 16
flexor digiti minimi, 10t–11t, 16
flexor digitorum profundus, 10t–11t, 15, 16

flexor pollicis brevis, 10t–11t, 15, 16
flexor pollicis longus, 10t–11t, 15
hypothenar
decremental response of, *191*
F-wave from, *361, 366*
M-response from, *361, 366*
inferior gemelli, 17t–18t
inferior oblique, 4t
inferior rectus, 4t
influences of nerve on, 223
infraspinatus, 10t–11t, 13
intercostal, 8
end-plates of, 173
innervation of, 9
interossei, 10t–11t, 17t–18t, 16
laryngeal, 4t, 291
lateral rectus, 4t
latissimus dorsi, 10t–11t, 298
levator palpebrae, 4t
levator scapulae, 10t–11t, 13
lumbrical, 10t–11t, 15, 16, 17t–18t
masseter, 4t, 5
voluntary contraction of
electromyographic recording of, *388*
medial rectus, 4t
multifidus, 298
non-limb
examination of, 289–304
normal
fasciculation in, 274
nuchal, 291
obturator externus, 17t–18t, 23
obturator internus, 17t–18t, 23
opponens digiti minimi, 10t–11t, 15–16
opponens pollicis, 10t–11t, 15
orbicularis oculi, 4t
blink reflex and, *347*
facial nerve conduction and, 193
R1 components from, *329*
orbicularis oris, 4t
blink reflex in, *337*
facial nerve conduction and, 193
palmaris longus, 10t–11t, 15
paraspinal, 8, 298–299
relaxation of
for electromyography, 299
pectoralis major, 10t–11t
pectoralis minor, 10t–11t
peroneus brevis, 17t–18t, 25
peroneus longus, 17t–18t, 25
peroneus tertius, 17t–18t, 25
platysma, 4t
blink reflex in
facial nerve disease and, *337*
pronator quadratus, 10t–11t, 15
pronator teres, 10t–11t, 15
injury to, 494
pterygoid, 4t, 5
quadratus femoris, 17t–18t

Myasthenia gravis—(continued)
  electrophysiologic tests for, 513–515
  end-plates in, 173
  etiologic considerations in, 511–512
  experimental autoimmune, 178
  fibrillation potentials and, 270
  immunologic changes in, 178
  ischemic test in, 208
  jitter and, 211
  morphologic changes in, 178
  motor unit potentials and, 280, 514
    fatigue of, 278
  muscle action potential and
    amplitude of, 199
  neonatal, 517
  ocular, 513
    electronystagmography and, 212
    ischemic test in, 208
    tonography and, 212
  ocular muscles in, 295
  pathophysiology of, 176–178
  polymyositis and, 539
  post-tetanic exhaustion and, 202, 514
  post-tetanic potentiation and, 201, 514
  quantum size and
    changes in, 185
  regional curare test and, 209–210
  repetitive stimulation and, 191, 195–196, 514
  single fiber electromyography and, 316
  stimulation in low rate of, 514
Myasthenic syndrome, 515–516
  acetylcholine quanta and
    defective release of, 179
  clinical symptoms of, 515–516
  compound muscle action potential and
    small amplitude of, 198
  cooling and, 191
  edrophonium test and, 516
  electrophysiologic tests for, 516
  end-plates in, 173
  etiologic considerations and, 515
  familial
    congenital
      deficient acetylcholine synthesis in,
        179
  motor unit potentials and, 280
  muscle action potential and
    amplitude of, 199
  pathophysiology of, 179
  post-tetanic exhaustion and, 201, 202
  post-tetanic potentiation and, 201, 202, 516
  quantum size and
    changes in, 185
  repetitive stimulation in, 197, 198
    amplitude decrement with, 196
  single fiber electromyography and, 316, 516
  small cell bronchogenic carcinoma and, 515
  stimulation in
    high rates of, 516

Mycobacterium leprae, 470
Myelin
  vs. axon involvement
    in nerve disease, 74–76
  thickness of
    conduction velocity and, 65
Myelin sheath
  degeneration of, 72
Myelinated fibers. See Fiber(s), myelinated.
Myelography
  in motor neuron disease, 433
  spontaneous activity following, 266
Myelopathy(ies)
  cervical spondylotic
    fasciculation potentials and, 272
Myoedema
  of hypothyroidism, 537
Myofibers. See Muscle fiber(s).
Myofibril(s), 219
  contraction of, 176
Myofilament(s), 219
Myogenic disorders
  repetitive stimulation in, 203
  typical findings in, 262, 263
  vs. lower motor neuron disorders, 280–282
Myoglobinuria, 534, 535
Myokymia, 555–556
  facial, 555
Myokymic discharge(s)
  fasciculation potentials and, 272
  radiation plexopathies and, 454
Myopathic disorders. See Myogenic disorders.
Myopathy(ies), 284–285, 527–548
  centronuclear, 532
  congenital, 531–532
    motor unit potentials and, 280
  endocrine, 536–538
  firing rates in, 229
  hereditary distal, 530
  hypokalemic, 553
  metabolic, 533–536
  myotubular, 532
  nemaline, 531–532
  ocular, 296
  thyroid, 536–537
Myophosphorylase deficiency, 534
Myosin filament(s), 219
Myosin-actin cross-bridges, 219
Myositis, 538–540
  inclusion body, 540
  infectious agents and, 540
  inflammatory
    classification of, 538
  motor unit potentials and, 280
  single fiber electromyography and, 316–317
Myotonia, 549–552
  decremental response in, 520
  electromyography in, 262–265, 552

hereditary
in goats, 263–264
percussion, 550
postactivation, 549
repetitive stimulation in, 203
Myotonia congenita, 262, 551–552
electromyography in, 552
Myotonia dystrophica. *See* Myotonic dystrophy.
Myotonic discharge, 262–265
in acid maltase deficiency, 533
in myotonic dystrophy, 265
in myotubular myopathy, 532
pathophysiology of, 263–265
positive vs. negative, 263
Myotonic dystrophy, 262, 550–551
congenital, 551
electromyography in, 551
multiple discharges and, 280
myotonic discharge in, 265
Myotonic phenomenon(a)
chloride conductance and, 264
Myotube(s)
fetal, 532
Myotubular myopathy
fibrillation potentials and, 270
Myxedema
complex repetitive discharges and, 274

Neck
muscles of, 291
Needle(s)
coaxial, 43, *43*
concentric
bipolar, 43, *44*
standard, 43, *43*
monopolar, 43, *44*
single fiber, 43, *44*
subcutaneous
stimulation with
artifacts and, 190
Needle electrodes, 86. *See also* Electrode(s).
exposed tip of
current flow and, 42
in recording nerve potentials, 94
insulation of
testing of, 42
nerve potentials and
recording of, 94
single fiber, 305
Needle insulation
testing of, 42
Negative after-potential, 33
Nemaline myopathy, 531–532
Neomycin
myasthenia gravis and, 520
post-tetanic exhaustion and, 186
presynaptic abnormalities and, 179–180
Neonatal myasthenia gravis, 517

Neostigmine
fibrillation potentials and, 267
Nernst equation, 28–30
Nerve(s)
abducens
muscles innervated by, 4t
accessory, 6–7, *7, 8, 9*
cranial
accessory nucleus and, 7
muscles innervated by, 4t
nucleus ambiguus and, 6
sternocleidomastoid and, 7
trapezius and, 7
spinal
injury to, 491
muscles innervated by, 4t
anterior thoracic, 10t–11t, *12*
assessment of, 105–141
autonomic
fibers of, 65
axillary
injury to, 492
muscles innervated by, 10t–11t, *15*
compression of
leg-crossing and, 501
conduction velocity of
in neurotmesis, 73
cranial, 3, 5–7
communication between, 7
mononeuropathy and, 489–491
muscles innervated by, 4t
cutaneous
A fibers in, 66
femoral
lateral, 20, *138, 139*
lesions of, 498
lateral
musculocutaneous nerve and, 13
sensory
conduction study of, *125*
dorsal cutaneous
intermediate, 128
medial, 128
dorsal scapular, 13, 10t–11t
entrapment of, 492
electrical properties of, 27–39
facial, 5, *5, 6*
acoustic neuromas and, 5
Bell's palsy and, 5
branching of, 6
cerebellopontine angle and, 5
course of, 5
excitability of, 323, 325
functional components of, 5
internal auditory meatus and, 5
involvement of
in Charcot-Marie-Tooth disease, 490
in Guillain-Barré syndrome, 490
muscles innervated by, 4t

Nerve graft
  autogenous, 73
    conduction velocity across, 73
Nerve potential(s)
  digital
    amplitude of, 95
  mixed, 94
  recording of, 86–88
  sural
    in vitro recording of, 66–68, 67
Nerve root(s). See Root(s).
Nerve stimulation
  techniques of
    errors in, 143–144
  unwanted
    blocking of, 144
Neuralgia
  brachial. See Idiopathic brachial neuritis.
  trigeminal
    blink reflex and, 333
Neuralgic amyotrophy. See Idiopathic bra-
    chial neuritis.
Neurapraxia, 70–71
  fibrillation potentials in, 71
  positive sharp waves in, 71
Neurapraxic lesions, 93
Neuritis
  brachial. See Idiopathic brachial neuritis.
Neurologic disease(s)
  unilateral
    blink reflex and, 333t
Neuroma(s)
  acoustic, 5
    blink reflex and, 336–337
  in neurotmesis, 73
Neuromuscular depression, 180–181
Neuromuscular facilitation, 180–181
Neuromuscular junction
  anatomy of, 171–188
  end-plate and, 172–173
Neuromuscular transmission
  acetylcholine molecules and, 180
  assessment of, 171–188
  calcium-dependent facilitation and,
    183
  cooling and, 191
  defects of, 520
  depressed
    antibiotic toxicity and, 200
    hypermagnesemia and, 200
    hypocalcemia and, 200
    snake poisoning and, 200
  disorders of, 511–525
    motor unit potentials and, 280
  effects of disease states on, 183–186
  in amyotrophic lateral sclerosis, 434
  neurosecretory potentiation and, 182
  paired stimuli and, 193–194
  physiology of, 171–188

recovery cycles of, 180–186
  normal, 181–183
Neuromyotonia, 554
  electromyography in, 554
Neuron(s)
  first order
    cell bodies of, 6
    main sensory nucleus and, 6
Neuropathy(ies)
  acrylamide, 74
  alcoholic, 464–466
    clinical symptoms of, 465
    electrophysiologic studies of, 465
    F-wave abnormalities and, 363
  amyloid, 467
  axonal
    paranodal demyelination in, 76
  axonal degeneration and, 74
  carcinomatous, 76
    electromyographic abnormalities in, 74
  compression, 489–508
    acute, 70
    chronic, 71
  conditions associated with, 74
  demyelinating
    diagnosis of
      reduced conduction velocity in, 76
  diabetic, 76, 464–465
    axon reflex and, 356
    classification of, 464
    electromyographic abnormalities in, 74
    F-waves and, 368–369
  diphtheric, 470
  dying back, 74
  entrapment
    F-wave abnormalities and, 363
  facial
    axon reflex and, 356
  familial amyloid, 467
  familial pressure-sensitive, 454
    brachial plexopathy and, 451
  femoral, 464
  giant axonal, 477
  hereditary ataxic, 475
  hereditary motor and sensory, 338, 338
  hereditary sensory, 477
  infective, 468–471
  inherited, 473–478
    classification of, 473
  lipoprotein, 477
  malignant conditions and, 466, 467
  metabolic, 471–473
  motor unit potentials and, 280
  multiple discharges and, 278
  myokymia associated with, 555
  nutritional, 74, 471–472
  paraproteinemia and, 468
  single fiber electromyography and, 315–316
  postinfective, 468–471

Paired discharges, 278
Paired shock technique, 158. *See also* Stimulation, paired.
Paired stimuli, *182, 183,* 184, 193–194. *See also* Stimulus, paired.
  blink reflex and, 344, *347*
  compound muscle action potentials and, *194*
  interstimulus intervals of, 160, 161*t,* 162, *162*
  neuromuscular transmission and, 193
  to median nerve, *181*
Palmar branch
  ulnar nerve conduction of, 497–498
Palmar stimulation
  median nerve conduction and, 110
  of median nerve, 148–149
Palmaris longus muscle. *See under* Muscle(s).
Palsy(ies)
  abducens, *340*
  extraocular
    neurogenic, 294–295
  facial
    peripheral, 490
  gaze, 295–296
  Erb-Duchenne, 451, 452
  Klumpke's, 450–451
  juvenile progressive bulbar palsy, 439
Pancoast's tumor, 452
Paralysis
  periodic. *See* Periodic paralysis.
Paramyotonia congenita, 262, 552
Paraproteinemia
  neuropathies associated with, 468
Paraspinal muscles. *See under* Muscle(s).
Parathyroid disease, 537
Paratrigeminal syndrome
  blink reflex and, 333
Parkinson's disease
  blink reflex and, 346–348
Parotid gland, 5
Patient(s)
  electrically sensitive, 617–618
Patient-lead leakage current, 616
Patient safety
  documents concerned with, 614–615
Pectoral nerve. *See* Nerve(s), anterior thoracic.
Pectoralis major muscle. *See under* Muscle(s).
Pectoralis minor muscle. *See under* Muscle(s).
Pellagra, 471
Pelvic girdle
  muscles of, 17*t–*18*t*
  nerves of, 498–500
Penicillamine
  myasthenia gravis and, 520
Percussion myotonia, 550
Perhexiline maleote
  toxic neuropathy and, 472
Periarteritis nodosa, 468

Perimysium, 217
Perineurium, 59–60, *60*
  in neurotmesis, 73
Periodic paralysis, 552–554
  classification of, 552
  decremental response in, 520
  hyperkalemic, 262, 553
    myotonia and, 550
    vs. paramyotonia congenita, 552
  hypokalemic, 553
  motor unit potentials and, 280
  normokalemic, 554
  repetitive stimulation in, 203
Peripheral facial paresis, 490
Peripheral nerve. *See under* Nerve(s).
Pernicious anemia, 471
Peroneal nerve
  common. *See* Nerve(s), peroneal, common.
  deep. *See* Nerve(s), peroneal, deep.
Peroneal sign, 558
Peroneus brevis muscle. *See under* Muscle(s).
Peroneus longus muscle. *See under* Muscle(s).
Peroneus tertius muscle. *See under* Muscle(s).
Pharynx
  muscles of
    accessory nerve and, 6
Phosphorylase-limit-dextrin, 533
Phrenic nerve. *See* Nerve(s), phrenic.
Pica, 472
Picket fence interference pattern, 282
Pinch sign
  anterior interosseous syndrome and, 494
Pituitary disease, 537–538
Plantar nerve, lateral. *See* Nerve(s), plantar, lateral.
Plasma resistance
  action potential and, 63
Plate(s)
  horizontal deflection, 47
  vertical deflection, 47
Plate endings
  muscle spindles and, 223
Platysma muscle. *See under* Muscle(s).
Plexopathy(ies), 449–462
  brachial
    familial, 454
  fibrillation potentials and, 267, 270
  F-wave and, 372
  secondary to radiation, 454
  vs. root avulsion, 95
Plexus(es)
  brachial, 116–117, 119, 122, 451–452
    anatomy of, *12*
    anterior divisions of, 9, *12*
    chronic compressive lesions of, 451
    diseases associated with, 451
    dorsal scapular nerve and, 13
    formation of, 9
    latencies of, 123*t*

Potassium conductance
   in intrinsic membranes, 31
Potassium equilibrium potential, 32
Potassium ions
   membrane channels for, 31
Potential(s)
   end-plate. *See* End-plate potential (EPP).
   equilibrium. *See* Equilibrium potential.
   miniature end-plate. *See* Miniature end-
      plate potentials (MEPP).
   motor unit. *See* Motor unit potential(s).
   sensory. *See* Sensory potential(s).
   somatosensory evoked. *See* Somatosensory
      evoked potentials.
   transmembrane. *See* Transmembrane po-
      tential.
Power, 582
Preamplifier
   averaging technique and, 87
   input impedance in, 45
Preconus, 17
Pressure-sensitive hereditary neuropathy, 476
Presynaptic abnormalities
   of neuromuscular junction, 179–180
Primary lateral sclerosis, 435–436
Progressive bulbar palsy, 435
Progressive muscular atrophy, 435
Progressive spinal muscular atrophy
   fasciculation potentials and, 272
Pronator quadratus muscle. *See under* Mus-
      cle(s).
Pronator teres muscle. *See under* Muscle(s).
Pronator teres syndrome, 494
Propagation velocity
   of muscle action potential, 307
Prostigmin
   fibrillation potentials and, 267
Pseudobulbar palsy
   blink reflex and, 345
   in amyotrophic lateral sclerosis, 433
Pseudofacilitation
   neuromuscular transmission and, 180
Pseudomeningocele(s), 451
Pseudomyotonia, 554
   complex repetitive discharges and,
      274
Pterygoid muscle. *See under* Muscle(s).

Quadratus femoris muscle. *See under* Mus-
      cle(s).
Quadratus plantar muscle. *See under* Mus-
      cle(s).
Quadriceps femoris muscles. *See under* Mus-
      cle(s).
Quantum(a)
   acetylcholine and, 174
      defective release of
         in myasthenic syndrome, 179
   mobilization store and, 174

Quantum size
   microelectrode recording and, 211
   of miniature end-plate potential, 174

Radial nerve. *See under* Nerve(s).
Radial nerve palsy, 492–493
   partial
      interference pattern in, *283*
      motor unit potentials in, *279*
Radiation
   plexopathy secondary to, 454
Radicular lesions
   diagnosis of, 8
   identification of, 298
   localization of, 455
Radiculopathy(ies), 8, 9, 455
   clinical assessment of, 450
   complex repetitive discharges and, 274
   fibrillation potentials and, 267, 270
   F-wave and, 363, 372, 457
   H-reflex in, 457
   multiple discharges and, 278
   paraspinal examination in, 457
   peripheral lesions vs., 130
   spontaneous activity in, 268
Radio frequency
   interference from, 53
Ramus(i)
   anterior
      abdominal muscles and, 8
      innervation of intercostal muscles by, 9
      of spinal nerve, 7–9
   posterior
      innervation of paraspinal muscles by, 9
      of spinal nerve, 7–9
      paraspinal muscles and, 8
Rate coding, 229
Raynaud's phenomenon
   dermatomyositis and, 538
R/D ratio, 327
   normal values of, 330–331, *332t*
Reactance, 591–593, *592*
Recorder
   magnetic tape, 48
Recording(s)
   multiple channel, 47–48
   portable
      precautions during, 617
Recording apparatus, 41–55
Recording system
   errors in, 144
Recovery curve
   of H-reflex, 383
   of neuromuscular transmission, 182
Recruitment
   motor unit and, 228–229
Recruitment frequency, 250
Recruitment patterns, 282, 284–285
   in dermatomyositis, *284*

in hysterical weakness, *283*
in radial nerve palsy, *283*
lower motor neuron disorders and, 282, 284
upper motor neuron disorders and, 282, 284
Rectification, 253
Rectifier(s), 593, *594*
Rectus femoris. *See under* Muscle(s).
Recurrent activation
motor neurons and, 355
Redundant ground, 619
Reflex(es). *See under individual names.*
Refractory period
absolute, 157
assessment of, 157–165
clinical limitations of, 164–165
clinical value of, 164–165
multiple sclerosis and, 164
physiologic basis for, 157–158
relative, 157
sodium conductance and, 158
subthreshold current and, 158
Refsum's disease, 475
Regeneration
aberrant, 290
Regional curare test, 209–210
Reinnervation
motor unit potentials during, 280
Relative refractory period, 157
Remyelination
conduction velocity and, 65
functional recovery and, 75
Renshaw cell(s), 355
Renshaw inhibition, 556
Repetitive discharge(s)
vs. axon reflexes, *360*
Repetitive stimulation. *See* Stimulation, repetitive.
Repolarization, 32
action potential and, 36
Resistance, 581–582
interference vs., 46
Resistors in parallel, 584–585, *585*
Resistors in series, 582, *583*
Response(s)
direct
blink reflex and, 334t
in facial diplegia, *327*
recording of
technique for, *326*
reflex
direct vs., 323, 325
Restless leg syndrome
myokymia and, 555
Reticulohistiocytosis
multicentric
myotonia and, 550
Reticulum
sarcoplasmic, 176
Rheobase, 63

Rheumatoid arthritis
carpal tunnel syndrome and, 494
myasthenia gravis and, 512
Rhomboid major muscle. *See under* Muscle(s).
Rhomboid minor muscle. *See under* Muscle(s).
Ring electrode, 96
Rise time, 38
of motor unit potentials, 243–244
Rise time constant, 587
Risus sardonicus, 556
Root(s)
anterior, 7
cervical 449–450
electrophysiologic studies of, 450
lesions of
histamine test and, 356
nerve conduction and, 115
stimulation of, 122, *123*
diseases of, 449–462
dorsal, 7
lumbosacral, 455–457
lesions of, 455
H-reflex and, 455
stimulation of, 134
posterior, 7
thoracic
stimulation of, 122
ventral, 7
Root avulsion
cervical, 112, 450–451
histamine test and, 451
lumbosacral, 457
preganglionic, 107
vs. plexopathy, 95
Root lesion(s). *See* Radicular lesions.
Root mean square, 593
Roussey–Levy syndrome, 474

SACRAL PLEXUS. *See* Plexus(es), sacral.
Saltatory conduction
in myelinated fibers, 64
Saphenous nerve. *See under* Nerve(s).
Sarcoid neuropathy, 468
Sarcoidosis
myositis associated with, 540
Sarcolemma, 218
Sarcomere, 219
Sarcoplasm
calcium in, 176
Sarcoplasmic reticulum, 176
Sartorius muscle. *See under* Muscle(s).
Saturday night palsy, 69, 70, 493
Scalenus anticus syndrome, 454–455
Scapula
winging of, 491
Scapuloperoneal spinal muscular atrophy, 439–440

Vincristine
  toxic neuropathy and, 472
Volar interossei muscle. *See under* Muscle(s).
Voltage, 581–582
  constant
    vs. constant current, 604–605
Voltage divider, 583–584, *584*
Voltanic pile, 570
Volume conduction
  clinical implications of, 36–38
  current density in, 34
  current flow in, 34
  effect of, 34–36
  solid angle and, 34
Volume conductor
  dipole and, 34
  wave fronts in, *37*

WALLENBERG SYNDROME
  blink reflex and, 341–342, 344

Wallerian degeneration, *72*
  nerve conduction during, 72
Waveform(s)
  analysis of
    clinical diagnosis and, 36
  calibration, *251*
  diphasic
    in action potential, 37
  of compound action potential
    in diseased nerves, 69
  of sensory nerve potentials, 95
  of spontaneous potentials, 38
  triphasic
    in action potential, 36
Werdnig-Hoffmann disease, 436
  vs. Pompe's disease, 533
Wood tick, 519

Z-LINES
  of muscle, 219